ESSENTIALS OF

Diagnostic Virology

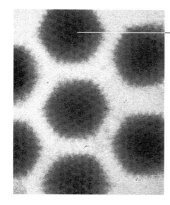

ESSENTIALS OF

Diagnostic Virology

GREGORY A. STORCH, M.D.

Professor of Pediatrics, Medicine, and Molecular Microbiology
Washington University School of Medicine
Director, Virology Laboratory
St. Louis Children's Hospital
St. Louis, Missouri

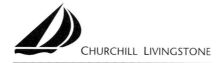

CHURCHILL LIVINGSTONE

A Division of Harcourt Brace & Company
New York, Edinburgh, London, Philadelphia, San Francisco

Library of Congress Cataloging-in-Publication Data

Essentials of diagnostic virology / [edited by] Gregory Storch. — 1st ed.

p.   cm.

Includes bibliographical references and index.

ISBN 0-443-07632-4

1. Diagnostic virology. I. Storch, Gregory. [DNLM: 1. Virus
    Diseases—diagnosis. 2. Infection—diagnosis. WC 500 E78 2000]

QR387.E85 2000 616.9′25075—dc21

DNLM/DLC   99–38986
for Library of Congress   CIP

ESSENTIALS OF DIAGNOSTIC VIROLOGY   ISBN 0-443-07632-4

Churchill Livingstone® is a registered trademark of Harcourt Brace & Company
is a trademark of Harcourt Brace & Company

Printed in the United States of America

Last digit is the print number: 9   8   7   6   5   4   3   2   1

Contributors

MAX Q. ARENS, PhD
Assistant Professor of Pediatrics
Washington University School of Medicine
Co-director, Retrovirus Laboratory
Associate Director, Clinical Virology Laboratory
St. Louis Children's Hospital
St. Louis, Missouri

TEDDY F. BADER, MD
Associate Clinical Professor
University of Colorado School of Medicine
Gastroenterologist
Kaiser Permanente
Exempla Hospital
Denver, Colorado

RICHARD S. BULLER, PhD
Research Instructor
Department of Pediatrics
Washington University School of Medicine
St. Louis, Missouri

GAIL J. DEMMLER
Associate Professor
Departments of Pediatrics and Pathology
Baylor College of Medicine
Houston, Texas
Active Staff, Pediatric Infectious Disease Service
Texas Childrens Hospital and Ben Taub General
    Hospital
Houston, Texas

ALEJO ERICE, MD
Associate Professor
Departments of Laboratory Medicine and Pathology,
    and Medicine, Infectious Disease Division
University of Minnesota Medical School
Minneapolis, Minnesota

KENNETH H. FIFE, MD, PhD
Professor of Medicine
Indiana University School of Medicine
Division of Infectious Diseases
Indianapolis, Indiana

CHARLES GROSE, MD
Professor of Pediatrics
Professor of Microbiology
University of Iowa College of Medicine
Director, Infectious Diseases and Rheumatology
    Division
Childrens Hospital of Iowa
Iowa City, Iowa

RICHARD L. HODINKA, PhD
Associate Professor
Departments of Pediatrics and Pathology
University of Pennsylvania School of Medicine
Director, Clinical Virology Laboratory
Children's Hospital of Philadelphia
Philadelphia, Pennsylvania

XI JIANG, PhD
Associate Professor
Eastern Virginia Medical School
Center for Pediatric Research
Children's Hospital Of The King's Daughters
Norfolk, Virginia

RUBEN LIM-BON-SIONG, MD
Associate Clinical Professor, Cornea, External Disease
    and Refractive Surgery Services
Department of Ophthalmology and Visual Sciences
Philippine General Hospital—College of Medicine
University of the Philippines, Manila

DAVID O. MATSON, MD, PhD
Professor of Pediatrics
Eastern Virginia Medical School
Associate Director, Head Infectious Diseases Section
Center for Pediatric Research
Norfolk, Virginia

DOUGLAS K. MITCHELL, MD
Assistant Professor of Pediatrics
Eastern Virginia Medical School
Center for Pediatric Research
Children's Hospital Of The King's Daughters
Norfolk, Virginia

KARYN L. MOSHAL, MRCP
Infectious Disease Fellow
Division of Immunologic and Infectious Diseases
Children's Hospital of Philadelphia
Philadelphia, Pennsylvania

JAY S. PEPOSE, MD, PhD
Bernard Becker Professor of Ophthalmology
    and Visual Sciences
Washington University School of Medicine
St. Louis, Missouri

JEROME YANKOWITZ, MD
Associate Professor
Director, Division of Maternal-Fetal Medicine and Fetal
    Diagnosis and Treatment Unit
Department of Obstetrics and Gynecology
University of Iowa College of Medicine
Iowa City, Iowa

This book is dedicated to my wife, Deborah;
my children, Rachel, Nathaniel, Emily, and Thomas;
and my parents, Sylvia and the late Harvey Storch.

Preface

*V*iral infections are among the most important causes of human disease. Until recently, however, they were relegated to the fringe of medical practice because they were difficult to diagnose in the laboratory and few specific treatments were available. Both these factors have changed. Rapid and accurate diagnosis of viral infections is now a reality, and effective treatments for a number of viral infections are widely used. The acquired immunodeficiency syndrome (AIDS) epidemic has had an enormous impact in this regard. Technologic developments related to diagnosis and treatment of human immunodeficiency virus (HIV) have been dramatic and have "spun off" to other viral infections. In addition, the AIDS epidemic and the increased success of organ transplantation have vastly increased the number of individuals at risk for serious opportunistic viral infections. Physicians caring for these and other patients depend on accurate and timely viral diagnosis to guide the appropriate use of powerful (and expensive) antiviral drugs.

The field of viral diagnosis is currently in a period of revolutionary change, brought about by the introduction of new molecular methods such as the polymerase chain reaction (PCR) that are rapidly expanding the capability to make specific viral diagnoses. The potential of these new methods is enormous, but their actual role in patient management is only beginning to become clear. For the foreseeable future, these methods will complement rather than replace conventional methods such as viral culture, antigen detection, and serology. The development of powerful new methods is welcome but has made the task of viral diagnosis more confusing for physicians caring for patients. Understanding of the capabilities of new molecular methods and their relationship to conventional methods is evolving.

The aim of *Essentials of Diagnostic Virology* is to provide practical guidance for those using the clinical laboratory to make specific viral diagnoses. Throughout the book, conventional and molecular techniques are fully integrated to help the clinician make best use of all available methods. The viewpoint is that of the clinician. If it succeeds in its aim as a useful guide for clinicians, this text should also be useful for clinical laboratory personnel, other allied health personnel, and researchers in the field of virology, especially those interested in the development of new diagnostic tests.

The scope of *Essentials of Diagnostic Virology* comprises all viral infections of humans, with emphasis according to clinical importance from the perspective of contemporary medical practice in the United States. Discussion is not limited to those tests traditionally performed in virology laboratories and includes tests that may be carried out in pathology, retrovirus, serology, blood bank, or even chemistry laboratories. Thus viral tests that are sometimes "carved out" from traditional virology laboratories are described, such as those involved in the diagnosis of hepatitis and HIV. Infections involving normal and immunocompromised hosts and adult and pediatric patients are covered comprehensively. The editor and authors have tried to create a book that is practical and that will be useful in real clinical situations, both common and unusual. The depth of coverage is much greater than that contained in a manual, but not so encyclopedic as to lose relevance to clinical practice. Where appropriate, authors have made concrete recommendations based on their understanding of their field of expertise.

An important aim of this book is to consolidate information pertaining to the diagnosis of common viral and unusual viral infections. The need for this type of information can arise suddenly, leaving the clinician and associated personnel searching through diverse sources for needed direction. Our hope is that *Essentials of Diagnostic Virology* will be a resource in these situations. For example, Chapter 16 details the diagnosis of viral hemorrhagic fevers and other geographically localized infections. Chapter 3 covers the diagnosis of rabies and B virus infections as well as central nervous system (CNS) pathogens such as the enteroviruses. Chapter 17 includes material relevant to patients who may have acquired their infection in Africa, where HIV-2 and unusual strains of HIV-1 may be found. Specialized testing may be required because some widely used tests cannot detect unusual strains.

The chapters of *Essentials of Diagnostic Virology* have been created and organized to emphasize clinical problems. Chapter 1 provides information on techniques used in diagnostic virology, including conventional cell culture, shell vial culture, antigen detection by fluorescent antibody staining and enzyme immunoassay, viral serology, electron microscopy, cytology, histology, immunohistochemistry, in situ hybridization, PCR, and other molecular techniques. Chapter 2 provides information on specimen selection, acquisition, and transport.

Chapters 3 to 11 are devoted to diagnosis of viral infection by organ system, including the CNS, respiratory and gastrointestinal tracts, skin and mucous membranes, genital tract, liver, heart, and eyes. Each of these chapters is written by a clinician expert in both clinical and laboratory aspects of viral infection of the specific organ system. Material is presented by organ system rather than by virus because patients present for medical care with symptoms directing attention to a specific organ system, rather than with an announcement that they are infected with a specific virus. The clinician must consider multiple different possibilities, and diagnostic testing must be organized to detect the most likely viruses. In each of these chapters, viral infections of the organ system are reviewed, and the approach to diagnosis is outlined based on the nature of the patient's illness.

Chapters 12 to 17 address clinical problems that are not limited to specific organ systems. These topics include infectious mononucleosis (as caused by Epstein-Barr virus, cytomegalovirus, and HIV), viral infections of childhood (measles, mumps, rubella, parvovirus B19, herpesviruses 6 and 7, non-CNS enterovirus infections), and congenital infections (in utero and postnatal diagnosis). Because the world is now highly interconnected with rapid travel across continents, Chapter 16 discusses such infections as Lassa, Ebola and Marburg viruses hantavirus, Colorado tick fever, and alphaviruses (e.g., Ross River virus) and includes maps to assist the clinician in determining relevant viral infections based on the patient's travels. Chapter 17 provides comprehensive information on numerous aspects of the diagnosis of HIV-1, as well as infections with HIV-2 and human T-cell lymphotropic viruses.

The last three chapters have a methodologic emphasis. Chapters 18 and 19 cover antiviral susceptibility testing and molecular typing of viruses. These chapters are included because the material is relevant to clinical virology but is typically found in diverse sources, often different from other sources of information about viral diagnosis. Chapter 20 is devoted to the discovery of new viral agents. One of the most exciting areas of medicine in recent years has been the discovery of new infectious agents. An advantage of specific viral diagnosis is that it highlights areas of current ignorance by defining infections for which no cause is known. For example, the existence of hepatitis agents other than hepatitis A and B viruses could be suspected only when accurate diagnostic tests for hepatitis A and B were developed, leading to the observation that many patients who apparently had viral hepatitis were not infected with either of these viruses. Chapter 20 reviews the methods that have been used to discover many human viruses, especially those discovered relatively recently, such as HIV, hepatitis C virus, and herpesvirus 8 (the Kaposi's sarcoma virus). It is hoped that this chapter will help in the ongoing effort to expand the realm of clinical virology through discovery of new, medically important viruses.

Finally, the appendices provide information in tabular format on (1) which diagnostic specimens to collect from patients with various clinical syndromes suggestive of viral infection, (2) collection requirements for various viral specimens, and (3) viral reference laboratories that perform viral diagnostic tests that may be outside of the scope of hospital-based virology laboratories.

I have received assistance from many sources in the preparation of this book. Special acknowledgment is due to the staff of the Virology Laboratory at St. Louis Children's Hospital in the Washington University Medical Center. Much of what I know about diagnostic virology has been derived from hands-on experience in this laboratory, where interactions with colleagues over the years have been especially important. Doctor Gerald Medoff guided my training in infectious diseases and has been a key role model. Doctors Patricia Charache and Mike Foreman at Johns Hopkins University oversaw my initial training in diagnostic virology. Doctor Milton Schlesinger graciously assisted me in learning selected techniques of molecular virology. Doctor Carl Smith has helped provide an environment in which new directions could be explored and new questions addressed. I have benefited enormously from collaborations with numerous clinical colleagues at Washington University Medical Center, especially those in the fields of infectious diseases, transplantation medicine, neurology, perinatal medicine, and ophthalmology. The invaluable facilities of the Bernard Becker Medical Library at Washington University provided materials for much of the research carried out in the writing of this book.

GREGORY A. STORCH

Communication with the editor

Readers of *Essentials of Diagnostic Virology* are invited to send queries about issues in *Diagnostic Virology* and comments about the book to the editor at STORCH@al.kids.wustl.edu.

Contents

Detailed Contents

ESSENTIALS OF

Diagnostic Virology

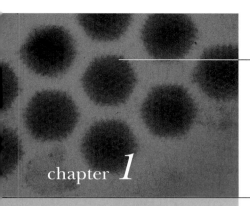

Gregory A. Storch

chapter *1*

Methodologic Overview

Outline continued

HISTORY OF DIAGNOSTIC VIROLOGY

The modern era of diagnostic virology began in 1948 with the report by Weller and Enders[1] of the first growth of pathogenic human viruses in *tissue culture*. Because the newly developed techniques for maintaining tissue cultures were beyond the scope of existing diagnostic laboratories, virology laboratories were established as distinct entities separate from traditional microbiology laboratories.

Cell culture, the growth of defined populations of cells not formed into discrete tissues, was a refinement of tissue culture, which had formed the basis of diagnostic virology for many years. Cell culture is now being gradually replaced by nonculture techniques based on immunologic or molecular methods.

The development of monoclonal antibodies in the 1970s[2] greatly increased the availability of immunologic reagents with well-defined specificity for individual viruses. Rapid viral diagnosis became a practical reality during the 1980s as diagnostic virology laboratories implemented monoclonal antibody–based assays to detect a wide variety of viral antigens directly in clinical specimens. The introduction of molecular techniques into the diagnostic virology laboratory accelerated with the development of the polymerase chain reaction (PCR), described in 1985.[3]

The laboratory diagnosis of viral infections currently employs multiple methods (Box 1–1). Not all these tests are used in every laboratory, and some are performed outside of traditional virology laboratories, in settings that include serology, blood bank, surgical pathology, specialized molecular diagnosis, retrovirology, and chemistry laboratories. This chapter discusses all the methods currently used for the laboratory diagnosis of viral infections, regardless of what type of laboratory performs the testing.

CELL CULTURE

The cultivation of viruses in cell culture is the activity that sets virology laboratories apart from other clinical laboratories. Although cell culture is routinely done in virology laboratories, it is still a craft surrounded by mystique. The success of cell culture depends on attention to multiple details, including the age and general health of the cells, the composition and freshness of the cell culture media, and the conditions of incubation.

Although it is gradually being replaced by immunologic and molecular procedures, cell culture retains the following advantages for viral diagnosis:

1. Viral culture can be an extremely sensitive diagnostic method, because one viable virion may be sufficient to initiate a positive culture.

2. Culture has the potential to yield many different viruses, whether or not their presence was suspected in the specimen submitted. This is in contrast to most rapid tests based on immunologic or nucleic acid reagents, which detect only the virus recognized by the test reagents.

3. Culture can detect multiple viruses present in the same specimen. The open-ended capability of culture for virus detection may lead to the discovery of new viral agents.

4. Culture provides a viral isolate that can be further characterized if necessary. This might include detailed typing, molecular fingerprinting, or antiviral susceptibility testing.

5. Apart from unusual episodes of laboratory contamination, the growth of a virus from a clinical sample provides incontrovertible evidence that the patient was infected with that virus. This does not necessarily mean, however, that the infection is clinically significant.

Box 1.1 Laboratory Techniques Used in Diagnosis of Viral Infections

Cell culture (conventional and shell vial)
Cytology
Histopathology
Electron microscopy
Antigen detection
  Fluorescent antibody (FA) staining of specimens
  Immunoperoxidase (IP) staining of specimens
  Enzyme immunoassay (EIA)
  Immunohistochemistry (IHC)
Nucleic acid detection
  Direct hybridization
  In situ hybridization (ISH)
  Target (template) amplification (polymerase chain reaction [PCR] and other techniques)
  Signal amplification (branched-chain DNA and hybrid capture assays)

Box 1.2   Viruses Detected in Cell Culture

Herpes simplex (HSV)
Varicella-zoster (VZV)
Cytomegalovirus (CMV)
Adenovirus
Enteroviruses (echoviruses,
    coxsackieviruses,
    polioviruses)
Respiratory syncytial (RSV)

Influenza
Parainfluenza
Rhinovirus
Measles
Rubella
Mumps

Viral culture also has significant shortcomings as a diagnostic method, primarily because it is expensive, relatively slow, and not applicable to all medically important viruses. In addition, successful culture depends on the viability of the virus in the specimen, which in turn depends greatly on the conditions and circumstances of specimen transport (see Chapter 2).

Viruses Detected and Time Required

Box 1–2 lists the main viruses frequently detected by viral culture. The time required to detect viruses by conventional cell culture varies widely. For example, herpes simplex virus (HSV) usually grows in 1 to 3 days, comparable to the time frame for bacterial cultures. On the other extreme, three weeks or more may be required for the conventional culture detection of cytomegalovirus (CMV). The shell vial culture method (see later discussion) is a modification of the conventional culture that detects CMV and some other viruses much more quickly. Table 1–1 shows the time required to detect viruses in cell culture.

Types

Many different types of cell cultures exist, but no method supports the growth of all medically important viruses. Therefore most specimens for viral culture are inoculated onto two or more different cell culture types. The different types of cell culture can be placed in one of three categories: primary, diploid (also called semi-continuous), and continuous.

Primary cell cultures are prepared directly from tissue, usually from an animal or an embryo. Preparation involves mincing the tissue, digesting with proteolytic enzymes to disperse the component cells further, and seeding the cells into an appropriate glass or plastic container with nutritive media that contain antimicrobial agents to inhibit bacterial and fungal overgrowth. A variant of the primary cell culture technique is the use of umbilical cord mononuclear cells, which are harvested from cord blood. Primary cell cultures can be "passaged" for a few generations before the cells die. *Passage* refers to the process of transferring a portion of the cells from a culture into a new container with fresh media and allowing the cells to multiply. Examples of primary cell cultures include monkey kidney cells, human amnion cells, and chick embryo cells.

Diploid (*semicontinuous) cell cultures* can be passaged for more generations than primary cultures. After approximately 50 to 100 passages, however, the cells become senescent and unable to survive further passage. Examples of diploid cultures include human embryonic lung fibroblast lines such as WI-38 and MRC-5.

Continuous cell cultures are transformed cell lines that are "immortalized" and can be passaged indefinitely. Examples include HEp-2, HeLa, and RK-13 cells. Table 1–2 lists cell cultures and the viruses they support.

Table 1.1   Time Required to Detect Viruses in Cell Culture

Virus	Number of isolates	Earliest day positive	Day when 50% positive	Day when 90% positive
Herpes simplex	512	1	1	3
Varicella-zoster	30*	3	7	13
Cytomegalovirus	116†	3	13	20
Adenovirus	125‡	1	4	11
Enteroviruses	85	1	4	10
Respiratory syncytial	70§	2	4	7
Influenza	61‖	2	4	7
Parainfluenza	104¶	1	6	12
Rhinovirus	130	1	6	12

Data from St. Louis Children's Hospital Virology Laboratory, 1997.
*12 of these were also detected on day 2 by shell vial assay.
†462 additional isolates were detected on day 1 or 2 by shell vial assay.
‡18 of these were detected on day 1 by fluorescent antibody (FA) staining.
§734 additional specimens were positive on day 1 by FA staining or enzyme immunoassay.
‖61 additional specimens were positive on day 1 by FA staining.
¶30 additional specimens were positive on day 1 by FA staining.

Table 1.2	Frequently Used Cell Culture Types
Culture type	**Viruses supported**
Primary	
Monkey kidney	Influenza
	Parainfluenza
	Enteroviruses
Rabbit kidney	Herpes simplex
Human embryonic kidney	Adenovirus
	Enteroviruses
Diploid	
Fibroblast	Cytomegalovirus
	Varicella-zoster
	Herpes simplex
	Rhinovirus
	Enteroviruses (some)
	Adenovirus
	Respiratory syncytial
Continuous	
HEp-2	Respiratory syncytial
	Adenovirus
	Herpes simplex
	Parainfluenza (some)
	Enteroviruses (some)
A549	Herpes simplex
	Adenovirus
	Enteroviruses
MDCK	Influenza
LLC-MK2	Parainfluenza
Rhabdomyosarcoma (RD)	Echoviruses
Buffalo green monkey kidney	Coxsackievirus

Growth

Cell cultures used in diagnostic virology laboratories are typically grown in *roller tubes* (Figure 1–1), but can also be grown in a variety of containers, including flasks, dishes, and microtiter trays. The cells are covered in culture media that contain essential nutrients, salts, vitamins, buffer, and antimicrobial agents. Fetal calf serum is included in most cell culture media but is omitted for cultures of respiratory viruses. Cells in culture usually adhere to the surface of the container. Shell vial cultures make use of cells grown on microscope coverslips that are placed within tubes and covered with culture media. Some cells do not adhere to surfaces; cultures of these cells are referred to as *suspension cultures.*

Culture Types Inoculated

Cell culture types used to grow viruses from a clinical specimen are selected based on which viruses are sought. When no specific information is provided, laboratories typically inoculate culture types that are useful for growing the viruses most often found in the specimen submitted. Therefore it is especially important to inform the laboratory if a virus is suspected that is unusual for the specimen being submitted, so that additional cell culture types can be used to maximize the chance of recovering that virus.

Inoculation of Specimens

The preparation of the specimen for inoculation depends on the nature of the specimen. Specimens such as throat swabs or stool specimens are treated with antibiotics before inoculation. Stool specimens are also homogenized and centrifuged to remove particulate matter. Cerebrospinal fluid is inoculated directly onto cell cultures. Before inoculation, many laboratories remove the media from cell cultures to allow closer contact of the inoculum with the cultured cells. After approximately 1 hour, media are replaced and cultures incubated. Incubating the cultures in rotating drums hastens the growth of several viruses. The typical temperature of incubation is 35° to 37°C, although some respiratory viral cultures may be incubated at 33°C because this temperature is optimal for some strains of influenza virus and rhinovirus.

Cytopathic Effect

The main method for detecting growth of viruses in cell culture is microscopic examination of the culture for morphologic changes in the cultured cells, referred to as *cytopathic effect* (CPE). CPE is detected by examination of the cultures under low-power microscopy at regular intervals, typically daily or every other day for the first week and less frequently thereafter. The time required for CPE to become evident varies from 1 day for some isolates of HSV to 21 days or more for some isolates of

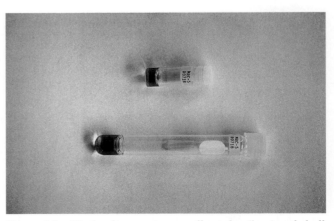

Figure 1.1   Viral culture systems: roller tube *(long)* and shell vial *(short).*

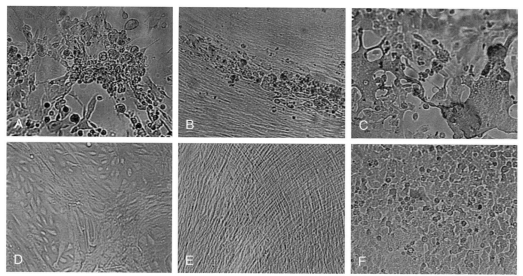

Figure 1.2 Cytopathic effect caused by viruses growing in cell culture. Herpes simplex virus growing in primary rabbit kidney cells (**A**); uninfected primary rabbit kidney cells (**D**). Cytomegalovirus growing in human embryonic lung fibroblast cells (**B**); uninfected human embryonic lung fibroblast cells (**E**). Respiratory syncytial virus growing in HEp-2 cells (**C**); uninfected HEp-2 cells (**F**).

CMV. The characteristics of the CPE usually allow the laboratory to make a tentative or even a definitive identification of the responsible virus. These characteristics include which cell culture types are affected, the shape assumed by the involved cells, whether the CPE is focal or diffuse, and how rapidly it appears and progresses. Examples of CPE caused by several different viruses are shown in Figure 1–2.

The viral identification is most often confirmed by fluorescent antibody (FA) staining of cells harvested from the culture. Confirmation of identification based on CPE is important because of the potential subjectivity of CPE-based identification but it may be omitted under selected circumstances. In my laboratory, for example, no confirmatory testing is performed when CPE typical for HSV is detected in a culture from an oral or genital site.

Hemadsorption

Certain viruses, notably influenza and parainfluenza, may grow to high titer in cell culture without producing CPE and therefore they require other methods for detection. Influenza and parainfluenza viruses growing in the culture can be detected by testing the inoculated culture for hemadsorption, or adherence of erythrocytes to the surface of the cultured cells. Hemadsorption is specific for the species from which the erythrocytes are derived. Guinea pig erythrocytes are widely used for detection of hemadsorption caused by influenza, parainfluenza, and mumps viruses.

To test for hemadsorption, the culture medium is removed from the inoculated cell culture, and a sus-

pension of guinea pig erythrocytes is added and incubated for 30 minutes. Low-power microscopy is used to evaluate the presence of hemadsorption (Figure 1–3). If hemadsorption is present, the laboratory can report that a hemadsorbing virus is present. The identity of the virus responsible for the hemadsorption can be determined by performing FA stains of cells from the cell culture using specific monoclonal antibodies. If no hemadsorption is present, the erythrocyte suspension can be removed and the culture reincubated after addition of fresh media.

Because influenza virus can grow very rapidly, it is advisable for laboratories to perform the first test for hemadsorption within the first 24 to 72 hours after inoculation. The hemadsorption test may be repeated two or three times during incubation of the culture.

Viral Interference

Some other viruses, notably rubella, also may grow without producing CPE and are detected by taking advantage of the phenomenon of interference. When an interfering virus grows in cell culture, it renders the cell culture resistant to other viruses to which it is ordinarily susceptible.

For example, when rubella virus grows in primary monkey kidney cells, those cells become resistant to infection with echovirus type 11. To test for interference in the laboratory, a culture in which rubella virus is being sought is "challenged" with a laboratory strain of echovirus type 11. If the echovirus fails to grow (but grows when inoculated into a companion cell culture that was not inoculated with the clinical sample), the

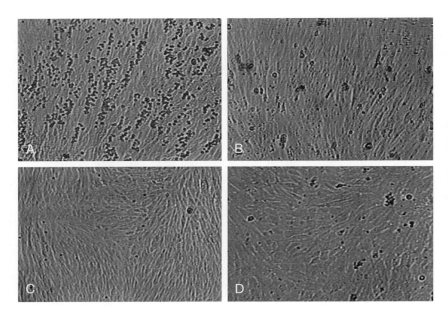

Figure 1.3 Hemadsorption of guinea pig erythrocytes associated with influenza virus infection. Rhesus monkey kidney cells infected with influenza virus (**A** and **B**) and uninfected (**C** and **D**). Guinea pig erythrocytes were added to A and C. Positive hemadsorption is shown in A.

culture is said to be *positive* for an interfering virus. FA staining or neutralization with a specific antiserum can be used to determine the identity of the interfering virus.

Pitfalls in Cell Culture

Several pitfalls can occur in carrying out cell culture. First, some cultures may be affected by toxins in the specimen, producing changes resembling viral CPE or destroying the cell culture so that viral CPE cannot be detected. For example, *Clostridium difficile* toxin present in a stool specimen disrupts the cell culture, making detection of viruses impossible. Other bacterial toxins, such as those produced by *Pseudomonas aeruginosa,* may have a similar effect. Serial passage of the cell culture exhibiting toxicity may dilute the toxin and allow viral growth to occur. Some virology laboratories have become skilled at recognizing *C. difficile* toxin and suggest this diagnosis when toxicity is observed.

Contamination with bacteria or fungi can also prevent detection of viruses. When contamination is detected, the cell culture supernatant can be filtered through a 0.45-micron filter and passed to a new cell culture. Cell cultures themselves can be contaminated with mycoplasma and become less sensitive for detection of viruses. An important part of the quality control of virology laboratories is regular checking of established cell lines for mycoplasma.

Finally, primary cell cultures may be infected with endogenous viruses, which can produce CPE that can be mistaken for the CPE of a virus in the clinical specimen. Immunologic confirmation of the virus suspected of causing the CPE can help avoid this pitfall. This is especially important if the CPE is observed only in primary cell cultures.

Shell Vial Culture

The shell vial culture combines components of traditional cell culture and antigen detection methods. This method was first applied to the detection of CMV and revolutionized the laboratory diagnosis of that virus by making it possible to detect a large proportion of positive cultures within 1 to 2 days of inoculation.[4, 5] Subsequently, the method has been applied to the detection of numerous other viruses, including HSV, varicella-zoster virus (VZV), and the human respiratory viruses (see Chapters 4 and 6).

Figure 1–4 illustrates the steps involved in the shell vial culture.[6] For the detection of CMV, human fibroblast cells are grown on a small, round coverslip placed at the bottom of a 1-dram vial (shell vial). The specimen is prepared for inoculation as for a conventional viral culture and inoculated into the shell vial. The vial is

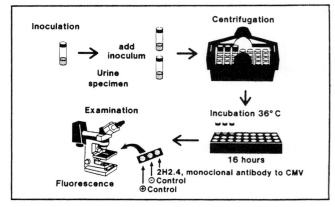

Figure 1.4 Shell vial assay for cytomegalovirus (CMV). (From Shuster EA, Beneke JS, Tegtmeier GE, et al: *Mayo Clin Proc* 60:577, 1985.)

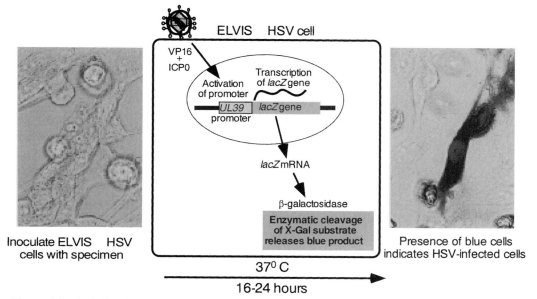

Figure 1.5   ELVIS HSV, a genetically engineered cell line for detection of herpes simplex virus (HSV) in clinical samples. ELVIS cells are baby hamster kidney cells that contain a β-galactosidase gene under control of the HSV promoter UL39. If HSV is present in the specimen, viral particles enter the cells, and the HSV proteins ICP0 and VP16 activate the UL39 promoter, leading to synthesis of β-galactosidase. Presence of β-galactosidase is detected by adding X-gal, a substrate for the enzyme. Activity of β-galactosidase on X-gal results in blue staining of ELVIS cells, visible microscopically. (Courtesy Paul Olivo, MD, PhD.)

then centrifuged at low speed (e.g., 700 × g) for 45 minutes. After centrifugation, additional medium is added and the culture incubated for 1 to 2 days. After the desired period of incubation, FA staining is performed on the cells on the coverslip, using a monoclonal antibody that recognizes an immediate early antigen of CMV expressed in the nucleus of infected cells. The presence of one or more fluorescent nuclei is evidence of a positive culture.

Sensitivity of the shell vial culture for CMV is comparable to or greater than that of conventional culture,[7, 8] although this varies considerably depending on the sensitivity of the shell vial culture and the conventional culture in the individual laboratory.

Genetically Engineered Cell Lines

Recently, genetically engineered cell lines have been constructed for the detection of viruses. An example is a detector cell line created by Stabell and Olivo[9] specifically directed at the detection of HSV (Figure 1–5). The cell line consists of baby hamster kidney cells that contain the *Escherichia coli* β-galactosidase gene placed under the control of a promoter from the herpes simplex gene UL39. The *promoter* is activated only by exposure to HSV proteins called ICP0 and VP16. If a specimen containing HSV is inoculated onto the detector cells, ICP0 and VP16 in the specimen will activate the promoter, causing production of β-galactosidase, which can

be detected by a simple histochemical stain of the culture performed 16 to 24 hours after inoculation.

A commercial version of this system called ELVIS HSV (Diagnostic Hybrids, Athens, Ohio), has been shown to have sensitivity comparable to conventional viral culture for detection of HSV in clinical specimens.[10] The system has also been adapted to the performance of HSV susceptibility assays.[11] A similar system is under development for detection of CMV.

A cell line called HeLa-CD4 has been used for the detection of human immunodeficiency virus (HIV). This cell line consists of HeLa cells that have been genetically engineered to express the CD4 surface marker, rendering them susceptible to infection with HIV, and to activate β-galactosidase as a marker of infection.[12] These cells have been conveniently adapted for quantitative cultures of HIV.

CYTOLOGY

Exfoliative cytology can provide important clues to the presence of viral infection. In general, cytologic findings implicate a group of viruses rather than a specific virus. Cytologic examination can be performed on smears prepared by applying a specimen directly to a microscope slide, on slides prepared by cytocentrifugation of fluids (e.g., bronchoalveolar lavage fluid), and on "touch preps" prepared from pieces of unfixed tissue. Figure 1–6 provides some examples of cytologic findings suggestive of viral infection.

The *Tzanck smear* is a technique for demonstrating the presence of HSV or VZV infection (see Chapter 6). Tzanck smears are prepared by applying material from the base of a lesion on a microscope slide, followed by air drying, fixation in acetone, and staining with Wright, Giemsa, or a variety of other stains. The presence of multinucleated giant cells or intranuclear inclusions suggests the presence of HSV or VZV. The technique is less sensitive than FA staining for the same viruses and does not distinguish between the two viruses. It is rapid, however, and can be performed without sophisticated equipment.

Another important application of cytology to viral diagnosis is *Papanicolaou staining* of cells obtained from the uterine cervix to screen for cervical cancer (*Pap smears*). These stains may provide evidence of human papillomavirus (HPV) infection. The presence of HPV is suggested by characteristic changes in keratinocytes, including a condensed nucleus with a prominent perinuclear clear zone. These changes are referred to as *koilocytosis*. More specific evidence of the presence of HPV can be provided by histochemical stains or molecular techniques (see Chapter 7).

Cytologic staining of cells present in urinary sediment may reveal intranuclear inclusions indicative of infection with either CMV or the polyomaviruses JC and BK. This finding is less sensitive than culture for detection of CMV. PCR is more sensitive for detecting BK virus (see Chapter 11) and can also differentiate it from the closely related JC virus, which can also be present in urine.

HISTOPATHOLOGY

As with cytology, histologic examination of tissue most often implicates a group of viruses rather than a specific virus. Histologic findings suggestive of viral infection include intranuclear and intracytoplasmic inclusions (Table 1–3), multinucleated giant cells, and syncytia. Histopathology can provide unique information about the role of viral infection in producing tissue inflammation and injury. It can be very useful in distinguishing between asymptomatic viral shedding and clinically significant infection, particularly for CMV infections in which prolonged viral shedding can occur without producing disease. The presence of cytomegalic inclusion cells in tissue obtained by biopsy or at autopsy is often considered the gold standard for diagnosing clinically significant CMV infection.

Histopathology can be enhanced by *immunohistochemistry* (IHC) to detect specific viral antigens and *in situ hybridization* (ISH) to detect specific viral nucleic acids. These methods can enhance the sensitivity of

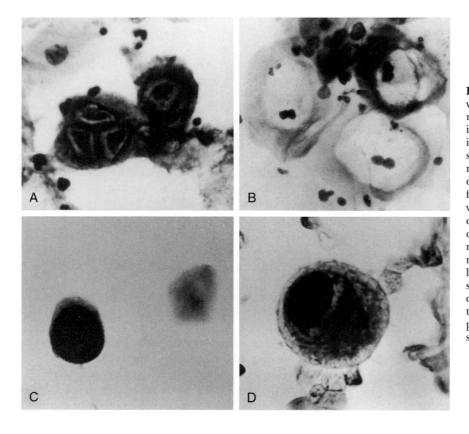

Figure 1.6 Cytologic findings suggestive of viral infection. **A,** Cervical smear shows multinucleated cells and Cowdry type A intranuclear inclusions of herpes simplex infection. **B,** Pap smear shows binucleate squamous epithelial cells with distinct perinuclear halos. These characteristics are described as "koilocytosis" and are cellular features associated with human papillomavirus infection. **C,** Urinary epithelial cell contains an enlarged nucleus with smudgy chromatin and a small, pale "glassy" intranuclear inclusion indicative of polyomavirus infection. **D,** Cell from bronchoalveolar lavage containing large intranuclear inclusion with perinuclear clear space (owl's eye cell) indicative of cytomegalovirus infection. (Courtesy Leslie Boucher, MD, Department of Pathology, Washington University, St. Louis.)

Table 1.3	Viruses Associated with Inclusions	
Virus	**Intranuclear**	**Intracytoplasmic**
Herpes simplex	X	
Varicella-zoster	X	
Cytomegalovirus	X	X
Adenovirus	X	
Polyomaviruses BK and JC	X	
Parvovirus B19	X	
Poxviruses		X
Measles	X	X
Parainfluenza		X
Rabies		X

detection and also allow identification of the presence of a specific viral agent.

IHC uses antiviral antibodies to stain tissue obtained by biopsy or at autopsy. The antiviral antibodies are usually linked to an enzyme such as horseradish peroxidase for immunoperoxidase (IP) staining or to a fluorescent label such as fluorescein isothiocyanate (FITC) for FA staining. IHC can often be performed on formalin-fixed tissue, but for some antigen-antibody combinations, sensitivity is better on fresh-frozen tissue. Consultation with a knowledgeable pathologist about specific applications is important. For some viruses such as the herpesviruses, whose life cycle includes latency, IHC can provide information about the presence of a particular virus and also which phase of the life cycle is involved in the disease process under study. For example, the presence of structural antigens of the virus indicates a productive cycle, whereas only a restricted number of nonstructural antigens may be present during the latent cycle.

ISH uses nucleic acid probes to detect specific viral nucleic acids, either deoxyribonucleic acid (DNA) or ribonucleic acid (RNA). Binding of the probe can be detected by radioisotopic or enzymatic labeling. Typically an enzyme such as horseradish peroxidase is chemically bound to the nucleic acid probe. After the enzyme-labeled probe has been incubated with the specimen, bound probe is detected by reaction with a substrate that undergoes a color change or emits light when acted on by the enzyme. Use of the enzymes deoxyribonuclease (DNase) and ribonuclease (RNase) can help distinguish which nucleic acid is being detected. Detection of specific viral RNAs provides information about the expression of individual viral genes. ISH can often be performed on formalin-fixed tissue but this depends on the characteristics of the probe and its target nucleic acid.

Recently the technique of in situ PCR has been developed that allows the reaction to be performed directly on tissue. In situ PCR can allow exquisitely sensitive detection of viral nucleic acid in tissues but it is currently available only in a limited number of laboratories with a special interest in the technique.

ELECTRON MICROSCOPY

Because it provides direct visualization of the infecting agent, electron microscopy has intuitive appeal as a technique for viral diagnosis. As with cell culture, electron microscopy is an "open" technique because it allows the visualization of multiple possible viruses, in contrast to immunologic or molecular techniques that detect only the virus to which specific reagents are directed. Electron microscopy is also useful for characterizing new viral agents (see Chapter 20).

Many viruses have distinctive appearances under electron microscopy that allow identification to the family level by a skilled electron microscopist. Two very different techniques are used in diagnostic electron microscopy, depending on the nature of the specimen: negative staining, used to visualize viruses in fluid samples, and thin sectioning, used to visualize viruses in tissue.

Negative Staining

Negative staining of fluid specimens can be performed quickly enough that it can be considered a rapid viral diagnostic technique. Negative-staining electron microscopy is especially useful for stool examination because (1) viral agents of gastroenteritis are often present in large numbers, allowing easy visualization; and (2) a number of these agents are noncultivable (see Chapter 5). In fact, rotavirus, the enteric adenoviruses, astroviruses, and caliciviruses were all discovered by electron microscopic examination of stool specimens.

To perform negative staining, the stool specimen is clarified by low-speed centrifugation, placed on a suitably prepared electron microscopy grid, and examined directly. When necessary, the procedure can be modified to increase the sensitivity of detection by concentrating viral particles in the specimen, either by physical methods such as ultracentrifugation or by reaction with appropriate antisera followed by centrifugation. The latter technique, *immune electron microscopy*, can also identify the virus based on the specificity of the antiserum employed.

Another application of negative staining is the analysis of blister fluid to distinguish rapidly between herpesviruses and poxviruses. These classes of viruses have characteristic appearances that allow them to be readily distinguished from one another. Negative staining has been used to visualize viruses in other fluids, especially serum (hepatitis A and B viruses, parvovirus B19) and urine (CMV, polyomaviruses JC and BK, and filoviruses such as Ebola and Marburg) but the low concentration of viral particles is often a limiting factor. Figure 16–2 is an example of a negative stain of Marburg virus.

Thin Sectioning

Thin sectioning is performed on tissue samples that have been fixed in specific fixatives suitable for electron microscopy, usually glutaraldehyde based. This technique is most useful for detailed examination of sections of tissue that have been identified as suspicious for viruses based on light microscopic findings, such as the presence of inclusion bodies. It is not suitable for scanning for viruses because only a very small field is visualized. Numerous viruses can be visualized, including herpesviruses, respiratory viruses, and rabies virus.[13-15]

ANTIGEN DETECTION

The detection of antigens directly in clinical specimens is an essential method for the laboratory diagnosis of viral infections. Antigen detection methods are widely used because they provide information rapidly, potentially within a few hours of receipt of the specimen in the laboratory. Also, antigen detection does not require the presence of viable virus. Therefore, when transport is delayed or is otherwise suboptimal, the sensitivity of antigen detection methods is affected less than culture. The techniques used most widely are fluorescent antibody (FA) staining, immunoperoxidase (IP) staining, and enzyme immunoassay (EIA). All these techniques are based on antibodies that specifically bind the virus being sought. Box 1–3 lists the viruses for which antigen detection is most successfully employed.

Fluorescent Antibody Staining

FA staining is the technique most widely used for viral antigen detection in specimens. The method involves use of an antibody, usually monoclonal, that is specific for the antigen being sought, and a fluorescent marker, usually fluorescein isothiocyanate (FITC). FITC pro-

duces "apple green" fluorescence when it is excited by light of the proper wavelength. Another widely used marker is tetramethylrhodamine isothiocyanate, which produces reddish orange fluorescence.

Two FA staining procedures are used: direct and indirect (Figure 1–7). In *direct* FA staining the antiviral antibody is conjugated with the fluorescent marker. In *indirect* FA staining the antiviral antibody is unlabeled and is detected with the use of a second antibody that binds to immunoglobulins from the species of origin of the first antibody (mouse in the case of most monoclonal antibodies). The second, or detector, antibody is conjugated with the fluorescent marker. The direct method is simpler to use but requires FITC conjugation of each antiviral antibody. The indirect method is slightly more sensitive and more versatile, because only the antiimmunoglobulin antibody is FITC conjugated.

The main applications of FA staining have been for the detection of respiratory, cutaneous, ocular, and bloodstream pathogens (see Chapters 4, 6, 10, and 15). Many different respiratory specimens can be used, including nasal swabs, nasal washes, nasal aspirates, tracheal aspirates, and bronchoalveolar lavage fluid. In each case the specimen is processed in the laboratory to prepare a pellet of cells, which is spotted onto one or more microscope slides. The cells are air dried, fixed in acetone, and stained with monoclonal antibodies to one or more viruses.

For ocular infections, material is scraped from the conjunctiva or cornea, placed on microscope slides, and processed as described for respiratory specimens. Staining is usually directed at detection of HSV and VZV antigens.

For cutaneous infections the lesion is scraped with a scalpel and cellular material is placed directly on one or more microscope slides. Alternatively, the base of the lesion can be rubbed vigorously with a swab and the swab submitted to the laboratory, where cellular material is washed from the swab and spotted onto a microscope slide. Staining is directed at detection of HSV and VZV.

In the CMV pp65 antigenemia assay, peripheral blood leukocytes are separated from anticoagulated blood, spotted onto a microscope slide, usually by cytocentrifugation, and stained using a monoclonal antibody specific for the pp65 antigen.

Immunoperoxidase Staining

IP staining is an alternative to FA staining. The difference is that horseradish peroxidase is used instead of a fluorescent marker. After the peroxidase-labeled antibody is incubated with the specimen, a substrate for peroxidase is added that changes color when acted on by the peroxidase. The advantage of this method is that the staining can be viewed by light microscopy, thus obviating the need for a fluorescent microscope. IP

Box 1.3 Viruses Identified by Antigen Detection Methods	
Respiratory syncytial	Varicella-zoster
Influenza	Cytomegalovirus
Parainfluenza	Rotavirus
Adenovirus	Hepatitis B
Herpes simplex	Measles

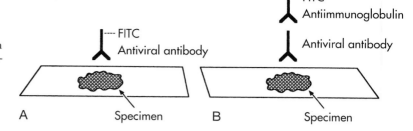

Figure 1.7   Fluorescent antibody stain for detection of viral antigen. **A,** Direct; **B,** indirect. *FITC,* Fluorescein isothiocyanate.

staining is particularly advantageous when performed on intact tissue, because the tissue can also be stained by histochemical stains, allowing examination of the spatial relationship between viral antigens and cellular structures.

The disadvantages of the IP method are that it is more cumbersome than FA staining, and endogenous peroxidases in some specimens can produce background staining.

Enzyme Immunoassay

EIA is a versatile and widely used method that can be applied to the detection of antibodies or antigens. When the antigen-antibody reaction takes place on a solid surface, the reaction is also known as *enzyme-linked immunosorbent assay* (ELISA).

Several versions of EIA have been used for antigen detection, including the frequently used double-antibody sandwich format (Figure 1–8). In this assay a "capture" antibody specific for the viral antigen being sought is bound to a reaction surface, such as the wells of a plastic microtiter tray or the surface of a plastic bead. When the specimen is added, viral antigen present in the specimen binds to the capture antibody. After washing to remove unbound specimen material, a

second antiviral antibody, the detector antibody, is added. The detector antibody can carry a chemically linked enzyme label (Figure 1–8, *A*), or can be detected by the addition of a third antibody with specificity for immunoglobulin of the species from which the second antibody was derived (Figure 1–8, *B*). After more washing to remove unbound antibody, the enzyme substrate is added and undergoes a color change if the enzyme is present (as a result of binding of the enzyme-labeled antibody). The resulting color change can be detected by eye or with the use of a spectrophotometer. Chemiluminescent reactions can also be employed and a luminometer used to detect emitted light.

The advantages of EIA for antigen detection are that it can be applied to diverse specimens, including fluids (which are not useful for FA staining and IP staining reactions) and even stool, and that it lends itself to automation. A number of laboratory instruments are now available that can carry out both antigen and antibody EIAs.

Membrane Immunoassays

In recent years, several commercial membrane immunoassays for viral antigens have been marketed (see Chapter 4). These assays are EIAs in which antigens or

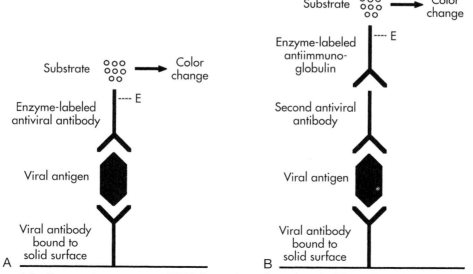

Figure 1.8   Enzyme immunoassay (EIA) for antigen detection. **A,** Direct; **B,** indirect. *E,* Enzyme.

antigen-antibody complexes are captured directly onto membranes. In the Directigen Flu A Test (Becton Dickinson, Cockeysville, Md), influenza A antigen is captured on a membrane and detected by reaction with an enzyme-labeled antibody against influenza A virus. In the TestPack (Abbott Laboratories, North Chicago), antigen in the specimen reacts with one antibody bound on microparticles and with a second antibody that is biotin labeled. The complexes are captured on a membrane, and an antibiotin antibody conjugated to the enzyme alkaline phosphatase is added, followed by an alkaline phosphatase substrate.

Both the Directigen Flu A Test and the Abbott TestPack are designed as self-contained cassettes for convenient testing of single specimens. They are simple enough to be used in physician's offices or in other outpatient facilities.

Limitations

Antigen detection methods are versatile but not applicable to all viruses. For example, the rhinoviruses are a diverse group with more than 90 serotypes, and cross-reacting antibodies suitable for use in antigen detection assays are not available. Some specimens are not suitable for antigen detection methods because of interfering substances. Finally, antigen detection methods are much less sensitive than nucleic acid amplification methods (e.g., PCR) and thus may lack the sensitivity necessary for some diagnostic applications.

MOLECULAR DIAGNOSIS

Diagnostic techniques based on the detection of specific viral nucleic acids are currently transforming the field of diagnostic virology. These techniques are based on the specific binding that occurs between single strands of nucleic acids having complementary nucleic acid sequences. The following characteristics make molecular diagnostic techniques advantageous for viral diagnosis:

1. Viral nucleic acids can be detected regardless of whether the virus being sought is capable of growing in cell culture. This is important because many medically important viruses are difficult or impossible to cultivate.

2. Nucleic acids are very stable to environmental conditions and can be detected even if no viable virus is present.

3. Each viral species has a unique nucleic acid sequence, providing the opportunity for virus-specific detection and identification.

4. Genus-specific or family-specific sequences provide the opportunity for broader-based detection.

Molecular diagnostic tests can be divided into three categories: direct hybridization; target (template) am-

plification, for which PCR is the paradigm; and signal amplification.

Direct Hybridization Assays

The most straightforward molecular diagnostic techniques are those based on direct detection of viral nucleic acid present in a specimen without amplification in the laboratory. Because of lack of sensitivity, few of these assays are currently used in diagnostic virology. An exception is a liquid hybridization assay used to detect hepatitis B DNA in serum (see Chapter 7).

All hybridization assays depend on an interaction between a nucleic acid reagent called a *probe* and the *target* viral nucleic acid present in the specimen. Different forms of direct hybridization assays include dot blot, slot blot, liquid hybridization, Southern blot, and ISH.

Nucleic acid probes. A nucleic acid probe is defined as a single-stranded segment of DNA or RNA with a defined sequence that is used as a reagent for the detection of nucleic acid segments having the complementary sequence. Probes can be as short as a 30–base oligonucleotide or as long as a viral genome consisting of thousands of nucleotides. To be visualized, probes must be labeled. Originally, probes were labeled with radioisotopes, usually ^{3}H, ^{35}S, or ^{32}P. Currently, nonisotopic enzymatic labels such as horseradish peroxidase and alkaline phosphatase are increasingly used. These enzymes act on a substrate to produce a color change or light emission.

Several systems for linking probes and detection labels are in use (Figure 1–9). Probes can be labeled with radioisotopes by several procedures and can be linked to enzymes through chemical reactions. An alternative method makes use of the high-affinity reaction between the coenzyme biotin and the molecule streptavidin. Biotin can be conveniently attached to nucleic acids, and streptavidin can be chemically coupled to enzymes. The resulting bond between biotin and streptavidin serves as a bridge linking the probe and the detection enzyme. A similar arrangement is achieved by attaching the molecule digoxigenin to the probe. Enzymes can be coupled to antidigoxigenin antibodies that bind to the biotin-labeled probe, forming the desired linkage.

Nucleic acid targets. The nucleic acid target for hybridization assays can be viral DNA or RNA. Any nucleic acid segment from the virus can potentially be used as a target but segments with sequences that are conserved among different strains and segments present in multiple copies are especially attractive as targets. DNA is more stable than RNA and generally easier to work with. The nucleic acid can be within viral particles, within virally infected cells, or free in the specimen. Before

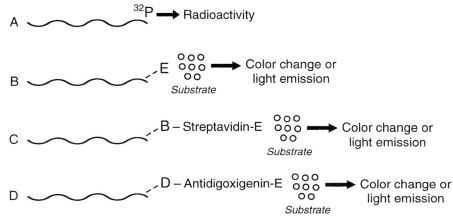

Figure 1.9 Systems for labeling nucleic acid probes. *A,* Radioisotopic label; **B,** enzymatic; **C,** biotin-streptavidin; **D,** digoxigenin-antidigoxigenin. Streptavidin and antidigoxigenin are coupled to enzymes such as horseradish peroxidase. Enzymatic substrate is chosen to undergo a color change or emit light when acted on by the enzyme. *E,* Enzyme; *B,* biotin; *D,* digoxigenin.

detection the target must be (1) released from viral particles or from within infected cells so that it is accessible to the probe and (2) denatured to separate the strands of nucleic acid so that binding with the probe can occur.

Dot blot and slot blot. In these assays the nucleic acid target is first released from virions or virally infected cells by digestive procedures. Nucleic acid is then denatured and immobilized or fixed on a membrane usually composed of nitrocellulose or nylon. Procedures used to fix nucleic acids on membranes include baking or ultraviolet (UV) irradiation. The dot or slot configuration of the target DNA on the membrane is achieved with the use of a specially designed apparatus that functions as a template. After fixation, the dot or slot is overlaid with the labeled probe. After allowing time for binding to occur, the membrane is washed to remove unbound probe. Bound isotopic probes are visualized by exposure of film or counting radioactivity in a counting chamber. Bound nonisotopic probes are detected by adding the appropriate enzyme substrate, yielding a color change or light emission. Binding of the probe is accepted as evidence that the target nucleic acid was present in the specimen. The sensitivity of the dot blot or slot blot reactions is approximately 10^4 to 10^5 molecules.[16]

Liquid hybridization. In the liquid or solution hybridization assay the hybridization between probe and target occurs in liquid phase. Binding of probe to target results in double-stranded nucleic acid, which can be detected by electrophoresis or by passage of the reaction mixture over a column that separates double-stranded nucleic acid from the unbound single-stranded probe. Liquid hybridization assays are generally more sensitive than dot blot or slot blot assays.

Southern blot. The Southern blot is a variation of direct hybridization that provides additional information about target DNA by virtue of prior digestion of the DNA with a restriction endonuclease. The steps involved in performing a Southern blot are as follows:

1. Target DNA is digested with a chosen restriction endonuclease to yield a set of fragments of variable size.
2. The digested target is subjected to electrophoresis to separate the fragments on the basis of size.
3. The separated fragments are transferred from the electrophoresis gel onto a membrane suitable for the performance of hybridization reactions.
4. The target DNA is denatured and immobilized on the surface of the membrane.
5. Labeled probe is added to the membrane under conditions that will allow binding to occur if segments complementary to the probe are present. The probe is chosen to match the sequence of one or more fragments of target DNA.
6. The membrane is washed to remove unbound probe.
7. The presence of bound probe is detected as described for dot blot and slot blot reactions.

Depending on the size of the probe and its location in relation to restriction endonuclease digestion sites, one or multiple target fragments will be revealed as bands on the membrane. Nucleotide sequence changes in the target that affect the digestion sites for the restriction endonuclease used to digest the target will change the size and number of fragments detected. Mutations in the probe binding site may also affect the ability of the probe to bind, affecting the intensity of the band. Thus the Southern blot has been used for molecular typing based on its ability to analyze differences among viral strains in the portion of the genome detected (see Chapter 19).

The advantage of the Southern blot is that the detection of a specific pattern of fragments makes the assay very specific. It is also sensitive, but less so than amplification-based techniques. The disadvantages of the Southern blot are that it is cumbersome, can be carried out only by a laboratory with specialized expertise, and requires a relatively large amount of target nucleic acid. Thus Southern blots can be performed on DNA extracted from tissue samples but not usually on other clinical specimens.

Polymerase Chain Reaction

The discovery of PCR by Kary Mullis in 1983 is the most important development in diagnostic virology since the development of cell culture. Mullis was awarded the 1993 Nobel Prize in Medicine for his accomplishment. PCR can detect as few as 1 to 10 copies of viral nucleic acid, providing a sensitivity comparable to or greater than viral culture and far exceeding that of other diagnostic tests. PCR has also proved to be very versatile, having the ability to detect DNA or RNA and to provide quantitative as well as qualitative information.

The power of PCR is magnified by linkage to nucleic acid sequencing of the PCR product, providing the capability for highly detailed analysis of the amplified portion of the viral genome. This capability has been used for the detection of antiviral drug resistance (see Chapter 18), for taxonomic analysis and molecular fingerprinting (see Chapter 19), and for the discovery of new viral agents (see Chapter 20).

Components. Several different components are essential to PCR. *Oligonucleotide primers* are short segments, usually 18 to 26 nucleotides, of single-stranded DNA that are complementary to opposite strands of DNA flanking a region to be amplified. The segment to be amplified is typically 100 to 1000 nucleotides but segments up to several thousand nucleotides in length can be amplified under special conditions.

Taq polymerase is a DNA polymerase that is stable at high temperatures. It was originally discovered in the bacterial species *Thermus aquaticus* found in thermal springs at Yellowstone National Park.

Nucleotides, Mg++ ions, and *buffer* must be present in the reaction mixture for the synthesis of new nucleic acid. *Template DNA* is the DNA segment being amplified by the PCR reaction; in the case of PCR to detect viral infection, the viral DNA serves as the template.

Cycles. PCR consists of multiple cycles, each consisting of three steps that occur at different temperatures (Figure 1–10). The reaction occurs in a thermal cycler, an instrument that accommodates tubes in which PCR takes place, and carries out a series of rapid temperature changes that cause the reaction to proceed through the steps of each cycle.

The first step in the cycle is *denaturation* of the double-stranded viral DNA template, achieved by elevating the reaction temperature to approximately 94°C. The second step is *annealing*, in which the oligonucleotide primers bind to template DNA. The annealing temperature is chosen to allow primer-template binding, typically 50° to 55°C, but sometimes other temperatures, depending on the nucleotide sequence of the primers and template. The final step of the cycle is *extension*, usually carried out at 72°C. During this step the primers are extended by the action of *Taq* polymerase, leading to the synthesis of new complementary strands of DNA.

At the end of the first cycle the amount of template DNA has been doubled. Cycles are repeated, leading to continued doubling of the DNA being amplified. The theoretic level of amplification exceeds 1 million–fold after 20 cycles and 1 billion-fold after 30 cycles. PCR reactions are typically carried out for 30 to 40 cycles because after approximately 30 cycles the efficiency of amplification declines and a plateau phase is reached.

Detection of products. After the PCR reaction is completed, the amplified DNA is detected by gel electrophoresis or by a hybridization reaction such as a Southern blot. Figure 1–11 shows an example of an agarose gel stained with ethidium bromide to allow visualization of PCR products.

More recently, PCR products have also been detected by EIAs modified to detect DNA rather than antigens. The Roche Amplicor Monitor assay used to detect HIV RNA in plasma provides an example of one such system (see Figure 17–7). In the Amplicor reaction, both the PCR primers are biotinylated, resulting in biotinylation of the amplified PCR product. After PCR is completed, the PCR products are transferred to microtiter trays with wells that are coated with a probe whose sequence is complementary to a segment of one strand of the amplified product. After the PCR product is denatured, the strand complementary to the probe is captured by annealing to the probe. After washing, streptavidin–horseradish peroxidase is added, followed by peroxidase substrate. The resulting color change is read in a spectrophotometer.

RNA detection. PCR itself detects only DNA, but RNA in a specimen can be detected by first converting the target RNA to its complementary DNA. This is accomplished using the enzyme *reverse transcriptase* (RT). This reaction can be carried out in the same reaction tube as the PCR simply by including RT and the appropriate buffer components in the reaction mixture, then initiating the reaction with a period of incubation at the appropriate temperature for the RT reaction to take place. Enzymes are also available that have RT activity as well as thermostable DNA polymerase activity, allowing both the RT reaction and the PCR to be performed

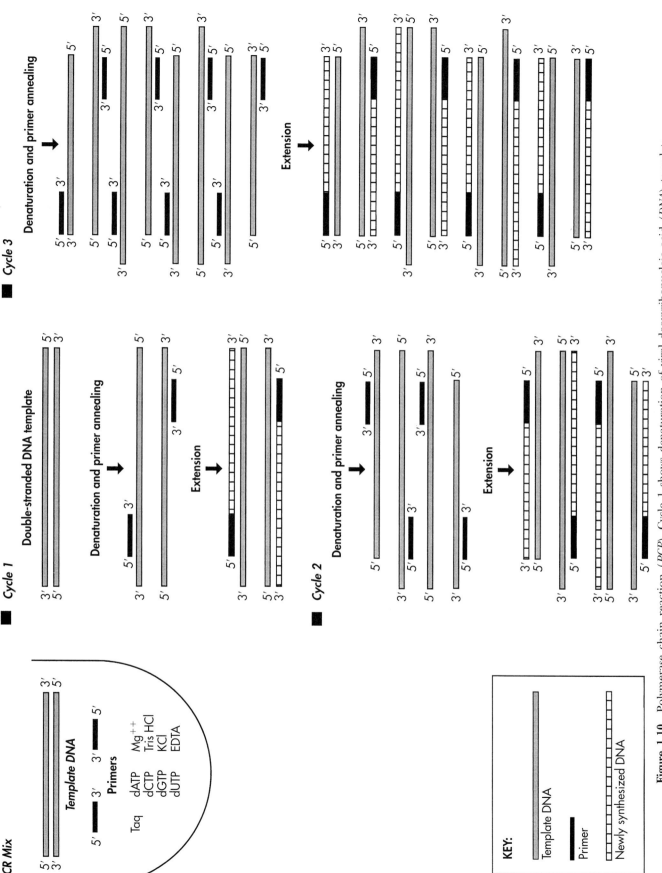

Figure 1.10 Polymerase chain reaction (*PCR*). Cycle 1 shows denaturation of viral deoxyribonucleic acid (*DNA*) template, annealing of PCR primers, and extension to form new complementary DNA strands. PCR product after cycle 1 consists of two new strands of DNA that are "long products" because extension has continued beyond downstream primer-binding site. Cycle 2 shows same steps as cycle 1. PCR product after cycle 2 consists of a total of six new strands (two from cycle 1 and four from cycle 2). Four of the new strands are "long strands" and two "short strands." PCR product after cycle 3 consists of 14 new strands (two from cycle 1, four from cycle 2, and eight from cycle 3), including six long strands and eight short strands. In subsequent steps, short strands will accumulate at an exponential rate, whereas long strands will accumulate at a linear rate.

15

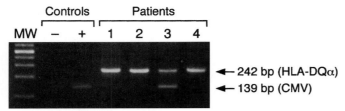

Figure 1.11 Detection of PCR products by agarose gel electrophoresis and ethidium bromide staining. The gel shown contains reaction products from PCR for cytomegalovirus *(CMV)*. Molecular weight *(MW)* standards and negative and positive controls are shown. Leukocyte samples from four patients show a band representing amplification of segment of HLA-DQα gene, used to demonstrate amplifiable human DNA in each patient sample. Patient 3 is positive for CMV. *bp*, base pairs.

using the same enzyme. Examples of widely used RT-PCR assays are the HIV and the hepatitis C plasma RNA assays.

Nested PCR. Nested PCR refers to a coordinated pair of PCRs carried out using two sets of oligonucleotide primers, an "outer" set and an "inner" set. The inner primers bind to sequences within the segment amplified by the outer set. Nested PCR is initiated by performing a standard PCR using the outer set of primers. After 10 to 30 cycles a small aliquot is removed and used as the template for a second PCR reaction using the inner primers. Nested PCR can achieve very high sensitivity and specificity. However, some laboratories avoid nested PCRs because the need to open the PCR tube after cycles of amplification have occurred introduces a risk of PCR contamination (see later discussion).

Multiplex PCR. Multiplex PCR refers to PCR assays in which two or more primer sets directed toward the amplification of different nucleic acid segments are incorporated into the same reaction mixture. Multiplex reactions are useful in detecting more than one agent in a clinical sample. For example, a multiplex reaction that detects the DNA of Epstein-Barr virus and *Toxoplasma gondii* is useful in evaluating CSF specimens from patients with acquired immunodeficiency syndrome (AIDS) who have mass lesions in the brain.[17] Another multiplex reaction has been used to detect all human herpesviruses and enteroviruses in the same reaction.[18]

Multiplex reactions can work only when the same set of PCR conditions allows amplification of each intended product. Interactions among primers can be a problem, especially as the number of sets of primers in the reaction increases.

Quantitative PCR. PCR can be modified so that the number of copies of target DNA (or RNA) in the specimen can be estimated. All quantitative methods require a method for measuring the amount of PCR product. This can be accomplished using instruments such as densitometers or video imaging systems.

In the simplest method for quantitation, a series of standards with known amounts of the target are amplified and a standard curve is constructed using the amount of PCR product measured in each tube. The amount of DNA in the specimen is estimated by comparing the strength of positivity of the reaction with the standard curve. A shortcoming of this method is that it does not account for tube-to-tube variation in the efficiency of PCR.

A method that is not affected by such variation is called *quantitative-competitive PCR* (Figure 1–12). This method uses a laboratory-constructed competitive standard that consists of a segment of DNA with the same primer binding sites as the target and thus is amplified by those primers. The standard is constructed so that its amplified product can be distinguished from the amplified target by virtue of its size or by differences in internal nucleotide sequence. A known amount of the competitive standard is included in each PCR reaction tube along with the template DNA. A standard curve is constructed using a series of PCRs to which the same amount of the competitive standard and an increasing amount of the target DNA are added. After the PCR is completed, the amounts of amplified target and amplified competitive standard products are measured, and the log of the ratio is plotted against the log of the amount of the target added to each tube. The amount of target DNA in an unknown sample is calculated from the standard curve.

Nucleotide sequencing. One of the most powerful attributes of PCR is that the nucleotide sequence of amplified products can be readily determined. This can be used to determine unknown sequences (provided sufficient sequence information is available to allow design of primers) and to study sequence heterogeneity within the amplified nucleic acid segment.

A variety of methods are available for sequencing the amplified products, some of which involve cloning the amplified product into a vector suitable for performing conventional sequencing reactions. Sequencing can also be performed directly on DNA or RNA present in the sample without cloning. This is accomplished by using a reaction known as *cycle sequencing*, which has the capability of determining nucleotide sequence from much smaller amounts of nucleic acid than are required by other sequencing methods. Cycle sequencing can use small amounts of template through the use of *Taq* polymerase and repetitive PCR-like cycles. Cycle sequencing can be used in conjunction with automated sequencing instruments to make nucleotide sequences available within 2 to 3 days.

Contamination. The problem of PCR contamination arises from two aspects of PCR itself: (1) the PCR reaction can detect the presence of a minute amount of a specific nucleic acid and (2) the end product of PCR is a large amount of the same nucleic acid sequence that the PCR is designed to detect. The danger is that PCR product may spread through the laboratory and "contaminate" other PCRs, causing them to be positive regardless of the presence of the nucleic acid target in the original material being analyzed by PCR. Aerosolization of liquid during the analysis of PCR products can lead to contamination of the laboratory environment or even of personnel working in the laboratory.

Numerous precautions can be undertaken in the laboratory to minimize the risk of contamination. The most basic precaution is the physical separation of areas of the laboratory devoted to specimen preparation, setup of the PCR, and analysis of the PCR products after amplification. Other precautions include the use of positive displacement pipettes or plugged pipette tips to block aerosols, UV irradiation of reaction components (not including *Taq* polymerase and PCR primers that can be inactivated by UV irradiation), use of small working aliquots, and frequent cleaning of equipment and laboratory surfaces with 10% bleach.

Two additional precautions employed by some laboratories are the use of uracil-*N*-glycosylase (UNG) or furocoumarin compounds in the PCR reaction mixture.[19] In the UNG method, deoxyuridine triphosphate (dUTP) is incorporated into the PCR reaction mixture in place of deoxythymidine triphosphate (dTTP), one of the four nucleotides required for DNA synthesis. *Taq* polymerase is able to use dUTP in place of dTTP; therefore, when PCR occurs, the resulting PCR product contains dUTP instead of dTTP. When subsequent PCRs are assembled, UNG is incorporated into the reaction mixture. At the start of PCR the tube is incubated at a temperature that permits UNG to cleave uracil residues from the DNA backbone. The site on the DNA backbone where the uracil was removed is vulnerable to scission during subsequent PCR. Any DNA present as a result of contamination from previous PCRs is eliminated as an effective PCR template.

The addition of furocoumarin compounds to the PCR reaction mixture accomplishes the same purpose by a different method. Furocoumarins such as psoralen and isopsoralen derivatives bind to DNA after exposure to light of the appropriate wavelength. One of these compounds can be included in the PCR reaction mix. After the PCR reaction has been completed, but before the tube is opened for analysis, the tube is exposed to light of the appropriate wavelength for a short period, leading to binding of the compound to the amplified PCR product. After binding occurs, the PCR product cannot serve as template for amplification, thus eliminating it as a source of contamination.

Other Amplification Methods

The success of PCR has stimulated the development of other amplification methods, several of which are undergoing commercial development for specific applications. Amplification methods can be divided into those that amplify the template (target) itself and those that amplify the signal. Examples of template amplification methods other than PCR are the *self-sustained sequence replication* (3SR) *method*, which is directed at amplification of RNA, the lipase chain reaction (LCR),

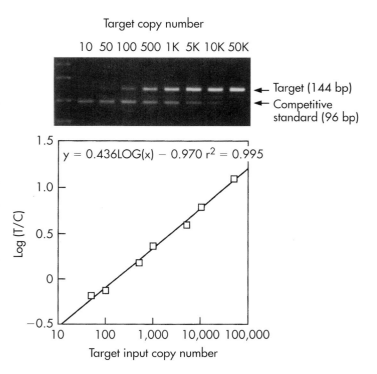

Figure 1.12 Quantitative-competitive PCR. In this reaction, increasing numbers of copies of 144– base-pair *(bp)* target have been added to a series of tubes; 250 copies of 96 base-pair competitor have also been added to each tube. Intensity of bands corresponding to 144– and 96–bp products is measured using a video imaging system, and log of ratio is plotted against log of number of copies of target added to each tube. Number of copies of target in an unknown sample is estimated by performing PCR after addition of 250 copies of competitor. Intensity of bands is measured, and number of copies of target is determined from standard curve produced using tubes to which known copies of target have been added. **A,** Ethidium bromide–stained gel; **B,** standard curve. *T/C,* Target/competitor.

and the *strand displacement assay* (SDA). A method similar to 3SR is being developed as the NucliSens assay by Organon Teknika (Durham, NC) for the detection of RNA from a variety of viruses, including HIV (see Figure 17–9). Another closely related method called transcription mediated amplification is being developed by Gen-Probe, Inc. (San Diego).

In *signal amplification assays*, DNA or RNA in the specimen is hybridized to a probe without amplification of the target. A high sensitivity of detection results from "amplification" of the signal achieved by the binding of many detector molecules to each target-probe hybrid. The *branched-chain DNA* (bDNA) *assay* is being developed by Bayer Diagnostics (Emeryville, Calif) for detection and quantitation of HIV RNA (see Figure 17–8), hepatitis C RNA (see Chapter 8), and several other viral nucleic acids. The *hybrid capture assay* (Figure 1–13), is being developed by Digene Corporation

(Beltsville, Md) for detection of the DNAs of HPV and CMV (see Chapters 7 and 15). Both the bDNA and the hybrid capture assays can be used to quantitate as well as detect specific viral nucleic acids.

SEROLOGY

The diagnosis of viral infections by measuring an antibody response to the virus was a landmark in the history of diagnostic virology. It remains important for the diagnosis of acute infection with certain viruses and for the determination of specific antiviral immunity. Serologic diagnosis depends on the kinetics of the antibody response to viral infection, (Figure 1–14).

Antiviral antibodies become detectable several weeks after infection. Virus-specific immunoglobulin M

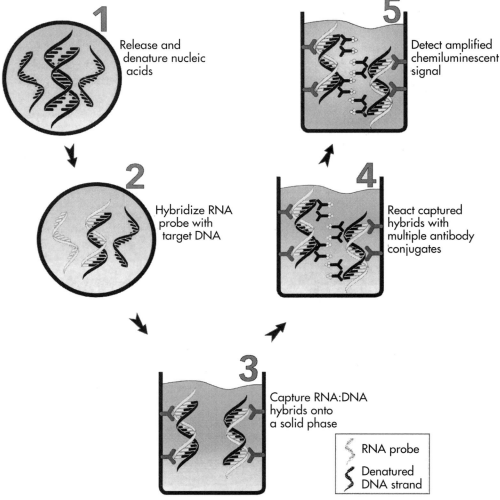

Figure 1.13 Steps in hybrid capture assay: *1,* target DNA is released and denatured; *2,* RNA probe hybridizes with target DNA; *3,* RNA:DNA hybrids are captured by antibody to RNA:DNA hybrids that is bound to sides of reaction vessel; *4,* enzyme-conjugated antibody that recognizes RNA:DNA hybrids binds to them; *5,* chemiluminescent substrate is added, and light is emitted if hybrids have been formed. (Courtesy Digene Corporation, Beltsville, Md.)

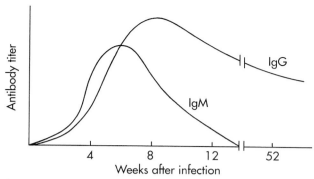

Figure 1.14 Kinetics of antiviral antibody response after acute infection. *IgM,* Immunoglobulin.

(IgM) antibodies are often detectable for a short period before virus-specific immunoglobulin G (IgG) antibodies. The IgM response tends to decline within approximately 1 to 2 months, although low levels may persist for one year or more in some viral infections. IgG antibodies are much more long lasting and may persist for the individual's life span.

Serologic evidence for acute infection consists of (1) *seroconversion* in serial specimens (absence of specific viral antibodies in a specimen obtained at the onset of illness and the presence of those antibodies in a specimen obtained several weeks later), (2) a rising or falling titer of virus-specific antibodies from the acute to the convalescent phase, or (3) the presence of virus-specific IgM antibodies in an acute phase specimen, which is particularly useful because it can provide a rapid diagnosis from a single specimen obtained early in the illness.

Serologic diagnosis is important for viruses that cannot be readily cultured or for which culture is slow or otherwise impractical. Box 1–4 lists viruses for which serology is useful in diagnosing acute infection. Among these are a special subset of viruses that typically cause chronic infection. The serodiagnosis of these infections is unusual because the presence of antibodies to the virus is diagnostic of currently active infection. Examples include HIV and the related retroviruses human T-cell lymphotropic (leukemia) virus types I and II (HTLV-I and II). For hepatitis C the presence of confirmed antibodies to the virus corresponds to active infection in approximately 85% of individuals.

Serology is uniquely useful for defining immunity with respect to specific viruses. It is important to use sensitive assays such as EIA for this purpose because antibody levels indicative of past infection may decline to very low levels years after the infection. The specific assay used must also be selected with care that it measures antibodies that correlate with immunity. Box 1–5 lists viruses for which serologic testing is used to determine immune status.

Serologic Assays

Several serologic assays are used for the detection of specific antiviral antibodies. Currently the most widely used are EIA and immunofluorescent assay (IFA). The neutralization assay remains an absolute gold standard in many instances.

Enzyme immunoassay. The EIA format used most often for detection of antibodies is termed the *indirect EIA* or *indirect ELISA* (Figure 1–15; see also Figure 1–8).

In this assay a viral antigen is bound to a solid phase, usually the inner surface of the well of a microtiter tray. Serum is added to the well and allowed to incubate. If present, antiviral antibodies bind to the surface-bound antigen. The serum is then removed and the well extensively washed. The next step is the addition of a

---

Box 1.4   Viral Infections Diagnosed by Serology

Epstein-Barr*
Cytomegalovirus (mononucleosis syndrome)*
Hepatitis (A to E)†
Measles*
Rubella*
Mumps*
Parvovirus B19*
Encephalitis viruses*
Rabies
Hemorrhagic fever viruses*
Dengue*
Human immunodeficiency (HIV)
Human T-cell lymphotropic (leukemia) virus types I and II (HTLV-I/II)

* Virus-specific IgM assays are used.
† Virus-specific IgM assays are used for hepatitis A and B (IgM anti-HBc [hepatitis B core antigen]).

Box 1.5   Serologic Determination of Immune Status

Varicella-zoster
Herpes simplex
Epstein-Barr (IgG antibodies to viral capsid antigen)
Rubella
Measles
Mumps
Parvovirus B19
Hepatitis A (total antibodies)
Hepatitis B (anti-HBs [hepatitis B surface antigen])

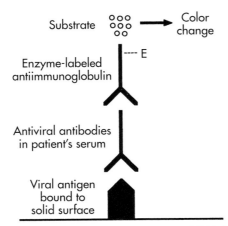

Figure 1.15 Indirect enzyme immunoassay (EIA). *E*, Enzyme.

second (detector) antibody with specificity for human immunoglobulins. The second antibody is typically a mouse monoclonal or a polyclonal antibody from a nonhuman species. It is linked to an enzyme such as horseradish peroxidase. The second antibody binds to any human antibody present (ideally because of specific binding to the viral antigen). The well is again extensively washed, and a substrate for the enzyme is added. If the second antibody is present, the enzyme to which it is linked will act on the substrate to induce a color change, which is measured by a spectrophotometer. An optical density cutoff of threefold greater than the absorbance of negative control specimens is often used to define a positive test. Cutoffs based on the standard deviation of negative controls are also sometimes used.

Advantages of the EIA method are that it is sensitive, versatile, and readily automated. In addition, it can be modified to detect virus-specific IgM or IgA antibodies through the use of isotype-specific second antibodies.

Immunofluorescent assay. IFA is conceptually similar to the indirect EIA. A viral antigen, which most often consists of fixed cells infected with the virus, is attached to microscope slides. Dilutions of serum to be tested are added to wells on the slide and allowed to incubate. After extensive washing, a detector antibody is added that consists of an antihuman immunoglobulin labeled with a fluorescent molecule, most often FITC. The slide is viewed under UV illumination, allowing visualization of bound antibody.

IFA is extremely versatile because any infected cell can be used as antigen. As in EIA, isotype-specific antibodies can be measured by using detector antibodies that are specific for IgM or IgA.

Neutralization assay. Neutralization assays measure the ability of antibodies to block viral infectivity. In these assays, serial dilutions of the serum to be tested are incubated with a standardized quantity of infectious virus. After a short incubation period the serum-virus mixtures are added to cells that support the growth of the virus, in parallel with a similar inoculum of virus that has not been incubated with serum. The neutralizing antibody titer is the highest serum dilution that prevents infection of the cells. The neutralization assay correlates well with protection from infection; it is sometimes considered the standard against which other serologic assays should be measured.

Because it is cumbersome and expensive, the neutralization assay is now rarely used in routine diagnostic laboratories.

Agglutination assay. Viral antigens can be bound to a variety of particles, including fixed erythrocytes and latex particles. Agglutination assays are performed by mixing dilutions of serum with a suspension of particles coated with the appropriate viral antigen. The agglutination titer is the highest serum dilution that results in visible agglutination of particles. The advantage of agglutination assays is simplicity; they are rapid and do not require sophisticated equipment. Therefore they are well suited for "stat" testing and for use under field conditions.

Hemagglutination inhibition. Certain viruses produce glycoproteins that hemagglutinate erythrocytes and are referred to as *hemagglutinins*. The hemagglutinin inhibition test is performed by determining the highest serum dilution that inhibits erythrocyte hemagglutination caused by a specific viral hemagglutinin. The test has been considered a reference test for antibodies to certain viruses such as rubella and dengue. It is not as sensitive as EIA, however, and is increasingly being replaced by EIA and IFA.

Complement fixation. The complement fixation test measures antibodies that bind, or "fix," complement and thus inhibit complement-mediated erythrocyte lysis. The advantage of the test is versatility; by substituting different viral antigens, the same test procedure can be used to measure antibodies against a wide variety of viruses. The test procedure is cumbersome, however, and less sensitive than other test formats, including EIA, IFA, and latex agglutination. For these reasons, the complement fixation test is used less often now than in the past.

Western blot and related assays. The Western blot has the ability to define the specific antigens to which an antibody response is directed. The test involves separation of individual viral proteins by *sodium dodecyl sulfate–polyacrylamide gel electrophoresis* (SDS-PAGE), usually performed on a partially purified viral preparation. The separated proteins are then transferred to a membrane, that is reacted with the patient's serum. The binding of antibodies to individual proteins is detected by an enzyme-labeled or radioisotope-labeled antihuman immunoglobulin.

The Western blot is cumbersome, but provides a very high level of specificity because of the ability to identify binding to individual viral proteins and the production of a characteristic blot fingerprint. Thus its main application in diagnostic laboratories is the confirmation of screening assays (e.g., EIA) that are less specific. For example, the Western blot is widely used to confirm a positive HIV EIA (see Figure 17–4). In the case of HIV, commercial availability of membrane strips that already contain HIV antigens makes the performance of Western blots practical and better standardized by obviating the need for laboratories to perform the electrophoresis and transfer steps.

Interpretation of Western blots requires considerable expertise. Other than for HIV, Western blots are rarely used in routine diagnostic laboratories because of their complexity and lack of commercial availability.

An assay that is similar conceptually to the Western blot is the recombinant *immunobinding (immunoblot) assay.* This assay differs from the Western blot in that specific viral antigens are produced within in vitro expression systems and artificially spotted onto membranes in a predetermined configuration, often in dots or in bands (see Figure 8–5). The membranes are then incubated with serum, and bound antibodies are detected as in the Western blot. The advantage of the immunoblot assay is that it allows detection of antibodies to specific viral antigens that are chosen for desired characteristics. Immunobinding assays are used widely to confirm positive hepatitis C ELISA results (see Chapter 8) and have also been used for the rapid diagnosis of hantavirus infections (see Chapter 16).

Virus-specific IgM Assays

Assays for virus-specific IgM antibodies are important because they often allow a specific diagnosis to be made based on analysis of a single serum specimen obtained during the acute phase of illness. These assays are most likely to be useful in diseases with incubation periods that are sufficiently long so that virus-specific IgM levels are present at detectable levels at the onset of illness. Hepatitis A provides an excellent example; because of its incubation period of 2 to 6 weeks, hepatitis A IgM antibodies are virtually always detectable at the time patients seek medical care. On the other hand, detection of specific IgM antibodies would not be expected to be useful in a disease such as influenza, in which the incubation period is too short for virus-specific IgM antibodies to reach a detectable level.

Longstanding methods used to measure virus-specific IgM antibodies include separating IgG and IgM fractions before performing the virus-specific antibody assay and performing the virus-specific assay before and after procedures (e.g., treatment with

β-mercaptoethanol) that selectively destroy IgM antibodies. Many modern virus-specific IgM antibody assays use IFA or the indirect EIA configuration (see Figure 1–15) with a detector antibody that binds only to human IgM.

An alternative assay configuration is the *IgM capture assay* (Figure 1–16), in which IgM antibodies in the serum are first "captured" using an antibody specific for human IgM. A preparation of viral antigen is added, followed by an enzyme-labeled antibody specific for the viral antigen. Binding is detected by the addition of the appropriate enzyme substrate.

Virus-specific IgM assays have several potential pitfalls. False-positive results can occur if the serum being tested contains *rheumatoid factor* (RF, IgM antibodies to human IgG) plus virus-specific IgG antibodies. If it does, complexes may form between the RF and the virus-specific IgG antibodies, and these complexes may be falsely detected by the assay as virus-specific IgM antibodies. This problem can be avoided by pretreatment of the serum to remove either RF or IgG antibodies. One of these pretreatments is included routinely in many commercial virus-specific IgM antibody assays.

False-negative results can occur if the serum being tested contains high levels of virus-specific IgG antibodies that may compete with the virus-specific IgM antibodies. The IgM capture assay configuration avoids this problem, as does serum pretreatment to remove IgG.

Complexities in the nature of the IgM antibody response must also be considered in interpreting virus-specific IgM antibody tests. In some patients the IgM antibody response is transient or low level, leading to failure to detect virus-specific IgM antibodies. In

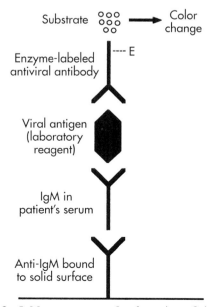

Figure 1.16 IgM capture assay for detection of virus-specific IgM antibodies. *E,* Enzyme.

others, low levels of IgM antibodies may persist for one year or longer, decreasing the specificity of the assay as an indicator of recent infection. In herpesvirus infections, IgM antibodies can sometimes be detected in reactivations as well as in primary infection.

Cerebrospinal Fluid Serology

Serologic testing can be applied to cerebrospinal fluid (CSF) for the diagnosis of central nervous system (CNS) infection (see Chapter 3). For unusual viruses such as rabies, the presence of any virus-specific antibodies within the CSF is diagnostic of active infection. For the diagnosis of encephalitis caused by the alphaviruses or flaviviruses, the presence of virus-specific antibodies is highly suspicious, and the presence of virus-specific IgM antibodies is diagnostic. For more common viruses such as the herpesviruses or the common respiratory viruses, the mere presence of virus-specific antibodies in CSF is not diagnostic of CNS infection because antibodies produced in the blood are present in the CSF even in the absence of CNS infection. The problem is further complicated because blood-brain barrier defects of many neurologic diseases can increase the passage of antibodies from blood to CSF.

Therefore, for the common viruses, *intrathecal antibody synthesis* must be demonstrated to provide evidence of CNS infection. Intrathecal synthesis of a specific antiviral antibody is evaluated by determining the quotient of two ratios: (1) the ratio of specific antiviral antibody level in CSF to serum and (2) the ratio of total IgG in CSF to serum:

$$CSF_{specific\ antibody}:serum_{specific\ antibody}/CSF_{IgG}:serum_{IgG}$$

A quotient greater than 1.5 is evidence of intrathecal antibody synthesis of the specific antibody. The antibody assay used to measure the specific antiviral antibody must have special characteristics. First, it must be very sensitive, since CSF antibody levels are usually low (approximately 1000-fold less than serum levels). Second, it must be capable of providing a quantitative result that allows calculation of the CSF/serum ratio of specific antibody level. EIAs are generally used but testing of a series of dilutions of CSF and serum is often required to obtain linear quantitative estimates of antibody level suitable for calculating the necessary ratio.

Because of the complexities involved, accurate determination of intrathecal antibody synthesis of specific antiviral antibodies is performed in only a limited number of reference laboratories.

Measurement of intrathecal antibody synthesis has been used in a variety of CNS infections. The most extensive experience is with HSV encephalitis, in which determinations of intrathecal antibody synthesis have limited clinical utility, because synthesis may not be detectable until 7 to 10 days after the onset of illness.

Interestingly, intrathecal antibody synthesis may persist for years after the acute infection. Therefore, the main utility of testing for intrathecal antibody synthesis is when specimens were not available early in the illness to allow a definitive diagnosis based on PCR. A caveat concerning diagnosis by demonstration of intrathecal antibody synthesis is that the clinician must consider evaluating its specificity by evaluating intrathecal synthesis of antibodies to at least one other virus, since in some diseases, most notably multiple sclerosis, polyclonal intrathecal antibody synthesis may occur.[20]

References

1. Weller RH, Enders JF: Production of hemagglutinin by mumps and influenza A viruses in suspended cell tissue cultures, *Proc Soc Exp Biol Med* 69:124, 1948.
2. Kohler G, Milstein C: Continuous cultures of fused cells secreting antibody of predefined specificity, *Nature* 256:495, 1975.
3. Saiki RK, Scharf S, Faloona F, et al: Enzymatic amplification of beta-globin genomic sequences and restriction site analysis of sickle cell anemia, *Science* 230:1350, 1985.
4. Gleaves CA, Smith TF, Shuster EA, Pearson GR: Rapid detection of cytomegalovirus in MRC-5 cells inoculated with urine specimens by using low-speed centrifugation and monoclonal antibody to an early antigen, *J Clin Microbiol* 19:917, 1984.
5. Griffiths PD, Panjwani DD, Stirk PR, et al: Rapid diagnosis of cytomegalovirus infection in immunocompromised patients by detection of early antigen fluorescent foci, *Lancet* 2:1242, 1984.
6. Shuster EA, Beneke JS, Tegtmeier GE, et al: Monoclonal antibody for rapid laboratory detection of cytomegalovirus infections: characterization and diagnostic application, *Mayo Clin Proc* 60:577, 1985.
7. Gleaves CA, Smith TF, Shuster EA, Pearson GR: Comparison of standard tube and shell vial cell culture techniques for the detection of cytomegalovirus in clinical specimens, *J Clin Microbiol* 21:217, 1985.
8. Arens M, Owen J, Hagerty CM, et al: Optimizing recovery of cytomegalovirus in the shell vial culture procedure, *Diagn Microbiol Infect Dis* 14:125, 1991.
9. Stabell EC, Olivo EC: Isolation of a cell line for rapid and sensitive histochemical assay for the detection of herpes simplex virus, *J Virol Methods* 38:195, 1992.
10. Stabell EC, O'Rourke SR, Storch GA, Olivo PD: Evaluation of a genetically engineered cell line and a histochemical beta-galactosidase assay to detect herpes simplex virus in clinical specimens, *J Clin Microbiol* 31:2796, 1993.
11. Tebas P, Stabell EC, Olivo PD: Antiviral susceptibility testing with a cell line which expresses beta-galactosidase after infection with herpes simplex virus, *Antimicrob Agents Chemother* 39:1287, 1995.
12. Rocancourt D, Bonnerot C, Jouin H, et al: Activation of a beta-galactosidase recombinant provirus: application to titration of human immunodeficiency virus (HIV) and HIV-infected cells, *J Virol* 64:2660, 1990.

13. Miller SE: Diagnosis of viral infections by electron microscopy. In Lennette EH, Lennette DA, Lennette ET, editors: *Diagnostic procedures for viral, rickettsial, and chlamydial infections*, ed 7, Washington, DC, 1995, American Public Health Association.

14. Doane FW, Anderson N: *Electron microscopy in diagnostic virology*, New York, 1987, Cambridge University Press.

15. Palmer EL, Martin ML: *Electron microscopy in viral diagnosis*, Boca Raton, Fl, 1988, CRC Press.

16. Persing DH: In vitro nucleic acid amplification techniques. In Persing DH, Smith TF, Tenover FC, White TJ, editors: *Diagnostic molecular microbiology: principles and applications*, Washington, DC, 1993, American Society for Microbiology.

17. Roberts TC, Storch GA: Multiplex polymerase chain reaction for diagnosis of AIDS-related central nervous system lymphoma and toxoplasmosis, *J Clin Microbiol* 35:268, 1997.

18. Casas I, Tenorio A, Echevarria JM, et al: Detection of enteroviral RNA and specific DNA of herpesviruses by multiplex genome amplification, *J Virol Methods* 66:39, 1997.

19. Persing DH, Cimino GD: Amplification product inactivation methods. In Persing DH, Smith TF, Tenover FC, White TJ, editors: *Diagnostic molecular microbiology: principles and applications*, Washington, DC, 1993, American Society for Microbiology.

20. Reiber H, Lange P: Quantitation of virus-specific antibodies in cerebrospinal fluid and serum: sensitive and specific detection of antibody synthesis in the brain, *Clin Chem* 37:1153, 1991.

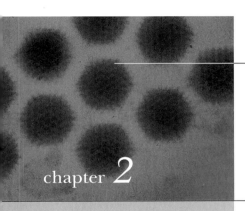

Richard Buller

Specimen Collection and *Transport*

chapter 2

OVERVIEW 26
GENERAL CONSIDERATIONS 26
VIRAL TRANSPORT MEDIA 26
COLLECTION SWABS 26
COLLECTION AND TRANSPORT TEMPERATURE 27
SPECIMENS FOR VIRAL ISOLATION AND ANTIGEN DETECTION 27
  Respiratory Specimens 27
    Nasopharyngeal swabs, aspirates, and washes 27
    Throat specimens 28
    Bronchoalveolar lavage and bronchial washes 29
    Sputum 29
  Blood 29
  Cerebrospinal Fluid 30
  Stool 31
  Biopsy Tissue 31
  Urine 31
  Ocular Specimens 32
  Vesicles and Other Skin Lesions 32
  Amniotic Fluid 32
SPECIMENS FOR MOLECULAR DIAGNOSTIC TESTS 33
  General Considerations 33
  Blood 33
  Cerebrospinal Fluid 33
  Tissue Specimens 34
  Ocular Fluid 34

OVERVIEW

Specimen collection and specimen transport are the first steps of the multistep process usually required for the laboratory diagnosis of viral infections. It is imperative, therefore, that this initial process be performed properly to ensure the integrity of laboratory results. The purpose of this chapter is to provide clinicians with the information necessary to collect and transport specimens that will yield useful laboratory results.

GENERAL CONSIDERATIONS

Clinicians are well advised to establish a rapport with the laboratory performing viral testing. Most virology laboratories will supply them with supplies for the collection and transport of specimens as well as information on the preferred method for obtaining specimens. All laboratories are under increased regulatory pressures, including attention to and documentation of quality control issues. As a part of a quality control program, a virology laboratory may have to refuse specimens that do not meet established criteria. By having an open line of communication with the laboratory, clinicians can avoid the possible disastrous loss of valuable specimen material through improper collection and transport.

Isolation of viruses in culture remains the mainstay of many viral diagnostic laboratories. The ability to grow a cultivable virus present in a clinical specimen depends on maintaining the infectivity of the virus from the time the specimen is obtained until it arrives in the laboratory and is inoculated into culture. Viruses vary greatly in their stability in regard to environmental factors such as temperature and pH. A simple model of viral structure is a nucleic acid surrounded by a proteinaceous capsid that, depending on the viral group, may or may not be surrounded by a lipid membrane derived from the infected cell. In general, nonenveloped viruses (those without a lipid membrane) are more stable than viruses surrounded by a lipid membrane. Thus, of the viruses most often isolated in culture, the nonenveloped viruses of the adenovirus and enterovirus groups are quite stable and generally do not present problems relative to maintaining infectivity. In contrast, enveloped viruses such as varicella-zoster virus (VZV) and respiratory syncytial virus (RSV) are considerably less stable, with significant losses of infectivity possible during specimen collection and transport.[1-4]

VIRAL TRANSPORT MEDIA

All viruses, regardless of stability, benefit from being transported in a medium that is prepared specifically to maintain viral infectivity. Numerous formulations exist for viral transport media, all of which generally contain (1) a *salt solution* to ensure proper ionic concentrations, (2) a *buffer* to maintain pH, (3) a source of *protein* for viral particle stability, and (4) *antibiotics* to prevent the overgrowth of bacteria and fungi that may be present in the specimen. Most clinical virology laboratories will provide their own viral transport media on request. For interested clinicians, many excellent references are available that contain "recipes" for making transport media.[5]

Our laboratory occasionally receives questions concerning the suitability of using bacterial transport media for viruses. Although the successful use of bacterial media to transport swabs for the isolation of herpes simplex virus (HSV) has been reported,[6] we recommend this only as a last resort.

COLLECTION SWABS

Certain collection procedures, including those for respiratory specimens, ocular specimens, specimens from lesions, and some rectal specimens, involve the use of swabs. The swab tip can be made of various materials, including cotton, rayon, Dacron, and calcium alginate.

A significant reduction in the titer of infectious HSV was reported after incubation of the virus in the presence of calcium alginate swab material.[7] This effect was not observed with other swab materials and was theorized to result from direct binding of the calcium alginate to the virus. Similarly, in another study in which herpetic lesions were swabbed with a calcium alginate and a cotton swab, a significant decrease in recovery of HSV in culture was noted when lesions were sampled with calcium alginate swabs relative to the cotton swab.[8] However, cotton as well as calcium alginate swabs were found to decrease the titer of infectious VZV when the swabs were incubated for 5 to 10 minutes in medium containing the virus.[4] Although similar effects of calcium alginate swabs have not been documented for other viruses, it seems prudent to avoid these swabs and use Dacron or rayon when obtaining any specimen for viral diagnosis.

Our laboratory does not supply or advise the use of swabs with wooden shafts, because this material has been implicated as a source of cell culture toxicity,[9] possibly because of the release of toxic resins from the wood.

Commercially available self-contained systems for viral specimen collection and transport include the Viral Culterette (Becton Dickinson, Cockeysville, Md) and Virocult (Medical Wire and Equipment, Cleveland). The *Viral Culturette* consists of a plastic tube containing a rayon-tipped swab and an ampule filled with a viral transport medium. After the sample has been obtained, the swab is inserted back into the tube and the ampule broken to release the transport medium. The *Virocult* system consists of a collection swab and a tube containing a sponge soaked with a transport medium. Both the Viral Culturette and the Virocult appear to perform well in published studies.[10-13] They have the added benefit of having shelf lives of 1 to 2 years.

Another commercially available transport medium is called *Multi-Microbe Media* (M-4, Micro Test, Snellville, Georgia). According to the manufacturer, M-4 can be used as a transport medium for chlamydiae and mycoplasmas and performs as well as any other commercial and standard transport media for maintaining viral infectivity.

COLLECTION AND TRANSPORT TEMPERATURE

For the diagnosis of acute viral infections, specimens should be collected as early as possible after symptoms appear and transported to the laboratory as quickly as possible. Collecting specimens early in the illness increases the chance of viral recovery because virus is generally present in highest titer at this time. When delays of more than an hour are anticipated in transporting specimens to the laboratory, specimens should be maintained at 4°C (the temperature of wet ice).[2, 3, 14, 15] Temperatures in excess of room temperature or unintentional freezing can render a virus noninfectious. Therefore, when courier or other transport services are used, specimens must be protected from the extremes of temperature possible in delivery vehicles or even in the open air under ambient conditions. Insulated containers and wet ice packs are adequate for this purpose.

Prolonged delays (longer than 24 hours) in specimen transport may significantly compromise the ability to isolate certain labile enveloped viruses such as RSV, VZV, and cytomegalovirus (CMV). As a last resort, it may be preferable to freeze such specimens and maintain them in a frozen state until they can reach the laboratory. It is important that they be quickly frozen at the lowest possible temperature. Flash freezing in liquid nitrogen is best but often not practical in clinical settings. Freezing in an ultra-low-temperature laboratory freezer at −70°C is preferable to a standard −20°C freezer; freezing at −20°C can seriously compromise the recovery of some viruses and is not recommended.[2, 4, 8, 16, 17] To maintain frozen specimens in transit, insulated containers and dry ice should be used.

SPECIMENS FOR VIRAL ISOLATION AND ANTIGEN DETECTION

Unless a specific virus is requested, identifying viruses in clinical specimens is a specimen-driven process. On receipt in the laboratory, the specimen type determines the type of cell cultures to be inoculated and the noncultural procedures (e.g., antigen detection) that may be performed. Therefore clinicians should be cognizant of the type of viruses that can be isolated from different specimen types, and the limitations of culture and other tests that may be performed.

This section discusses the different types of specimens typically submitted for viral isolation and viral antigen detection. The information includes data from published reports on the performance of different specimen types for the recovery of viruses in culture. Data from the virology laboratory at Washington University Medical Center in St. Louis and other laboratories provide the range of viruses detected in clinical specimens.

Respiratory Specimens

Specimens collected for the recovery of viruses causing respiratory illnesses include upper respiratory samples such as nasopharyngeal (NP) swabs, nasal washes and aspirates, and throat swabs, and lower respiratory specimens such as sputum, bronchial washings, and bronchoalveolar lavage (BAL) fluids.

When an upper respiratory specimen is collected, it is important to ensure the recovery of *respiratory epithelial cells*, especially when FA stain studies are to be performed. These cells serve as the site of viral replication in the upper respiratory tract and contain the viral antigens that are visualized by the staining procedures.

Nasopharyngeal swabs, aspirates, and washes. NP swabs, aspirates, and washes are the specimens submitted most often for the recovery of respiratory viruses. Figure 2–1 provides detailed instructions for their collection.

Depending on the preference of the laboratory, the NP swab can be inserted into a vial of transport medium or applied directly to a slide for antigen detection studies. The direct application of the swab to slides can work well and tends to have less interfering mucus than aspirates.[18] In our laboratory, personnel collect two NP swabs, place them in a vial of transport medium, and cut the metal shafts so the swabs remain in the vial. By having the swabs remain in the transport medium, the vials can be vigorously mixed in the laboratory, thereby ensuring recovery of an adequate number of epithelial cells.

Nasal wash: syringe method

Materials: Saline
 3-5 ml syringe*
 2" 18-20 gauge tubing*
 Viral Transport Medium (VTM)
 Specimen container

1. Fill syringe with saline; attach tubing to syringe tip.
2. Quickly instill saline into nostril.
3a. Aspirate the recoverable nasal specimen. Recovery must occur immediately, as the instilled fluid will rapidly drain.
3b. (alternate) In appropriate cases, patients may tilt head forward to allow specimen to drain into suitable sterile container.
4. (if aspirated) Inject aspirated specimen from syringe into suitable dry, sterile specimen container or one containing VTM, according to virology laboratory requirements.

Nasal wash: bulb method

Materials: Saline
 1-2 oz. tapered rubber bulb*
 Viral Transport Medium (VTM)
 Specimen container

1. Suction 3-5 ml saline into a new sterile bulb.
2. Insert bulb into one nostril until nostril is occluded.
3. Instill saline into nostril with one squeeze of the bulb and immediately release bulb to collect recoverable nasal specimen.
4. Empty bulb into suitable dry, sterile specimen container or one containing VTM, according to virology laboratory requirements.

*Length and diameter of syringe, tube or bulb as appropriate for infant, child, or adult.

Nasopharyngeal swab method

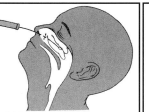

Materials: Mini-Tip **Culturette** Brand
 Collection and Transport
 System or
 Nasopharyngeal swab with
 synthetic fiber tip
 1-2 ml Viral Transport Medium (VTM)
 Specimen container

1. Insert swab into one nostril.
2. Press swab tip on the mucosal surface of the mid-inferior portion of the inferior turbinate (see sketch), and rub the swab tip several times across the mucosal surface to loosen and collect cellular material.
3. Withdraw swab; insert into **Culturette** or container with VTM.

Figure 2.1 Procedures for obtaining nasal and nasopharyngeal specimens. (Courtesy Becton Dickinson Microbiology Systems, Sparks, Md.)

Vacuum-assisted nasal aspirate method

Materials: Portable suction pump
 Sterile suction catheter
 Mucus trap (i.e., Luken's tube)
 Viral Transport Medium (VTM)

1. Attach mucus trap to suction pump and catheter, leaving wrapper on suction catheter; turn on suction and adjust to suggested pressure.
2. Without applying suction, insert catheter into nose, directed posteriorly and toward the opening of the external ear. **NOTE:** depth of insertion necessary to reach posterior pharynx is equivalent to distance between anterior naris and external opening of the ear.
3. Apply suction. Using a rotating movement, slowly withdraw catheter. **NOTE:** catheter should remain in nasopharynx no longer than 10 seconds.
4. Hold trap upright to prevent secretions from going into pump.
5. Rinse catheter (if necessary) with approximately 2.0 ml VTM; disconnect suction; connect tubing to arm of mucus trap to seal.

Patient age	Catheter size (French)[†]	Suction pressure
Premature infant	6	80-100 mm Hg
Infant	8	80-100 mm Hg
Toddler/Preschooler	10	100-120 mm Hg
School age	12	100-120 mm Hg
Adolescent/Adult	14	120-150 mm Hg

[†]To determine length of catheter tubing, measure distance from tip of nose to external opening of ear.

Most studies indicate that washes and aspirates have higher rates of respiratory virus recovery than NP swabs.[1, 19, 20] In at least one study, however, NP swabs performed as well as aspirates, possibly because only two individuals collected all the NP swabs following a standardized procedure.[21] Collection of NP washes and aspirates, even in inexperienced hands, will most likely produce better viral recovery than NP swabs but NP swabs can perform well if two swabs are collected and collectors are appropriately trained. Lastly, some patients tolerate NP wash or aspirate collection better than swab procedures.[1, 19]

Throat specimens. Throat specimens are sometimes submitted to rule out infections with respiratory viruses even though they are not the optimal source for these viruses. Recovery of respiratory viruses from throat specimens probably represents the presence of virus-containing secretions that have drained into the throat from the NP area. Of the 190 throat swab specimens for viral culture received in 1996 by our laboratory, 33 yielded virus; most were HSV of unknown significance, with only 11 respiratory viruses (Table 2–1). Another drawback is that throat specimens typically do not yield sufficient numbers of respiratory epithelial cells to allow viral antigen detection studies.

Bronchoalveolar lavage and bronchial washes. BAL and bronchial washing specimens are rich sources of respiratory epithelial cells from the lower respiratory tract and thus are excellent specimens for culture and antigen detection studies for the diagnosis of viral respiratory disease. Our laboratory noted no significant increase in viral recovery from bronchial washing relative to BAL fluid, and bronchial washings were associated with a higher rate of cell culture toxicity. Therefore, when both BAL and bronchial washings are available from the same patient, BAL fluid may be preferable for viral culture. Because viruses isolated from these specimens may not truly reflect lower respiratory infection, their presence only resulting from contamination with upper airway secretions, BAL specimens are preferred because of a lower likelihood of such contamination relative to bronchial washings.

Of BAL and bronchial washing specimens submitted in 1996 to our laboratory, 25% yielded a virus (see Table 2–1). Most isolates were HSV or CMV, but a significant number of respiratory viruses were also isolated, many of which likely represented significant lower respiratory tract infection. Similar results were seen in a report on the recovery of viruses in BAL fluid from immunosuppressed patients. Although CMV and HSV made up a majority of viral isolates in this study, several respiratory viruses were also recovered.[22]

Sputum. Although not often thought of as a specimen for viral diagnosis, sputum is occasionally submitted.

Kimball et al.[23] reported 20 viral isolations (six influenza A viruses, two RSVs, three rhinoviruses, nine HSVs) from 100 stored frozen sputum samples obtained from patients hospitalized with pneumonia and originally submitted for bacterial culture only. Thus, even though specimen handling was not optimal (i.e., the sputum was frozen), a number of respiratory viruses were recovered. Interestingly, the finding of RSV and influenza virus had not been previously known or expected. In another report, sputum from children with acute wheezy bronchitis had a higher rate of viral isolation than did nasal or throat swabs.[24]

Induced sputum has also been found to be an adequate specimen for the culture of CMV- from HIV-infected individuals, with the sensitivity of CMV recovery from induced sputum reported to be 68% relative to BAL fluid.[25] For 1996, 45 of the 131 sputum specimens cultured in our laboratory yielded a virus but only seven represented respiratory viruses, with most isolates being CMV and HSV. Thus for patients in whom a lower respiratory specimen is desired but for whom BAL or bronchial washing specimens are not possible, sputum may be an option.

Blood

For blood specimens, 5 to 10 ml of anticoagulated blood is usually adequate for adults. For children the laboratory will generally accept smaller volumes, if necessary. Acceptable anticoagulants include ethylenediaminetetraacetic acid (EDTA), acid citrate dextrose (ACD), and heparin, although heparin should be avoided if molecular diagnostic methods will be used because heparin can interfere with some assays.

Table 2.1   Viruses Isolated from Clinical Specimens (Number Tested)

Virus	NP (3025)	BAL/ br wsh (1412)	Throat (190)	Tracheal aspirate (209)	Sputum (131)	Blood (3439)	CSF (744)	Skin (1128)	Stool (637)	Biopsy (541)	Urine (494)	Ocular (276)	TOTAL (12,226)
Respiratory syncytial	425	8	0	1	1	—	—	—	—	1	—	—	436
Influenza A	252	6	4	1	2	—	—	—	—	0	—	—	265
Influenza B	56	9	1	1	2	—	—	—	—	0	—	—	69
Parainfluenza 1	7	0	0	0	0	—	—	—	—	0	—	—	7
Parainfluenza 2	5	3	0	0	0	—	—	—	—	0	—	—	8
Parainfluenza 3	48	9	1	3	0	—	—	—	—	0	—	—	61
Parainfluenza 4	4	0	0	0	0	—	—	—	—	0	—	—	4
Rhinovirus	65	16	1	4	4	—	—	—	—	0	—	—	90
Adenovirus	59	2	4	0	0	0	0	—	25	0	1	7	98
Herpes simplex	17	32	20	8	12	2	0	348	19	9	0	12	479
Cytomegalovirus	44	272	1	13	24	255	0	—	1	12	43	—	665
Varicella-zoster	0	0	0	0	0	0	0	42	—	0	0	—	42
Enterovirus	27	1	1	1	0	0	18	0	33	0	0	0	81
TOTAL (% positive)	1009 **(33)**	358 **(25)**	33 **(17)**	32 **(15)**	45 **(34)**	257 **(7.5)**	18 **(2.4)**	390 **(35)**	78 **(12)**	22 **(4.1)**	44 **(8.9)**	19 **(6.9)**	2,305 **(19)**

Specimens submitted to virology laboratory of St Louis Children's Hospital during 1996.
BAL, Bronchoalveolar lavage; *NP,* nasopharyngeal swab; *CSF,* cerebrospinal fluid; *br wsh,* bronchial wash.

For CMV, infectious virus is associated almost exclusively with the white blood cell (WBC) fraction. Therefore specimens from leukopenic patients may contain an inadequate number of WBCs to rule out reliably the presence of virus.[26] Options for these patients include submitting a larger volume of blood or testing the specimen by a method that requires fewer cells, such as nucleic acid amplification.

A number of viral infections have a viremic phase, including CMV, enteroviruses, HSV, VZV, rubeola, and certain arboviruses. In reality, however, most blood specimens are submitted to virology laboratories to rule out CMV viremia. This is reflected in our own experience in 1996, where of 257 blood viral isolates, 255 were CMV and two HSV (see Table 2–1). The two HSV isolates were from an infant with neonatal infection and an adult with systemic HSV disease. Because most blood specimens are submitted for CMV detection, many laboratories, including ours, optimize their blood culture procedures for the recovery of CMV. Therefore, if another virus is suspected, the laboratory should be notified.

Infectious CMV in blood specimens appears to be quite labile. Data from our laboratory suggested that the ability to detect CMV in culture from blood specimens was severely compromised when 24 hours or longer passed before processing and inoculation.[27] Also, the stability of the virus was not enhanced by transport at 4°C relative to room temperature. This lack of stability has also been reported for the CMV antigenemia test, with some authors recommending that blood submitted for CMV antigenemia testing be transported and processed within 6 hours, especially if the test will be used to report a quantitative result.[28, 29] In contrast to culture and antigen detection assays, detection of CMV deoxyribonucleic acid (DNA) by molecular diagnostic testing appears to be acceptably robust (see later discussion).[27, 29]

Other viral agents are not usually isolated from blood because the infections are uncommon or the viremic phase occurs before symptoms. Thus, although varicella disease includes a viremic stage, virus is usually not isolated or sought from the blood because the viremia precedes the onset of the systemic manifestations.

Blood is a potentially useful and possibly underappreciated specimen for culture of the enteroviruses. Enteroviruses have been isolated from the blood of infants with enteroviral disease,[30, 31] in some cases as the only specimen yielding virus when throat, stool, and cerebrospinal fluid (CSF) were also cultured.

Another group of viral agents can be found in the blood but do not grow in culture, including the agents of viral hepatitis and human parvovirus B19. For other viruses, such as human immunodeficiency virus (HIV), Epstein-Barr virus (EBV), and human herpesvirus 6 (HHV-6), culture is possible but not performed in most diagnostic virology laboratories. Diagnosis for these agents usually relies on serologic or nucleic acid detection methods.

The collection of blood specimens for molecular tests is discussed later.

Cerebrospinal Fluid

CSF is most often submitted to rule out a viral cause of aseptic meningitis or encephalitis. Other than collection of an adequate volume (most laboratories prefer a minimum of 1 ml but will accept less) and prompt transport in a sterile container, no other special procedures are required.

Although several viruses can cause central nervous system (CNS) infections, enteroviruses represent the largest group of viruses isolated from CSF in routine virology laboratories. During 1996 in our laboratory, a virus was isolated from only 2% of CSF specimens submitted, with enteroviruses accounting for 100% of the isolates (see Table 2–1). An estimated 15% to 20% of reported cases of aseptic meningitis are caused by enteroviruses, with most cases due to unknown causes.[32]

Clinicians should be aware of the limitations of viral culture for the diagnosis of viral CNS infections. Polymerase chain reaction (PCR) testing of CSF for enteroviruses has resulted in significantly higher rates of positivity than culture.[33, 34] Culture misses some cases of enteroviral meningitis because of low titers of virus in the CSF, and because some coxsackie A viruses do not grow in culture. Members of the herpesvirus group (e.g., HSV, CMV, VZV) are only rarely isolated from CSF cultures, once again likely because they are present in the CSF in very low titers.

The extreme sensitivity of DNA amplification methods such as PCR allows laboratories to offer meaningful assays for the detection of nonenteroviral agents in CSF. Clinicians desiring a laboratory diagnosis for viral CNS infections caused by agents such as HSV, VZV, CMV, EBV, HHV-6, and JC virus (human polyomavirus) should consider sending specimens to a reliable laboratory capable of applying nucleic acid amplification methods to CSF specimens. In contrast to our experience with culture of CSF for 1996, PCR allowed for detection of a variety of CNS viruses from CSF specimens submitted to our molecular diagnostic laboratory.

Detection of rabies virus or arboviruses in CSF is usually not performed in routine, hospital-based virology laboratories. Rather, the testing for these agents is usually under the purview of state or federal laboratories. Local routine virology laboratories usually are able to assist in transporting the specimen to the appropriate laboratory.

Although the range of viruses that is routinely isolated in culture from CSF is limited, exceptions exist when unusual or unexpected viruses are isolated, such as a recently reported case of an unusual arbovirus that was first detected when it produced cytopathic effect in cell culture inoculated with CSF from a patient with a severe unexplained illness.[35]

Stool

Collection of a stool specimen for viral diagnosis involves placing 2 to 4 g of formed or liquid stool in a sterile container and transporting it to the laboratory. If transport is delayed, the sample should be refrigerated at 4°C to prevent the overgrowth of bacteria. Rectal swabs are a poor substitute for a stool specimen because the volume of material may be inadequate, especially if fecal material is not visible on the swab. Rectal swabs are most useful for diagnosis of proctitis due to HSV. Swabs should be placed in viral transport media before transport.

Stool specimens and rectal swabs are routinely submitted to virology laboratories for isolation or detection of viral agents, but currently, none of the common agents of viral gastroenteritis can be grown in culture. Thus no practical culture systems exist for any of these agents, including Norwalk-related viruses, astroviruses, rotaviruses, and enteric adenoviruses. Although some cultivable enteroviruses have been implicated in gastroenteritis,[36] submission of stool specimens for culture to rule out viral gastroenteritis rarely yields clinically useful information and is not recommended.

Current assays available for the routine laboratory diagnosis of viral gastroenteritis are limited to antigen detection assays for rotaviruses and enteric adenoviruses. Some laboratories have developed antigen detection and nucleic acid–based assays for other noncultivable agents of viral gastroenteritis, but these tests currently are not widely available. Another option for the demonstration of virus in stool specimens is electron microscopy, although the number of laboratories possessing an electron microscope and the expertise needed for preparing and interpreting specimens for viral diagnosis are limited. A clinician wanting to identify a cause of viral gastroenteritis should confer with the laboratory on the types and limitations of the tests available, including those performed on site and available from reference laboratories.

Stool culture can be beneficial in support of a diagnosis of enteroviral disease when the virus cannot be isolated from the site of disease. Thus it has been shown that submission of a stool culture, in addition to a specimen from a specific site, such as CSF in cases of suspected enteroviral meningitis, can allow for a presumptive diagnosis of enteroviral disease when the primary site does not yield a virus.[37, 38] Two important considerations apply, however, as follows:

1. Vaccine strains of poliovirus remain in stool for a prolonged period after administration of live attenuated vaccine. A review of the patient's vaccination history usually resolves interpretation of the significance of poliovirus isolation from stool specimens.

2. Enteroviruses may be shed in the stool for several months after an acute infection or by individuals who had completely asymptomatic infection.

During 1996 our laboratory recovered 33 enteroviruses, 25 adenoviruses, and 19 isolates of HSV from stool. Clinical judgement would be necessary to determine the clinical significance of most of these isolates. Adenoviruses isolated in culture from stool do not include types 40 and 41, which are responsible for gastroenteritis.

Biopsy Tissue

Tissue specimens obtained at biopsy or autopsy should be placed in a sterile container and covered with an adequate volume of viral transport medium to ensure that the specimen does not dry out during transport. If viral transport medium is not available at the time the specimen is collected, normal sterile saline is an acceptable substitute.

Depending on the tissue site, almost any virus can be isolated from a biopsy specimen. Despite the relatively low recovery of viruses observed during a typical year (see Table 2–1), the isolation of a virus from a tissue source can represent a significant infection at that site. Ideally, viral isolation from tissue should be correlated with histologic findings for best understanding of the role of the virus in the disease process.

Urine

Collection of 5 to 10 ml of clean voided urine in a sterile leak-proof container is adequate for viral studies. In infants from whom it may be difficult to collect this volume, 1 to 2 ml is often sufficient because viruses, if present, tend to be in high titer. Once collected, the urine should be refrigerated at 4°C to maintain viral viability and to prevent the overgrowth of bacteria or fungi.

Viruses that can be isolated from urine include CMV, adenoviruses, mumps, rubeola, rubella, and enteroviruses. Mumps, rubeola, and rubella are uncommon in the United States at present, and they require special culture techniques for detection. It is therefore important to notify the laboratory when it is necessary to rule out the presence of one of these viruses in a urine specimen.

The majority of urine specimens are tested to rule out the presence of CMV, either to diagnose in utero infection of a newborn or to monitor immunosuppressed patients for viral shedding. This is reflected in urine isolates from our laboratory, where from a culture algorithm optimized for recovery of CMV, 43 of 44 urine isolates from 1996 were CMV, with a single isolate of an adenovirus (see Table 2–1). When testing urine to diagnose congenital CMV infection, it is important to collect the specimen as early in life as possible. After 2 weeks of life, detection of CMV in urine may reflect postnatal infection with the virus and not true in utero infection. In contrast to our 1996 experience, viral isolation data from 1972 show that mumps virus made up 22 of 27 urine isolates and CMV only two isolates.[39]

Ocular Specimens

Conjunctival swabs, corneal scrapings, and ocular fluid are the usual ocular specimens submitted for viral studies. To ensure recovery of an adequate number of cells from the conjunctival surface, it is advisable first to remove any exudate with an initial swab. A second swab is then rolled on the conjunctiva and immediately placed in viral transport medium. The same specimen can often be used for antigen detection tests and viral culture, although consultation with the laboratory is recommended if both tests are desired. Collection of corneal scrapings and ocular fluid is generally limited to an ophthalmologist.

Corneal scrapings may be applied directly to a microscope slide for antigen detection studies for HSV and adenoviruses or immediately placed in viral transport medium if culture is desired. It is not advisable to submit ocular fluid specimens for viral culture because the extremely small volumes that can be collected compromise the ability to isolate virus. Rather, viral detection in ocular fluids is best accomplished with nucleic acid amplification methods such as PCR. If culture is desired, the fluid should be transported in a sterile tube at 4°C.

Agents of viral conjunctivitis and keratitis include adenoviruses, HSV, VZV, enteroviruses, influenza, mumps, measles, Newcastle disease virus, and certain poxviruses such as vaccinia and molluscum contagiosum. HSV and adenoviruses constitute the majority of day-to-day ocular isolates in our experience. A 1972 study reported 16 virus isolations, all HSV and adenoviruses, from 296 specimens.[39] Laboratories generally have no difficulty detecting adenovirus, HSV, and enterovirus infections using standard methods. If influenza, mumps, measles, Newcastle disease virus, or a poxvirus is suspected, however, the laboratory should be notified because special techniques may be necessary to detect these viruses.

Agents of viral endophthalmitis include members of the herpesvirus group, including HSV, VZV, and CMV, as well as rubella and measles viruses. Because only very small volumes of ocular fluid are usually available for testing, when submitting these specimens for diagnosis of viral endophthalmitis, clinicians should attempt to rank the agents suspected in terms of likelihood. This allows the laboratory to test for the most likely agent(s) first, thereby lessening the chance of wasting the small volumes of these valuable specimens on testing for viruses less likely to be involved.

Vesicles and Other Skin Lesions

For vesicular lesions, it is best to sample fresh, fluid-filled lesions because more viruses are recovered from these lesions than from older, crusted vesicles. For sample collection, a 26- or 27-gauge needle and a tuberculin syringe are used to aspirate liquid from the vesicle. The fluid should then be expressed into a vial of viral transport medium and the syringe and needle rinsed and flushed with transport medium. The vesicle can then be unroofed and swabbed vigorously to obtain cells from the base of the lesion. Dacron or rayon swabs are recommended, since both VZV and HSV have been inactivated by cotton and calcium alginate swabs.[4, 7, 8] The swab should be immediately placed into a vial of transport medium or, if FA antigen detection studies are desired, rolled onto the surface of a clean microscope slide. Separate swabs should be used; one is placed in transport medium and the second used for depositing cells on a glass slide.

Although HSV, VZV, enteroviruses, and poxviruses can cause vesicular skin lesions, HSV and VZV usually account for most isolates. This is reflected in our 1996 data (see Table 2–1) and in 1972 data, where HSV and VZV accounted for 384 of 390 viral skin isolates.[39]

When collecting lesion specimens, clinicians should be aware that VZV is one of the more labile of the commonly isolated viruses. Because of this, direct detection of VZV by immunofluorescent staining of cells from vesicles is more sensitive than culture and is therefore the recommended test for detecting VZV from skin lesions.[40]

Human papillomavirus (HPV) is the causative agent of warts. Culture is not an option for the laboratory diagnosis of HPV lesions. Rather, DNA hybridization or amplification performed on nucleic acid extracted from tissue specimens is the test of choice. This assay is usually performed only in reference laboratories experienced in the techniques. Local virology or pathology laboratories probably can assist in the collection and transport of specimens to the appropriate testing facility.

Amniotic Fluid

Amniotic fluid may be collected and sent to the virology laboratory for culture to rule out intrapartum infections due to CMV and rubella. Since both these agents are enveloped viruses and thus somewhat labile, amniotic fluid specimens must be transported to the laboratory as quickly as possible. If delays are unavoidable, the specimen should be kept at wet ice temperatures. For culture, 2 ml of amniotic fluid should be sufficient. Although culture generally has adequate sensitivity for detection of CMV and rubella, if a laboratory with culture capabilities is not available or transport time will be prolonged, molecular testing should be considered. For cases of suspected parvovirus B19 infection, molecular testing is the only option for this noncultivable agent.

SPECIMENS FOR MOLECULAR DIAGNOSTIC TESTS

General Considerations

The application of PCR and other nucleic acid amplification techniques to the diagnosis of certain viral infections is having a profound effect on the laboratory diagnosis of viral illnesses. Because these assays rely on the detection of specific viral nucleic acid sequences, either DNA or ribonucleic acid (RNA), specimen collection and transportation must be done in a manner that ensures the stability and amplifiability of nucleic acids.

DNA is a relatively stable molecule, but RNA is unstable and especially susceptible to degradation by enzymes (RNases) that are ubiquitous in the environment. Therefore specimen requirements for molecular testing for RNA viruses such as HIV, hepatitis C virus (HCV), and enteroviruses are generally more stringent than those for DNA viruses such as CMV and HSV. To ensure the amplifiability of nucleic acids, it is important to avoid substances or practices that can result in the inhibition of amplification assays. Examples include the use of blood collection tubes containing heparin as an anticoagulant and freezing of whole blood specimens, which results in release of heme from red blood cells (RBCs). Since heparin and heme are known inhibitors of PCR reactions, their presence could result in false-negative results.

Molecular diagnostics is a rapidly evolving field. Currently, only a handful of kits are available and approved by the Food and Drug Administration (FDA) for the detection of virus by nucleic acid amplification. These kits have explicit instructions for collection and transport of specimens that must be followed for the results to be valid. In contrast to kits, most nucleic acid amplification assays currently available for viruses were developed in individual clinical laboratories ("home brew" assays). Thus a PCR assay for the detection of HSV DNA in CSF from patients suspected of having herpes encephalitis offered by one laboratory may differ from the same test performed at another site. For clinicians planning to submit specimens for molecular diagnostic testing, it is advisable to contact the laboratory before obtaining the specimen. Laboratories should have detailed verbal or written instructions that outline the correct specimen collection and transport procedures for their assays. Having this information before specimen collection will avoid the loss of valuable specimen material and delays in result reporting.

The information presented here on specific specimen types for molecular diagnostics represents recommended guidelines and data from published studies. Clinicians should contact the testing laboratory for specific instructions.

Blood

Data suggest that DNA is quite stable in blood specimens if the specimens are not subjected to extremes of temperature.[41] Intact DNA has been extracted from blood specimens held at room temperature for 8 to 30 days.[42] Data from our laboratory and others have shown that CMV DNA is stable in whole blood stored at room temperature for up to 3 days.[27, 29] Presumably, DNA from other DNA viruses would be equally stable under these conditions. Blood specimens submitted for detection of DNA viruses can therefore be safely transported at room temperature. Since temperatures above room temperature are found to reduce the amount of intact extractable DNA from blood specimens,[43] however, specimens should be insulated to protect them if ambient temperatures exceed 25°C.

Viral RNA is generally considered to be much less stable than DNA in blood specimens, thereby requiring expedited transport to the laboratory. For example, the package insert for the Roche Amplicor HIV-1 Monitor test, which is used to quantitate levels of HIV-1 RNA in patient blood, states that EDTA blood collection tubes must be used and that, once collected, the blood can be stored for no longer than 6 hours at 2° to 25°C before processing. Therefore, when submitting specimens for testing for RNA viruses such as HCV and HIV, the clinician must be aware of transport requirements before drawing the specimen. This would preclude practices such as collecting specimens so late in the day that they could not be received and processed within the recommended time limits.

Cerebrospinal Fluid

CSF is a common specimen submitted for detection of viruses by molecular methods. During 1996, our laboratory tested 817 CSF specimens by PCR for different viral agents, including HSV, CMV, EBV, VZV, parvovirus B19, and JC virus (human polyomavirus), mostly to rule out encephalitis or meningitis caused by HSV or opportunistic viruses in patients with AIDS (Table 2–2).

Minimal data exist on the stability of viral nucleic acids in CSF, despite it being a common specimen. One study showed that purified HSV DNA added to pooled CSF specimens was suitable for PCR amplification after storage for up to 30 days at room temperature, at 4°C, or frozen at −20° to −72°C.[44] The authors concluded that it would not be necessary to collect a second CSF

Table 2.2 Viruses Detected by PCR Testing of Clinical Specimens: Number Tested (Number Positive)

Virus	CSF	Blood	Amniotic fluid	Ocular fluid	Serum/plasma
Herpes simplex	478 (19)	13 (2)	—	13 (0)	—
Cytomegalovirus	136 (24)	1447 (314)	15 (2)	9 (0)	—
Epstein-Barr	102 (34)	140 (111)	—	10 (1)	11 (2)
JC (polyomavirus)	49 (8)	—	—	—	—
Parvovirus B19	3 (0)	1 (0)	15 (1)	—	37 (6)
Varicella-zoster	49 (5)	1 (0)	—	11 (1)	—

Specimens submitted to molecular virology laboratory of St Louis Children's Hospital during 1996.
CSF, Cerebrospinal fluid.

specimen for PCR testing when an initial specimen had been collected for other studies and then subsequently tested for HSV, even if the specimen had been left at room or refrigerator temperatures for several days. No reason exists to expect that other DNA viruses would be significantly less stable than HSV. When CSF is submitted for detection of HSV DNA, it is advisable to obtain the specimen before the administration of antiviral agents, or as early in the course as possible, since DNA may drop to undetectable levels after a week of treatment.[45]

Data on the stability of amplifiable RNA from RNA viruses in CSF are lacking. A study performed before the advent of nucleic acid amplification assays examined the effect of different storage conditions of CSF spiked with known amounts of enteroviruses and then tested for the presence of enteroviral RNA by a nonamplified hybridization reaction. Results indicated no effect on the ability to detect enteroviral RNA after storage for up to 96 hours at room temperature, 4°, −20°, and −70°C,[46] probably because of the known stability of enteroviruses. It is reasonable to assume that enteroviruses in CSF would exhibit similar stability for PCR or other nucleic acid amplification assays.

Tissue Specimens

Current recommendations for tissue specimens submitted for nucleic acid detection of viral RNA or DNA state that specimens should be "snap" frozen in liquid nitrogen or in a −70°C bath such as dry ice/alcohol as quickly as possible after collection.[42] The longer a specimen sits at room temperature or refrigerator temperatures, the more likely that endogenous proteases and nucleases could render any viral nucleic acid present nonamplifiable. Once frozen, the tissue specimen can be stored at −70° or −20°C before testing for DNA viruses. Because of the lability of RNA, frozen tissue should be stored only at −70°C or lower when RNA viruses are being considered.

Ocular Fluid

As stated earlier, the small volumes of ocular fluid usually available for testing give nucleic acid amplification tests a clear advantage over other methods for the laboratory diagnosis of viral endophthalmitis. No data are available on collection and transport of these specimens. It is probably prudent to place the specimen on wet ice and transport it as rapidly as possible to the laboratory, or to freeze and transport on dry ice if more than 24 hours will be required for transport. Ocular fluid specimens have been found to contain PCR inhibitors.[47] Clinicians should be sure that the testing laboratory is aware of this fact and has procedures to remove or control for these inhibitors.

References

1. Hall CV, Douglas G Jr: Clinically useful method for the isolation of respiratory syncytial virus, *J Infect Dis* 131:1, 1975.
2. Hambling MH: Survival of the respiratory syncytial virus during storage under various conditions, *Br J Exp Pathol* 45:647, 1964.
3. Baxter BD, Couch RB, Greenberg SB, Kasel JA: Maintenance of viability and comparison of identification methods for influenza and other respiratory viruses of humans, *J Clin Microbiol* 6:19, 1977.
4. Levin MJ, Leventhal S, Masters HA: Factors influencing quantitative isolation of varicella-zoster virus, *J Clin Microbiol* 19:880, 1984.
5. Johnson FB: Transport of viral specimens, *J Clin Microbiol Rev* 3:120, 1990.
6. Rodin P, Hare MJ, Barwell CF, Withers MJ: Transport of herpes simplex virus in Stuart's medium, *Br J Vener Dis* 47:198, 1971.
7. Crane LR, Gutterman, PA, Chapel T, Lerner AM: Incubation of swab materials with herpes simplex virus, *J Infect Dis* 141:531, 1980.
8. Bettoli E, Brewer PM, Oxtoby MJ, et al: The role of temperature and swab materials in the recovery of her-

pes simplex virus from lesions, *J Infect Dis* 145:399, 1982.

9. Schachter J, Stamm WE: *Chlamydia.* In Murray PR, editor: *Manual of clinical microbiology,* ed 7, Washington DC, 1999, ASM Press.

10. Perez TR, Mosman PL, Juchau SV: Experience with Virocult as a viral collection and transportation system, *Diagn Microbiol Infect Dis* 2:7, 1984.

11. Stanley TV, Leask BGS: A new virus transport system assessed, *Practitioner* 225:204, 1981.

12. Johnson FB, Leavitt RW, Richards DF: Evaluation of the Virocult transport tube for isolation of herpes simplex virus from clinical specimens, *J Clin Microbiol* 20:120, 1984.

13. Huntoon CJ, House RF, Smith TF: Recovery of viruses from three transport media incorporated into culturettes, *Arch Pathol Lab Med* 105:436, 1981.

14. Bromberg K, Daidone B, Clarke L, Sierra MF: Comparison of immediate and delayed inoculation of HEp-2 cells for isolation of respiratory syncytial virus, *J Clin Microbiol* 20:123, 1984.

15. Feldman RA: Cytomegalovirus in stored urine specimens: a quantitative study, *J Pediatr* 73:611, 1968.

16. Macasaet FF, Smith TF, Holley KE: Effect of storage on recovery of cytomegalovirus from necropsy tissue, *J Clin Pathol* 29:1077, 1976.

17. Yeager AS, Morris JE, Prober CG: Storage and transport of cultures for herpes simplex virus, type 2, *Am J Clin Pathol* 72:977, 1979.

18. Mackie PLK, Madge PJ, Getty S, Paton JY: Rapid diagnosis of respiratory syncytial virus infection by using perinasal swabs, *J Clin Microbiol* 29:2653, 1991.

19. Ahluwalia G, Embree J, McNicol P, et al: Comparison of nasopharyngeal aspirate and nasopharyngeal swab specimens for respiratory syncytial virus diagnosis by cell culture, indirect immunofluorescence assay and enzyme-linked immunosorbant assay, *J Clin Microbiol* 25:763, 1987.

20. Treuhaft MW, Soukup JM, Sullivan BJ: Practical recommendations for the detection of pediatric respiratory syncytial virus infection, *J Clin Microbiol* 22:270, 1985.

21. Frayha H, Castriciano S, Mahony J, Chernesky M: Nasopharyngeal swabs and nasopharyngeal aspirates equally effective for the diagnosis of viral respiratory disease in hospitalized children, *J Clin Microbiol* 27:1387, 1989.

22. Connolly MG, Baughman RP, Dohn MN, Linnemann CC Jr: Recovery of viruses other than cytomegalovirus from bronchoalveolar lavage fluid, *Chest* 105:1775, 1994.

23. Kimball AM, Foy HM, Cooney MK, et al: Isolation of respiratory syncytial and influenza viruses from the sputum of patients hospitalized with pneumonia, *J Infect Dis* 147:181, 1983.

24. Horn MEC, Reed SE, Taylor P: Role of viruses and bacteria in acute wheezy bronchitis in childhood: a study of sputum, *Arch Dis Child* 54:587, 1979.

25. Rush JD, Ng VL, Hopewell PC, et al: Comparative recovery of cytomegalovirus from saliva, mucolysed induced sputum, and bronchoalveolar lavage fluid from patients at risk for or with acquired immunodeficiency syndrome, *J Clin Microbiol* 27:2864, 1989.

26. Buller RS, Bailey TC, Ettinger NA, et al: Use of a modified shell-vial technique to quantitate CMV viremia in a population of solid-organ transplant recipients, *J Clin Microbiol* 30:2620, 1992.

27. Roberts TC, Buller RS, Gaudreault-Keener M, et al: Effects of storage temperature and time on qualitative and quantitative detection of cytomegalovirus in blood specimens by shell vial culture and PCR, *J Clin Microbiol* 35:2224, 1997.

28. Landry ML, Ferguson D, Cohen S, et al: Effect of delayed specimen processing on cytomegalovirus antigenemia test results, *J Clin Microbiol* 33:257, 1995.

29. Schafer P, Tenschert W, Gutensohn K, Laufs R: Minimal effect of delayed sample processing on results of quantitative PCR for cytomegalovirus DNA in leukocytes compared to results of antigenemia assay, *J Clin Microbiol* 35:741, 1997.

30. Dagan R, Jenista JA, Prather SL, et al: Viremia in hospitalized children with enterovirus infections, *J Pediatr* 106:397, 1985.

31. Prather SL, Dagan R, Jenista JA, Menegus MA: The isolation of enteroviruses from blood: a comparison of four processing methods, *J Med Virol* 14:221, 1984.

32. Hammer SM, Connolly KJ: Viral aseptic meningitis in the United States: clinical features, viral etiologies, and differential diagnosis, *Curr Clin Top Infect Dis* 12:1, 1992.

33. Rotbart HA: Enzymatic RNA amplification of the enteroviruses, *J Clin Microbiol* 28:438, 1990.

34. Rotbart HA, Sawyer MH, Fast S, et al: Diagnosis of enteroviral meningitis by using PCR with a colorimetric microwell detection assay, *J Clin Microbiol* 32:2590, 1994.

35. Sexton DJ, Rollin PE, Breitschwerdt EB, et al: Life-threatening Cache Valley virus infection, *N Engl J Med* 336:547, 1997.

36. Morens DM, Pallansch MA, Moore M: Polioviruses and other enteroviruses. In Belshe RB, editor: *Textbook of human virology,* ed 2, St. Louis, 1991, Mosby.

37. Chonmaitree T, Menegus MA, Powell KR: The clinical relevance of CSF viral culture, *JAMA* 247:1843, 1982.

38. Mintz L, Drew WL: Relation of culture site to the recovery of nonpolio enteroviruses, *Am J Clin Pathol* 74:324, 1980.

39. Herrmann EC Jr: Rates of isolation of viruses from a wide spectrum of clinical specimens, *Am J Clin Pathol* 57:188, 1972.

40. Coffin SE, Hodinka RL: Utility of direct immunofluorescence and virus culture for detection of varicella-zoster virus in skin lesions, *J Clin Microbiol* 33:2792, 1995.

41. Cushwa WT, Medrano JF: Effects of blood storage time and temperature on DNA yield and quality, *BioTechniques* 14:204, 1993.

42. Farkas DH, Kaul KL, Wiedbrauk DL, Kiechle FL: Specimen collection and storage for diagnostic molecular pathology investigation, *Arch Pathol Lab Med* 120:591, 1996.

43. Madisen L, Hoar DI, Holroyd CD, et al: DNA banking:

the effects of storage of blood and isolated DNA on the integrity of DNA, *Am J Med Genet* 27:379, 1987.

44. Wiedbrauk, DL, Cunningham W: Stability of herpes simplex virus DNA in cerebrospinal fluid specimens, *Diagn Molec Pathol* 5:249, 1996.

45. Lakeman FD, Whitley RJ, National Institute of Allergy and Infectious Diseases Collaborative Antiviral Study Group: Diagnosis of herpes simplex encephalitis: application of polymerase chain reaction to cerebrospinal fluid from brain-biopsied patients and correlation with disease, *J Infect Dis* 171:857, 1995.

46. Rotbart HA, Levin MJ, Villarreal LP, et al: Factors affecting the detection of enteroviruses in cerebrospinal fluid with coxsackievirus B3 and poliovirus 1 cDNA probes, *J Clin Microbiol* 22:220, 1985.

47. Wiedbrauk DL, Werner JC, Drevon AM: Inhibition of PCR by aqueous and vitreous fluids, *J Clin Microbiol* 33:2643, 1995.

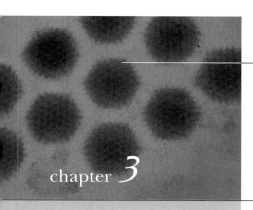

chapter *3*

Gregory A. Storch

Central Nervous System Infections

OVERVIEW

Viruses are prominent causes of nervous system infection, accounting for the great majority of cases of acute encephalitis and meningitis. Although these two entities may overlap clinically, the virologic approach differs, and therefore each is discussed separately in this chapter. Opportunistic infections of the central nervous system are included with encephalitis because of similarities in the virologic approach. The spinal cord syndromes of acute transverse myelitis and Guillain-Barré syndrome are discussed in a separate section. Although controversy surrounds the cause of the spongiform encephalopathies such as Creutzfeldt-Jakob disease, these entities are discussed here for historic reasons since at times authorities have thought (and some still think) that they are caused by viruses.

ENCEPHALITIS

Encephalitis is a clinical/pathological syndrome characterized by inflammation of the brain. Viruses are the most important causes. The cardinal feature of encephalitis is alteration of consciousness. Headache and fever are virtually always present, and some patients have other manifestations, including seizures, stiff neck, weakness, abnormal movements, and focal neurologic signs. Encephalitis is linked to viral infection in two pathogenetically distinct ways that have different implications for diagnosis: *acute viral infection*, in which the viral agent is present in the brain at the time the patient is ill, and *postinfectious demyelinating encephalitis*, also referred to as *acute disseminated encephalomyelitis*, in which direct evidence of viral invasion is not present.

Many viruses cause encephalitis in the United States (Box 3–1, see Figure 3–2). The first step in using the laboratory to establish a viral etiology is to consider clues provided by the patient's history and clinical findings (Table 3–1). Unless the clinical clues point strongly in another direction, the first task in diagnostic approach is usually to determine whether or not the patient has herpes simplex virus (HSV) encephalitis. The reason is that early treatment of HSV encephalitis with acyclovir improves the outcome. Because acyclovir is relatively nontoxic, treatment is often started as diagnostic studies are being initiated and continued unless another diagnosis is established. If the patient is immunocompromised, viruses such as cytomegalovirus (CMV), varicella-zoster virus (VZV), and polyomavirus JC, which are unusual causes of central nervous system (CNS) infection in immunocompetent individuals, must also be considered.

Table 3–2 lists manifestations of opportunistic CNS infections in patients with acquired immunodeficiency syndrome (AIDS). The polymerase chain reaction (PCR) has dramatically improved the capability for recognizing these infections during life. Table 3–3 correlates the results of PCR performed on cerebrospinal fluid (CSF) and autopsy findings in AIDS patients.

Herpes Simplex Encephalitis

The most important clinical manifestation that distinguishes HSV encephalitis from other forms of viral encephalitis is the presence of focal neurologic findings, usually resulting from damage to one or both temporal lobes, where the virus tends to localize. Other important clinical manifestations are progression over several days, fever, and CSF mononuclear pleocytosis. Red blood cells may be present as well, but their

---

Box 3.1 Viruses that Cause Encephalitis in United States

Herpesviruses

Herpes simplex (HSV)
Varicella-zoster (VZV)
Epstein-Barr (EBV)
Cytomegalovirus (CMV)
Human herpesvirus 6 (HHV-6)
B virus

Arthropod-borne viruses

St. Louis encephalitis
Eastern equine encephalitis
Western equine encephalitis
California encephalitis group
Powassan encephalitis
Colorado tick fever

Rabies

Enteroviruses

Echovirus
Coxsackievirus
Poliovirus

Viruses associated with "childhood diseases"

Mumps
Measles
Rubella

Viruses primarily causing respiratory disease

Influenza
Parainfluenza
Adenovirus

Lymphocytic choriomeningitis (LCM) virus

Human immunodeficiency virus (HIV)

JC virus (polyomavirus)

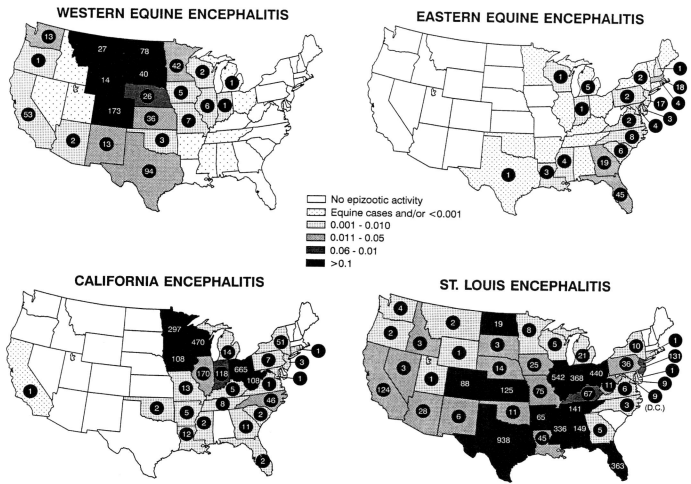

Figure 3.1 Reported cases and incidence of encephalitis caused by eastern equine, western equine, St. Louis, and California serogroup viruses, 1973 to 1993. (From Tsai TF: In Long SS, Pickering LK, Prober CG, editors: *Principles and practice of pediatric infectious diseases*, New York, 1997, Churchill Livingstone.)

absence does not rule out the diagnosis. Behavioral changes, seizures, and decreased level of consciousness (LOC) are common but not universal findings.

Although these findings increase the level of suspicion for HSV encephalitis, they can be present in other forms of viral encephalitis as well. The presence or absence of cutaneous herpetic lesions, either concurrent with encephalitis or in the past, is not helpful. Neuroimaging techniques may reveal evidence of a focal process, especially in the temporal lobe, but may be negative early in the disease. Magnetic resonance imaging (MRI) is the most sensitive technique for detecting early changes. HSV encephalitis is unusual in immunocompromised patients and can have atypical clinical manifestations. A number of cases in patients with AIDS have occurred in association with CMV ventriculoencephalitis.[1]

Laboratory diagnosis. Except during the newborn period, CSF cultures are rarely positive for HSV in patients with HSV encephalitis. Until recently, laboratory diag-

nosis depended on brain biopsy (see later discussion) to obtain tissue for culture and other studies. Although still considered the "gold standard," brain biopsy is rapidly being replaced by PCR performed on CSF. Demonstration of intrathecal production of HSV antibodies can be used to confirm the diagnosis, but this is cumbersome to perform and is not positive until late in the illness.

Polymerase chain reaction. The relative simplicity of making a diagnosis by using a test performed on CSF rather than brain tissue makes PCR extremely appealing for the diagnosis of HSV encephalitis. In a landmark study that compared PCR and brain biopsy, the sensitivity and specificity of PCR were 98% and 96%, respectively.[1] The true specificity may actually be higher, since some of the cases that were positive by PCR but negative by brain biopsy may have actually been cases of HSV encephalitis. In a recent metaanalysis that included data from all studies in which PCR was compared with either brain biopsy or demonstration of intrathecal HSV

Table 3.1 Important Clues for Establishing Etiology of Viral Encephalitis

Clue	Viral agent(s)
Temporal lobe localization	Herpes simplex virus
Mosquito exposure	Arboviruses (see Figure 3–1)
Animal bite or exposure to bats	Rabies
Exposure to mice or hamsters	Lymphocytic choriomeningitis virus
Summer or fall onset	Arboviruses, enteroviruses
Fall or winter onset	Lymphocytic choriomeningitis virus
Travel	Regional arboviruses (see Figure 3–1), Colorado tick fever
Rash	Enteroviruses, HHV-6, measles, rubella, varicella-zoster virus
Parotitis/orchitis	Mumps
Concurrent or recent chickenpox or shingles	Varicella-zoster virus
Recent respiratory illness	Influenza, parainfluenza, adenovirus
Mononucleosis-like illness	Epstein-Barr virus, cytomegalovirus, HIV
HIV risk factors	HIV, herpesviruses, JC virus
Immunosuppression	Herpesviruses, JC virus, measles, adenovirus

HHV-6, Human herpesvirus 6; *HIV*, human immunodeficiency virus.

antibody production, the sensitivity of PCR was 96% and the specificity 99%.[2]

An important caveat is that HSV PCR assays are not currently standardized, and the performance of assays devised in individual laboratories may differ in sensitivity and specificity. Some confidence in a laboratory's ability to perform the assay can be gained if the laboratory participates in the HSV PCR proficiency testing program of the College of American Pathologists (CAP). CAP certification of the laboratory also ensures that precautions are in place to prevent PCR contamination, which can result in false-positive tests.

The clinician must be aware of the *type specificity* of the PCR assay used in the diagnosis of HSV encephalitis. HSV exists in two distinct types, HSV-1 and HSV-2. *HSV-1* accounts for almost all cases of encephalitis beyond the newborn period, whereas *HSV-2* accounts for the majority of neonatal HSV infection as well as most cases of HSV meningitis in adults (see later discussion). PCR assays may be designed to detect HSV-1 only,[3] HSV-2 only, or both simultaneously.[1, 2] If the assay used to test CSF is specific for HSV-1, rare cases of HSV-2 encephalitis may be missed.

Another important caveat is that even sensitive PCR assays are occasionally negative in true cases of HSV-1

encephalitis.[1, 4] This unfortunate result is most likely to occur early in the disease. Thus, if the PCR is negative when the clinical suspicion is high, the PCR should be repeated on a different CSF specimen obtained 1 to 2 days later. If the second PCR is negative, it is very unlikely that the patient has HSV encephalitis. A short period of antiviral therapy appears to have little effect on the sensitivity of PCR (Figure 3–1). In published studies, up to 5 days of acyclovir therapy has not caused the PCR to become negative.[1, 3, 5]

A key clinical question is whether a negative PCR can be used as the basis for discontinuing acyclovir therapy. If clinical suspicion is high, it is prudent to continue acyclovir therapy even though the PCR is negative; other causes of the encephalitis should be sought. If the clinical suspicion is intermediate or low, however, and if the PCR assay has sensitivity comparable to that of the assay used in the landmark study (capability to detect 20 copies of a plasmid containing gene segment detected by PCR assay), a negative PCR has a very high negative predictive value and is useful for ruling out the diagnosis. For example, a recent decision analysis showed that if the pretest probability was 5% (corresponding to a low level of clinical suspicion), a negative PCR had a negative predictive value of 99.8%.[2] Thus, when clinical suspicion is not high and the PCR is negative, it appears reasonable to discontinue acyclovir therapy. Table 3–4 shows the relationship between the pretest probability and the predictive values of positive and negative tests.

Brain biopsy. The role of brain biopsy in the diagnosis of HSV encephalitis has been controversial ever since acyclovir was licensed to treat the disease. Some suggest that all suspected cases should be confirmed by brain biopsy because the gain from enhanced diagnostic information outweighs the morbidity of brain biopsy.[6] Others argue that noninvasive testing and empiric acyclovir therapy is a more effective approach.[7] This debate is still not entirely resolved, although the

Table 3.2 Viral Opportunistic Infections in Patients with AIDS

Virus	Manifestation(s)
Cytomegalovirus	Encephalitis, radiculomyelitis, peripheral neuritis
Epstein-Barr	Primary central nervous system lymphoma
JC	Progressive multifocal leukoencephalopathy (PML)
Varicella-zoster	Encephalitis, myelitis, multifocal leukoencephalopathy
Herpes simplex	Myelitis, encephalitis (rare)

Table 3.3	Polymerase Chain Reaction (PCR) for Diagnosis of Opportunistic Infections of Central Nervous System in Patients with AIDS*				
Virus	Cases	Sensitivity (%)	Specificity (%)	Positive predictive value (%)	Negative predictive value (%)
Cytomegalovirus	45	82	98	92	95
Epstein-Barr	36	97	98	90	99
JC	39	72	99	93	95
Herpes simplex	6	100	99.5	86	100

From Cinque P, Vago L, Dahl H, et al: *AIDS* 10:951, 1996.
*Based on 217 cases, with autopsies and PCR performed on cerebrospinal fluid within 180 days of death.

increasing use of PCR may be decreasing the frequency with which brain biopsy is performed.

Brain biopsy performed for the diagnosis of possible HSV encephalitis can be carried out either by an open approach or by stereotactic-guided closed needle aspiration. Regardless of technique used, the most definitive means for documenting HSV infection is viral culture. The rate of false-negative cultures is approximately 5%, and can be accounted for by sampling error or problems in handling the specimen before it reaches the laboratory. Acyclovir therapy before the biopsy can also reduce the yield of culture.

The other main techniques for documenting the herpetic etiology of the encephalitis are summarized in Table 3–5. The most important methods are histopathology, electron microscopy, and immunofluorescence. These techniques may have significant shortcomings in sensitivity, and with the exception of fluorescent antibody (FA) staining, do not provide a unique virologic diagnosis. The use of HSV PCR on brain tissue is not advised at this time because of reports that HSV deoxyribonucleic acid (DNA) can be detected in a substantial proportion of normal-autopsy brain specimens.[8]

Histopathologic examination of the brain in HSV encephalitis may reveal hemorrhagic necrosis, an acute and chronic inflammatory cell infiltrate, and thrombosis and fibrinoid necrosis of vessels. These changes are not specific for HSV encephalitis and can be present in other forms of encephalitis. More specific findings are the presence of "ground glass" nucleic and eosinophilic intranuclear inclusions, termed *Cowdry type A*, present in approximately 50% of cases. These intranuclear inclusions are highly suggestive of HSV infection but are not absolutely diagnostic, since they can also be seen in other forms of viral encephalitis.

Electron microscopy (EM) may reveal the presence of viral capsids consistent with HSV. The yield on EM examination of tissue is not high unless intranuclear inclusions are seen by light microscopy.

A specific and rapid diagnosis can be made by performing FA staining of impression smears of brain tissue made at biopsy. FA staining can also be performed on formalin-fixed paraffin-embedded tissue. The availability of monoclonal antibodies to HSV provides high specificity. Shortcomings of FA staining are the need for considerable experience and relatively low sensitivity (70% in one large series[9]).

Serology. HSV encephalitis represents a primary infection in approximately 30% of patients and secondary reactivation of previously latent infection in the remain-

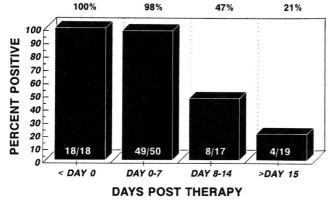

Figure 3.2   Duration of positive PCR: day 0, brain biopsy, and initiation of therapy. (From Lakeman FD, Whitley RJ: *J Infect Dis* 171:860, 1995.)

Table 3.4	Polymerase Chain Reaction (PCR) for Herpes Simplex Encephalitis: Positive and Negative Predictive Values for Different Pretest Probabilities*

	Predictive value (%)	
Pretest probability	Positive test	Negative test
0.05	87.4	0.2
0.35	98.6	2.3
0.60	99.3	6.2

From Tebas P, Nease R, Storch GA: *Am J Med* 105:287, 1998.
*Based on a PCR sensitivity of 96% and specificity of 99% for the diagnosis of HSV encephalitis.

Table 3.5	Handling of Brain Tissue for Diagnosis of Herpes Simplex Encephalitis	
Test	**Instructions**	**Sensitivity***
Viral culture	Place tissue in sterile container. Transport immediately to laboratory on ice. Freeze at −70°C if more than 24 hours will elapse before receipt by laboratory.	95%
Histopathology	Fix tissue in formalin (Bouin's fixative may improve visualization of inclusions).	85% (56% for presence of inclusions)
Fluorescent antibody (FA) staining	Prepare impression smears by touching tissue to clean microscope slides; can also be performed on formalin-fixed, paraffin-embedded tissue.	70%
Electron microscopy	Fix tissue in glutaraldehyde.	45%

*Data from Namahias AJ, Whitley RJ, Visintine AN, et al: *J Infec Dis* 45:829, 1982; and Soong S-Y, Watson NE, Caddell GR, et al: *J Infect Dis* 163:17, 1991.

ing 70%. In one large series, however, 28% of patients failed to seroconvert or have an increase in antibody titer.[9] In addition, some patients with CNS diseases not caused by HSV may experience HSV reactivation with an accompanying increase in antibody titer. For these reasons, measurement of antibody titers in blood has no role in the diagnosis of HSV encephalitis.

Intrathecal antibody synthesis. The preferred serologic approach is the demonstration of intrathecal synthesis of HSV-specific antibodies. This is accomplished by measuring HSV antibodies in serum and CSF specimens (obtained together) and comparing the ratio of HSV antibody levels with the ratio of albumin or globulin in the same CSF and serum samples. Comparison with the albumin ratio serves to control for blood-brain barrier (BBB) leakage, which could allow HSV antibodies to be present in CSF in the absence of intrathecal synthesis. Comparison with the globulin ratio also demonstrates that the increased production of HSV antibodies occurred in response to HSV infection rather than as a reflection of polyclonal stimulation. Specific standards are used to determine whether these ratios are elevated (see Chapter 1).[10-12]

A diagnostic serologic response may not be present until more than 7 days have elapsed since onset. Testing for intrathecal synthesis of specific antibodies is available only in reference laboratories and should generally be reserved for problematic patients in whom diagnostic testing is still required relatively late after onset.

Varicella-zoster Virus

Infection with VZV is nearly universal in the United States and other countries in the temperate zones. *Varicella* refers to the clinical syndrome associated with primary VZV infection; *zoster* (or *shingles*) refers to the syndrome associated with viral reactivation from latency. The diagnosis of these entities is discussed in Chapter 6. Box 3–2 lists CNS complications of VZV

infection. Table 3–6 summarizes diagnostic testing for CNS complications of VZV infection.

Varicella. *Cerebellar ataxia* is the most familiar CNS complication of varicella, with an estimated incidence of 1 : 4000 cases. Because ataxia typically occurs in close temporal association with varicella (usually from several days before to 2 weeks after the onset of rash) and because the syndrome is so characteristic, specific diagnostic testing is usually unnecessary. The CSF may be normal or may have a modest mononuclear pleocytosis with mild to moderate elevation of protein and normal level of glucose. The pathogenesis of the syndrome is uncertain, with some evidence of direct viral invasion and other evidence suggesting a parainfectious process. Viral cultures have been uniformly negative and are therefore not recommended.

Box 3.2 Neurologic Syndromes Associated with Varicella-zoster Virus

Varicella associated
Acute cerebellar ataxia
Diffuse encephalitis
Aseptic meningitis
Transverse myelitis
Reye's syndrome

Zoster associated
Encephalitis
Aseptic meningitis
Contralateral hemiplegia (ophthalmic zoster)
Multifocal leukoencephalitis
Myelitis
Ramsay Hunt syndrome, other cranial nerve palsies
Guillain-Barré syndrome

Table 3.6   Diagnosis of Central Nervous System Complications of Varicella-zoster Infection

Syndrome	Pleocytosis	Culture	Intrathecal antibody synthesis	Polymerase chain reaction
Cerebellar ataxia	Variable	No	Yes	?
Varicella encephalitis	Yes	No	Yes	?
Zoster encephalitis	Yes	Yes	Yes	Probably yes
Reye's syndrome	No	No	No	Probably no

Other approaches to diagnosis have been described in case reports, including FA staining to detect VZV antigen in CSF mononuclear cells,[13] detection of VZV antibodies, perhaps reflecting intrathecal antibody synthesis,[14, 15] and PCR to detect VZV DNA.[16] PCR appears the most promising, but more experience is required to define its sensitivity and specificity in this syndrome.

Diffuse encephalitis is a more serious but fortunately less common neurologic complication of varicella than cerebellar ataxia, also occurring shortly before or within several weeks after the onset of the varicella rash. It is distinguished from acute cerebellar ataxia by evidence of altered sensorium, sometimes accompanied by seizures and focal neurologic findings. The CSF findings are similar to those in acute cerebellar ataxia, although the cell count tends to be higher. As with acute cerebellar ataxia, the pathogenesis is not well known, and insufficient experience exists to recommend specific diagnostic tests. The use of PCR is appealing, but further experience is required to define sensitivity and specificity.

Zoster. The CNS complications of zoster occur most often in immunocompromised patients. The varied clinical manifestations include diffuse or focal encephalitis, aseptic meningitis, multifocal leukoencephalopathy, ventriculitis, and vasculopathy.[17-19] Encephalitis usually occurs during or within several months of an episode of zoster. Cases can occur without concomitant rash and are referred to as *zoster sine herpete*. The CSF in cases of zoster-associated encephalitis typically has a mononuclear cell pleocytosis, elevated protein, and normal glucose. These findings can also be seen in up to 40% of cases of uncomplicated zoster.[20]

In contrast to the neurologic syndromes associated with varicella, VZV has been cultured from the CSF of patients with zoster-associated encephalitis. PCR can be very useful, especially in patients without simultaneous cutaneous involvement.[18, 19] The interpretation of CSF PCR when cutaneous zoster is present is problematic because at least one study has shown the presence of VZV DNA in CSF in patients with uncomplicated zoster.[20a] VZV DNA has also been detected in the CSF of some patients with AIDS and the progressive outer retinal necrosis (PORN) syndrome, even in the absence of overt CNS disease,[18] as well as in some patients without recognizable CNS disease.[19]

Reye's syndrome is now rarely seen since the recognition of its association with aspirin. Before that, varicella and influenza were the viral infections most closely linked to the entity. Reye's syndrome is characterized by acute fatty degeneration of the liver and an encephalopathy with prominently increased intracranial pressure (ICP). The virus that initiates the process cannot be cultured from the CSF, and the diagnosis is based on the presence of fatty degeneration of the liver, increased ICP, and a preceding viral infection.

Epstein-Barr Virus

EBV causes encephalitis and other diverse neurologic syndromes (Table 3–7). EBV is closely associated with most cases of primary CNS lymphoma in patients with AIDS. Neurologic complications of EBV infection have been identified mainly by their occurrence during or immediately after an episode of acute mononucleosis. However, neurologic manifestations of EBV infection can also occur without clinically recognizable infectious mononucleosis.[21, 22]

As with varicella, the relative pathogenetic roles of direct viral invasion and immunologically mediated damage are uncertain. Laboratory evidence implicating EBV as the cause of neurologic syndromes has consisted of detection in CSF of atypical lymphocytes, EBV

Table 3.7   Neurologic Syndromes Associated with Epstein-Barr Virus (EBV) and Cytomegalovirus(CMV)

Syndrome	EBV	CMV
Encephalitis	Yes	Yes
Aseptic meningitis	Yes	Yes
Transverse myelitis	Yes	Yes
Bell's palsy, other cranial nerve palsies	Yes	Yes (?)
Guillain-Barré syndrome	Yes	Yes
Mononeuritis multiplex	Yes	Yes
Primary central nervous system lymphoma	Yes	No

antibodies, a positive culture for EBV, or EBV DNA. None of these methods is fully satisfactory. Criteria for establishing a diagnosis based on the presence of EBV antibodies are not clear, and therefore diagnoses based on CSF serology should be considered only presumptive. Culturing of EBV is very cumbersome and not performed in routine diagnostic virology laboratories. PCR is promising, but more information is required concerning whether EBV DNA may be detectable in CSF during uncomplicated infectious mononucleosis, in other neurologic illnesses, or even apart from any illness.

At present the best approach is to use serologic testing of the patient's blood to document acute EBV infection (see Chapter 12), combined with CSF PCR to provide evidence of viral CNS involvement.

AIDS-associated primary CNS lymphoma. PCR to detect EBV DNA in CSF has proved very useful for the diagnosis of AIDS-associated primary CNS lymphoma in patients with AIDS, with reported sensitivity of 83% to 100% and specificity of 88% to 100%.[23-26] EBV PCR may be helpful in distinguishing lymphoma from cerebral toxoplasmosis or other contrast-enhancing brain lesions that occur in patients with AIDS. However, PCR should not be considered a routine replacement for brain biopsy. A negative result does not rule out lymphoma, especially if the lesion is small and located at some distance from the ventricles. In addition, occasional patients have detectable EBV but no evidence of lymphoma. It is unknown at this time whether these patients have lymphoma that is not evident on imaging studies or at postmortem examination or, alternatively, have EBV infection of the CNS without lymphoma.

Cytomegalovirus

CMV is an extremely rare cause of encephalitis in nonimmunocompromised individuals but is an important cause of encephalitis in patients with AIDS.[27] Interestingly, very few cases have been diagnosed in patients with any form of immunocompromise other than AIDS. Approximately 20% to 30% of patients dying from AIDS have evidence of CMV infection of the brain, although not all have clinical manifestations attributable to this infection.[28]

Most cases of CMV encephalitis can be classified pathologically as ventriculoencephalitis or focal microglial nodular encephalitis. *Ventriculoencephalitis* is characterized by extensive necrosis of the ventricular lining cells, infiltration of neutrophils, and multiple CMV intranuclear inclusions. The corresponding clinical manifestations are a rapidly progressive disorder of cognition, often accompanied by cranial nerve palsies and serum electrolyte abnormalities. The rapidity of progression distinguishes this entity from HIV dementia, which may be present simultaneously. The CSF may

be normal or may have an elevated leukocyte count, sometimes with an increased percentage of neutrophils, and an elevated protein. The glucose is typically normal or slightly low. Neuroimaging studies may reveal periventricular enhancement and ventricular enlargement but may also be normal.

Focal microglial nodular encephalitis is characterized by multiple small glial nodules located in gray matter, often containing CMV inclusion bodies but usually with no surrounding inflammatory response. The clinical correlation of microglial nodular encephalitis is unknown.

The diagnosis of CMV infection of the CNS is based on PCR, which is much more sensitive than culture or antigen detection for this purpose. A positive PCR correlates with the presence of CMV infection of the CNS. Quantitation of the level of CMV DNA in CSF is helpful because patients with ventriculoencephalitis have very high levels.[27] Patients with low levels of CMV DNA in CSF who are not currently symptomatic are at risk of developing CMV encephalitis, but the level of risk is unknown. Following the level of CMV DNA in CSF can be useful for monitoring therapy.[29]

Human Herpesvirus 6

HHV-6 is a recently recognized member of the herpesvirus family now known to be the cause of *roseola infantum* (*exanthem subitum*), a common illness of childhood (see Chapter 13). It is also neurotropic, and its role in neurologic disease is the subject of ongoing investigation. As with other herpesviruses, HHV-6 is thought to have clinical manifestations associated with both primary and reactivation disease. CNS invasion has been demonstrated, both through detection of HHV-6 in brain tissue[30] and by detection of HHV-6 DNA in CSF by PCR.[31, 32]

Neurologic manifestations associated with HHV-6 infection include febrile seizures and meningoencephalitis in infants with roseola[31] and encephalitis and encephalopathy in adults. Reports of encephalitis in adults include a fatal case in a bone marrow transplant recipient[30] and a case that resembled Devic's variant of multiple sclerosis (MS).[33] A highly provocative report suggested a link between HHV-6 and MS, based on the demonstration of HHV-6 antigens in oligodendrocytes of MS patients but not in controls.[34] HHV-6 DNA has also been detected in the CSF of some patients with focal encephalitis.[35]

The diagnosis of HHV-6 disease of the CNS is problematic because HHV-6 DNA can be found in normal brain tissue[36] and in CSF from some children without acute neurologic disease.[32] The occurrence of encephalitis in temporal association with acute HHV-6 infection is suggestive of but not definitive evidence for a causal relationship. In these cases, acute HHV-6 infection can be documented by viral culture of peripheral blood or by the finding of HHV-6 DNA in peripheral blood by PCR in a patient who is seronegative for HHV-6 and subsequently undergoes seroconversion (see Chapter 13). The detection of HHV-6 DNA in CSF using PCR provides further supportive evidence. However, only demonstration of HHV-6 antigen or nucleic acid by immunohistochemistry (IHC) or in situ hybridization (ISH) in association with histologic evidence of encephalitis can be considered definitive evidence.

B Virus

B virus, also known as *Herpesvirus simiae* or *cercopithecine herpesvirus*, is a pathogen of Old World monkeys that rarely infects humans who have contact with infected monkeys or their tissues. At least one secondary case has occurred in contact of a person infected via contact with a monkey. As with HSV and VZV, B virus is an alpha herpesvirus with a tendency to infect mucosal epithelial and CNS cells. Infected monkeys may be asymptomatic or may have intermittent mucosal lesions that resemble human cold sores. Asymptomatic shedding of the virus by infected monkeys can occur. Most cases of human disease begin peripherally at the site of a bite or other inoculation, then spread to involve the CNS, causing an ascending encephalomyelitis with a mortality rate of 70%.[37] Acyclovir may be effective in treating the disease.

Laboratory evaluation is needed in two settings: at the time of exposure and for evaluation of suspect cases. Detailed guidelines are available for the prevention and treatment of B-virus infections in exposed persons.[37] Laboratory tests that can be useful include serologic assays for anti–B-virus antibodies, cell culture, and PCR. Isolation of the virus in cell culture is the mainstay of diagnosis. The virus grows in a variety of cell culture types, including African green monkey kidney, rabbit kidney, BSC-1, and LLC-RK-1 cells.[38] Although these cell culture types are widely available, attempts to culture B virus should be made only by specialized laboratories capable of implementing the appropriate biosafety precautions (level 4).

Once the virus grows in culture, identification as B virus can be accomplished by sodium dodecyl sulphate–polyacrylamide gel electrophoresis (SDS-PAGE) of viral proteins and by restriction endonuclease analysis of viral DNA. Serologic testing for anti–B-virus antibodies can be useful, both for determining whether monkeys are infected and for making the diagnosis in humans with negative cultures. Interpretation of serologic results can be problematic, however, because of cross-reactions with other human and simian herpesviruses.

At the time of a possible human exposure, serum samples for serologic testing should be collected both from the monkey implicated in the exposure and from the exposed person. Swab cultures from the monkey's buccal mucosa, conjunctivae (bilateral), and urogenital area (if contamination by urine suspected) should also be obtained.[37] Dacron swabs with wooden or paper (not metal) shafts should be used and should be placed in standard viral transport media and stored cold until they can be frozen at −20°C or colder. These specimens are useful for evaluating the likelihood that exposure to B virus occurred. The utility of specimens from the bite wound obtained immediately after the bite is controversial. The highest priority is thorough cleansing of the wound, and cultures should be obtained only after cleansing.

Early clinical manifestations include vesicular lesions at the site of the bite or other inoculation, followed by signs of encephalomyelitis. The specimens that should be obtained to evaluate symptomatic individuals include serum for convalescent antibody titers, swabs for culture from any suspicious mucocutaneous lesions, and CSF for culture and CSF antibody titers.[37] Full-thickness skin biopsies of suspicious lesions provide useful material for culture. Specimens collected for culture can also be used for PCR. Several PCR assays for B virus have been described[39, 40] but are still under evaluation.

Cases of B virus are rare, and expert consultation is always advisable. The following laboratories conduct B-virus identification and serologic testing:

Julia K. Hilliard, PhD
Southwest Foundation for Biomedical Research
Department of Virology and Immunology
7620 Northwest Loop 410
San Antonio, Texas 78228
Telephone: (210) 258-9400, ext 280; or (210) 673-3269
Pager: 1-800-443-7243; ID 068746

Seymour S. Kalter, PhD
Virus Reference Laboratory
7540 Louis Pasteur Dr.
San Antonio, Texas 78229

David Brown, MRC Path
Virus Reference Division
Central Public Health Laboratory
61 Colindale Ave.
London NW9 5HT, England
Telephone: 081-200-4400

Arthropod-borne Viruses (Arboviruses)

The arboviruses are viruses from within the families Togaviridae, Bunyaviridae, and Flaviviridae that have insect or tick vectors and bird or animal reservoirs. The individual viruses most closely identified with encephalitis are eastern, western, and Venezuelan equine encephalitis viruses and St. Louis, La Crosse (California serogroup), and Japanese encephalitis viruses (Table 3–8).

Table 3.8	Arthropod-borne Viruses (Arboviruses) that Cause Encephalitis			
Family	**Genus**	**Virus**	**Principal vector(s)**	**Primary host(s)**
Togaviridae	*Alphavirus*	Eastern equine encephalitis	*Culex melanura**	Birds
		Western equine encephalitis	*Culex tarsalis*	Birds
		Venezuelan equine encephalitis	Multiple mosquito species	Rodents, aquatic birds, horses, burros
Flaviviridae	*Flavivirus*	St. Louis encephalitis	*Culex tarsalis* *Culex nigripalpus* *Culex quinquefasciatus* *Culex pipiens*	Birds
		Powassan	*Ixodes* spp.	Squirrels, ground hogs
		Tick-borne encephalitis	*Ixodes persulcatus*	Rodents, goats
		Japanese encephalitis	*Culex tritaeniorhynchus*	Pigs
		Murray Valley encephalitis	*Culex annulirostris*	Birds
Bunyaviridae	*Bunyavirus*	California encephalitis group (includes La Crosse, Jamestown Canyon, snowshoe hare, and Cache Valley viruses)	*Aedes triseriatus*†	Woodland mammals
Reoviridae	*Coltivirus*	Colorado tick fever	*Dermacentor andersoni* (Western dog tick)	Ground squirrels, chipmunks

*Other species may be involved in transmission to humans.
†La Crosse encephalitis.

Diseases caused by these viruses have been unusual in the United States in recent years. Of 100 cases reported in 1994, there were 76 cases of California serogroup encephalitis, 20 of St. Louis encephalitis, two of western equine encephalitis, one of eastern equine encephalitis, and one of Powassan encephalitis.[41] Because of the difficulties in making a specific diagnosis, reported cases undoubtedly underestimate the true number of cases.

The clinical features of arthropod-borne encephalitis overlap and include fever, malaise, headache, seizures, and abnormal mental status with lethargy or coma. Focal neurologic findings occur in some patients. Neuroimaging may be normal or may reveal diverse abnormalities. In a recent study of neuroimaging findings in eastern equine encephalitis, abnormalities in the basal ganglia, thalami, and brain stem were prominent.[42] The electroencephalogram (EEG) is often abnormal and can reveal *periodic lateralizing epileptiform discharges* (PLEDs), often considered suggestive of HSV encephalitis.[43]

Although no specific treatment exists, a specific diagnosis should be made whenever possible because of the public health implications. The occurrence of human cases triggers health departments to implement vector control measures and to educate the public regarding avoidance of mosquitoes.

The first factor to consider in identifying an arboviral cause of encephalitis is *where* the patient was exposed. Figure 3–1 shows the distribution of cases in the United States in recent years. The incubation periods are 5 to 10 days for western equine encephalitis, 5 to 7 days for eastern equine encephalitis, 1 to 6 days for Venezuelan equine encephalitis, 4 to 21 days for St. Louis encephalitis, 7 days for La Crosse virus,[44] and 1 to 14 days for Colorado tick fever.[45]

The diagnostic test of choice for diagnosing arboviral encephalitis is immunoglobulin M (IgM) serology.[44] Seroconversion or a rising titer of virus-specific IgG antibodies is also diagnostic but less practical because of the interval required between acute and convalescent specimens. A variety of techniques have been used to detect arboviral antibodies, including enzyme immunoassay (EIA), hemagglutination inhibition, indirect immunofluorescence, neutralization, and complement fixation. Indirect immunofluorescence and IgM capture EIA are the techniques most often used to detect arboviral IgM antibodies. Specimens for testing should include both CSF and serum. Approximately 40% of patients have arboviral IgM antibodies detectable in serum or CSF by 4 days after onset, and this percentage increases by approximately 10% per day, so that by day 10 nearly all cases are positive.[46] These antibodies are detected in CSF only for a short period during and immediately after the illness but may persist at low levels in serum for up to 1 year.[44] Therefore the presence of arboviral IgM antibodies in CSF is considered diagnostic of recent infection, whereas the presence in serum is considered presumptive evidence. Cross-reactions among different arboviruses can occur, especially between closely related viruses. Therefore serologic testing is not always able to implicate a specific causative virus. This can be a problem in areas of the world such as the Far East, where closely related arboviruses such as Japanese B encephalitis and dengue virus coexist.

Other diagnostic techniques have limited role in the diagnosis of arboviral encephalitis. Cultures of blood and CSF are rarely positive, except from autopsy specimens. In addition, most diagnostic virology laboratories have little experience with these viruses and may lack reagents to identify them if they do grow in available cell cultures. Finally, culture of these viruses without adequate precautions may be hazardous, as shown by a number of laboratory-acquired infections. PCR assays for the arboviruses have been developed, but experience with human cases is limited. These assays may prove to be useful in arboviral screening of mosquitoes for surveillance purposes.

Colorado tick fever. The diagnostic approach to Colorado tick fever (see also Chapter 16) differs from that just described. The Colorado tick fever virus is present in circulating erythrocytes and can be detected during the acute infection and for many weeks afterward.[47] The virus can be cultured from a blood clot and has also been detected by FA staining. Recently a PCR assay has been developed that can be performed on the same blood clot specimen submitted for culture.[48] If early positive experience with this assay continues, it will likely become the test of choice for establishing a rapid diagnosis. Serologic tests to detect IgG and IgM antibodies to Colorado tick fever virus can also be performed as an alternative approach to diagnosis. These antibodies may not be detectable until the second week of illness.[49]

The reference center in the United States for arboviral diagnosis is the Arbovirus Disease Branch of the Division of Vector-Borne Infections of the Centers for Disease Control and Prevention (CDC) at Fort Collins, Colorado. That unit can provide expert consultation and assistance in making a specific laboratory diagnosis. State health department laboratories may also be helpful in providing advice regarding local distribution of arboviral infections and procedures for sending specimens for diagnostic studies.

Enteroviruses

Rarely, patients with enteroviral infection have encephalitis rather than or in addition to meningitis. A special group is patients with congenital hypogammaglobulinemia, who are susceptible to chronic enteroviral meningoencephalitis. The diagnostic studies undertaken to document enteroviral encephalitis are the same as those used to document enteroviral meningitis (see later discussion).

Rabies

Although currently rare in the United States, cases of human rabies continue to occur, including troublesome cases with onset more than 1 year after exposure and others with no clear patient history of an animal bite. Although most patients have a history of exposure and the clinical manifestations are often distinctive, the diagnosis of rabies should be considered in any case of encephalitis of unknown etiology. No specific treatment is available, but accurate diagnosis may be important for minimizing exposures of caregivers and providing appropriate postexposure prophylaxis for exposed patients.

Rabies diagnostic tests are typically carried out in state health department laboratories and the CDC Rabies Laboratory rather than in hospital diagnostic laboratories. The state health department laboratory should be consulted in all cases; some state laboratories can analyze specimens, whereas others ship specimens directly to the CDC. The CDC Rabies Laboratory recently prepared a set of instructions for collection and processing of samples for rabies diagnosis (Box 3–3). Several approaches are used for the diagnosis of human rabies (Table 3–9). None is positive in all cases, so each should be used in all possible cases. In addition, rabies diagnostic tests may be negative early in the illness and should be repeated if clinical suspicion still exists.

Early in the illness, tests should be performed to detect rabies antigen, to culture the virus, and to detect rabies ribonucleic acid (RNA) by reverse-transcription PCR (RT-PCR). Rabies antigen is detected by FA staining performed on skin biopsy, usually obtained from the nape of the neck. Rabies antigen is found in cutaneous nerves surrounding the follicles. Sidebar provides specific instructions for obtaining and transporting this specimen. False-negative tests can occur early in the illness.[50] The use of corneal impression smears for rabies antigen detection is less sensitive than skin biopsy and is no longer recommended.[51]

Saliva should be submitted for viral isolation in all cases. Rabies virus can be isolated using murine neuroblastoma cells or by intracerebral mouse inoculation. Virus can also be isolated in some cases from CSF. RT-PCR can also be performed on these specimens.[51, 52] Nucleotide sequencing of PCR products can identify the animal source of the rabies virus strain.

After the eighth day of illness, rabies antibodies are present and should be tested for in specimens of serum and CSF. Samples from earlier in the illness may be useful for comparison purposes. Rabies antibodies appear in the CSF a few days after they are detectable in serum. The presence of rabies antibodies in serum is diagnostic of rabies only in those who have not been vaccinated, since the vaccine induces a detectable level of rabies antibodies. The presence of rabies antibodies in CSF is diagnostic regardless of vaccination status, since rabies antibodies have not been detected in the CSF of vaccinated individuals.[51]

Brain tissue obtained by biopsy or at postmortem can be examined using FA staining. Sections from the medulla, cerebellum, and hippocampus should be

Box 3.3   Collection of Samples for Diagnosis of Rabies in Humans

A diagnosis of rabies should be considered for patients with signs or symptoms of encephalitis or myelitis. The course of the illness, additional history, and laboratory tests for other more common etiologies can determine if samples specific for rabies should be collected. The following instructions should be used to collect samples only after a consultation with your state health department or with the Rabies Laboratory at the Centers for Disease Control and Prevention (CDC, 404-639-1050).

Patient history

Complete the form detailing the patient's clinical history and provide the name and phone number of the physician who should be contacted with the test results.

Samples

Consider all samples as potentially infectious. Test tubes and other sample containers must be securely sealed (tape around the cap will ensure that the containers do not open during transit). If immediate shipment is not possible, samples should be stored frozen at $-20°C$ or below. Samples should be shipped frozen on dry ice by an overnight courier in watertight primary containers and leak-proof secondary containers that meet the guidelines of the International Air Transport Association. The CDC Rabies Laboratory should be telephoned at the time of shipment and given information on the mode of shipment, expected arrival time, and courier tracking number. Shipment address is as follows:

Rabies Laboratory
DASH, Bldg 4, Room B32
Centers for Disease Control and Prevention
1600 Clifton Road, NE
Atlanta, GA 30333

Saliva

Using a sterile eyedropper pipette, collect saliva and place in a small sterile container which can be sealed securely. No preservatives or additional material should be added. Laboratory tests to be performed include detection of rabies RNA (by reverse-transcription polymerase chain reaction [RT-PCR] of extracted nucleic acids) and isolation of infectious virus in cell culture. Tracheal aspirates and sputum are not suitable for rabies tests.

Neck biopsy

A section of skin 5 to 6 mm in diameter should be taken from the posterior region of the neck at the hairline. The biopsy specimen should contain a minimum of 10 hair follicles and be of sufficient depth to include the cutaneous nerves at the base of the follicle. Place the specimen on a piece of sterile gauze moistened with sterile water and place in a sealed container. Do not add preservatives or additional fluids. Laboratory tests to be performed include RT-PCR and immunofluorescent staining for viral antigen in frozen sections of the biopsy.

Serum and cerebrospinal fluid (CSF)

At least 0.5 ml of serum or CSF should be collected; no preservatives should be added. Do not send whole blood. If no vaccine or rabies immune serum has been given, the presence of antibody to rabies virus in the serum is diagnostic and tests of CSF are unnecessary. Antibody to rabies virus in the CSF, regardless of the immunization history, suggests a rabies virus infection. Laboratory tests for antibody include indirect immunofluorescence and virus neutralization.

Brain biopsy

The rarity of rabies and the lack of an effective treatment make the collection of a brain biopsy unwarranted; however, biopsy samples negative for herpes encephalitis should be tested for evidence of rabies infection. The biopsy is placed in a sterile sealed container; do not add preservatives or additional fluids. Laboratory tests to be performed include RT-PCR and immunofluorescent staining for viral antigen in touch impressions.

Modified from Jean Smith, MS, Centers for Disease Control and Prevention, Atlanta, 1997.

Table 3.9   Specimens and Tests for Rabies

Specimen	Test performed	Comments
Skin biopsy	Fluorescent antibody stain, PCR*	Best specimen for establishing an early diagnosis. Sensitivity is higher in late disease. Second biopsy should be obtained if first is negative and clinical suspicion still exists.
Saliva	Viral isolation, PCR*	May provide early diagnosis.
Serum	Antibody detection	Not positive until day 8 of illness. Not diagnostic in vaccinated individuals.
Cerebrospinal fluid (CSF)	Antibody detection	Antibodies in CSF appear a few days later than in serum. Presence of rabies antibodies in CSF is diagnostic, even in vaccinated individuals.

*Polymerase chain reaction is considered a supplementary technique to other tests performed on the same specimen.

examined. Although rabies can be diagnosed during life by examination of brain tissue, brain biopsy is not recommended as a primary diagnostic technique because the diagnosis can usually be established using the other techniques just described.

Serologic tests for rabies antibodies in serum can also be used to determine the rabies immune status of an individual. Because current rabies vaccines are highly effective, measurement of antibody titers is not recommended to confirm vaccine efficacy unless the individual is immunocompromised. In individuals with ongoing exposure, rabies antibody titers can be used to determine the need for booster doses of vaccine. Techniques for measurement of rabies antibodies include neutralization, indirect immunofluorescence, and enzyme-linked immunosorbent assay (ELISA). Rabies antibody testing is performed only in reference laboratories.

Mumps

Before the widespread use of mumps vaccine, mumps virus was the most common cause of encephalitis in the United States. In recent years, however, mumps has been uncommon.

CNS manifestations are a frequent complication of mumps. CSF pleocytosis occurs in approximately 50% of patients with mumps parotitis without clinical evidence of CNS involvement. Conversely, approximately 10% of patients with recognized mumps infections of the CNS have no clinical evidence of parotitis. Meningitis is a much more common manifestation of CNS involvement than encephalitis.

Encephalitis can be divided into early-onset cases that occur simultaneously with parotitis and late-onset cases that occur 7 to 10 days later. The latter group may be caused by demyelination rather than direct viral infection of the brain. In general, the clinical features of either form are those of a nonfocal encephalitis. High fever may be present. The CSF shows a mononuclear pleocytosis in most patients, although a minority have a predominance of polymorphonuclear neutrophil leukocytes (PMNS). The protein concentration is generally mildly elevated, and the glucose level is normal or decreased. A useful clue is that serum amylase is typically elevated.[53, 54]

The specific laboratory diagnosis of mumps encephalitis may be made by viral culture or serology. The virus can be cultured from CSF, saliva, or urine. Saliva and CSF are generally positive for approximately 8 days after onset, whereas viral shedding can continue in the urine for 2 weeks. The laboratory should be notified that mumps virus is suspected because mumps virus may not produce obvious cytopathic effect (CPE) when it grows in cell culture, and the hemadsorption technique (see Chapter 1) must be used to detect viral growth. In patients with meningitis or encephalitis, culture of the virus from CSF provides the most unequivocal diagnosis of mumps infection of the CNS.

Because of the current rarity of mumps in the United States, many virology laboratories have little recent experience culturing the virus, and serologic diagnosis may be more practical. A variety of serologic tests can be used to detect an antibody response, including ELISA, hemagglutination inhibition, and complement fixation. The ELISA is the most widely available at this time and can be used to detect virus-specific IgM antibodies, thus giving a diagnosis of current infection from a single acute-phase specimen. Mumps-specific IgM antibodies are present in all patients by the fifth day of illness and persist for at least 60 days. Documentation of acute infection through a rise in titer can also be used, but this may be difficult using ELISA because titers are sometimes already high at the time of clinical illness. Measurement of mumps antibodies in CSF can also be helpful. The presence of mumps-specific IgG or especially IgM antibodies in CSF is strong evidence for mumps as the cause of disease. The interpretation of IgG but not IgM antibody titers may be clouded by cross-reactions with closely related parainfluenza viruses.

Measles

Infection of the CNS is a well-known complication of measles. Three different forms of measles encephalitis have been recognized (Table 3–10). The approach to the diagnosis of each varies.

Table 3.10	Measles Encephalitis			
Form	**Host**	**Timing**	**Incidence**	**Pathogenesis**
Postinfectious encephalitis	Normal	Within 3 weeks of rash	$1:10^3$	Immune-mediated demyelination
Subacute measles encephalitis	Immunocompromised	Weeks to months after acute measles	Rare	Uncontrolled infection
Subacute sclerosing panencephalitis (SSPE)	Normal*	Years after infection	$1:10^6$	Defective virus

*Recently, cases have been recognized in children with congenital HIV infection.[59]

The first form, known as *postinfectious encephalomyelitis*, typically occurs within 2 to 3 weeks of onset of rash and is marked by return of high fever, obtundation, seizures, and decreased LOC. The diagnosis is typically presumptive, based on the recent occurrence of measles (see Chapter 13). Most tests for the presence of measles virus in the brain have been negative, and this disease is thought to be immunologically mediated. Recently, several cases have been diagnosed using PCR to demonstrate measles virus RNA in CSF.[55, 56]

Subacute measles encephalitis, also known as *inclusion body encephalitis*, occurs in individuals with depression of cell-mediated immunity. This entity tends to occur within 6 months of acute measles[57] and is rapidly progressive with variable manifestations. Measles virus is present in the brain, although some studies have suggested that the virus is defective, as in SSPE[57] (see next), leading to suggestions that this entity is a variant form of SSPE. Diagnosis in the past has been accomplished by examination of brain tissue, looking for characteristic inclusions and evidence of measles virus, including selected measles proteins (demonstrated by IHC), nucleic acids (demonstrated by ISH), or viral particles (visualized by EM). More recently, a few cases have been diagnosed by PCR performed on brain tissue.[58]

Subacute sclerosing panencephalitis (SSPE) is a characteristic syndrome that typically arises years after acute measles. Recently, cases of an SSPE-like syndrome have also been described in young children with HIV infection.[59] The manifestations include myoclonus, clumsiness, and progressive intellectual deterioration, progressing to death. Often the episode of acute measles occurred before age 2 years. Male gender and rural residence have been epidemiologic risk factors. Since the control of measles through vaccination, the incidence of SSPE has declined greatly. The pathogenesis is thought to involve defective replication of measles virus in the brain, such that complete viral particles are not produced and released.

The diagnosis of SSPE is based on the characteristic clinical features and the demonstration of high measles antibody titers in CSF. Specimens of CSF and serum obtained within 24 hours of each other should be submitted to the laboratory for measles antibody measurements. The criteria for determining whether the CSF antibody titer is diagnostic are not well defined. One suggestion has been that the ratio of CSF to serum measles antibody titer is 1:5 to 1:50 in SSPE patients compared with 1:200 to 1:500 in normal individuals.[60] It is also important to determine a similar ratio for antibodies to another virus, to ensure that the increased CSF to serum antibody ratio is specific for measles virus and not the result of BBB leakage. A more sophisticated study available in selected research laboratories is the demonstration of an increased rate of intrathecal synthesis of measles-specific antibodies.[61]

Rubella

Encephalitis is an unusual complication of rubella, estimated to occur in 1 per 6000 cases.[62] The onset of encephalitis is usually within six days of the rash, with symptoms including headache, stiff neck, vomiting, seizures, and a decreased LOC. Typically the CSF has a moderate increase in mononuclear cells. The pathogenesis is not well defined. Although the illness has some features of postviral demyelination, extensive demyelination has not been observed in postmortem examinations.[62] In one case, rubella virus has been isolated from CSF.[63]

A presumptive diagnosis is based on the close temporal relationship to acute rubella (see Chapter 13). Efforts should also be made to isolate the virus from CSF or brain tissue if available. At least 1 ml of CSF should be submitted for culture. A specific request to look for rubella virus is necessary, since usual procedures would not be adequate for detecting that virus. PCR has been used successfully for the diagnosis of other manifestations of rubella,[64] but there is only a single case report to date of its application to the diagnosis of encephalitis.[65]

A different form of rubella encephalitis is *progressive rubella panencephalitis*.[66] This syndrome occurs without obvious temporal relationship to acute rubella. Some cases have occurred in individuals with evidence of congenital rubella. The clinical manifestations resemble those of SSPE, with gradual mental deterioration, seizures, and other evidence of cerebral dysfunction. The diagnosis has been made by detection of high levels of rubella antibodies in CSF. In one case, rubella virus was isolated from brain, suggesting that efforts to isolate the virus from CSF or brain tissue should be made. The role of PCR has not been evaluated.

Adenovirus

Adenovirus has been identified as the cause of encephalitis in a small number of patients. Several cases have been in individuals with immunosuppression from a variety of causes, including HIV, bone marrow transplantation, and hypogammaglobulinemia. Other cases have occurred in patients with simultaneous adenovirus pneumonia.

Efforts to diagnose adenovirus encephalitis should include viral cultures of CSF and brain tissue if available. Notification of the virology laboratory that adenovirus is suspected is important so that specimens can be inoculated onto cell cultures with optimal sensitivity for adenoviruses. The role of PCR has not been evaluated, but this technique is potentially useful because of its sensitivity and the difficulty in culturing some adenovirus serotypes.

Influenza

Encephalitis and encephalopathy have been associated with influenza. Cases include an encephalopathy that may accompany the acute illness, an inflammatory postinfectious encephalitis, and Reye's syndrome.[67] The latter has become extremely rare since the recognition of the etiologic link to aspirin consumption.

No well-defined diagnostic criteria exist for establishing influenza as the etiology of a case of encephalitis. At present, suspicion should be directed to influenza as the cause when the neurologic disease occurs in association with documented influenza, and when a patient has respiratory manifestations during an outbreak of influenza in the community (see Chapter 4). CSF and brain tissue should be cultured for influenza virus if these specimens are available. The laboratory should be notified to look specifically for influenza virus, because like mumps virus, influenza virus may grow in culture without producing CPE. Both of these viruses can be detected by the hemadsorption technique performed upon monkey kidney cell cultures that have been inoculated with the patient's specimen.

The mechanism of the CNS complications of influenza has not been established. Cultures have been positive only in rare cases, possibly because active viral infection is not responsible for the clinical manifestations.

JC Virus

The JC virus is a polyomavirus that has been associated with virtually all cases of *progressive multifocal leukoencephalopathy* (PML) in patients with AIDS. PML is present in approximately 4% of patients dying from AIDS. Its manifestations are varied and include difficulties with cognition, motor function, vision, and speech. The pathologic lesions are foci of demyelination which contain oligodendrocytes with enlarged nuclei that contain inclusions composed of polyomavirus virions.

Culture of JC virus requires special techniques that are not available in routine diagnostic virology laboratories. Until recently, the diagnosis could be made only by pathologic examination of biopsy or autopsy tissue, but several studies have now shown that PCR can be used to detect JC virus DNA in the CSF of AIDS patients with PML. In most series the sensitivity has been 70% to 90%, and the specificity has usually been greater than 95%.[68] Therefore a positive test strongly supports the diagnosis, but a negative result does not rule it out. Repeating the PCR on a specimen obtained later in the course of the disease may lead to a diagnosis in some patients in whom the initial PCR is negative.

MENINGITIS

The term *aseptic meningitis* is often used to refer to *nonbacterial meningitis*. Viruses are by far the most common cause of this syndrome, although other infectious agents and some medications can produce it as well (Box 3–4). The symptoms of *viral meningitis* are similar to those of bacterial meningitis and include fever, headache, stiff neck, nausea, and vomiting. Typically the CSF examination reveals a leukocytosis with a predominance of mononuclear cells. The CSF protein concentration is usually normal or moderately elevated, and the glucose level is normal or moderately decreased. Routine bacterial cultures are negative. The outcome of viral meningitis is usually benign. Important clues suggest a specific viral etiology (Table 3–11).

Enteroviruses

The enteroviruses are single-stranded RNA viruses that include the coxsackie A and B viruses, the echoviruses,

---

Box 3.4 Causes of Aseptic Meningitis

Viral
Enteroviruses
    Echoviruses
    Coxsackie A and B
    Polioviruses
Herpes simplex virus
Epstein-Barr virus
Varicella-zoster virus
Cytomegalovirus (rare)
Lymphocytic choriomeningitis virus
Mumps virus
Arboviruses
Human immunodeficiency virus

Nonviral
Medications
    Nonsteroidal antiinflammatory agents (NSAIDs)
    Trimethoprim (TMP)-sulfamethoxazole (SMX)
      (co-trimoxazole)
    OKT3 and other immunoglobulins
Partially treated bacterial infection
Parameningeal infection
Tuberculosis
Fungal infection
    Cryptococcus neoformans
    Histoplasma capsulatum
Leptospirosis
Syphilis
Lyme disease
Rocky Mountain spotted fever
Ehrlichiosis

Table 3.11	Clues for Establishing the Etiology of Viral Meningitis	
Clue	**Virus**	**Diagnostic test (specimen)**
Summer-fall onset	Enteroviruses	Culture (CSF)
		RT-PCR (CSF)
Fall-winter onset	Lymphocytic choriomeningitis virus	Culture (CSF)
		Serology (serum)
Genital lesions	Herpes simplex type-2	PCR (CSF)
Recurrent episodes	Herpes simplex type-2	PCR (CSF)
Contact with mice or hamsters	Lymphocytic choriomeningitis	Culture (CSF)
		Serology (serum)
Parotitis or orchitis	Mumps	Culture (CSF, saliva, urine)
Infectious mononucleosis	Epstein-Barr	Serology (serum)
HIV risk factors	Human immunodeficiency	p24 antigen (serum)
		HIV RNA (plasma)

RT-PCR, Reverse-transcription polymerase chain reaction; *CSF*, cerebrospinal fluid; *RNA*, ribonucleic acid.

and the polioviruses. In all, 67 distinct serotypes have been identified. The primary site of replication of these viruses is the gastrointestinal tract, and they are transmitted primarily by the fecal-oral route. They cause a wide variety of infections in addition to meningitis (see Chapters 9 and 13). In temperate countries they are highly seasonal, with a summer-fall predominance. Multiple serotypes are usually present during an enteroviral season, but one may be predominant. A limited number of serotypes, including coxsackieviruses B2 and B5 and echoviruses 4, 6, 9, 11, 16, and 30, account for a large proportion of all cases of enteroviral meningitis.[69] Cases of meningitis are most common in infants and young children but can occur at any age. The great majority of patients recover without sequelae.

Certain clinical features suggest the diagnosis of enteroviral meningitis. After a prodrome of fever and malaise lasting 1 to 2 days, patients typically experience headache, photophobia, and stiff neck. Infants usually show marked irritability. Fever is present in most cases. Typical CSF findings include pleocytosis, usually with less than 500 leukocytes/mm^3, although counts of several thousand occur occasionally. A mononuclear predominance is typical, but PMNs may predominate, especially early in the illness. In these patients, the percentage of PMNs is usually less than 90%. In occasional patients, no cells are present in the CSF even though an enterovirus is grown in culture. The protein concentration is usually normal or slightly elevated, most often less than 100 mg/dl. The glucose level is usually normal, but may be slightly depressed. Neuroimaging studies are usually normal.

The conventional approach to laboratory diagnosis of enteroviral infection is to culture the causative agent, although RT-PCR most likely will become the preferred approach as soon as assays become widely available (see following discussion). For the diagnosis of enteroviral meningitis by culture, the specimen of choice is CSF, since a positive viral culture of the CSF is diagnostic of enteroviral meningitis. Unfortunately, the sensitivity of this technique is no more than 50% to 70%, probably because of low titers of virus in CSF. In addition, some enteroviruses, especially the coxsackie A viruses, may not grow in cell culture. Isolation of these serotypes requires suckling mouse inoculation, a procedure that is not performed in most diagnostic virology laboratories. A recent study suggests that viruses of these serotypes are not common causes of meningitis.[70] To maximize sensitivity, the CSF should be obtained as early in the illness as possible. At least 1.0 ml should be submitted whenever possible to allow several different cell culture types to be inoculated. Cultures of the throat or nasopharynx and the stool have higher sensitivity than the stool, but these must be interpreted with the understanding that viral excretion in the stool may continue for weeks after an enteroviral infection. In addition, asymptomatic shedding of enteroviruses may occur during the months when these viruses are prevalent.[71]

Viral cultures suffer from certain other limitations that decrease their utility. In addition to suboptimal sensitivity, cultures are relatively slow. The usual time required for a culture of CSF to become positive for an enterovirus is approximately 3 to 4 days, but 7 to 10 days can be required in some cases. Since the course of the disease is rapid, a delay of 3 to 4 days often means that clinical decisions are made before the culture result is available. A further limitation that applies to cultures of the nasopharyngeal secretions or stool in young children is possible confusion between pathogenic enteroviruses and the polio vaccine virus. After administration of the live attenuated (Sabin) polio vaccine, the vaccine strain may be cultured from the nasopharynx for several weeks and from the stool for several months. The polio vaccine virus grows well in cell culture, and the CPE that it produces in the culture may be indistinguishable from CPE produced by pathogenic enteroviruses. If alerted, many laboratories can perform FA stains or neutralization assays to distinguish between the polio vaccine virus and nonpolio enteroviruses. It should also be possible soon to adapt molecular assays to distinguishing between the two. The polio vaccine strain is not found in CSF in normal children.

If the clinical features of a case of aseptic meningitis are typical and it occurs in the midst of a community outbreak of enteroviral infections, specific viral diagnosis may not be necessary. However, viral cultures are useful in certain clinical situations (Box 3–5). Even though several days may be required for the cultures to become positive, a positive CSF culture in the patient who has received antibiotics before having a lumbar puncture may save a number of days of hospitalization and antibiotic therapy.

Serologic assays have very limited application to enteroviral diagnosis for several reasons. First, the antigenic diversity of the enteroviruses renders serologic testing impractical. Second, the need to detect a rise in antibody titer means that several weeks must elapse before a convalescent specimen is available. Assays to detect IgM antibodies have been reported but are not widely available. Tests to detect enterovirus antigens have not been developed because of the antigenic diversity of the enterovirus group.

RT-PCR shows great promise for improving enteroviral diagnosis. A number of RT-PCR assays for enteroviruses have been described. For most of these, the target for amplification has been a segment of the 5′ noncoding region of the enterovirus genome, which is conserved in almost all serotypes. One recent enterovirus RT-PCR assay was shown to detect 60 of the 67 known enterovirus serotypes.[72] The seven serotypes not detected were coxsackieviruses A11, A17, and A24 and echoviruses 16, 22, and 23; coxsackievirus A15 was not available for testing. None of these accounts for a large proportion of cases of enteroviral meningitis.[70] Because the enteroviruses have an RNA genome, the first step in the assay is synthesis of the complementary strand of DNA (cDNA) using the enzyme reverse transcriptase (RT). Some RT assays are performed using a specific enzyme to perform the RT and a different enzyme to perform PCR. Enzymes are also available that carry out both reverse-transcription and thermostable DNA polymerization under different conditions.

Studies have reported that enterovirus PCR performed on CSF is more sensitive than culture.[73, 74] Because PCR can be carried out in 1 day, it offers the prospect of rapid and accurate laboratory diagnosis of enteroviral infection and should be useful in providing a specific diagnosis in patients who have been pretreated with antibiotics and in atypical cases. If PCR assays can be made sufficiently convenient to allow frequent testing, they could become useful in all patients with enteroviral infection serious enough to require hospitalization.

Herpes Simplex Virus

HSV accounts for approximately 1% to 5% of cases of viral meningitis. HSV meningitis differs from HSV encephalitis in the following respects:

1. HSV meningitis is usually caused by HSV type 2 rather than type 1, the usual cause of HSV encephalitis.
2. The clinical course is a self-limited meningitis, usually not associated with permanent neurologic sequelae, rather than a necrotizing encephalitis.
3. The causative virus can sometimes be cultured from CSF, in contrast to HSV encephalitis, in which the virus is only rarely cultured from CSF.

The role of antiviral therapy in HSV meningitis is not clearly established, but it may hasten the resolution of symptoms.

The predominant clinical findings of HSV meningitis are typical of viral meningitis: headache, nausea, vomiting, photophobia, and stiff neck. CSF findings are also typical of viral meningitis. The simultaneous presence of genital herpetic lesions can be a clue to the etiology of the meningitis. The clinician must be aware, however, that HSV meningitis can occur without evident genital lesions.[75] One of the salient features of this clinical entity is that *it may recur*. Recurrent episodes are often separated by years. Some patients with the diagnosis of Mollaret's meningitis have been found actually to have recurrent HSV meningitis.[76]

The diagnostic test of choice for confirming the diagnosis of HSV meningitis is PCR. PCR is superior to culture because although the virus can be cultured from CSF of patients with primary episodes, it cannot be recovered from those with recurrent episodes.[77] The PCR assay must have the capability for detecting HSV-2. The sensitivity of PCR for making the diagnosis of HSV meningitis is not well defined at present, but in my experience it appears to be high.

Varicella-zoster Virus

Recent studies indicate that VZV is a common cause of viral meningitis, especially in adolescents and

---

Box 3.5   Indications for Cultures/PCR in Aseptic Meningitis

Prior treatment with antibiotics
Unusual clinical features
   Marked neutrophilic pleocytosis
   Hypoglycorrhachia
   Focal neurologic findings
Occurrence outside enteroviral season
Previous history of aseptic meningitis
Immunocompromised patient

adults.[77a, 77b] VZV meningitis can occur as a complication of varicella or zoster. Cases can also occur without cutaneous lesions.[77a] The symptoms of VZV meningitis are the same as in meningitis caused by other viruses. PCR performed on CSF appears to be much more sensitive than culture of CSF. Reported cases have resolved rapidly without sequelae.

Lymphocytic Choriomeningitis Virus

Lymphocytic choriomeningitis (LCM) virus is an RNA virus in the Arenaviridae family, which also includes Lassa fever virus and viruses (e.g., Junin, Machupo) that cause South American hemorrhagic fever. Humans are infected by contact with infected mice or hamsters, although the history of contact may not always be recognized. Cases have been rare in the United States in recent years.

Most patients have the clinical features of aseptic meningitis, with few having findings of encephalomyelitis. The illness is often biphasic, with an incubation period of 5 to 10 days, followed by an initial illness phase of several days characterized by fever, myalgias, headache, and constitutional symptoms. Orchitis and parotitis may occur in some patients. Leukopenia and thrombocytopenia may also occur. The fever subsides but then reappears 2 to 4 days later with severe headache, stiff neck, and in some patients, findings indicative of encephalitis.

The CSF typically contains several hundred to a few thousand mononuclear cells, moderately elevated protein concentration and normal or decreased glucose level. In addition to the possible history of contact with mice or hamsters, an additional epidemiologic clue is a tendency for cases to occur in the fall or winter, when enteroviral infection, which the illness may resemble, is less common.[78-80]

The laboratory diagnosis of LCM can be accomplished by viral culture or serology. The virus can be cultured from blood or CSF by inoculation into the brains of weanling mice or by inoculation of Vero cell cultures.[78] Most diagnostic virology laboratories are not prepared to isolate LCM virus, and therefore the specimens are usually sent to a reference laboratory. Serum and CSF should be frozen at −70°C and shipped on dry ice. Often, serologic diagnosis may be more practical. Acute and convalescent serum samples should be collected 2 or more weeks apart and tested for antibodies to LCM virus. An immunofluorescent antibody (IFA) assay for IgM antibodies to LCM can provide a diagnosis from a single specimen obtained during the acute phase of illness. IFA assay can also be performed on CSF and is diagnostic if positive.[78] Serologic testing is available through some commercial reference laboratories and the CDC. A PCR assay for LCM has been described,[81] but clinical experience to date is minimal.

Other Viruses

As shown in Box 3–4, a variety of other viruses can cause meningitis, although all are unusual. The most important are EBV, VZV, mumps, and HIV. Most of these viruses also cause encephalitis, and the distinction between encephalitis and meningitis may not be clear. Diagnostic testing for cases of meningitis is the same as discussed for those viruses in the section on encephalitis. The diagnosis of HIV meningitis or meningoencephalitis is usually made presumptively in a patient with aseptic meningitis and evidence of early HIV infection (see Chapter 17). HIV p24 antigen or HIV RNA can be detected in the CSF, but this does not absolutely establish that the CNS illness is caused by HIV, since these tests can also be positive in HIV-infected individuals who do not have HIV meningitis.

TRANSVERSE MYELITIS AND GUILLAIN-BARRÉ SYNDROME

Acute transverse myelitis and Guillain-Barré syndrome (acute idiopathic [febrile] polyneuritis, acute inflammatory demyelinating polyneuropathy) are disorders of the spinal cord associated with a variety of infectious and noninfectious causes. In both syndromes, patients typically have a history of antecedent symptoms suggestive of viral infection. A wide variety of specific viruses has been associated with each, but these associations are often poorly documented. The viruses most clearly associated with *acute transverse myelitis* are CMV, EBV, VZV, and a variety of enteroviruses. Cases have also been reported in association with hepatitis A virus (HAV), parvovirus B19, rubella virus, adenovirus, and HIV.[82] The virus most clearly associated with Guillain-Barré syndrome is CMV, with EBV, VZV, and HIV having less well-defined associations.[83]

The pathogeneses of acute transverse myelitis and Guillain-Barré syndrome are not well defined. Some cases occur following symptoms indicative of viral infection, suggesting an immunopathogenic mechanism. Viruses have rarely been isolated from CSF of patients with acute transverse myelitis, supporting a role for direct viral invasion in some cases. The reported experience with PCR is minimal to date. In most patients with transverse myelitis or Guillain-Barré syndrome in whom viruses have been implicated, the viral diagnosis has been established by serologic testing of blood, with very few cases documented using CSF serology.

Because isolation of a virus from CSF or detection of viral nucleic acid in CSF would be the strongest evidence linking a particular virus to one of these syndromes, these techniques are recommended, even though the yield of culture is low and the utility of PCR unknown. Acute and convalescent serum samples should be obtained for serologic tests against the most likely causative agents. More specific suggestions for documenting infection with specific agents are contained in the sections on encephalitis or meningitis caused by the same viruses.

SPONGIFORM ENCEPHALOPATHIES

The spongiform encephalopathies are a group of transmissible diseases of the central nervous system with long incubation periods that share characteristics of both infectious and neurodegenerative processes. The human diseases include *Creutzfeldt-Jakob disease, kuru, Gerstmann-Sträussler-Scheinker disease,* and *familial fatal insomnia.* Several similar diseases that occur in animals include scrapie, bovine spongiform encephalopathy, transmissible mink encephalopathy, and chronic wasting disease of elk and deer.

For many years these diseases were thought to be slow viral infections, and therefore they are included in this chapter. In 1982, Prusiner[84] suggested that they are caused by a new class of infectious agents termed *prions,* which are unique in that they are composed of a single protein with no nucleic acid. The prion protein designated PRP^{sc} is thought to be derived by a conformational change from a normal cellular protein designated PRP^{c}. The normal function of PRP^{c} is unknown.

Creutzfeldt-Jakob disease (CJD, CJ syndrome, Jakob-Creutzfeldt disease, Jakob's disease) is the most common of this class of diseases in humans. CJD is suspected based on the occurrence of rapidly progressive dementia with myoclonus, typically occurring in middle or advanced age. Although most cases are sporadic, specific modes of transmission are sometimes identified, including neurosurgical procedures, corneal grafts, dural mater grafts, and treatment with cadaveric human growth hormone. Recently, atypical cases have been reported in adolescents and young adults in the United Kingdom, raising concern about transmission from cows with bovine spongiform encephalopathy ("mad-cow disease").[85]

The CSF of patients with CJD is typically normal or may contain a mildly elevated protein concentration. The EEG may reveal a characteristic pattern of periodic sharp wave complexes. No neuroimaging findings are diagnostic, and no diagnostic test exists currently other than examination of brain tissue. Brain examination is diagnostic when the typical findings of neuronal loss, reactive gliosis, and neuronal vacuolation, described as *spongiform change,* are present. The diagnosis is further confirmed by using the Western blot technique to demonstrate the presence of PRP^{sc} in brain.

A recent report used an immunoassay to detect a protein designated 14-3-3 in CSF from patients with CJD.[86] The presence of the protein in CSF had sensitivity of 95% and specificity of 96% for the diagnosis of CJD. The test was positive in several patients with recent cerebrovascular accidents (CVAs, strokes), leading the authors to emphasize that the test should be performed only in the appropriate clinical setting of the patient with dementia who has not had a cerebral infarct within the preceding month. Because the test was positive in one patient with Alzheimer's disease, further evaluation of specificity may be required. This report represents the first possibility for confirming the diagnosis of CJD without a brain biopsy, but the assay should be considered a research approach until further evaluation has been done.

The handling of specimens suspected of containing the agents responsible for the spongiform encephalopathies has been the subject of much discussion. Although not transmissible from person to person, parenteral exposures apparently have resulted in transmission. The transmissible agents are relatively resistant to ordinary forms of disinfection. Within the laboratory, gloves should be worn when working with specimens possibly containing these agents, and the use of needles and other sharp objects should be avoided. Recommendations for disinfection are steam autoclaving for 2 hours at 132°C or exposure to 5.25% sodium hypochlorite (undiluted household bleach) or 2M sodium hydroxide.[87]

References

1. Lakeman FD, Whitley RJ, National Institute of Allergy and Infectious Diseases Collaborative Antiviral Study Group: Diagnosis of herpes simplex encephalitis: application of polymerase chain reaction to cerebrospinal fluid from brain-biopsied patients and correlation with disease, *J Infect Dis* 171:857, 1995.
2. Tebas P, Nease R, Storch GA: Decision analysis of PCR for the diagnosis of herpes simplex encephalitis, *Am J Med* 105:357, 1998.
3. Aurelius E, Johansson B, Skoldenberg B, et al: Rapid diagnosis of herpes simplex encephalitis by nested polymerase chain reaction assay of cerebrospinal fluid, *Lancet* 337:189, 1991.
4. Aurelius E, Johansson B, Skoldenberg B, Forsgren M: Encephalitis in immunocompetent patients due to herpes simplex virus type 1 or 2 as determined by type-specific polymerase chain reaction and antibody assays of cerebrospinal fluid, *J Med Virol* 39:179, 1993.
5. Aurelius E: Herpes simplex encephalitis: early diagnosis and immune activation in the acute stage and during long-term follow-up, *Scand J Infect Dis* 89 (suppl):3, 1993.
6. Whitley RJ, Cobbs CG, Alford CAJ, et al: Diseases that mimic herpes simplex encephalitis: diagnosis, presentation, outcome, *JAMA* 262:234, 1989.
7. Wasiewski WW, Fishman MA: Herpes simplex encephalitis: the brain biopsy controversey, *J Pediatr* 113:575, 1988.

8. Jamieson GA, Maitland NJ, Wilcock GK, et al: Latent herpes simplex virus type 1 in normal and Alzheimer's disease brains, *J Med Virol* 33:224, 1991.

9. Nahmias AJ, Whitley RJ, Visintine AN, et al: Herpes simplex virus encephalitis: laboratory evaluations and their diagnostic significance, *J Infect Dis* 145:829, 1982.

10. Reiber H, Lange P: Quantitation of virus-specific antibodies in cerebrospinal fluid and serum: sensitive and specific detection of antibody synthesis in the brain, *Clin Chem* 37:1153, 1991.

11. Monteyne P, Albert F, Weissbrich B, et al: The detection of intrathecal synthesis of anti–herpes simplex IgG antibodies: comparison between an antigen-mediated immunoblotting technique and antibody index calculations, *J Med Virol* 53:324, 1997.

12. Cinque P, Cleator GM, Weber T, et al: The role of laboratory investigation in the diagnosis and management of patients with suspected herpes simplex encephalitis: a consensus report, *J Neurol Neurosurg Psychiatry* 61:339, 1996.

13. Peters AC, Versteeg J, Lindeman J, Bots GT: Varicella and acute cerebellar ataxia. *Arch Neurol* 32:77, 1978.

14. Gershon A, Steinberg S, Greenberg S, Taber L: Varicella-zoster–associated encephalitis: detection of specific antibody in cerebrospinal fluid, *J Clin Microbiol* 12:764, 1980.

15. Echevarría J, Téllez A, Martínez-Martín P: Subclass distribution of the serum and intrathecal IgG antibody response in varicella-zoster virus infections, *J Infect Dis* 162:621, 1990.

16. Puchhammer-Stockl E, Popow-Kraupp T, Heinz FX, et al: Detection of varicella-zoster virus DNA by polymerase chain reaction in the cerebrospinal fluid of patients suffering from neurological complications associated with chicken pox or herpes zoster, *J Clin Microbiol* 29:1513, 1991.

17. Gray F, Belec L, Lescs MC, et al: Varicella-zoster virus infection of the central nervous system in the acquired immune deficiency syndrome, *Brain* 117:987, 1994.

18. Burke DG, Kalayjian RC, Vann VR, et al: Polymerase chain reaction detection and clinical significance of varicella-zoster virus in cerebrospinal fluid from human immunodeficiency virus–infected patients, *J Infect Dis* 176:1080, 1997.

19. Cinque P, Bossolasco S, Vago L, et al: Varicella-zoster virus (VZV) DNA in cerebrospinal fluid of patients infected with human immunodeficiency virus: VZV disease of the central nervous system or subclinical reactivation of VZV disease, *Clin Infect Dis* 25:634, 1997.

20. Gold E: Serologic and virus-isolation studies of patients with varicella-zoster infection, *N Engl J Med* 274:181, 1966.

20a. Haanpää M, Dastidar P, Weinberg A, et al: CSF and MRI findings in patients with acute herpes zoster, *Neurology* 51:1405, 1998.

21. Grose C, Henle W, Henle G, Feorino P: Primary Epstein-Barr virus infections in acute neurologic diseases, *N Engl J Med* 292:392, 1975.

22. Domachowske JB, Cunningham CK, Cummings DL, et al: Acute manifestations and neurologic sequelae of Epstein-Barr virus encephalitis in children, *Pediatr Infect Dis J* 15:871, 1996.

23. Cinque P, Vago L, Dahl H, et al: Polymerase chain reaction on cerebrospinal fluid for diagnosis of virus-associated opportunistic diseases of the central nervous system in HIV-infected patients, *AIDS* 10:951, 1996.

24. Cinque P, Brytting M, Vago L, et al: Epstein-Barr virus DNA in cerebrospinal fluid from patients with AIDS-related primary lymphoma of the central nervous system, *Lancet* 342:398, 1993.

25. Arribas JR, Clifford DF, Fichtenbaum DJ, et al: Detection of Epstein-Barr virus DNA in cerebrospinal fluid for diagnosis of AIDS-related central nervous system lymphoma, *J Clin Microbiol* 33:1580, 1995.

26. De Luca A, Antinori A, Cingolani A, et al: Evaluation of cerebrospinal fluid EBV-DNA and IL-10 as markers for *in vivo* diagnosis of AIDS-related primary central nervous system lymphoma, *Br J Hematol* 90:844, 1995.

27. Arribas JR, Storch GA, Clifford DB, Tselis AC: Cytomegalovirus encephalitis, *Ann Intern Med* 125:577, 1996.

28. Morgello S, Cho ES, Nielsen S, et al: Cytomegalovirus encephalitis in patients with acquired immunodeficiency syndrome: an autopsy study of 30 cases and a review of the literature, *Hum Pathol* 18:289, 1987.

29. Cinque P, Baldanti F, Vago L, et al: Ganciclovir therapy for cytomegalovirus (CMV) infection of the central nervous system in AIDS patients: monitoring by CMV DNA detection in cerebrospinal fluid, *J Infect Dis* 171:1603, 1995.

30. Drobyski WR, Knox KK, Majewski D, Carrigan DR: Brief report: fatal encephalitis due to variant B human herpesvirus-6 infection in a bone marrow-transplant recipient, *N Engl J Med* 330:1356, 1994.

31. Yoshikawa T, Nakashima T, Suga S, et al: Human herpesvirus-6 DNA in cerebrospinal fluid of a child with exanthem subitum and meningoencephalitis, *Pediatrics* 89:888, 1992.

32. Caserta M, Hall C, Schnabel K, et al: Neuroinvasion and persistence of human herpesvirus in children, *J Infect Dis* 170:1586, 1994.

33. Novoa LJ, Nagra RM, Nakawatase T, et al: Fulminant demyelinating encephalomyelitis associated with productive HHV-6 infection in an immunocompetent adult, *J Med Virol* 52(3):301, 1997.

34. Challoner PB, Smith KT, Parker JD, et al: Plaque-associated expression of human herpesvirus 6 in multiple sclerosis, *Proc Natl Acad Sci USA* 92:7440, 1995.

35. McCullers JA, Lakeman FD, Whitley RJ: Human herpesvirus 6 is associated with focal encephalitis, *J Infect Dis* 21:571, 1995.

36. Luppi M, Barozzi P, Maiorana A, et al: Human herpesvirus 6 infection in normal human brain tissue, *J Infect Dis* 169:943, 1994 (letter).

37. Holmes G, Chapman L, Stewart J, et al: Guidelines for the prevention and treatment of B-virus infections in exposed persons, *J Infect Dis* 20:421, 1995.

38. Whitley R: B virus. In Scheld W, Whitley R, Durack D, editors: *Infections of the central nervous system,* ed 2, Philadelphia, 1997, Lippincott-Raven.

39. Scinicariello F, Eberle R, Hilliard J: Rapid detection of B virus (Herpesvirus simiae) DNA by polymerase chain reaction, *J Infect Dis* 168:747, 1993.

40. Slomka M, Brown D, Clewley J, et al: Polymerase chain reaction for detection of herpesvirus simiae (B virus) in clinical specimens, *Arch Virol* 131:89, 1993.

41. Centers for Disease Control: Arboviral disease—United States, 1994, *MMWR* 44:641, 1995.

42. Deresiewicz RL, Thaler SJ, Hsu L, Zamani AA: Clinical and neuroradiographic manifestations of eastern equine encephalitis, *N Engl J Med* 336:1867, 1997.

43. McJunkin JE, Khan RR, Tsai TF: California-La Crosse encephalitis, *Emerg Infect Dis* 12:83, 1998.

44. Calisher CH: Medically important arboviruses of the United States and Canada, *Clin Microbiol Rev* 7:89, 1994.

45. Goodpasture HC, Poland JD, Francy DB, et al: Colorado tick fever: clinical, epidemiologic, and laboratory aspects of 228 cases in Colorado in 1973-1974, *Ann Intern Med* 88:303, 1978.

46. Tsai TF: Arboviruses. In Murray PR, Baron EJ, Pfaller MA, et al, editors: *Manual of clinical microbiology*, ed 7, Washington, DC, 1999, ASM Press.

47. Emmons RW, Oshiro LS, Johnson HN, Lennette EH: Intra-erythrocytic location of Colorado tick fever virus, *J Gen Virol* 17:185, 1972.

48. Johnson AJ, Karabatos N, Lanciotti RS: Detection of Colorado tick fever virus by using reverse transcriptase PCR and application of the technique in laboratory diagnosis, *J Clin Microbiol* 35:1203, 1997.

49. Calisher CH, Poland JD, Calisher SB, Warmoth LA: Diagnosis of Colorado tick fever virus infection by enzyme immunoassays for immunoglobulin M and G antibodies, *J Clin Microbiol* 22:84, 1985.

50. Blenden DC, Creech W, Torres-Anjel MJ: Use of immunofluorescence examination to detect rabies virus antigen in the skin of humans with clinical encephalitis, *J Infect Dis* 154:698, 1986.

51. Smith JS: Rabies virus. In Murray PR, Baron EJ, Pfaller MA, et al, editors: *Manual of clinical microbiology*, ed 7, Washington, DC, 1999, ASM Press.

52. Kamolvarin N, Tirawatnpong T, Rattanasiwamoke R, et al: Diagnosis of rabies by polymerase chain reaction using nested primers, *J Infect Dis* 167:207, 1993.

53. Baum SG, Litman N. Mumps virus. In Mandell GM, Bennett JE, Dolin R, editors: *Principles and practice of infectious diseases,* ed 4, New York, 1995, Churchill Livingstone.

54. Wolinsky JS: Mumps virus. In Fields BN, Knipe DM, Howley PM, editors: *Virology,* ed 3, Philadelphia, 1996, Lippincott-Raven.

55. Nakayama T, Mori T, Yamaguchi S, et al: Detection of measles virus genome directly from clinical samples by reverse transcriptase–polymerase chain reaction and genetic variability, *Virus Res* 35:1, 1995.

56. Matsuzono Y, Narita M, Tshiguro N, Togashi T: Detection of measles virus from clinical samples using the polymerase chain reaction, *Arch Pediatr Adolesc Med* 148:289, 1994.

57. Griffin D: Measles. In Scheld W, Whitley R, Durack D, editors: *Infections of the central nervous system,* ed 2, Philadelphia, 1997, Lippincott-Raven.

58. Mustafa M, Weitman S, Winick N, et al: Subacute measles encephalitis in the young immunocompromised host: report of two cases diagnosed by polymerase chain reaction and treated with ribavirin and review of the literature, *Clin Infect Dis* 16:654, 1993.

59. Koppel B, Poon T, Khandji A, et al: Subacute sclerosing panencephalitis and acquired immunodeficiency syndrome: role of electroencephalography and magnetic resonance imaging, *J Neuroimag* 6:122, 1996.

60. Griffin DE, Bellini WJ: Measles virus. In Fields BN, Knipe DM, Howley PM, editors: *Virology,* ed 3, Philadelphia, 1996, Lippincott-Raven.

61. Conrad A, Chiang E, Andeen L, et al: Quantitation of intrathecal measles virus IgG antibody synthesis rate: subacute sclerosing panencephalitis and multiple sclerosis, *J Neuroimmunol* 54:99, 1994.

62. Wolinsky JS: Rubella. In Fields BN, Knipe DM, Howley PM, editors: *Virology,* ed 3, Philadelphia, 1996, Lippincott-Raven.

63. Squadrini F, Taparelli F, DeRienzo B, et al: Rubella virus isolation from cerebrospinal fluid in postnatal rubella encephalitis, *Br Med J* 2:1329, 1977.

64. Bosma T, Corbett K, O'Shea S, et al: PCR for detection of rubella virus RNA in clinical samples, *J Clin Microbiol* 33:1075, 1995.

65. Date M, Gondoh M, Kato S, et al: A case of rubella encephalitis: rubella virus genome was detected in the cerebrospinal fluid by polymerase chain reaction, *No to Hattatsu* 27:286, 1995.

66. Asher DM. Slow viral infections. In Scheld WM, Whitley RJ, Durack DT, editors: *Infections of the central nervous system,* ed 2, Philadelphia, 1997, Lippincott-Raven.

67. Murphy BR, Webster RG: Orthomyxoviruses, In Fields BN, Knipe DM, Howley PM, editors: *Virology,* ed 3, Philadelphia, 1996, Lippincott-Raven.

68. Cinque P, Scarpellini P, Vago L, et al: Diagnosis of central nervous system complications in HIV-infected patients: cerebrospinal fluid analysis by the polymerase chain reaction, *AIDS* 11:1, 1997.

69. Modlin JF: Enteroviruses: coxsackieviruses, echoviruses and newer enteroviruses. In Long SS, Pickering LK, Prober CG, editors: *Principles and practice of pediatric infectious diseases,* New York, 1997, Churchill-Livingstone.

70. Berlin LE, Rorabaugh ML, Heldrich F, et al: Aseptic meningitis in infants less than 2 years of age: diagnosis and etiology, *J Infect Dis* 168:888, 1993.

71. Gelfand HM, Holguin AH, Marchetti GE, Feorino PM: A continuing surveillance of enterovirus infections in healthy children in six United States cities, *Am J Hyg* 78:358, 1963.

72. Rotbart HA: Enteroviruses. In Murray PR, Baron EJ, Pfaller MA, et al, editors: *Manual of clinical microbiology,* ed 7, Washington, DC, 1999, ASM Press.

73. Rotbart HA: Diagnosis of enteroviral meningitis with the polymerase chain reaction, *J Clin Microbiol* 117:85, 1990.

74. Sawyer MH, Holland D, Aintablian N, et al: Diagnosis of enteroviral central nervous system infection by polymerase chain reaction during a large community outbreak, *Pediatr Infect Dis J* 13:177, 1994.

75. Schlesinger Y, Buller RS, Brunstrom JE, et al: Expanded spectrum of herpes simplex encephalitis in childhood, *J Pediatr* 126:234, 1995.

76. Tedder DG, Ashley R, Tyler R, Levin MJ: Herpes sim-

plex virus infection as a cause of benign recurrent lymphocytic meningitis, *Ann Intern Med* 121:334, 1994.

77. Bergström T, Vahlne A, Alestig K: Primary and recurrent herpes simplex virus type 2–induced meningitis, *J Infect Dis* 162:322, 1990.

77a. Echevarria JM, Casas I, Martinez-Martin P: Infections of the nervous system caused by varicella-zoster virus: a review, *Intervirology* 40:72, 1997.

77b. Reed SJ, Kurtz JB: Laboratory diagnosis of common viral infections of the central nervous system by using a single multiplex PCR screening assay, *J Clin Microbiol* 37:1352, 1999.

78. Jahrling PB: Filoviruses and arenaviruses. In Murray PR, Baron EJ, Pfaller MA, et al, editors: *Manual of clinical microbiology*, ed 7, Washington, DC, 1999, ASM Press.

79. Peters CJ, Johnson KM: Lymphocytic choriomeningitis virus, Lassa virus, and other arenaviruses. In Mandell GM, Bennett JE, Dolin R, editors: *Principles and practice of infectious diseases*, ed 4, New York, 1995, Churchill Livingstone.

80. Peters CJ, Buchmeier M, Rollin PE, Ksiazek TG: Arenaviruses. In Fields BN, Knipe DM, Howley PM, editors: *Virology*, ed 3, Philadelphia, 1996, Lippincott-Raven.

81. Park JY, Peters CJ, Rollin PE, et al: Development of a reverse transcription–polymerase chain reaction assay for diagnosis of lymphocytic choriomeningitis virus infection and its use in a prospective surveillance study, *J Med Virol* 51:107, 1997.

82. Miles C, Hoffman W, Lai CW, Freeman JW: Cytomegalovirus-associated transverse myelitis, *Neurology* 43:2143, 1993.

83. Mussell HG, Percy AK, Benton JW: Guillain-Barré syndrome. In Scheld WM, Whitley RJ, Durack DT, editors: *Infections of the central nervous system*, ed 2, Philadelphia, 1997, Lippincott-Raven.

84. Prusiner SB: Novel proteinaceous infectious particles cause scrapie, *Science* 216:136, 1982.

85. Will RG, Ironside JW, Zeidler M, et al: A new variant of Creutzfeldt-Jakob disease in the UK, *Lancet* 347(9006):921, 1996.

86. Hsich G, Kenney K, Gibbs CJ, et al: The 14-3-3 brain protein in cerebrospinal fluid as a marker for the transmissible spongiform encephalopathies, *N Engl J Med* 335:924, 1996.

87. Asher DM: Spongiform encephalopathies. In Murray PR, Baron EJ, Pfaller MA, et al, editors: *Manual of clinical microbiology*, ed 6, Washington, DC, 1995, ASM Press.

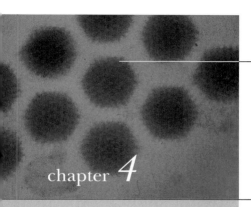

Gregory A. Storch

chapter *4*

Respiratory Infections

OVERVIEW

Viruses are the most common cause of human respiratory tract infection. Most viral infections of the respiratory tract are limited to the upper airways, but lower respiratory tract involvement is also common, especially in young children, elderly persons, and immunocompromised patients. The severity of viral respiratory tract infection ranges from trivial to life threatening. Powerful methods are now available that can reveal the specific virus causing respiratory tract infection, sometimes within a few hours.

Laboratory diagnosis is not needed for viral respiratory infections that are mild and self-limited. Specific viral diagnosis may be helpful in patients with serious infections and should be undertaken when one or more of the following conditions is met:

1. A therapeutic decision (e.g., use of an antiviral agent) will be affected by the diagnostic result.
2. Hospital infection control decisions (e.g., patient room placement) will be affected.
3. Information useful for understanding the patient's illness is obtained, possibly providing valuable prognostic information and decreasing the need for other diagnostic tests.
4. Information is required for public health purposes (e.g., to identify a strain of influenza virus in the community).

This chapter is divided into four sections. The first section describes the major viruses that produce respiratory tract infection and provides clinical and epidemiologic clues that can be helpful in diagnosis. The second section provides a general description of the laboratory methods used to detect respiratory viruses. The third section describes the laboratory detection of individual agents. The final section focuses on clinical syndromes of viral respiratory infection and describes the approach to making a specific virologic diagnosis in these patients.

RESPIRATORY VIRUSES

A limited number of viruses accounts for a large proportion of all viral respiratory tract infections (Box 4–1). Although these viruses produce overlapping clinical syndromes, they are virologically diverse. *Influenza virus, parainfluenza virus,* and *respiratory syncytial virus* (RSV) are members of related families of ribonucleic acid (RNA) viruses, the Orthomyxoviridae and Paramyxoviridae. The *rhinoviruses* and *coronaviruses* are members of the Picornaviridae and Coronaviridae, very different families of ribonucleic acid (RNA) viruses that bear little taxonomic relationship to the other common respiratory viruses. *Herpes simplex virus* (HSV), *cytomega-*lovirus (CMV), *varicella-zoster virus* (VZV), and the *Epstein-Barr virus* (EBV) are members of the family Herpesviridae, deoxyribonucleic acid (DNA) viruses whose life cycle includes a latent phase.

Clinical Syndromes

The common respiratory viruses are often associated with specific clinical syndromes (Table 4–1). For example, rhinovirus and coronavirus cause the *common cold,* adenovirus and EBV tend to cause *pharyngitis,* parainfluenza virus is associated with *croup,* influenza virus with a characteristic syndrome of febrile *tracheobronchitis* with headache and myalgias, and RSV with *bronchiolitis.* Although these associations are important, clinicians should remember that the syndromes overlap and that any of the common respiratory viruses can occasionally produce infection at any level of the respiratory tract. Other important associations are HSV with tracheobronchitis and occasionally pharyngitis, CMV with *pneumonia* in immunocompromised individuals, and VZV and EBV with rare cases of pneumonia.

Epidemiologic Clues to Diagnosis

In addition to clinical findings, epidemiologic patterns may provide important clues regarding the viral etiology of specific episodes of illness (Figure 4–1). RSV, influenza virus, and the parainfluenza viruses have the most characteristic epidemiologic patterns. In temperate zones, RSV outbreaks begin in late fall and last until early to middle spring. During these periods a large proportion of all infants with viral-like respiratory disease are infected with RSV.

Box 4.1 Viruses that Produce Respiratory Disease

Common

Influenza
Parainfluenza
Respiratory syncytial (RSV)
Rhinovirus
Adenovirus
Coronavirus
Enteroviruses

Unusual or restricted to special patient populations

Herpes simplex (HSV)
Cytomegalovirus (CMV)
Varicella-zoster (VZV)
Epstein-Barr (EBV)
Measles

Table 4.1	Respiratory Viruses and Clinical Syndromes
Virus	**Syndrome***
Rhinovirus	Common cold
Coronavirus	Common cold
Adenovirus	Pharyngitis
	Conjunctivitis
Parainfluenza, 1-4	Croup
	Laryngitis
Influenza, A-C	Tracheobronchitis (influenza syndrome)
Respiratory syncytial	Bronchiolitis
Enteroviruses	Herpangina
	Oral ulcers (hand, foot, and mouth disease)
Herpes simplex	Tracheobronchitis
Cytomegalovirus	Pneumonia (immunocompromised hosts)
Varicella-zoster	Pneumonia (unusual)
Epstein-Barr	Pharyngitis (common)
	Pneumonia (rare)
Measles	Croup and bronchiolitis (common in children under 2 years)
	Pneumonia (less than 10% of cases)

*Syndrome characteristically associated with each virus. Individual viral agents can also be associated with syndromes other than those indicated.

Influenza outbreaks also occur in the winter but have a more abrupt onset and decline, usually lasting 6 to 8 weeks. During these outbreaks, influenza-like illness is widespread in the affected community and accounts for a high proportion of all respiratory illness. Influenza outbreaks have dramatic effects on school and workplace attendance. School closings resulting from epidemic respiratory illness almost always signal the presence of influenza virus in the community. Influenza outbreaks may have second waves, sometimes occurring well after the first wave has subsided. The second wave may be associated with a different strain and may be a harbinger of the strain that will be dominant in the next influenza season.

Parainfluenza outbreaks occur in the fall (*types 1 and 2*) or the late spring (*type 3*). Parainfluenza types 1 and 2 outbreaks are associated with cases of croup, whereas type 3 outbreaks may produce a mixture of croup and lower respiratory tract illness such as bronchiolitis.

DIAGNOSTIC METHODS

The major laboratory methods for establishing the etiology of viral respiratory infections are antigen detection and culture. *Antigen detection methods* such as fluorescent antibody (FA) staining and enzyme immunoassay (EIA) are rapid and can identify an etiologic agent within a few hours. An advantage of these methods, especially when conditions of specimen transport are not ideal, is that viable virus within the specimen is not required. Although slower than antigen detection, *viral culture* continues to be useful because (1) it is the most sensitive method for detecting some viruses, (2) antigen detection methods are not available for all the respiratory viruses, and (3) culture provides an isolate that can be further characterized if necessary.

Serology has little role in the diagnosis of acute respiratory infections in clinical practice because the other methods are widely available and provide results more rapidly. Serology can be useful in epidemiologic studies, however, and helpful in establishing a gold standard against which other methods can be compared. The polymerase chain reaction (PCR) has been applied to the detection of a number of respiratory viruses but is still a research tool.

Table 4–2 summarizes the methods in widespread use for detecting each of the major respiratory viruses.

Specimens

Maximum viral shedding occurs during the first few days of acute viral respiratory infection. Therefore specimens to determine the etiology of those illnesses should be obtained as early in the illness as possible. After the first 3 to 5 days, virus levels decrease, but viral shedding may continue for 1 to 2 weeks depending on the virus, age of the patient, and severity of the infection. A variety of specimens can be used for culture and antigen detection procedures (Box 4–2).

Because most viral respiratory infections involve the upper respiratory tract with or without involvement of the lower respiratory tract, specimens from the nose and throat are often useful. Nasal wash and nasal pharyngeal (NP) aspirate specimens contain the highest titers of virus and can provide large numbers of cells for FA staining.[1-5] NP swabs are easier to obtain and, if collected carefully, can also provide suitable specimens for culture and FA staining.[6-8]

Other approaches include the use of a nasal curette (Rhinoprobe scraper, 3M Diagnostic Systems, Santa Clara, Calif) to obtain respiratory epithelial cells from the nose[9] and a cytology brush to obtain posterior nasal swabs.[10] In a direct comparison with NP aspirates, the brush yielded fewer respiratory epithelial cells, although the overall detection of positive FA stains was comparable.[10] Throat swabs have been widely used for recovery of influenza virus and are also useful for adenovirus infections. They are less useful for FA staining, however, because they may yield large numbers of squamous epithelial cells rather than the respiratory epithelial cells needed for antigen detection.[11] The yield of viral cultures may be maximized by

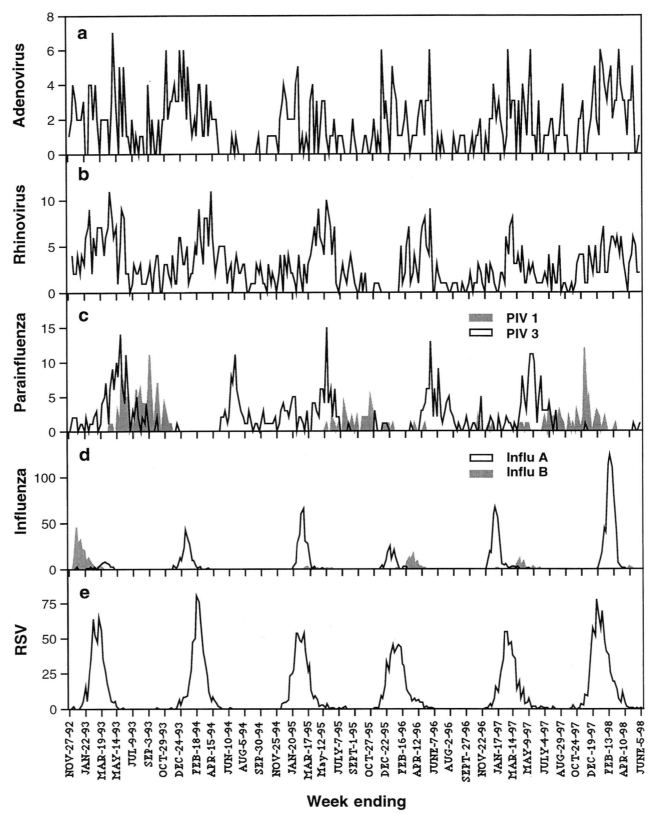

Figure 4.1   Epidemiologic patterns of common respiratory viruses detected by culture and antigen detection procedures at St. Louis Children's Hospital Virology Laboratory, 1992 to 1998. *RSV*, Respiratory syncytial virus; *PIV*, parainfluenza virus.

Table 4.2	Methods Used for Detection of Respiratory Viruses	
Virus	**Culture**	**Antigen detection**
Rhinovirus	Yes	No
Coronavirus	Research only	Yes (not widely available)
Adenovirus	Yes	Yes
Parainfluenza types 1, 2, and 3	Yes	Yes
Parainfluenza type 4	Yes	Yes (not widely used)
Influenza types A and B	Yes	Yes
Influenza C	Yes	No
Respiratory syncytial	Yes	Yes

combining a throat swab with an NP specimen in the same transport tube.[12]

Special considerations apply to the choice of specimen in adult patients, since none of the techniques used for obtaining NP specimens in young children is ideal for adults. The relative yield of various types of NP specimens has not been systematically studied in adults. Nasal washing provides a useful specimen, but this procedure requires patient cooperation, which may be difficult to achieve in some functionally impaired patients. Obtaining an NP aspirate requires an available source of suction, an appropriate trap, and tubing. NP swabs are the simplest NP specimen to obtain, but patients dislike them. In the absence of definitive data, the best advice is to obtain the specimen that is most appropriate for the individual patient and for which appropriate materials are available.

For patients with lower respiratory tract involvement, tracheal aspirates and bronchoscopy specimens, especially bronchoalveolar lavage (BAL) fluid, can be very useful for both culture and antigen detection. BAL fluid is a better specimen than bronchial washings, partly because bronchial washings produce more extraneous fluorescence in FA stains and are more likely to produce cytotoxicity in cell cultures. Sputum has not been widely used for viral studies because its mucoid composition makes it difficult to work with in the laboratory. In one small study, sputum was insensitive for detecting CMV in renal transplant patients with CMV pneumonia.[13] However, another study has reported good results using sputum to detect CMV in patients with acquired immunodeficiency syndrome (AIDS).[14] Recovery of respiratory viruses from sputum has also been reported.[15] In our laboratory, sputum has also been useful for the detection of influenza virus and for HSV in patients with tracheobronchitis (see later discussion).

All specimens for culture or respiratory viruses should be transported to the laboratory on ice unless arrival in less than 1 hour is ensured. Chapter 2 provides additional information on procedures for obtaining and transporting respiratory specimens.

Cultures for Respiratory Viruses

Because of the variety of viruses potentially involved and differences in methods required for growth and detection, the respiratory viral culture is the most complex of any routine viral culture. Methods used to culture the respiratory viruses include conventional cell culture, shell vial culture, and egg inoculation. The latter method has been used extensively for influenza virus isolation but is not currently used in most diagnostic laboratories for reasons of convenience and because cell cultures provide comparable or nearly comparable sensitivity for influenza A and better sensitivity for influenza B virus.[12]

Conventional cell culture. The conventional cell culture can detect all the common respiratory viruses, except coronavirus, but must incorporate several cell culture types and procedures to optimize recovery of each virus. Primary monkey kidney cells are usually used because of their sensitivity for influenza and parainfluenza viruses. *Continuous cells* that can be used as alternatives are Madin-Darby canine kidney (MDCK) cells for influenza A and B viruses and LLC-MK2 cells (a continuous cell line derived from rhesus monkey kidney cells) for parainfluenza viruses.[16] HEp-2 cells, a continuous line of human epithelial-like cells originally derived from a laryngeal tumor, greatly enhance the recovery of RSV. Human fibroblast cells such as MRC-5 or WI-35 are required for growth of rhinoviruses. Human embryonic kidney cells can maximize the yield of adenoviruses. Incubation at 33° to 34°C may facilitate the growth of influenza and rhinoviruses, and therefore some laboratories set up cultures for incubation at this temperature as well as at 35° to 37°C. Serum-free media is required for the optimal growth of the influenza and parainfluenza viruses. Growth of most of the respiratory viruses in cell culture is revealed by detection of cytopathic effect (CPE), but hemadsorption or hemagglutination assays performed on the inoculated cultures

Box 4.2	Specimens Used for Diagnosis of Viral Respiratory Tract Infection

Nasopharyngeal aspirate
Nasopharyngeal swab
Nasal wash
Throat swab
Tracheal aspirate
Bronchoalveolar lavage fluid

are required for maximum detection of influenza and parainfluenza viruses.

Because of the varied procedures required for the detection of different respiratory viruses, laboratories may adjust their culture "setup" and battery of reagents used for rapid antigen detection based on which viruses are currently circulating in the community. Therefore communication with the laboratory is important, particularly when seeking to detect a particular virus at times other than its normal seasonal occurrence. The time required to detect the common respiratory viruses in conventional cell culture varies from 1 to 14 days.

Shell vial culture. The shell vial culture method combines elements of cell culture and antigen detection to achieve rapid culture-based detection. This method, which has been widely used for detection of CMV, has also been employed to detect respiratory viruses in some virology laboratories. Chapter 2 describes the shell vial method.

Practical considerations in applying the shell vial method to the detection of respiratory viruses are (1) at least two different cell culture types must be used to achieve detection of the important respiratory viruses, and (2) detection reagents must have the capability to detect each of the viruses being sought. A combination of rhesus monkey kidney cells or MDCK cells paired with human fibroblast or A549 cells provides the potential to detect RSV, influenza and parainfluenza viruses, and adenoviruses. Pools of monoclonal antibodies have been used for FA staining of cultures. Rhinoviruses and coronaviruses are not detected by the shell vial method because of lack of appropriate antibodies for FA staining.

The sensitivity of the shell vial culture compared with conventional culture for detection of respiratory viruses varies widely in published studies (see following sections on individual viruses). Generalizations regarding comparative sensitivity of these techniques are difficult because of methodologic differences in performing both types of culture.

Antigen Detection

Antigen detection using FA staining or EIA performed on the specimen itself without culture amplification is widely used for the laboratory diagnosis of RSV, influenza, parainfluenza, and adenovirus infections. The major advantages are rapidity and lack of requirement for viable virus in the specimen, which allows greater latitude in conditions of transport than is possible for viral culture.

Fluorescent antibody staining. Reagents are commercially available for FA staining for the common respiratory viruses other than rhinovirus and coronavirus. Commercial EIAs are available for RSV and influenza A.

FA staining is directed primarily at the detection of viral antigens expressed in respiratory epithelial cells. Accordingly, specimens must provide adequate cells for examination. The best specimens are obtained by NP aspirate, nasal wash, or NP swab. Tracheal aspirates and BAL fluid can also be used. On arrival in the laboratory, respiratory epithelial cells in the specimen are washed by centrifugation, pelleted, and then spotted onto one or more microscope slides. Mucolytic agents are sometimes used when thick mucus is present that cannot be removed by centrifugation and washing. Some laboratories use the NP swab to smear cells directly onto clean glass microscope slides, either at the patient's bedside or in the laboratory.

After drying and fixation, slides are stained using antibodies specific for the viruses being sought. Monoclonal antibodies for the common respiratory viruses are commercially available and used in most laboratories. The final step is examination of the slides using a fluorescent microscope with ultraviolet epiillumination. Characteristic patterns of nuclear and cytoplasmic staining are seen, depending on the virus and the antibody in use. An advantage of FA staining compared with EIA is that microscopic examination allows the quality of the specimen to be evaluated. Although the minimum number of cells that must be evaluated is not standardized, most laboratories require at least 50 to 100 respiratory epithelial cells. When the number of cells available for examination is lower than that number and no viral antigen is detected, the specimen can be reported as "inadequate" rather than negative. The presence of characteristic staining of even one cell is usually considered *positive*. Recently, innovative assays have been described in which more than one viral antigen can be detected simultaneously by using monoclonal antibodies with different fluorescent labels.[17]

For pediatric patients, FA staining tends to be more sensitive than viral culture for RSV and less sensitive for the other respiratory viruses.[18] Statements about the sensitivity of FA staining or other antigen detection techniques in actual practice may be misleading, however, because they are affected by numerous variables. These include the virus under investigation, type and quality of the specimen, timing in relation to onset of illness, age of the patient, quality of the reagents used, experience and care of the laboratory, and technical factors that affect test performance. Experience with antigen detection techniques performed on specimens from adult patients is much more limited. High sensitivity for detecting influenza virus antigens in adult specimens has been reported,[8, 19-21] but the sensitivity of tests for detecting RSV antigen in specimens from adults has been very low.[22-24a]

Enzyme immunoassay. EIA techniques have also been widely applied for the detection of respiratory viral antigens. These assays detect cell-free antigen as well as antigen in infected cells. A major practical advantage of commercially available EIAs for RSV and influenza A virus is that they can be performed by personnel with less specialized training than required for fluorescent microscopy. EIAs can also be adapted to automated instruments, and at least one instrument-based assay for RSV is currently available. In the most widely used configuration for antigen detection, a "capture antibody" is attached to the sides of plastic tubes or wells in plastic microtiter trays and is used to capture antigen present in the specimen. Captured antigen is then detected using an enzyme-labeled second antibody. Commercial membrane immunoassays that employ binding or capture on a membrane are also available (see sections on RSV and influenza). The major disadvantage of all EIAs relative to FA staining is the lack of a simple method for evaluating the quality of the specimen.

Use of antigen detection and culture. Laboratories currently vary widely in how they employ antigen detection procedures and culture. Some laboratories have used antigen detection to supplant viral culture, whereas others perform both procedures. An important consideration is that culture tends to be more sensitive than antigen detection methods for all viruses other than RSV.[18] Even with RSV, the virus may grow from some specimens that are negative by antigen detection methods.[25] Thus maximum yield is achieved by using both antigen detection and culture. In our laboratory the total number of specimens positive for RSV is increased by approximately 5% if culture is performed in addition to an antigen detection method. Another consideration is that more than one virus is present in 5% to 10% of respiratory specimens.[26]

The approach used in our laboratory is to first perform antigen detection assay for the viruses prevalent in the community. If the antigen detection procedure is positive for RSV or influenza, culture is not performed because these viruses tend to have dominant clinical manifestations, and detection of a second virus would rarely have implications for treatment. If RSV or influenza is not detected by the antigen detection procedure, the specimen is cultured.

Polymerase Chain Reaction

The application of PCR to the diagnosis of viral respiratory tract infections is complicated by the following:

1. Most of the viral respiratory tract pathogens are RNA viruses; therefore a reverse-transcription reaction to synthesize a DNA copy of the viral RNA must be performed before PCR can occur.
2. Respiratory tract specimens pose greater potential problems of PCR inhibition than more homogeneous specimens such as cerebrospinal fluid.
3. Antigen detection has been quite successful for

detection of some respiratory tract infections, especially RSV, and is simpler and less expensive to perform than PCR.
4. The possibility that the sensitivity of PCR may produce a positive test for an extended time after acute infection has not yet been investigated.

For these reasons, PCR for detection of respiratory tract pathogens remains largely a research tool. An intriguing prospect is the possibility of using PCR to detect multiple respiratory agents, either through a panel of PCR reactions[27] or by a multiplex PCR that can detect multiple agents with a single reaction.[28] PCR may also prove to be particularly advantageous for specimens from adult patients when the quantity of virus may be low and antigen detection tests may be insensitive.

DETECTION OF SPECIFIC RESPIRATORY VIRUSES

Rhinovirus

Rhinoviruses are the most important cause of the common cold. Although most rhinovirus infections are mild and self-limited, they can cause substantial morbidity in vulnerable patients such as neonates or adults with chronic lung disease. An important role for rhinoviruses as a cause of asthma exacerbations is under investigation.[28a]

The rhinoviruses are positive-sense, single-stranded RNA viruses that are members of the family Picornaviridae. They are closely related to the enteroviruses, which are in the same family. The salient characteristic of the rhinoviruses that has affected the diagnostic approach is *antigenic diversity.* Approximately 102 serotypes are known, and a single common antigen that would be a useful target for diagnostic reagents has not been identified. Therefore antigen detection methods are not available, and culture is the only method currently in widespread use.

Rhinoviruses grow readily in cell culture. Optimal growth occurs in human diploid fibroblast cell lines (e.g., MRC-5, WI-38). Rhinoviruses can also be grown in human embryonic kidney cells. Cell lines can vary greatly in their sensitivity to rhinoviral growth, and a laboratory interested in detecting rhinoviruses should monitor the performance of it's lines. A temperature of 33° to 34°C is required for optimal growth, and cultures should be kept in motion by incubation in a roller drum. Rhinoviruses are generally detected in cell culture by the production of a characteristic CPE, which usually becomes apparent 3 to 10 days after inoculation. The CPE of rhinoviruses can resemble that produced by enteroviruses. When necessary, the two viruses can be distinguished by performing FA staining of the culture using enterovirus-specific monoclonal antibodies or by performing the acid lability test. Rhinoviruses are inactivated by exposure to acid, whereas the enteroviruses are acid stable.

Coronavirus

Studies suggest that the human coronaviruses are second only to the rhinoviruses as causes of the common cold, accounting for up to 35% of mild upper respiratory infections in adults.[29] They may also cause some lower respiratory tract disease and may be a precipitating cause of asthma in some patients. The coronaviruses are positive-sense, single-stranded RNA viruses that are members of the family Coronaviridae. Two different coronavirus groups represented by the prototype strains 229E and OC43 have been found to produce human infection. Other members of the family are important animal pathogens.

The human coronaviruses are the most difficult of the human respiratory viral pathogens to detect in the laboratory. They do not grow well in cell culture and are not detected in most routine diagnostic virology laboratories. In research studies they have been grown in organ cultures of human embryonic trachea. FA staining has been applied but was insensitive,[30] and reagents are not widely available. Serologic methods have also been used but are currently available only in research laboratories. Experience with PCR is still very limited,[31] but this technique has the potential for greatly improving coronavirus diagnosis.

Adenovirus

The human adenoviruses are nonenveloped, double-stranded DNA viruses that are members of the family Adenoviridae. A total of 49 serotypes are currently recognized as causes of human disease. Serotypes 1 to 7 are most often associated with respiratory tract infection.[32-34] The adenovirus virion consists of an icosahedral capsid composed of structural units (*capsomers*) referred to as *hexons* and *pentons*. The hexons contain a common antigenic determinant that is useful as a target for diagnostic reagents. Adenovirus infections are most common in young children and are estimated to cause approximately 5% of respiratory infections in children less than 5 years of age.[32, 33]

The respiratory syndromes linked to adenoviruses include the common cold, pharyngitis and tonsillitis, pharyngoconjunctival fever, and pneumonia. Severe cases of adenoviral pneumonia have occurred in infants, military recruits, and immunocompromised patients. Most adenoviral respiratory infections occur as endemic infections, but outbreaks of disease also occur.

Adenoviral respiratory infection can be diagnosed by culture, antigen detection, or serology. Adenoviruses are stable and grow well in culture, but culture detects only about 50% of respiratory adenoviral infections compared with serology.[32] During acute respiratory infection, adenoviruses can be isolated from respiratory secretions and from stool. The optimal cell culture type for culturing adenoviruses is human embryonic kidney.[33, 35] Other sensitive cell culture types are A549, KB, HeLa, and HEp-2.[36] Viral cultures may be positive as early as 1 day after inoculation, but 10 to 14 days may be required to recover some isolates. The shell vial technique has been used to decrease the time required for detection. The sensitivity of shell vial cultures for adenoviruses compared with conventional culture has varied in published reports from 48% to 100%.[37-39]

The interpretation of a positive culture for adenovirus is complicated because adenoviruses can cause persistent or latent infection,[36, 40, 41] and can be associated with prolonged viral shedding, especially in the stool.[41] In one large study, adenoviruses were recovered from 2.7% of pharyngeal and 6.4% of anal swabs taken from children without respiratory illness.[33] In a more recent study, adenoviruses were recovered from nasal wash specimens of only 0.6% of asymptomatic children attending day care.[34] Because of the more limited duration of respiratory shedding, recovery of an adenovirus from a respiratory specimen is considered presumptive evidence for adenoviral respiratory tract disease. A positive stool culture is much weaker evidence, and thus stool cultures are not recommended for the diagnosis of acute adenoviral respiratory infection.

Rapid diagnosis of adenoviral respiratory infections can be accomplished by FA staining. Cross-reacting monoclonal antibodies that recognize all adenovirus serotypes are commercially available and widely used. FA staining for adenovirus is less sensitive than culture, with reported sensitivities varying between 28% and 68%.[7, 18, 42] These studies were done using polyclonal antisera; sensitivity may be higher with monoclonal antibody reagents, but published data are not available. PCR has been applied to the diagnosis of adenoviral respiratory infections[43] but is not yet in routine clinical use. Serology is impractical for patient management because of the need for convalescent phase specimen.

Influenza

The influenza viruses are negative-sense, single-stranded viruses classified in the family Orthomyxoviridae. Influenza strains are divided into types A, B, and C based on differences in the core proteins.

Influenza A strains are subdivided according to their hemagglutinin and neuraminidase proteins. Three hemagglutinin subtypes and two neuraminidase subtypes account for virtually all human infections.[44] The influenza A strains circulating in recent years have been of subtypes H3N2 and H1N1, although recently, H5N1 strains were recovered from an outbreak in Hong Kong.[45] Influenza strains are also named according to the city in which they were first isolated, the laboratory number of the isolate, and the year of isolation. For example, recent strains of influenza A were A/Texas/36/91 (H1N1) and A/Wuhan/359/95 (H3N2). Influenza A strains can be associated with worldwide pandemics. *Influenza B* also produces epidemic disease, but the clinical illness tends to be milder and the overall impact on the community is less than that associated with influenza A. *Influenza C* is much less common and has not been associated with large epidemics. It accounts for less than 1% of cases of influenza in children[46] and has rarely been associated with illness in adults.

Specific measures are available to prevent and treat infections caused by influenza A virus. The drugs *amantadine* and *rimantadine* inhibit viral entry into cells and are licensed in the United States for prevention and treatment of influenza A infections. These drugs have no activity against influenza B or C or other respiratory viruses. Ribavirin has activity against influenza A and B but is not currently licensed to treat these infections. *Neuraminidase inhibitors* are a new class of drugs that are under active development for use in treating influenza A or B.[47]

Influenza vaccine is effective at preventing influenza virus infections. The currently licensed vaccine is an inactivated vaccine that must be given annually and is effective only against the serotypes included in the vaccine. Live influenza virus vaccines are under active development.[48]

Influenza viruses can be detected either by culture or by antigen detection techniques. Influenza A and B strains grow well in cell culture. The most sensitive cell culture types are primary monkey kidney cells and MDCK cells. Special conditions required for optimal recovery of influenza viruses include use of cell culture media with no serum and incubation at 33° to 34°C. When MDCK cells are used, the cell culture medium must include trypsin to cleave the influenza hemagglutinin. Influenza viruses also grow well in embryonated hen's eggs. Inoculation of the allantoic and amniotic cavities of 11-day-old eggs has been widely performed in the past to detect influenza viruses. However, this procedure is no longer used in most diagnostic laboratories because cell culture isolation provides comparable or greater sensitivity for influenza A and B and is more convenient. Influenza C virus grows in some cell culture types, including primary monkey kidney, primary chicken embryo, LLC-MK2, and MDCK cells. Recently, a human malignant melanoma cell line designated (HMV-II) has been reported to be sensitive for influenza C virus,[49] but optimal recovery requires egg inoculation.[12]

The growth of influenza viruses in cell culture is detected in several ways. Many, but not all, strains produce CPE that is visible by routine microscopy. Influenza viruses are more uniformly detected by hemadsorption or hemagglutination assays on the inoculated culture. The *hemadsorption technique* involves adding a suspension of erythrocytes, usually derived from a guinea pig, to the inoculated cell culture and observing for adsorption of the erythrocytes to the cultured cells (see Figure 1–3). The *hemagglutination reaction* involves testing cell culture media for the ability to agglutinate guinea pig erythrocytes. Other viruses that produce hemadsorption and hemagglutination of guinea pig erythrocytes are parainfluenza viruses and mumps virus. Therefore, after a positive hemadsorption or hemagglutination reaction is detected, additional procedures such as FA staining of the cell culture must be performed to identify the responsible virus.

Because CPE may not be an early finding (or may not occur at all, even when influenza virus is growing in the culture) and is not always visible to allow detection of viral growth, the speed of detection of influenza viruses in culture depends on the frequency of hemadsorption or hemagglutination testing. In one study in which hemadsorption was performed daily, nearly 100% of isolates were detected by the third day of incubation.[50] Many laboratories perform hemadsorption or hemagglutination two or three times during the life of a culture. Influenza C virus produces hemadsorption with rat or chicken but not guinea pig erythrocytes.[12, 49] Thus growth of influenza C virus in culture may not be detected by many laboratories that use guinea pig erythrocytes for the hemadsorption assay.

The shell vial assay has been applied to the detection of influenza virus. Influenza shell vial cultures require the use of either rhesus or other primary monkey kidney cells or MDCK cells. The sensitivity reported for this procedure compared with conventional tube culture varies widely. In nine studies comparing shell vial and conventional cultures for influenza virus detection,[37, 51-58] the average percentage of all isolates detected by shell vial culture was 81.4%, compared with 87.9% for conventional culture.

Influenza virus antigen detection tests are now widely available. FA staining, which is employed by many laboratories, generally requires separate reagents for detection of influenza A and B. Reagents for detection of influenza C are not available. Published reports on the sensitivity of FA staining for influenza virus compared with culture vary greatly. Some laboratories have reported sensitivity close to or equal to 100% compared with culture,[8, 21, 59-61] but sensitivity with FA staining is lower in other reports. In most laboratories a negative FA stain does not rule out influenza and should be supported by a culture to achieve maximum detection.

EIA is also widely used for detection of influenza viruses. A new test called FLU OIA (Biostar, Boulder, Co.) that uses the optical immunoassay method also employed for group A streptococcal antigen detection has recently been licensed by the Food and Drug Administration.

The commercial test currently most widely used is the Directigen Flu A Test (Becton Dickinson, Cockeysville, Md), a membrane immunoassay that detects influenza A virus only. To perform the test, the specimen is washed over a membrane contained in a test device, and influenza antigen present in the specimen is trapped on the membrane. Trapped antigen is detected by an enzyme-conjugated monoclonal antibody specific for the influenza A virus nucleoprotein. The test is simple to perform and requires only 15 minutes. It can be used on NP aspirates, washes, and swabs and on throat swabs, although the manufacturer states that NP aspirates and washes are the specimens of choice. The sensitivity compared with culture has varied from 60% to 100%.[8, 60, 62, 63] One study found that some weak positive reactions were false positives. Freezing and thawing of specimens before testing has been found to decrease the sensitivity.[60] Despite its limitations, the Flu A Test may be useful in some settings by allowing rapid diagnosis of influenza A without the need for laboratory personnel with specialized virology training.

Recently a new rapid assay based on detection of neuraminidase activity was licensed for detection of influenza A and B infections (ZstatFlu, Zymetx, Oklahoma City). This assay is not an EIA; rather, it employs a neuraminidase substrate conjugated to a chromogen, which is cleaved and undergoes a color change when acted on by influenza neuraminidase. The test does not detect influenza C. Parainfluenza virus neuraminidases are not detected because the substrate is specific for the neuraminidase of influenza A and B viruses. The test uses a throat swab and requires approximately 1 hour. The manufacturer reports a sensitivity of 60% to 65% compared with viral culture.

Both FA staining and EIA can be useful in adult as well as pediatric patients. Leonardi et al.[8] performed multiple tests for influenza A antigens on combined NP and throat swabs from residents of geriatric care centers and found a sensitivity of 92.5% for FA staining compared with culture and 86.8% to 92.5% for two commercial EIAs. Staynor et al.[19] reported a high sensitivity for FA staining performed on nasal swabs obtained from nursing home residents. Both studies reported that rapid diagnosis of influenza infections was useful in controlling the spread of influenza in institutions for elderly patients. Gardner and McQuillin[20] reported lower sensitivity for influenza FA staining in adults compared with children.

RT-PCR has been used to detect influenza virus RNA in respiratory specimens, with sensitivity comparable to or greater than culture.[64, 65] Because of its greater complexity compared with antigen detection, influenza RT-PCR is not currently used in standard diagnostic virology laboratories.

Parainfluenza

The parainfluenza viruses are negative-sense, single-stranded RNA viruses that are classified in the family Paramyxoviridae. Four antigenic types have been recognized and are designated 1 to 4. Infection with parainfluenza viruses is extremely common and usually results in upper respiratory infection. Young children, especially those experiencing primary infection, may also develop lower respiratory tract disease. Parainfluenza viruses are the main causes of *croup*, which occurs in young children, especially those between the ages of 6 months and 3 years.

Some clinical and epidemiologic differences among the four types have been recognized. Parainfluenza *types 1 and 2* tend to occur in the fall and may occur in an every other year pattern. In recent years in St. Louis, outbreaks of parainfluenza *type 3* have occurred in the late spring and early summer. Infants with parainfluenza type 3 often develop lower respiratory tract infection that presents as bronchiolitis or pneumonia. Less is known about parainfluenza *type 4* because it can be difficult to culture, but it appears to cause both upper and lower respiratory tract infection.[66, 67]

Parainfluenza virus infections can be diagnosed by culture or antigen detection. These viruses grow best in primary monkey kidney cells. They also can grow well in the LLC-MK2 continuous line of monkey kidney cells. Parainfluenza viruses are detected in cell culture either by production of CPE or by hemadsorption or hemagglutination reactions performed on the cell culture. The nature of the CPE differs for the different parainfluenza types. Types 1 and 3 may produce only minimal or nonspecific CPE and are often detected by hemadsorption before CPE is evident. Type 2 produces a syncytial CPE that is more easily detectable. Type 4 is the most difficult to recover in culture, often requiring 10 days or more to produce CPE or hemadsorption, which may be weak.[68]

Growth of parainfluenza viruses in cell culture is generally slower than for the influenza viruses, although more than 50% of type 1 and type 3 isolates can be detected by hemadsorption within 48 hours of inoculation.[50] The specific identification of the parainfluenza type present in a cell culture is usually based on FA staining of the infected culture using specific monoclonal antibodies. The shell vial technique has been used to detect parainfluenza viruses and can provide faster detection than conventional culture. Published experience is inadequate to evaluate the sensitivity compared with conventional culture.

FA staining is now widely available for detection of parainfluenza antigens in specimens. The specimen of choice is an NP aspirate, wash, or swab. Specific monoclonal antibody reagents allow detection of any of the parainfluenza types. Most studies report lower sensitivity with FA staining than with culture.[7, 18, 69-71] For optimal detection a viral culture should be performed if the FA stain is negative. EIAs have also been used for the rapid detection of parainfluenza antigens in clinical specimens, but none is commercially available. RT-PCR has been used in research studies[72] but is not yet in routine use.

Respiratory Syncytial Virus

RSV is considered to be the most important viral respiratory pathogen of infants. As with the parainfluenza viruses, RSV is a negative-sense, single-stranded RNA virus that is classified in the family Paramyxoviridae. Two groups designated A and B are recognized. Infection with RSV group A is more common and may be more severe.[73] Cross-reacting reagents that detect both subtypes are available for diagnostic use.

Virtually all children are infected with RSV by age 2 years, and approximately 90,000 hospitalizations occur yearly in the United States.[74] RSV is highly seasonal, causing yearly outbreaks that typically begin in the late fall or early winter and last for 4 to 5 months. During RSV outbreaks, most children with acute respiratory infection have RSV infection. The characteristic clinical syndrome associated with the virus is *bronchiolitis*. Other patients have pneumonia, croup, a cold-like illness, or a nonspecific viral respiratory tract syndrome.

The only specific therapeutic agent currently available is *ribavirin*, which is licensed by the Food and Drug Administration (FDA) for the treatment of serious RSV infections. The drug is administered by small-particle aerosol and is expensive. Questions about its efficacy and difficulties involved in its administration have led to decreased use. RSV immunoglobulin preparations are licensed for prevention of RSV disease in children less than 24 months of age with bronchopulmonary dysplasia or for infants up to 6 months of age with a history of premature birth at less than 35 weeks of gestation. These preparations are also expensive but may be effective in reducing hospitalizations.[75, 75a]

The laboratory diagnosis of RSV infection is based on detection of the virus by culture or antigen detection. The best specimen is an NP aspirate or wash, but NP swabs are also used successfully by some laboratories. The infectivity of RSV is labile, and the ability to recover the virus in culture is compromised by suboptimal conditions of specimen transport.[4, 24] Thus, for culturing RSV, rapid transport to the laboratory is important. Specimens should be kept on ice if transport requires more than 1 hour. The cell culture type of choice is HEp-2 cells, a continuous line of human epithelial-like cells derived from a laryngeal carcinoma. RSV also grows in a variety of other cell culture types,

including HeLa cells, primary monkey kidney cells, human embryonic fibroblasts, and A549 cells. One report indicated that use of primary monkey kidney and human fibroblast cells in addition to HEp-2 cells increased the overall recovery of virus and decreased the time required for detection.[76]

RSV produces CPE in infected cells and is usually detected after 2 to 8 days of incubation. The CPE in infected cells is distinct and usually sufficient for confident identification of the virus in the laboratory. When necessary, however, the presence of RSV in culture can be confirmed by FA staining of cells from the culture using an RSV-specific monoclonal antibody. The shell vial technique has been used to decrease the time required for detection of RSV in culture. It has comparable sensitivity to conventional culture[53, 57, 77-80] but is less sensitive than FA staining performed directly on the specimen.[77, 78, 81]

RSV represents the best example in diagnostic virology of the utility of antigen detection techniques. Both FA staining and EIA are widely used. Results of FA staining can be available 1 to 2 hours after the specimen reaches the laboratory. The sensitivity of the FA stain is greater than culture in many laboratories,[18, 82] partly because antigen detection does not require the virus to be viable. The difference in sensitivity between FA staining and culture becomes greater later in the illness, when the titer of viable virus decreases but viral antigens are still detectable.[21] Occasionally, FA staining performed on tracheal aspirates and BAL specimens is positive when NP specimens from the same patient are negative.[83] The specificity of the FA stain is high when high-quality monoclonal antibody reagents are used. Further generalization about the specificity of the procedure is difficult because this parameter is determined not only by the quality of reagents, but also by the skill of the personnel performing the test.

EIA represents an alternative to FA staining for detection of RSV antigens. Two EIAs, Abbott TESTPACK (Abbott Laboratories, North Chicago) and Directigen RSV (Becton Dickinson) are notable because of their convenience and ease of performance. These tests require only 15 to 20 minutes to perform. Two studies have shown that they could be performed accurately by house officers without extensive laboratory training.[84, 85]

TESTPACK RSV uses microparticles coated with anti-RSV antibodies that are mixed with the specimen, followed by the addition of biotin-labeled RSV antibodies. If RSV antigen is present, complexes composed of the antibody-coated microparticles, RSV antigen in the specimen, and biotin-labeled antibodies are formed. These complexes are captured on a reaction disk within a test device and subsequently detected using an antibiotin–alkaline phosphatase conjugate. The TESTPACK RSV should be performed only on NP aspirate, wash, or swab specimens. Swabs should be cotton, rayon, or Dacron tipped.

As in the Directigen Flu A Test, the Directigen RSV test captures RSV antigen directly on a membrane enclosed in a test device. The captured antigen is detected using monoclonal antibodies to the RSV nucleocapsid and fusion proteins. The Directigen RSV test can be performed on NP aspirate, wash, or swab or tracheal aspirate specimens. NP aspirates and washes are the preferred specimens. If an NP swab is used, the tip should not be calcium alginate. Excessively bloody specimens should not be tested because results may be uninterpretable or falsely positive. Excessively mucoid specimens may require dilution or sonication in the laboratory before testing.

TESTPACK has been more extensively evaluated than Directigen. The sensitivity of TESTPACK compared with culture has varied from 83%[59] to greater than 100%.[85-90] The sensitivity compared with FA staining has varied from 77% to 100%.[59, 84, 85, 87, 90-93] False-positive tests have not been a problem. Evaluations of Directigen yielded poorer results in that more culture-positive specimens were negative by Directigen, and some weakly positive Directigen tests were false positives.[94, 95] Although the manufacturer cautions against testing frozen specimens, one report suggested that freezing and thawing of the specimen before testing might increase the sensitivity of the Directigen test.[94]

The performance of RSV antigen tests on specimens from adult patients has been disappointing. This may be related to decreased titers of virus in adults with RSV compared with infants. Limited information on comparative titers is available. In one study, however, the geometric mean viral titer in nasal wash–throat swab specimens from immunocompromised adult patients was 35 plaque-forming units per milliliter (PFUs/ml), compared with 1.45 million PFUs/ml in nasal wash specimens from pediatric patients. Compared with culture, a commercial RSV EIA performed on the nasal wash–throat swab specimens obtained from adult patients had a sensitivity of only 15%.[22] Data on titers in nonimmunocompromised adults are not available, but it is unlikely that viral titers or the sensitivity of antigen detection would be higher in such patients.

Falsey et al.[24] compared bedside-inoculated and routine cultures of throat swabs with FA staining and a commercial EIA of nasal specimens from a cytology brush. Acute and convalescent serology for RSV was also performed. Of 11 adult patients with RSV infection demonstrated by serology, bedside-inoculated culture was positive in six, routine culture in four, FA staining in one, and EIA in none. These results further support that antigen detection techniques for RSV are not useful in adult patients. This experience is limited, however, and the subject requires further investigation.

RT-PCR has been used to detect RSV in specimens, and sensitivity comparable to or greater than culture has been reported.[96-98] In addition to detecting viral RNA, one RT-PCR assay was also able to type the virus as group A or B directly in the specimen.[98] These assays are not currently employed in routine diagnostic virology laboratories.

Herpes Simplex Virus

In addition to causing lesions of the lips and mouth, HSV is also associated with pharyngitis, tracheobronchitis, and pneumonia. HSV can produce an *exudative pharyngitis*, recognized most often in young adults, that cannot be distinguished from other causes of exudative pharyngitis.[99, 100] The presence of herpetic lesions of the anterior mouth, lips, or gingiva can provide a diagnostic clue, but these lesions are not present in all cases. In some patients, careful inspection may reveal shallow, ulcerated lesions on the tonsils and posterior pharynx.[99] The diagnosis can be confirmed by culture, but growth of HSV from the oropharynx must be interpreted cautiously, since asymptomatic excretion of HSV is present in up to 20% of children 7 months to 2 years of age and up to 5% of those over 15 years.[99, 101]

HSV also causes two lower respiratory tract syndromes: tracheitis/bronchopneumonia and interstitial pneumonia (Table 4–3). *HSV tracheobronchitis* was originally described as occurring primarily in burn patients and immunocompromised patients.[102] More recently, it has also been recognized in immunocompetent patients, including those with endotracheal intubation because of recent surgery[103] or respiratory failure[104] and elderly individuals without preexisting respiratory disease.[105] The most prominent clinical finding is bronchospasm.[104-106] When bronchoscopy is performed, the airways typically appear erythematous. Discrete vesicles or ulcerations involving the airways are unusual. Instead, the airways are often covered by a thick, fibrinopurulent membrane that can cause obstruction.[104, 105] The virus associated with these infections is virtually always HSV-1, and most cases represent reactivation of previous infection. Treatment with acyclovir can lead to rapid improvement.[105, 106]

HSV interstitial pneumonia is a different syndrome that is unusual and occurs mainly in profoundly immunosuppressed individuals such as bone marrow transplant recipients[107] and in newborns with disseminated infection.[108]

The diagnosis of HSV disease of the lower respiratory tract is complicated by asymptomatic shedding of HSV from the oropharynx occurring in 1% to 5% of adults.[101] In addition, HSV shedding may increase with other stresses. For example, one study found that 74% of patients with adult respiratory distress syndrome (ARDS) had positive cultures of oropharyngeal and

Table 4.3	Risk Factors for Herpes Simplex Bronchitis or Pneumonia	
Syndrome	**Risk factors**
Tracheobronchitis	Immunosuppression
	Thermal injury
	Endotracheal intubation
	Surgery
	Elderly age group
Interstitial pneumonitis	Profound immunosuppression
	Neonatal age group

tracheobronchial secretions.[109] This situation creates a diagnostic quandary because the finding of HSV in a respiratory specimen may be the result of asymptomatic shedding but may also be a sign of clinically significant HSV tracheobronchitis. Cytology can be helpful in recognizing clinically significant infection because the presence of respiratory epithelial cells with intranuclear inclusions and multinucleated giant cells is evidence of invasive disease, especially if the specimen comes from the lower respiratory tract. A biopsy of the bronchial epithelium provides the most specific diagnosis.

The diagnostic utility of bronchoscopy has been emphasized[104, 105] because it allows visualization of the bronchial mucosa and provides the opportunity to obtain specimens for cytology, histopathology, and culture. Viral serology is of no value, since most patients are seropositive at the onset because of previous infection. HSV interstitial pneumonitis can be definitively diagnosed only by lung biopsy showing consistent pathologic changes plus a positive culture of the biopsy specimen or demonstration of HSV antigens by immunohistochemistry.

Cytomegalovirus

CMV is a well-known cause of pneumonia in immunocompromised individuals, especially bone marrow transplant recipients. It is also common in lung transplant recipients but is less common in recipients of other solid organs. CMV is frequently present in the lungs of patients with AIDS but infrequently causes clinically significant pneumonia.

Histology and culture of lung tissue represent the gold standard for the diagnosis of CMV pneumonia. Transbronchial lung biopsy is useful but can be falsely negative because of sampling error. Detection of CMV in other respiratory specimens (e.g., BAL fluid) is consistent with CMV pneumonia but nonspecific because CMV can be present in the respiratory tract when pneumonia is not present.[110, 111]

CLINICAL SYNDROMES

The Common Cold

The main causes of the common cold are the rhinoviruses and the coronaviruses. RSV and the parainfluenza viruses are also implicated, especially in children. Specific viral diagnosis is not usually indicated. When viral diagnosis is required because of unusual clinical features or for other reasons, the optimal specimen is an aspirate, swab, or wash obtained from the deep nasal passages. *Rhinoviruses* but not coronaviruses are detected readily in culture. Reagents for antigen detection are not available in most virology laboratories for either virus. For these reasons, some specimens from patients with viral colds will yield negative results when tested by routine viral culture and antigen detection methods.

Pharyngitis

Most cases of pharyngitis are caused by viruses. Viruses are particularly likely to be the cause when pharyngitis is accompanied by nasal or ocular findings and when oral ulcerations are present. Table 4–4 summarizes the viral agents most often associated with pharyngitis.

Adenovirus (especially types 1, 2, 3, 5, and 7),[40, 112] *EBV*, and rarely *HSV* can produce an exudative tonsillitis with clinical manifestations that resemble those of group A streptococcal infection.[113] With all three viral agents, fever and lymphadenopathy are common. Coexisting conjunctivitis occurs with adenovirus types 3 and

Table 4.4	Viruses that Cause Pharyngitis	
Virus	**Comments**
Adenovirus	May produce exudative tonsillitis. Conjunctivitis may also be present (pharyngoconjunctival fever).
Epstein-Barr	Infectious mononucleosis
Other respiratory viruses (rhinovirus, influenza, parainfluenza, respiratory syncytial)	Coexisting nasal symptoms or influenza-like illness
Coxsackieviruses	Herpangina (small vesicles/ulcers with surrounding erythema involving soft palate)
	Hand-foot-and-mouth disease (vesicles within mouth, on lips, and on hands, feet, and buttocks)
Herpes simplex	Vesicles and ulcers, lips and gingiva may be involved, adenopathy often present

7 and may be a clue that one of these viruses is responsible for the illness. A prolonged systemic illness and the presence of atypical lymphocytes in the peripheral blood should raise suspicion for EBV (see Chapter 12). An exudative pharyngitis with vesicles or ulcers involving the lips or gingiva should suggest the possibility of HSV.

Herpangina is a syndrome characterized by small vesicles on the soft palate, sometimes also involving the tonsils and pharynx. The vesicles frequently ulcerate, leaving small ulcers with surrounding erythema. Most cases are caused by *coxsackie A viruses*, although *coxsackie B viruses* and *echoviruses* have also been implicated.[114] *Hand-foot-and-mouth disease* involves vesicular lesions within the mouth that may also involve the lips, hand, feet, and buttocks. It is also associated with coxsackie A viruses, especially A16.

Sore throat is often present in infections with other respiratory viruses, including *rhinoviruses, influenza, parainfluenza,* and *RSV,* but is usually not the primary manifestation of the illness. Other findings, such as the presence of an influenza-like syndrome, may suggest one of these viruses as the cause.

The specimen of choice for detecting viral agents causing pharyngitis is a throat swab for culture. If nasal findings are also present, sensitivity of detection may be maximized by submitting both throat and NP specimens, which can be combined in the laboratory. The NP swab or aspirate can also be used for FA staining to yield a rapid diagnosis. Caution must be used in interpreting the results of viral cultures of the pharynx, especially when HSV is recovered, because it may sometimes be recovered from asymptomatic individuals.

Croup and Laryngitis

Croup is a clinical syndrome characterized by airway obstruction at the subglottic level. Most cases occur in children between ages 6 months and 3 years. Almost all cases are caused by viruses, especially *parainfluenza.* Other viruses occasionally implicated are *RSV, influenza, adenovirus, rhinovirus,* and *measles.* Affected children have inspiratory stridor, hoarseness, and a barking cough. The illness may be punctuated by exacerbations; patients respond to reassurance and moist humidified air. Radiographs of the neck reveal subglottic narrowing. Onset of disease coincides with occurrence of parainfluenza virus in the community: early fall for parainfluenza types 1 and 2 and spring and summer for parainfluenza type 3. Croup caused by viruses is sometimes confused with bacterial tracheitis caused by *Staphylococcus aureus* and acute epiglottitis, usually caused by *Haemophilus influenzae* type B.

Because of the strong association between croup and the parainfluenza viruses, specific viral diagnosis is not routinely necessary. When needed, the best specimen for laboratory diagnosis is an NP aspirate, wash, or swab

for FA staining of NP epithelial cells for parainfluenza and other respiratory viruses. Sensitivity of this test varies but in many laboratories is less than 100%. Therefore a negative FA stain does not rule out the presence of parainfluenza viruses, and a culture should be performed for optimal detection. A culture will also allow the detection of parainfluenza type 4, which is often not included in the panel of antibodies used to perform FA staining of specimens.

Tracheobronchitis and Influenza Syndrome

Tracheobronchitis can be a manifestation of infection with any of the respiratory viruses. It is frequently the predominant respiratory manifestation of *influenza virus* infection. Infection with influenza viruses often produces a characteristic clinical syndrome of nonproductive cough, high fever, headache, and myalgias, lasting 3 to 7 days. The illness often has a stereotypical presentation, but a substantial number of cases are less easily recognized. Myositis can be a prominent manifestation, especially in children with influenza B. In infants, high fever may be the predominant manifestation. In elderly patients or those with chronic cardiac or respiratory disease, decompensation of the chronic illness may be the dominant clinical manifestation.

Laboratory diagnosis of influenza is not necessary for individuals with a stereotypical influenza-like illness during an influenza outbreak but may be useful when clinical features are not clear-cut. In elderly patients, specific diagnosis may lead to treatment of influenza A infections with amantadine or rimantadine. One study reported that the extent of influenza outbreaks was decreased in nursing homes where specific viral testing was performed for patients with respiratory infection.[8]

In infants and young children, specimens of choice for detection of influenza viruses are NP aspirate, wash, or swab. In adults, recommended specimens for antigen detection and culture include NP wash, aspirate, or swab; throat swab; sputum if available; tracheal aspirate; and BAL fluid. A nasal specimen and throat swab can also be combined and sent together to the laboratory. The laboratory should be notified that influenza is suspected so that procedures can be optimized for its detection. Specimens should be transported promptly to the laboratory, but influenza viruses are stable for 3 to 5 days when held at 4°C.[115]

Bronchiolitis

Bronchiolitis is the most characteristic manifestation of infection with *RSV* in infants less than 1 year of age. Other viruses, such as *parainfluenza type 3* or *measles,* can also produce bronchiolitis. The illness caused by RSV characteristically begins with coryza followed promptly by cough. The temperature is elevated but usually less than 39°C. As the illness progresses, the infant develops tachypnea and other signs of labored respirations, such as nasal flaring and intercostal rib retractions. Wheezing may be audible. The illness may be difficult to distinguish from asthma, although bronchiolitis occurs at a younger age than most cases of asthma, and many patients have not had previous episodes of wheezing. The duration of illness is typically 7 to 14 days. Young infants, especially those with a history of prematurity and respiratory instability, may experience apnea with RSV infection.

Specific viral diagnosis is not necessary for infants with a typical bronchiolitis-like illness when RSV is common in the community. For less clear-cut cases, specific viral diagnosis may assist in management. During the RSV season, many hospitals determine patient location based on RSV infection status. Physicians and parents place a high value on knowing the specific diagnosis in children hospitalized with respiratory infection.[116] As for the other respiratory viruses, the best specimen for detecting RSV is the NP aspirate or wash, but nasal swabs can be used successfully as well (see earlier section on RSV).

It is sometimes useful to submit a second specimen when the clinical impression strongly suggests a diagnosis of RSV infection and the first specimen submitted is negative. Likewise, in patients who are severely ill and have an endotracheal tube in place, tracheal aspirate or bronchoscopy specimens are sometimes positive even when RSV has not been detected in an NP specimen.

Pneumonia

Viral pneumonia is unusual in healthy adults but is important in young children and in immunocompromised patients of any age (Table 4–5). Viral pneumonia in young children is usually caused by the common respiratory viruses, especially *RSV* and the *parainfluenza*

viruses. These cases represent an extension from bronchiolitis, and often the distinction between bronchiolitis and pneumonia is not clear, especially because bronchiolitis is frequently complicated by areas of atelectasis. The diagnostic approach to these cases is the same as for bronchiolitis.

Most cases of viral pneumonia in healthy adults are caused by *influenza viruses.* These patients present with an interstitial pneumonia that is distinct from bacterial superinfection that may complicate influenza. The diagnosis of influenza pneumonia depends on ruling out bacterial superinfection with organisms such as *Streptococcus pneumoniae, S. aureus,* and *H. influenzae.* The unequivocal determination that influenza virus is responsible for the patient's pneumonia requires a lung biopsy with demonstration of influenza virus antigen or nucleic acid in areas of involved lung.

Adenoviruses have also been responsible for some cases of pneumonia in adults, especially military recruits. Some of these cases are accompanied by sore throat and conjunctivitis. A presumptive diagnosis is based on the detection of adenovirus in respiratory secretions and the elimination of other possible causes. As for influenza, definitive attribution of the pneumonia to adenovirus requires demonstration of adenovirus in involved lung tissue samples.

The diagnosis of other, more unusual causes of pneumonia (e.g., VZV, measles virus, hantaviruses) is discussed elsewhere (e.g., see Chapters 6, 13, and 16). The diagnosis of pneumonia in immunocompromised patients is discussed next after adult considerations.

Special Considerations in Adults

All the major respiratory viruses produce infections in adults. The role of influenza viruses as causes of morbidity and mortality in adults is well appreciated.

Table 4.5   Viruses that Cause Pneumonia

Virus	Children	Adults	Immunocompromised patients
Respiratory syncytial (RSV)	++	+	+
Influenza	+	+	+
Parainfluenza	++	+	+
Adenovirus	+	+	+
Cytomegalovirus (CMV)	Rare*	–	++
Herpes simplex (HSV)	Rare*	–†	+
Varicella-zoster (VZV)	Rare	+	Rare
Epstein-Barr (EBV)	Rare	Rare	–‡
Measles	+§	+§	+§
Hantavirus	Rare§	+§	–

*May occur in congenital infection.
†HSV is associated with tracheobronchitis in normal adults.
‡EBV lymphoproliferative disease may involve the lung.
§Appropriate epidemiologic setting.

Likewise, the impact of rhinoviruses in producing the common cold in adults is well known.

The role of *RSV* as an important cause of respiratory disease in adults, especially elderly patients, is being increasingly recognized. The clinical manifestations of RSV infection overlap with those of influenza, although bronchospasm may be more common in patients with RSV and fever more common in influenza.[23, 117, 118] In a study by Falsey et al,[23] RSV was found in 10% and influenza in 11% of elderly individuals with influenza-like illnesses or acute cardiopulmonary conditions. Despite their frequency, RSV infections in adults are significantly underrecognized. The diagnosis often is not considered, and the virus is difficult to detect in adults because of low titers[22] and RSVs lability.

Specimens to submit from adults with upper respiratory infection include one of the following: a nasal wash, NP swab, or aspirate or a combined nasal specimen and throat swab. Sputum (if available), tracheal aspirate, or BAL fluid are also useful specimens. Influenza A antigen tests have sufficient yield to justify performing them if available, but the yield of RSV antigen detection tests is very low. Culture should always be performed unless an antigen detection test is positive. BAL fluid should be submitted for antigen detection and viral culture if the illness is sufficiently severe to require bronchoscopic evaluation.

Immunocompromised Patients

CMV has long been recognized as a major cause of pulmonary infection in immunocompromised patients. *HSV* is an unusual cause of pneumonia in immunocompromised patients discussed earlier. CMV or HSV pneumonitis presents typically as an interstitial pneumonia without other distinguishing clinical characteristics. A presumptive diagnosis of CMV pneumonia is based on the detection of CMV in respiratory secretions in the appropriate setting when other pathogens have been ruled out. Because asymptomatic shedding of CMV from the respiratory tract can occur and can coexist with other pulmonary pathogens, caution must be used in interpreting the significance of CMV. The detection of CMV antigen in respiratory cells obtained by tracheal aspirate or BAL is suggestive but not definitive evidence of CMV pneumonia. A definitive diagnosis is based on detection of CMV inclusions, CMV antigen, or CMV nucleic acid in involved lung tissue obtained by biopsy.

Recent studies indicate that the major respiratory viruses, especially *RSV, influenza,* and *parainfluenza,* are also important causes of pneumonia in immunocompromised patients. As in nonimmunocompromised patients, antigen detection methods and culture each can provide diagnostic information. Particularly in adult immunocompromised patients, however, the yield of antigen detection tests for viruses other than influenza virus has been disappointing.[22, 119] The same specimens described earlier for pediatric and adult patients can be tested and may yield the causative agent. Some oncologists consider NP swabs to be contraindicated in patients with thrombocytopenia.

The highest virologic yield has come from bronchoscopy with BAL. BAL fluid is an excellent specimen for both antigen detection tests and culture, and the fluid can be used to detect other nonviral agents that could be present as alternative or additional agents of disease. A respiratory virus detected in a BAL specimen could be introduced into the lower airway during insertion of the bronchoscope, but in practice such isolates have usually been clinically significant. Histologic evidence of viral infection is the ultimate proof of the role of the virus as the etiologic agent, but the additional yield from obtaining tissue may not justify the risk involved in obtaining a biopsy, particularly if thrombocytopenia or coagulopathy is present.

References

1. Ahluwalia G, Embree J, McNicol P, et al: Comparison of nasopharyngeal aspirate and nasopharyngeal swab specimens for respiratory syncytial virus diagnosis by cell culture, indirect immunofluorescence assay, and enzyme-linked immunosorbent assay, *J Clin Microbiol* 25:763, 1987.
2. McIntosh K, Hendry RM, Fahnestock ML, Pierik LT: Enzyme-linked immunosorbent assay for detection of respiratory syncytial virus infection: application to clinical samples, *J Clin Microbiol* 16:329, 1982.
3. Treuhaft MW, Soukup JM, Sullivan BJ: Practical recommendations for the detection of pediatric respiratory syncytial virus infections, *J Clin Microbiol* 22:270, 1985.
4. Hall CB, Douglas RG Jr: Clinically useful method for the isolation of respiratory syncytial virus, *J Infect Dis* 131:1, 1975.
5. Masters HB, Weber KO, Groothuis JR, et al: Comparison of nasopharyngeal washings and swab specimens for diagnosis of respiratory syncytial virus by EIA, FAT, and cell culture, *Diagn Microbiol Infect Dis* 8:101, 1987.
6. Frayha H, Castriciano S, Mahony J, Chernesky M: Nasopharyngeal swabs and nasopharyngeal aspirates equally effective for the diagnosis of viral respiratory disease in hospitalized children, *J Clin Microbiol* 27:1387, 1989.
7. Minnich L, Ray CG: Comparison of direct immunofluorescent staining of clinical specimens for respiratory virus antigens with conventional isolation techniques, *J Clin Microbiol* 12:391, 1980.
8. Leonardi GP, Leib H, Birkhead GS, et al: Comparison of rapid detection methods for influenza A virus and their value in health-care management of institutionalized geriatric patients, *J Clin Microbiol* 32:70, 1994.

9. Jalowayski AA, Walpita P, Puryear BA, Connor JD: Rapid detection of respiratory syncytial virus in nasopharyngeal specimens obtained with the Rhinoprobe scraper, *J Clin Microbiol* 28:738, 1990.

10. Barnes SD, Leclair JM, Forman MS, et al: Comparison of nasal brush and a nasopharyngeal aspirate techniques in obtaining specimens for detection of respiratory syncytial viral antigen by immunofluorescence, *Pediatr Infect Dis J* 8:598, 1989.

11. American Society for Microbiology: Specter S, coordinating editor, Cumitech 24: *Rapid detection of viruses by immunofluorescence,* Washington, DC, 1988.

12. Couch RB, Kasel JA: Influenza. In Lennette EH, Lennette DA, Lennette ET, editors: *Diagnostic procedures for viral, rickettsial, and chlamydial infections,* ed 7, Washington, DC, 1995, American Public Health Association.

13. Behrens HW, Quick CA: Bronchoscopic diagnosis of cytomegalovirus infection, *J Infect Dis* 130:174, 1974.

14. Rush JD, Ng VL, Hopewell PC, et al: Comparative recovery of cytomegalovirus from saliva, mucolysed induced sputum, and bronchoalveolar lavage fluid from patients at risk for or with acquired immunodeficiency syndrome, *J Clin Microbiol* 27:2864, 1989.

15. Kimball AM, Foy HM, Cooney MK, et al: Isolation of respiratory syncytial and influenza viruses from the sputum of patients hospitalized with pneumonia, *J Infect Dis* 147:181, 1983.

16. Frank AL, Couch RB, Griffis CA, Baxter BD: Comparison of different tissue cultures for isolation and quantitation of influenza and parainfluenza viruses, *J Clin Microbiol* 10:32, 1979.

17. Murphy P, Roberts ZM, Waner JL: Differential diagnosis of influenza A, influenza B, and respiratory syncytial virus infections by direct immunofluorescence using mixtures of monoclonal antibodies of different isotypes, *J Clin Microbiol* 34:1798, 1996.

18. Ray CG, Minnich LL: Efficiency of immunofluorescence for rapid detection of common respiratory viruses, *J Clin Microbiol* 25:355, 1987.

19. Staynor K, Foster G, McArthur M, et al: Influenza A outbreak in a nursing home: the value of early diagnosis and use of amantadine, *Can J Infect Control* 9:109, 1994.

20. Daisy JA, Lief FS, Friedman HM: Rapid diagnosis of influenza A infection by direct immunofluorescence of nasopharyngeal aspirates in adults, *J Clin Microbiol* 9:688, 1979.

21. Gardner PS, McQuillin J: Rapid virus diagnosis. *Application of immunofluorescence,* ed 2, London, 1980, Butterworths.

22. Englund JA, Piedra PA, Jewell A, et al: Rapid diagnosis of respiratory syncytial virus infections in immunocompromised adults, *J Clin Microbiol* 34:1649, 1996.

23. Falsey AR, Cunningham CK, Barker WH, et al: Respiratory syncytial virus and influenza A infections in hospitalized elderly, *J Infect Dis* 172:389, 1995.

24. Falsey AR, McCann RM, Hall WJ, Criddle MM: Evaluation of four methods for the diagnosis of respiratory syncytial virus infection in older adults, *J Am Geriatr Soc* 44:71, 1996.

25. Waner JL, Whitehurst NJ, Jonas S, et al: Isolation of viruses from specimens submitted for direct immunofluorescence test for respiratory syncytial virus, *J Pediatr* 108:249, 1986.

26. Subbarao EK, Griffis J, Waner JL: Detection of multiple viral agents in nasopharyngeal specimens yielding respiratory syncytial virus (RSV): an assessment of diagnostic strategy and clinical significance, *Diagn Microbiol Infect Dis* 12:327, 1989.

27. Gilbert LL, Dakhama A, Bone BM, et al: Diagnosis of viral respiratory tract infections in children by using a reverse transcription–PCR panel, *J Clin Microbiol* 34:140, 1996.

28. Fan J, Henrickson KJ, Savatski LL: Rapid simultaneous diagnosis of infections with respiratory syncytial viruses A and B, influenza viruses A and B, and human parainfluenza virus types 1, 2, and 3 by multiplex quantitative reverse transcription–polymerase chain reaction–enzyme hybridization assay (Hexaplex), *Clin Infect Dis* 26:1397, 1998.

28a. Gern JE, Busse WW: Association of rhinovirus infections with asthma, *Clin Microbiol Rev* 12:9, 1999.

29. McIntosh K: Coronaviruses. In Richman DD, Whitley RJ, Hayden FG, editors: *Clinical virology,* New York, 1997, Churchill Livingstone.

30. McIntosh K, McQuillin J, Reed SE, Gardner PS: Diagnosis of human coronavirus infection by immunofluorescence: method and application to respiratory disease in hospitalized children, *J Med Virol* 2:341, 1978.

31. Myint S, Johnston S, Sanderson G, Simpson H: Evaluation of nested polymerase chain methods for the detection of human coronaviruses 229E and OC43, *Mol Cell Probes* 8:357, 1994.

32. Fox JP, Hall CE, Cooney MK: The Seattle Virus Watch. VII. Observations of adenovirus infections, *Am J Epidemiol* 105:362, 1977.

33. Brandt CD, Kim HW, Vargosco AJ, et al: Infections in 18,000 children in a controlled study of respiratory tract disease. I. Adenovirus pathogenicity in relation to serologic type and illness syndrome, *Am J Epidemiol* 90:484, 1969.

34. Edwards KM, Thompson J, Paolini J, Wright P: Adenovirus infections in young children, *Pediatrics* 76:420, 1985.

35. Krisher KK, Menegus MA: Evaluation of three types of cell culture for recovery of adenovirus from clinical specimens, *J Clin Microbiol* 25:1323, 1987.

36. Wadell G, Allard A, Hierholzer JC: Adenoviruses. In Murray PR, Baron EJ, Pfaller MA, et al, editors: *Manual of clinical microbiology,* ed 7, Washington, DC, 1999, ASM Press.

37. Olsen MA, Shuck KM, Sambol AR, et al: Isolation of seven respiratory viruses in shell vials: a practical and highly sensitive method, *J Clin Microbiol* 31:422, 1993.

38. Trabelski A, Pozzetto B, Mbida AD, et al: Evaluation of four methods for rapid detection of adenovirus, *Eur J Clin Microbiol Infect Dis* 11:535, 1992.

39. Espy MJ, Hierholzer JC, Smith TF: The effect of centrifugation on the rapid detection of adenovirus in shell vials, *Am J Clin Pathol* 88:358, 1987.

40. Ruuskanen O, Meurman O, Akusjärvi G: Adenoviruses. In Richman DD, Whitley RJ, Hayden FG, editors: *Clinical virology*, New York, 1997, Churchill Livingstone.

41. Fox JP, Brandt C, Wassermann FE, et al: The Virus Watch Program: a continuing surveillance of viral infections in metropolitan New York families. VI. Observations of adenovirus infections: virus excretion patterns, antibody response, efficiency of surveillance, patterns of infections, and relation to illness, *Am J Epidemiol* 89:25, 1969.

42. Lehtomäki K, Julkunen I, Sandelin K, et al: Rapid diagnosis of respiratory adenovirus infections in young adult men, *J Clin Microbiol* 24:108, 1986.

43. Morris DJ, Cooper RJ, Barr T, Bailey AS: Polymerase chain reaction for rapid diagnosis of respiratory adenovirus infections, *J Infect* 32:113, 1995.

44. Hayden FG, Palese P: Influenza virus. In Richman DD, Whitley RJ, Hayden FG, editors: *Clinical virology*, New York, 1997, Churchill Livingstone.

45. Claas EC, Osterhaus AD, van Beek R, et al: Human influenza A H5N1 virus related to a highly pathogenic avian influenza virus, *Lancet* 351(9101):472, 1998.

46. Moriuchi H, Katsushima N, Nishimura H, et al: Community-acquired influenza C virus infection in children, *J Pediatr* 118:235, 1991.

47. Hayden FG, Osterhaus AD, Treanor JJ, et al: Efficacy and safety of the neuraminidase inhibitor zanamivir in the treatment of influenzavirus infections, *N Engl J Med* 337:874, 1997.

48. Belshe RB, Mendelman PM, Treanor J, et al: The efficacy of live attenuated, cold-adapted, trivalent, intranasal influenzavirus vaccine in children, *N Engl J Med* 338:1405, 1998.

49. Moriuchi H, Oshima T, Nishimura H, et al: Human malignant melanoma cell line (HMV-II) for isolation of influenza C and parainfluenza viruses, *J Clin Microbiol* 28:1147, 1990.

50. Minnich LL, Ray CG: Early testing of cell cultures for detection of hemadsorbing viruses, *J Clin Microbiol* 25:421, 1987.

51. Espy MJ, Smith TF, Harman MW, Kendal AP: Rapid detection of influenza virus by shell vial assay with monoclonal antibodies, *J Clin Microbiol* 24:677, 1986.

52. Stokes CE, Bernstein JM, Kyger SA, Hayden FG: Rapid diagnosis of influenza A and B by 24h fluorescent focus assay, *J Clin Microbiol* 26:1263, 1988.

53. Rabalais GP, Stout GG, Ladd KL, Cost KM: Rapid diagnosis of respiratory viral infections by using a shell vial assay and monoclonal antibody pool, *J Clin Microbiol* 30:1505, 1992.

54. Guenther SH, Linnemann CC Jr: Indirect immunofluorescence assay for rapid diagnosis of influenza virus, *Lab Med* 19:581, 1988.

55. Johnston SLG, Siegel CS: A comparison of direct immunofluorescence, shell vial culture, and conventional cell culture for the rapid detection of influenza A and B, *Diagn Microbiol Infect Dis* 14:131, 1991.

56. Mills RD, Cain KJ, Woods GL: Detection of influenza virus by centrifugal inoculation of MDCK cells and staining with monoclonal antibodies, *J Clin Microbiol* 27:2505, 1989.

57. Lee SHS, Boutileir JE, MacDonald MA, Forward KR: Enhanced detection of respiratory viruses using the shell vial technique and monoclonal antibodies, *J Virol Meth* 39:39, 1992.

58. Bartholoma NY, Forbes BA: Successful use of shell vial centrifugation and 16- to 18-hour immunofluorescent staining for the detection of influenza A and B in clinical specimens, *Am J Clin Pathol* 92:487, 1989.

59. Todd SJ, Minnich L, Waner JL: Comparison of rapid immunofluorescence procedure with TestPack RSV and Directigen FLU-A for diagnosis of respiratory syncytial virus and influenza A virus, *J Clin Microbiol* 33:1650, 1995.

60. Waner JL, Todd SJ, Shalaby J, et al: Comparison of Directigen FLU-A with viral isolation and direct immunofluorescence for the rapid detection and identification of influenza A virus, *J Clin Microbiol* 29:479, 1991.

61. Dominguez EA, Taber LH, Couch RB: Comparison of rapid diagnostic techniques for respiratory syncytial and influenza A virus respiratory infections in young children, *J Clin Microbiol* 31:2286, 1993.

62. Ryan-Poirier KA, Katz JM, Webster RG, Kawaoka Y: Application of Directigen FLU-A for the detection of influenza A virus in human and nonhuman specimens, *J Clin Microbiol* 30:1072, 1992.

63. Johnston SLG, Bloy H: Evaluation of a rapid enzyme immunoassay for detection of influenza A virus, *J Clin Microbiol* 31:142, 1993.

64. Claas ECJ, van Milaan AJ, Sprenger MJW, et al: Prospective application of reverse transcription polymerase chain reaction for diagnosing influenza infections in respiratory samples from a children's hospital, *J Clin Microbiol* 31:2218, 1993.

65. Cherian T, Bobo L, Steinhoff MC, et al: Use of PCR-enzyme immunoassay for identification of influenza A virus matrix RNA in clinical samples negative for cultivable virus, *J Clin Microbiol* 32:623, 1994.

66. Lindquist SW, Darnule A, Istas A, Demmler GJ: Parainfluenza virus type 4 infections in pediatric patients, *Pediatr Infect Dis J* 16:34, 1997.

67. Rubin EE, Quennec P, Mcdonald JC: Infections due to parainfluenza virus type 4 in children, *Clin Infect Dis* 7:998, 1993.

68. Henrickson KJ. Human parainfluenza viruses. In Lennette EH, Lennette DA, Lennette ET, editors: *Diagnostic procedures for viral, rickettsial, and chlamydial infections*, ed 7, Washington, DC, 1995, American Public Health Association.

69. Stout C, Murphy MD, Lawrence S, Julian S: Evaluation of a monoclonal antibody pool for rapid diagnosis of respiratory viral infections, *J Clin Microbiol* 27:448, 1989.

70. Wong DT, Welliver RC, Riddlesberger KR, et al: Rapid diagnosis of parainfluenza virus infection in children, *J Clin Microbiol* 16:164, 1982.

71. Waner JL, Whitehurst NJ, Downs T, Graves DG: Production of monoclonal antibodies against parainfluenza 3 virus and their use in diagnosis by immunofluorescence, *J Clin Microbiol* 22:535, 1985.

72. Fan J, Hendrickson KJ: Rapid diagnosis of human parainfluenza virus type 1 infection by quantitative re-

verse transcription–PCR–enzyme hybridization assay, *J Clin Microbiol* 34:1914, 1996.

73. Walsh EE, McConnochie KM, Long CE, Hall CB: Severity of respiratory syncytial virus infection is related to virus strain, *J Infect Dis* 175:814, 1997.

74. Institute of Medicine. Appendix N. In *New vaccine development: establishing priorities.* Vol 1. *Diseases of importance in the United States,* Washington, DC, 1985, National Academy Press.

75. Groothuis JR, Simoes EA, Levin MJ, et al: Prophylactic administration of respiratory syncytial virus immune globulin to high-risk infants and young children: the Respiratory Syncytial Virus Immune Globulin Study Group, *N Engl J Med* 329:1524, 1993.

75a. IMpact RSV Study Group: Palivizumab, a humanized respiratory syncytial virus monoclonal antibody, reduces hospitalization from respiratory syncytial virus infection in high-risk patients, *Pediatrics* 102:531, 1998.

76. Arens MQ, Swierkosz EM, Schmidt RR, et al: Enhanced isolation of respiratory syncytial virus in cell culture, *J Clin Microbiol* 23:800, 1986.

77. Smith MC, Creutz C, Hung YT: Detection of respiratory syncytial virus in nasopharyngeal secretions by shell vial technique, *J Clin Microbiol* 29:463, 1991.

78. Matthey S, Nicholson D, Ruhs S, et al: Rapid detection of respiratory viruses by shell vial culture and direct staining by using pooled and individual monoclonal antibodies, *J Clin Microbiol* 30:540, 1992.

79. Pedneault L, Robillard L, Turgeon JP: Validation of respiratory syncytial virus enzyme immunoassay and shell vial assay results, *J Clin Microbiol* 32:2861, 1994.

80. Mendoza J, Navarro JM, Rojas A, de la Rosa M: Evaluation of immunofluorescence, two enzyme immunoassays and the shell-vial assay for detection of respiratory syncytial virus, *Eur J Clin Microbiol Infect Dis* 10:40, 1991.

81. Schirm J, Luijt DS, Pastoor GW, et al: Rapid detection of respiratory viruses using mixtures of monoclonal antibodies on shell vial cultures, *J Med Virol* 38:147, 1992.

82. Kellogg JA: Culture vs direct antigen assays for detection of microbial pathogens from lower respiratory tract specimens suspected of containing the respiratory syncytial virus, *Arch Pathol Lab Med* 115:451, 1991.

83. Derish MT, Kulhanjian JA, Frankel LR, Smith DW: Value of bronchoalveolar lavage in diagnosing severe respiratory syncytial virus infections in infants, *J Pediatr* 119:761, 1991.

84. Subbarao EK, Dietrich MC, De Sierra TM, et al: Rapid detection of respiratory syncytial virus by a biotin-enhanced immunoassay: test performance by laboratory technologists and housestaff, *Pediatr Infect Dis J* 8:865, 1989.

85. Krilov LR, Lipson SM, Barone SR, et al: Evaluation of a rapid diagnostic test for respiratory syncytial virus (RSV): potential for bedside diagnosis, *Pediatrics* 93: 903, 1994.

86. Wren CG, Bate BJ, Masters HB, Lauer BA: Detection of respiratory syncytial virus antigen in nasal washings by Abbott TestPack enzyme immunoassay, *J Clin Microbiol* 28:1395, 1990.

87. Halstead DC, Todd S, Fritch G: Evaluation of five methods for respiratory syncytial virus detection, *J Clin Microbiol* 28:1021, 1990.

88. Michaels MG, Serdy C, Barbadora K, et al: Respiratory syncytial virus: a comparison of diagnostic modalities, *Pediatr Infect Dis J* 11:613, 1992.

89. Olsen M, Shuck KM, Sambol AR: Evaluation of Abbott TestPack RSV for the diagnosis of respiratory syncytial virus infections, *Diagn Microbiol Infect Dis* 16:105, 1993.

90. Swierkosz EM, Flanders R, Melvin L, et al: Evaluation of the Abbott TESTPACK RSV enzyme immunoassay for detection of respiratory syncytial virus in nasopharyngeal swab specimens, *J Clin Microbiol* 27: 1151, 1989.

91. Miller H, Milk R, Diaz-Mitoma F: Comparison of the VIDAS RSV assay and the Abbott Testpack RSV with direct immunofluorescence for detection of respiratory syncytial virus in nasopharyngeal aspirates, *J Clin Microbiol* 31:1336, 1993.

92. Thomas EE, Book LE: Comparison of two rapid methods for detection of respiratory syncytial virus (RSV) (TestPack RSV and Ortho RSV ELISA) with direct immunofluorescence and virus isolation for the diagnosis of pediatric RSV infection, *J Clin Microbiol* 29:632, 1991.

93. Hite SA, Huang YT: Microwave-accelerated direct immunofluorescent staining for respiratory syncytial virus and influenza A virus, *J Clin Microbiol* 34:1819, 1996.

94. Waner JL, Whitehurst NJ, Todd SJ, et al: Comparison of Directigen RSV with viral isolation and direct immunofluorescence for the identification of respiratory syncytial virus, *J Clin Microbiol* 28:480, 1990.

95. Kok T, Barancek K, Burrell CJ: Evaluation of the Becton Dickinson Directigen Test for respiratory syncytial virus in nasopharyngeal aspirates, *J Clin Microbiol* 28:1458, 1990.

96. Paton AW, Paton JC, Lawrence J, et al: Rapid detection of respiratory syncytial virus in nasopharyngeal aspirates by reverse transcription and polymerase chain reaction amplification, *J Clin Microbiol* 30:901, 1992.

97. Freymuth F, Eugene G, Vabret A, et al: Detection of respiratory syncytial virus by reverse transcription–PCR and hybridization with a DNA enzyme immunoassay, *J Clin Microbiol* 33:3352, 1995.

98. van Milaan AJ, Sprenger MJW, Rothbart PH, et al: Detection of respiratory syncytial virus by RNA–polymerase chain reaction and differentiation of subgroups with oligonucleotide probes, *J Med Virol* 44:80, 1994.

99. Glezen WP, Fernald GW, Lohr JA: Acute respiratory disease of university students with special reference to the etiologic role of *Herpesvirus hominis, Am J Epidemiol* 101:111, 1975.

100. McMillan JA, Weiner LB, Higgins AM, Lamparella VJ: Pharyngitis associated with herpes simplex virus in college students, *Pediatr Infect Dis J* 12:280, 1993.

101. Whitley RJ, Roizman B: Herpes simplex viruses. In Richman DD, Whitley RJ, Hayden FG, editors: *Clinical virology,* New York, 1997, Churchill Livingstone.

102. Nash G: Necrotizing tracheobronchitis and bronchopneumonia consistent with herpetic infection, *Hum Pathol* 3:283, 1972.

103. Klainer AS, Oud L, Randazzo J, et al: Herpes simplex virus involvement of the lower respiratory tract following surgery, *Chest* 106(suppl):8S, 1994.

104. Graham BS, Snell JD Jr: Herpes simplex virus infection of the adult lower respiratory tract, *Medicine* 62:384, 1983.

105. Sherry MK, Klainer AS, Wolff M, Gerhard H: Herpetic tracheobronchitis, *Ann Intern Med* 109:229, 1988.

106. Legge RH, Thompson AB, Linder J, et al: Acyclovir-responsive herpetic tracheobronchitis, *Am J Med* 85:561, 1988.

107. Ramsay PG, Fife KH, Hackman RC, et al: Herpes simplex pneumonia: clinical, virologic, and pathologic features in 20 patients, *Ann Intern Med* 97:813, 1982.

108. Hubbell C, Dominguez R, Kohl S: Neonatal herpes simplex pneumonia, *Rev Infect Dis* 10:431, 1988.

109. Tuxen DV, Wilson JW, Cade JF: Prevention of lower respiratory herpes simplex virus infection with acyclovir in patients with the adult respiratory distress syndrome, *Am Rev Respir Dis* 136:402, 1987.

110. Schmidt GM, Horak DA, Niland JC, et al: A randomized, controlled trial of prophylactic ganciclovir for cytomegalovirus pulmonary infection in recipients of allogeneic bone marrow transplants, *N Engl J Med* 324:1005, 1991.

111. Storch GA, Ettinger NA, Ockner D, et al: Quantitative cultures of the cell fraction and supernatant of bronchoalveolar lavage fluid for the diagnosis of cytomegalovirus pneumonitis in lung transplant recipients, *J Infect Dis* 168:1502, 1993.

112. Hammond GW: Adenoviruses. In Long SS, Pickering LK, Prober CG, editors: *Principles and practice of pediatric infectious diseases*, New York, 1997, Churchill Livingstone.

113. Glezen WP, Clyde WAJ, Senior RJ, et al: Group A streptococci, mycoplasmas, and viruses associated with acute pharyngitis, *JAMA* 202:119, 1967.

114. Cherry JD, Jahn CL: Herpangina: the etiologic spectrum, *Pediatrics* 36:632, 1965.

115. Baxter BD, Couch RB, Greenberg SB, Kasel JA: Maintenance of viability and comparison of identification methods for influenza and other respiratory viruses of humans, *J Clin Microbiol* 6:19, 1977.

116. Adcock PM, Stout GG, Hauck MA, Marshall GS: Effect of rapid viral diagnosis on the management of children hospitalized with lower respiratory tract infection, *Pediatr Infect Dis J* 16:842, 1997.

117. Dowell SF, Anderson LJ, Gary HDJ, et al: Respiratory syncytial virus is an important cause of community-acquired lower respiratory infection among hospitalized adults, *J Infect Dis* 174:456, 1996.

118. Wald TG, Miller BA, Shult P, et al: Can respiratory syncytial virus and influenza A be distinguished clinically in institutionalized older persons? *J Am Geriatr Soc* 43:170, 1995.

119. Wendt CH, Fox JMK, Hertz MI: Paramyxovirus infections in lung transplant recipients, *J Heart Lung Transplant* 14:479, 1995.

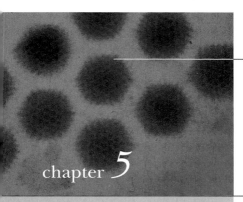

Douglas K. Mitchell, Xi Jiang, David O. Matson

chapter *5*

Gastrointestinal Infections

Outline continued

OVERVIEW

Most cases of acute gastroenteritis are caused by viruses. Few are confirmed in the laboratory, however, because many cases are relatively mild and self-limited and laboratory detection of the most common agents is difficult. Great progress has been made in the past two decades in defining four groups of viruses that account for most cases of viral gastroenteritis: *rotaviruses, astroviruses, caliciviruses,* and the *enteric adenoviruses.* All are either difficult or impossible to culture. Therefore laboratory diagnosis is based on other methods, including electron microscopy, antigen detection, and nucleic acid detection. Antigen detection assays for rotavirus and the enteric adenoviruses are widely available, and an antigen detection assay for astrovirus is available in research laboratories. Nucleic acid detection assays are under development. This chapter provides an overview of viral gastroenteritis and discusses the evolving approach to detecting each of these agents.

VIRAL GASTROENTERITIS

History

In 1910, Ito[1] in Japan described "pseudocholera infantum," a "winter vomiting syndrome" also described in 1929 by Zahorsky,[2] a physician practicing in St. Louis. The syndrome occurred predominantly in children and accounted for a major portion of clinical practice in winter months. The timing of recognition of this syndrome may reflect public health improvements attributable to a cleaner water supply and better sewage handling, resulting in an overall reduction in gastroenteritis cases caused by bacteria and parasites, both with a summer predominance. Such improvements have greatly affected the occurrence of summer diarrhea. A study in Sweden found that the overall seasonal predominance of diarrhea in children switched from the summer in the 1930s to the winter in the 1980s.[3]

In retrospect, Ito and Zahorsky were probably describing rotavirus gastroenteritis, but little progress in diagnosis occurred over the next 50 years. Studies in the 1930s and 1940s failed to prove that the presumed agent(s) of the winter vomiting syndrome was transmissible to animals.[4] Cell culture techniques applied successfully to poliovirus in the 1940s failed when applied to the cultivation of the agents of gastroenteritis. By 1970 a definitive review of these studies concluded that no agent could be implicated as a cause of the common, annual winter vomiting syndrome.[5]

At the same time, however, the first breakthrough studies were being conducted. In 1972, Kapikian et al[6] reported the application of *immune electron microscopy* (IEM) to the investigation of an outbreak of gastroenteritis among schoolchildren and their teachers in Norwalk, Ohio. The agent they discovered has since proved to be the prototype human calicivirus.[7] In 1973, Bishop et al[8] followed leads provided by the study of diarrhea in infant mice and reported visualization of viral particles in duodenal biopsy specimens of children hospitalized for gastroenteritis. These particles have since been named rotaviruses.

The technique permitting these breakthrough studies was the application of electron microscopy (EM) to study fecal matter from diarrhea cases in carefully controlled cases and situations. Subsequent surveys using EM for particle visualization yielded a number of candidate agents in diarrhea stool specimens, many of which were identified because they were already known diarrhea agents in animals.[9, 10] Researchers have yet to develop alternative detection techniques for some of these viruses.

Clinical Manifestations

Gastroenteritis describes a clinical syndrome consisting of a constellation of symptoms and signs with multiple causes. Affected individuals typically have diarrhea, vomiting, fever, abdominal cramps, dehydration, irritability, and anorexia. The manifestations vary among individual patients and also depend on the duration and severity of symptoms (Table 5–1). Many patients develop metabolic acidosis caused by bicarbonate loss and dehydration. These symptoms can result from enteric infection by viral, bacterial, fungal, or parasitic organisms.

Table 5.1	Symptoms in Hospitalized Children with Gastroenteritis*

Symptom†	Incidence (%)
Vomiting	76
Fever	69
Dehydration	61
Irritability	43
Lethargy	31

*Modified from Rodriguez WJ, Kim HW, Arrobio JO, et al: *J Pediatr* 91:188, 1977.
†Anorexia, headache, abdominal cramps, and myalgia typically occur in adults with gastroenteritis but are difficult to assess in children.

Table 5.2	Comparison of Viral Enteropathogens			
Genus/group	**Family**	**Genome**	**Types**	
Rotavirus	Reoviridae	Double-stranded RNA	Groups A-F 14 G types (serotypes) 21 P types	
Astrovirus	Astroviridae	Single-stranded RNA	8 antigenic types	
Calicivirus	Caliciviridae	Single-stranded RNA	4 antigenically distinct genera	
Adenovirus	Adenoviridae	Double-stranded DNA	Serotypes 40 and 41; serotype 31?	

Most viral infections are of short duration (less than 7 days) and sudden onset, with watery, nonmucous, and nonbloody stools. Asymptomatic infections or very mild illnesses (e.g., loose stools, single vomiting episode, mild malaise) are much more common than the infections seen by physicians.

Epidemiology

Viral gastroenteritis occurs in all age groups, with the peak incidence of severe illness in children 6 to 24 months of age. Viral infections account for 50% to 90% of the cases of acute gastroenteritis that result in hospitalization in the United States. Viral gastroenteritis results in approximately 220,000 hospitalizations each year among children younger than 5 years of age in the United States. These hospitalizations account for 3% to 10% of all pediatric hospital days. About 70% of the hospitalizations occur during a 2- to 4-month winter peak, during which rotavirus is the predominant cause.

Rotavirus is the major cause of acute viral gastroenteritis, and its epidemiology is well defined; the epidemiology of other agents is less well defined. Transmission of all the agents is by the fecal-oral route, by intermediary fomites, or by contaminated food or water. Rotaviruses, astroviruses,[11] caliciviruses,[12] and enteric adenovirus,[13] have been reported as causes of nosocomial outbreaks of diarrhea.

Differential Diagnosis

The viruses that are proven causes of acute gastroenteritis are rotaviruses, astroviruses, caliciviruses, and enteric adenoviruses (Table 5–2). Several other virus families are suspected but unproven causes of gastroenteritis. Commercial assays are available to diagnose rotavirus and enteric adenovirus infections, but other enteric viruses cannot be detected easily in the clinical laboratory. The most widely used assays for detecting viral enteropathogens directly are EM, IEM, enzyme immunoassay (EIA), latex agglutination, gel electrophoresis, cell culture, polymerase chain reaction (PCR), and reverse-transcription PCR (RT-PCR) (Table 5–3). EM is the only method that can simultaneously detect

Table 5.3	Diagnostic Methods for Enteric Viral Pathogens	
Organism	**Preferred methods**	**Alternative methods**
Rotaviruses	EM, EIA*	RT-PCR, electrophero-typing, genotyping, culture, antibody EIA
Astroviruses	EM	EIA, RT-PCR, culture, genotyping, antibody EIA
Caliciviruses	EM	EIA, RT-PCR, genotyping, antibody EIA
Enteric adenoviruses	EM, EIA*	PCR, culture, restriction enzyme analysis

EM, Electron microscopy; *EIA*, enzyme immunoassay; *PCR*, polymerase chain reaction; *RT-PCR*, reverse-transcription polymerase chain reaction.
*These EIAs are commercially available (see Table 5–6).

and identify each of the important viral agents in the same specimen.

Attempts to determine the viral cause of a gastroenteritis episode from historic information are generally discouraging. A few trends in the patterns of illness onset and duration provide a relative clue that a gastroenteritis illness episode was caused by a particular virus (Table 5–4). A stepwise approach to an episode or outbreak of diarrhea facilitates the clinician's identification of an etiologic agent. The clinical history is helpful in differentiating bacterial, parasitic, and viral causes.

Rotaviruses and astroviruses have peak incidence in the winter. Among sporadic cases, rotaviruses are more common by more than 20:1. The viral gastroenteritis agents are more likely to cause illness between 4 and 24 months of age. Enteric adenoviruses are most likely to cause illness lasting more than 7 days. Viral diarrhea stools rarely contain blood or mucus. History of child care center attendance in a child less than 2 years old implicates viral gastroenteritis agents over *Giardia* and bacterial causes of illness. Caliciviruses, and less so

Table 5.4	Clues in Differential Diagnosis of Pediatric Diarrhea		
Factor	**Differential clue**	**Likely viruses***	**Strength of clue**
Season	Winter	R	++++
		As	+
Age	6-24 months	R, As, C	++
	<6 months	Ad	+
Duration	>7 days	Ad	+
Stool characteristics	Nonbloody, nonmucous	R, As, C, Ad	+
Exposures	Child care center	R, As, C, Ad	++
Fecal leukocytes	Absent	R, As, C, Ad	++

R, Rotaviruses; *As*, astroviruses; *C*, caliciviruses; *Ad*, adenoviruses.

astroviruses, are strongly associated with water and food contamination. The association between caliciviral infection and seafood consumption is particularly strong.

The least expensive and most rapid laboratory method for differentiating probable viral acute gastroenteritis from nonviral causes is the test for *fecal leukocytes*. The presence of fecal leukocytes, detected by a Wright or methylene blue stain of a fecal smear, indicates that inflammation is occurring in the bowel wall. Most bacteria cause a polymorphonuclear inflammation. *Salmonella typhi* and *Entamoeba histolytica* frequently cause a mononuclear reaction (Table 5–5). Fecal leukocytes are typically absent or present only in minimal numbers in viral gastroenteritis.

Investigation of Outbreaks

Outbreaks of viral gastroenteritis are common in hospitals, child care centers, and other settings where

Table 5.5	Value of Fecal Leukocytes in Distinguishing Viral and Nonviral Gastroenteritis
Cause	**Frequency of leukocytes in fecal smear (%)**
Viruses	0-10
Vibrio cholerae, EHEC, ETEC, EPEC, *Giardia lamblia*	0-10
Shigella spp, *Salmonella* spp, (not *typhi*), *Campylobacter jejuni*, *Clostridium difficile*	90-100
Yersinia enterocolitica, *Vibrio parahaemolyticus*	Variable
Salmonella typhi	100
Entamoeba histolytica (amebic dysentery)	100
Ulcerative colitis	100

EHEC, Enterohemorrhagic *Escherichia coli*; *ETEC*, enterotoxigenic *Escherichia coli*; *EPEC*, enteropathogenic *Escherichia coli*.

susceptible individuals have a common exposure. Timing of stool and blood collection is crucial to detecting an etiologic agent of such outbreaks. In general, the same diagnostic clues apply to both sporadic and outbreak-associated cases of viral gastroenteritis (see Table 5–4).

Stool specimens should be collected as early as possible after illness onset, stored at 4°C, and transported on wet ice until examined. Acute and convalescent serum pairs should be collected and stored for testing together. As many individuals in the outbreak as feasible should submit samples, with a practical upper limit being 30. The first test to apply to the stool specimens is EM, followed by EIAs, then culture, PCR, and RT-PCR, depending on which diagnostic clues are present. All available stool specimens should be tested to increase the likelihood of detecting the etiologic agent and linking it to the outbreak. Assays for multiple agents should be applied to identify polymicrobial outbreaks.

ROTAVIRUSES

Description

Rotaviruses are frequent pathogens in humans and other mammalian and avian hosts (Box 5–1). Rotaviruses are among the few human pathogens with a segmented genome (11 segments) of double-stranded ribonucleic acid (RNA) (see Table 5–2). The virus is 70 to 75 nm in diameter when visualized by negative-stain EM (Figure 5–1). Two surface neutralization proteins, *VP4* and *VP7*, form the outer capsid, and the major capsid protein, *VP6*, forms the inner capsid. Six serologic groups (A through F) have been identified based on antigenic heterogeneity; groups A, B, and C occur in humans.

Group A rotavirus causes infantile gastroenteritis worldwide. *Group B* rotaviruses have caused epidemics in mainland China affecting all ages and sporadic infections elsewhere. *Group C* rotaviruses occasionally

History: known animal pathogens since early 1960s; first human infections recognized in 1973 when virus was visualized in duodenal biopsy specimens from children with acute diarrhea

Epidemiology: most common cause of severe diarrhea in children worldwide

Clinical manifestations: explosive diarrhea and vomiting (up to 40 times daily), rapidly dehydrating, with fever, abdominal pain, and malaise

Diagnosis: commercial EIA and latex agglutination assays, including office versions; electron microscopy

Case occurrence: 50%-60% of hospital cases; 10%-20% of office cases

cause outbreaks of infection in children; studies in North America are limited. Group B and C serogroups probably circulate primarily in animals. The VP4 and VP7 of group A rotaviruses each have distinct antigenic types, called *P and G types,* respectively; 21 potential P types are known from distinct genetic variants, and 14 G types are known. Unless otherwise indicated, group A rotaviruses are the subject of the remainder of this section.

Rotaviruses have a distinct winter peak of occurrence and are detected more often as the severity of illness increases. For example, rotaviruses account for about 10% of diarrhea episodes in young children that result in medical treatment but are associated with about 40% of episodes that require in-hospital care. Therefore in the United States and similar temperate countries, as many as 90% of diarrhea episodes requiring in-hospital care during the peak of the winter diarrhea season can be attributed to rotavirus. During the winter peak a child between 3 and 24 months of age with acute, nonbloody, nonmucous diarrhea is much more likely to have rotavirus infection than not.

Rotaviruses may be excreted in stools at up to 10^{11} particles per gram of feces. Stools collected during the first several days of illness have the highest concentration of virus, whereas stools collected 8 or more days after onset of illness usually test negative for virus. Stool specimens should be stored at 4°C and tested within 3 days of collection. Otherwise, samples should be frozen at −70°C until tested. For some methods of identification, such as latex agglutination and EIA, rectal swabs provide sufficient sample. For electropherotyping, genotyping, antigenic typing, and cell culture, a specimen of stool is preferred.

Preferred Detection Methods

Most diagnostic virology laboratories use antigen detection by EIA or latex agglutination for detection of rotavirus. A number of commercial assays are available, including EIA and latex agglutination assays.[14] All antigen assays are directed toward detection of the group antigens. Commercially available EIAs have comparable specificity and sensitivity (greater than 95% for each) when used to test specimens from children with symptomatic infection. Latex agglutination assays tend to be somewhat less sensitive. Differences among assays of one type relate primarily to the choice of host for antibody production and in the manual manipulations and time required for assay performance.

Figure 5.1 Electron micrographs of four viruses known to cause pediatric gastroenteritis, visualized by negative staining in diarrhea stool specimens from children. *Top left,* Rotaviruses are 70-nm particles with a double shell and a characteristic "wagon wheel" appearance. *Top right,* Enteric adenoviruses are 70- to 90-nm particles with a characteristic icosahedral structure. *Bottom left,* Astroviruses (located here around head of bacteriophage) are 26 to 28 nm, have a smooth edge, and have five- or six-pointed stars in some particles. *Bottom right,* Caliciviruses with "typical" appearance are 30 to 35 nm and have distinctive "Star of David" appearance or 10 surface spikes apparent in some particles, depending on the orientation. Particle staining is variable among stool specimens, and characteristic features are not always seen. (Bar = 50 nm.) (Courtesy W. David Cubitt, Institute of Child Health, London; from Matson DO: In Long, SS, Prober, CG, Pickering, LK, editors: *Principles and practice of pediatric infectious diseases,* New York, 1996, Churchill Livingstone.)

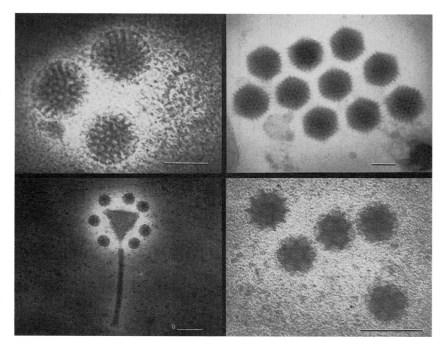

Alternative Detection Methods

A variety of other laboratory methods can be applied for detection of rotavirus infection (see Table 5–3). Most of these are research methods, but two methods, EM and electropherotyping, are used in some diagnostic centers.

Electron microscopy. A rapid method of negative staining for viral particle identification in fecal samples by EM was developed by Dr. W. David Cubitt.[15] A small portion of stool specimen is placed on an EM grid and stained with phosphotungstic acid. EM has sensitivity comparable to that of commercial assays, with a lower limit of detection of about 10^6 particles/g of stool specimen. IEM and solid-phase IEM can enhance detection sensitivity. EM cannot distinguish rotavirus groups.

Electropherotyping. Electropherotyping refers to the analysis of the migration pattern of the 11 rotavirus genome segments in polyacrylamide gels[16] (see Chapter 19). The viral RNA can be extracted with phenol-chloroform from viral particles in stool specimens and applied to a polyacrylamide gel. The segments then are driven by current into the gel and resolved by size. Rotaviruses generate a characteristic pattern of migration with the bands arranging into groups of 4, 2, 3, and 2, in that order, from the top of the gel to the bottom. Groups A, B, and C each have unique electrophoretic profiles. Similar migration patterns occur among strains from outbreaks of infection, and differences in migration patterns are helpful in distinguishing whether or not infections are epidemiologically related. In addition, this method is convenient for identifying simultaneous infections with multiple rotavirus strains. Finally, until other assays are available, electropherotyping is the simplest method for determining whether a particular strain is in group A or another group.

Cell culture. Rotaviruses are difficult to cultivate from clinical specimens. A variety of cell lines may be used. Lines derived from African green monkey kidney (e.g., MA104), human liver (HEp-G2), and human colonic carcinoma (CaCo-2) cells all may be used. Success varies from 30% to 90% depending on experience of the laboratory, freshness of the sample, and utilization of multiple blind passages. This technique is not used in routine diagnostic virology laboratories.

Antigenic typing. P and G types can be determined for infecting strains by EIA using monoclonal antibodies.[17] G-typing monoclonals are available in research laboratories for all the common human G types, and experimental P-typing monoclonals have been developed for a few P types. G-typing success rates usually are 70% to 90% depending on the freshness of the sample

and the monoclonal antibodies used. These typing methods are useful for epidemiologic and immunologic investigations.

Reverse-transcription PCR. RT-PCR is useful for detecting rotaviruses in certain situations.[18] Environmental surfaces and fluids can be sampled and virus detected when infectious virus might be difficult to recover or concentrations are less than those usually observed in clinical specimens. RT-PCR also is used to amplify gene segments for genotyping reactions.[19, 20] In most clinical situations, sufficient virus is present in a sample to use the commercial antigen detection assays to determine whether an illness is caused by rotavirus.

Genotyping. Genotyping based on RT-PCR provides an alternative typing method that can be used when antigenic typing is unsuccessful or impossible because of lack of serologic reagents.[19] Using appropriate primers, genotyping correlates very well with antigenic typing results and is considered an acceptable alternative method for designating the G type of an infecting strain. Genotyping is often used in research investigations.

Serology. A variety of assay formats have been applied to detection of antibody to rotaviruses. These methods are available in research laboratories for application in special situations.

ASTROVIRUSES

Description

Human astroviruses are nonenveloped, single-stranded RNA viruses that were first identified in 1975 by EM studies of diarrhea stool specimens from children (Box 5–2). Eight human astrovirus antigenic types have been

---

Box 5.2   Summary of Astroviruses

History: detected by electron microscopy in stool samples of children with diarrhea in 1975

Epidemiology: common cause of pediatric gastroenteritis; large outbreaks associated with food and water contamination

Clinical manifestations: gastroenteritis indistinguishable from that caused by other agents; illness lasts approximately 4 days

Diagnosis: electron microscopy; rapid EIAs in research laboratories

Case occurrence: 8%-10% of hospital and office cases

identified, and the complete genomic sequences of several types are known.[21, 22] The genomic organization of astroviruses is sufficiently different from other positive-strand RNA viruses to warrant classification of astroviruses as a new virus family, the Astroviridae.[23]

Human astrovirus infections occur worldwide. Astroviruses have been detected by EIA in the stools of 1.5% to 9% of children with diarrhea and in 1% to 2% of stools from asymptomatic control children.[24] Astrovirus-associated illness occurs predominantly in the winter. Astrovirus causes endemic diarrhea.[25] In addition, outbreaks of diarrhea associated with astroviral infection have been reported in schools,[26] geriatric care facilities and hospitals,[27] pediatric hospitals,[11] and child care centers.[28]

Astrovirus *type 1* has been the prevalent type in the United Kingdom, accounting for more than 65% of cases.[29] Recent surveys indicate that other types are increasing in the United Kingdom; this change in types may be associated with an increase in the number of outbreaks.[30] Multiple types co-circulate in the United States and Mexico.[21, 31] Reports of large outbreaks of food-borne astrovirus *type 6* in Japan involving thousands of children and adults provide further evidence of the need to evaluate differences in geographic and temporal distribution of types.[26]

Antibodies to astrovirus are acquired by 75% of children by 5 to 10 years of age.[32] Myint et al[33] demonstrated that 93% of surfers had serologic evidence of exposure to astrovirus antigenic *type 4*, whereas a control group had only 22% seroprevalence to the same type. This report implicated water exposure as a risk factor for infection by astroviruses in surfers. Midthun et al[34] reported an antibody prevalence to antigenic *type 5* of 13% in children 6 months to 3 years of age and 41% in older children.

Preferred Detection Methods

Usually detected by EM, astroviruses are 28 nm in diameter, have a distinctive five- or six-pointed star on the surface of the particle (giving the virus its name), and have a smooth particulate edge (Figure 5–1). Only a few virions on an EM grid have the typical star.[35]

Alternative Detection Methods

Alternative methods for astrovirus now include most methods available for other viruses.

Cell culture. Astroviruses grow in CaCo-2 cells and monkey kidney (LLC-MK2) cells in the presence of trypsin.[36] Astrovirus can be cultivated from fresh or frozen stool samples. The presence of virus in cell culture requires confirmation by other methods, such as EM, EIA, or RT-PCR. Astrovirus culture is not performed in most routine diagnostic virology laboratories.

Enzyme immunoassay. Astrovirus antigen can be detected in stool specimens by EIA using a group-specific monoclonal antibody in combination with polyclonal sera.[28, 37] These assays are not currently commercially available. The EIA is suitable for detection of astroviruses from symptomatic patients in outbreaks or with sporadic illness. Its sensitivity is considerably less than that of RT-PCR for the detection of astrovirus in asymptomatic infections.[38]

Reverse-transcription PCR. RT-PCR has been applied for detection of all eight types of astrovirus (group specific) and of specific types (type specific).[22, 38, 39] Group-specific detection of astrovirus was more sensitive than EIA to define the extent of outbreaks in child care centers and a nosocomial outbreak in a bone marrow transplant unit.[38, 39a] RT-PCR was not a significant advantage over EIA detection in community surveillance studies.[39b] RT-PCR will be of greatest utility in genotyping and sequityping astroviruses for epidemiologic purposes.

Typing. Antigenic typing and genotyping methods still are in development, but some success has been reported. Polyclonal rabbit typing sera have been used to identify the eight astrovirus antigenic types, but these antisera now are depleted. Type-specific sequences within the capsid gene of astroviruses have permitted the design of genotyping primers for RT-PCR.[21] In preliminary experiments the genotype and antigenic typing methods have yielded congruent results.

Serology. Assays for antibody to astrovirus are in development in research laboratories. The most recent seroprevalence studies have used type-specific capsid protein produced in a baculovirus system as recombinant antigen in microimmunofluorescence and EIA formats to detect human antiastrovirus antibody.[40] Comparable assays for all astrovirus types will be useful for further definition of the epidemiology of astroviruses.

CALICIVIRUSES

Description

Caliciviruses (CVs) are nonenveloped, single-stranded, positive-sense RNA viruses that have been implicated as causes of acute gastroenteritis (Box 5–3). Among the CVs that cause gastroenteritis, two morphologic types, termed *typical CV* and *small round structured virus* (SRSV), can be discerned by negative-stain EM. *Norwalk virus* (NV) is the prototype SRSV infecting humans. Most other human CVs (HuCVs) are morphologically similar and have been called *NV-like* or *NV-related viruses*. Many individual strains have been described, including

---

Box 5.3   Summary of Caliciviruses

History: known animal pathogens since 1930s; first human infections recognized in 1970s

Epidemiology: most common cause of outbreaks of gastroenteritis in adults in North America; frequently associated with water and food contamination

Clinical manifestations: in children, indistinguishable from rotavirus infections; in adults, usually explosive vomiting

Diagnosis: research assays; electron microscopy

Case occurrence: 3%-10(?)% of hospital and office cases

NV,[6] Snow Mountain virus (SMV),[41] Hawaii virus,[42, 43] Taunton agent,[43] Montgomery County agent,[44] "mini-reovirus,"[45] Sapporo calicivirus,[46] and many recently characterized strains.[47-59] Multiple antigenic types of HuCVs exist, but lack of specific reagents has precluded meaningful antigenic classification.

Based on genomic organization and phylogenetic analysis of the genomes, CVs are separated into four genera designated Norwalk-like viruses, Sapporo-like viruses, *Vesivirus,* and *Lagovirus.*[58] The first three are known to infect humans. Most of the SRSVs are included in the genus *Norwalk-like virus,* which contains distinguishable genetic groups, the NV-like and the SMV-like genogroups. The genus *Sapporo-like virus* is composed of most typical HuCVs, including the prototype Sapporo/82 strain. Genetic and antigenic variants also are found in the Sapporo-like viruses, but classification of these variants into genetic clusters will require characterization of additional strains.[59]

Although HEV is currently classified as a CV based on the morphology and genomic organization, the primary genomic sequence reveals little similarity to any other CV. Recently accumulated evidence suggests that it should be removed from the CV family.

HuCVs infect all age groups and have a worldwide distribution. Early studies showed that up to 42% of outbreaks of nonbacterial gastroenteritis in the United States during the 1970s were caused by HuCVs.[60] Recent studies using RT-PCR showed that 85% of such outbreaks in the Netherlands were associated with HuCVs. Large-scale serosurveys of HuCVs have been conducted using new assays developed after molecular characterization of HuCVs.[48, 49, 61-75] These studies found that children in both developed and developing countries acquire serum antibodies to HuCVs early in life (generally by 3 years of age),[53, 61-63] which reinforces the need to understand why outbreaks of HuCV illness appear to affect adults more often than children. Also, predominant HuCV antigenic types may change over time. Currently, among strains in the genus *Norwalk-like virus,* SMV-like strains are predominant, whereas the strains in the NV-like cluster that were common in the 1970s and 1980s are rarely detected. Further studies are needed to confirm such changes in prevalence of antigenic types and to describe pressures that drive such changes, such as acquisition of herd immunity.

The gastroenteritis of the Norwalk-like and Sapporo-like viruses is clinically indistinguishable from that caused by other enteric viruses.[71, 76] Outbreaks of infection in adults are notable for the sudden onset of illness in many patients. In adults, vomiting is frequently a prominent feature of illness. Symptoms occur 12 to 24 hours after infection and last for 24 to 48 hours. Patients being excreting HuCVs in stools as early as 15 hours after infection, with peak excretion 24 to 48 hours postinfection and continue excreting for as long as 14 days after illness onset.

The major public health concern about HuCVs has been their ability to cause large outbreaks of gastroenteritis in school-age children and adults. Such outbreaks usually have high attack rates, occurring in schools, restaurants, summer camps, hospitals, nursing homes, and cruise ships.[41, 45, 46, 60] Exposure to a common source of the virus, such as contaminated food or water, usually can be identified. Outbreaks resulting from consumption of uncooked shellfish are common. HuCVs also can be spread by person-to-person transmission.

Preferred Detection Methods

Commercial assays for CVs are not available. EM remains a useful technique for detection of HuCV in stools but has limited sensitivity. IEM is more sensitive than direct EM but requires the availability of specific antibody as a reagent. Testing is sometimes performed using paired acute and convalescent sera from an outbreak patient. Other assays include EIA, radioimmunoassay (RIA), and Western blot. These assays currently are available only in academic research laboratories.

Electron microscopy. CVs are rough-edged, round particles, about 35 nm in diameter. Typical CVs have a "Star of David" on the surface of the virion in some orientations; the star has a dark center. SRSV particles lack the "Star of David" and simply appear to be round particles with rough edges (Figure 5-1). HuCV particle concentrations usually are low in stool specimens; only a few particles may have a typical CV appearance, and the duration of virus excretion is short. Successful detection of CVs in stool specimens by direct EM requires optimal timing of sample collection.

Immune electron microscopy. IEM has been widely used since it first detected NV in 1972.[6] IEM is specific because specific antibodies are used to bind target viruses before EM examination. In the traditional IEM method the antibody-antigen reaction is performed in solution.[6, 77] An alternative method uses specific antibody bound to the EM grid to capture viral particles.[7, 76] An advantage of *solid-phase immune electron microscopy* (SPIEM) is that particle morphology is retained; in the traditional IEM method, particles are coated with antibody, obscuring surface details. Antibodies used for IEM can be raised in animals or derived from infected patients. Paired acute and convalescent sera from infected patients are essential for comparative testing to identify an unknown pathogen. By using specific antigens, IEM is also used to measure serum antibody. Both IEM and SPIEM are useful for antigenic typing of HuCVs.

Alternative Detection Methods

EM and IEM are cumbersome methods and relatively insensitive for CVs. Other methods are being developed and are variably applicable to different CV genera.

Cell culture. Most animal CVs, but no HuCVs, can be cultivated in cell culture. Current research efforts focus on cultivation methods for HuCVs.

Enzyme immunoassay. In addition to IEM and SPIEM, other immunologic methods were described for detection of HuCV infection before molecular cloning of the HuCV genome. These methods include RIA,[78] EIA, and Western blot.[79] The recent expression of HuCV capsid antigens in the baculovirus system has facilitated the development of EIAs for diagnosis of HuCV.* Expression of the viral capsid gene in baculovirus of several strains of HuCVs resulted in a single viral capsid protein that self-assembled into virion-like particles.[49, 65] These particles do not contain viral RNA but are morphologically and antigenically identical to authentic virions from human stool specimens. Antigen detection EIAs use hyperimmune antisera generated with the virion-like particles and antibody detection EIAs use the baculovirus-expressed particles as capture antigens.[67, 71] These assays have been type specific; that is, they detect only the specific virus used to generate the hyperimmune antiserum.

Reverse-transcription PCR. The determination of full-length and partial HuCV genome sequences led to development of RT-PCR to detect viral RNA in stool specimens. Oligonucleotide primers based on conserved genome regions have been designed for broad detection of HuCVs, although more than one pair of primers is necessary for detection of all strains in different HuCV genera.[50, 54, 56, 67, 79a] Methods for extraction of viral RNA from stool specimens and removal

*References 48, 49, 65, 66, 68-70, 75.

of inhibitors for the reverse transcriptase and Taq polymerases have been developed.[64] RT-PCR followed by sequencing the amplified cDNA products provided a powerful tool in molecular epidemiology to describe the genetic variation of the family.[47, 50, 52, 54, 56-58] RT-PCR has also been used to detect CVs in shellfish and other environmental samples.[80a-80e] Because multiple steps are involved in extraction of viral RNA and because RT-PCR requires sophisticated reagents and equipment, RT-PCR is currently performed only in research laboratories.

Genotyping. The same sequence information that enabled HuCV detection by RT-PCR has been used to establish genotyping methods.[47, 49-52, 58, 59, 80]

Serology. Detection of antibodies to HuCVs is complicated by two factors: the antigenic specificity of antibody detection assays is still uncertain, and the presence of preexisting serum or fecal antibody to NV is a risk factor for illness and infection in adults, but not in children.[49, 81-84]

Choice of assay. The diversity of strains detected by these assays differs considerably. The antigen detection EIAs detect strains very closely related to the strain used to generate the detector antibody. The degree of relatedness for predicting whether an antigen detection EIA will detect a strain appears to be greater than 95% nucleotide identity in the most conserved region of the CV genome (3D or polymerase region). Such strains are in the same genetic cluster within a genus. Strains that share about 70% or more nucleotide identity in the 3D region have cross-reacting epitopes that can be detected in antibody detection assays. Nucleotide identity greater than 70% in the 3D region places a strain in the same CV genus. RT-PCR using certain 3D region primers detects strains across CV genera.

ENTERIC ADENOVIRUSES

Description

Adenoviruses are DNA viruses with 49 distinct serotypes that cause disease in humans. *Types 40 and 41*, and rarely 31, have been associated with gastroenteritis[85] (Box 5–4). The adenoviruses are 70 to 90 nm in diameter, nonenveloped, and contain double-stranded DNA (see Table 5–2). Types 40 and 41 are difficult or impossible to cultivate in cell cultures used to grow other adenovirus types but can be grown in specialized cell lines (e.g., Graham 293).

Enteric adenoviruses types 40 and 41 are widespread and cause endemic diarrhea and outbreaks of diarrhea in hospitals, orphanages, and child care centers.[86, 87]

Enteric adenoviruses cause 2% to 22% of pediatric diarrhea in inpatients and outpatients.[13, 85, 88] Adenoviruses infect all age groups, with antibody prevalence studies showing that more than 50% of children are seropositive by the third or fourth year of life.[13, 89] Enteric adenoviruses are a more important cause of viral gastroenteritis in infants less than 6 months of age than in older children. These viruses have been implicated in severe infections in infants with necrotizing enterocolitis and, as with other viral gastroenteritis agents, have been shown to cause severe infections in immunocompromised individuals.[90] Infections appear to occur year-round, the mode of transmission is fecal-oral, and the incubation period is 3 to 10 days. Asymptomatic infection is common, and asymptomatic excretion after illness may last for several weeks.[86]

Enteric adenoviruses cause diarrhea that lasts 6 to 9 days and may be associated with emesis and fever. Children admitted with enteric adenoviral infection are more likely to have diarrhea for more than 5 days but less likely to be febrile or dehydrated than children with rotavirus infection.[13, 86, 91, 92] The diarrhea is watery without blood or fecal leukocytes. Persistent lactose intolerance also has been reported.[92]

Preferred Detection Methods

Unlike the adenoviruses that cause respiratory infection, enteric adenoviruses are difficult to culture. EM and EIA have been the preferred methods for detection.

Electron microscopy. EM initially was used to detect enteric adenoviruses.[85, 91] As with all adenoviruses, they have icosahedral symmetry and are 70 to 90 nm in diameter, nonenveloped, and not distinguishable from respiratory adenoviruses that may occur in stool specimens (Figure 5–1).

Enzyme immunoassay. Commercially available EIAs using monoclonal antibodies with specificity for enteric adenovirus serotypes are available (Table 5–6).[93] The sensitivity compared with EM is 78% to 98%, with a reported specificity of 95%.

Alternative Detection Methods

EM and EIA generally are preferred for enteric adenoviruses because the alternative methods are slow or require considerable laboratory resources and expertise.

Cell culture. Enteric adenoviruses were initially called "fastidious adenoviruses" because they were difficult to cultivate in tissue culture. Enteric adenoviruses can be cultivated in HEp-2 and Graham 293 cell lines, but this is usually performed only in research settings.[85, 94, 95]

Restriction enzyme analysis. This is the definitive method for typing adenovirus isolates.[96] For restriction enzyme analysis, viral DNA is extracted directly from a stool sample and digested by selected restriction en-

Table 5.6 Commercially Available Diagnostic Assays for Viral Enteropathogens

Virus	Assay name	Assay	Manufacturer
Rotavirus	Rotaclone	Monoclonal EIA	Cambridge Biotech
	Pathfinder	Monoclonal EIA	Sanofi Diagnostics Pasteur
	Rotavirus EIA	Polyclonal EIA	International Diagnostics
	Wellcozyme	Polyclonal EIA	Wellcome Diagnostics
	Rotazyme II	Polyclonal EIA	Abbott Laboratories
	TestPack	Monoclonal and polyclonal EIA	Abbott Laboratories
	Rotastat	Latex agglutination	International Diagnostics
	Meritec Rotavirus	Latex agglutination	Meridian Diagnostics
	Virogen Rotatest	Latex agglutination	Wampole Laboratories
	Wellcome RV Latex	Latex agglutination	Wellcome Diagnostics
Enteric adenovirus	Adenoclone	EIA	Cambridge Biotech

zymes (see Chapter 19). The digested DNA fragments then are resolved by electrophoresis and visualized by ethidium bromide. Enteric adenovirus types 40 and 41 have distinctive migration patterns of the digested fragments.

References

1. Ito S: Pseudocholera infantum, *Jikazasshi* 751, 1910.
2. Zahorsky J: Hyperemesis hiemis or winter vomiting disease, *Arch Paediatr* 46:391, 1929.
3. Persson LA, Samuelson G, Sjolin S: Nutrition and health in Swedish children, 1930-1980: three nutrition surveys in a northern Swedish county, *Acta Paediatr Scand* 78:865, 1989.
4. Hodes HL: Viral gastroenteritis, *Am J Dis Child* 131:729, 1977.
5. Yow MD, Melnick JL, Blattner RJ, et al: The association of viruses and bacteria with infantile diarrhea, *Am J Epidemiol* 92:33, 1970.
6. Kapikian AZ, Wyatt RG, Dolin R, et al: Visualization by immune electron microscopy of a 27-nm particle associated with acute infectious non-bacterial gastroenteritis, *J Virol* 10:1075, 1972.
7. Jiang X, Graham DY, Wang K, Estes MK: Norwalk virus genome cloning and characterization, *Science* 250:1580, 1990.
8. Bishop RF, Davidson GP, Holmes IH, Ruck BJ: Virus particles in epithelial cells of duodenal mucosa from children with acute nonbacterial gastroenteritis, *Lancet* 2:1281, 1973.
9. Flewett TH, Bryden AS, Davies H: Diagnostic electron microscopy of faeces. I. The viral flora of the faeces as seen by electron microscopy, *J Clin Pathol* 27:603, 1974.
10. Appleton H, Higgins PG: Viruses and gastroenteritis in infants, *Lancet* 1:1297, 1975.
11. Esahli H, Breback K, Bennet R, et al: Astroviruses as a cause of nosocomial outbreaks of infant diarrhea, *Pediatr Infect Dis J* 10:511, 1991.
12. Middleton PJ, Szymanski MT, Petric M: Viruses associated with acute gastroenteritis in young children, *Am J Dis Child* 131:733, 1977.
13. Kotloff KL, Losonsky GA, Morris JG, et al: Enteric adenovirus infection and childhood diarrhea: an epidemiologic study in three clinical settings, *Pediatrics* 84:219, 1989.
14. Dennehy PH, Gauntlett DR, Tente WE: Comparison of nine commercial immunoassays for the detection of rotavirus in fecal specimens, *J Clin Microbiol* 26:1630, 1988.
15. Barrish JP, Hicks MJ, Cubitt WD, et al: A rapid staining method for negative staining of fecal samples for diagnosis of viral-induced gastroenteritis by transmission electron microscopy. Presented at the 52nd Annual Meeting of the Microscopy Society of America, 1994.
16. Estes MK, Graham DY, Dimitrov DH: The molecular epidemiology of rotavirus gastroenteritis, *Prog Med Virol* 29:1, 1984.
17. Taniguchi K, Urasawa T, Morita Y, et al: Direct serotyping of human rotavirus in stools by an enzyme-linked immunosorbent assay using serotype 1-, 2-, 3-, and 4-specific monoclonal antibodies to VP7, *J Infect Dis* 155:1159, 1987.
18. Wilde J, Van R, Pickering LK, et al: Detection of rotaviruses in the day care environment: detection by reverse transcriptase polymerase chain reaction, *J Infect Dis* 166:507, 1992.
19. Gouvea V, Glass RI, Woods P, et al: Polymerase chain reaction amplification and typing of rotavirus nucleic acid from stool specimens, *J Clin Microbiol* 28:276, 1990.
20. Gentsch JR, Glass RI, Woods P: Identification of group A rotavirus gene 4 types by polymerase chain reaction, *J Clin Microbiol* 30:1365, 1992.
21. Noel JS, Lee TW, Kurtz JB, et al: Typing of human astroviruses from clinical isolates by enzyme immunoassay and nucleotide sequencing, *J Clin Microbiol* 33:797, 1995.
22. Jonassen TO, Monceyron C, Lee TW, et al: Detection of all serotypes of human astrovirus by the polymerase chain reaction, *J Virol Methods* 52:327, 1995.
23. Monroe SS, Jiang B, Stine SE, et al: Subgenomic RNA sequence of human astrovirus supports classification of *Astroviridae* as a new family of RNA viruses, *J Virol* 67:3611, 1993.
24. Glass RI, Noel J, Mitchell D, et al: The changing epidemiology of astrovirus-associated gastroenteritis: a review, *Arch Virol* 12 (suppl):287, 1996.
25. Herrmann JE, Taylor DN, Echeverria P, Blacklow NR: Astroviruses as a cause of gastroenteritis in children, *N Engl J Med* 324:1757, 1991.
26. Oishi I, Yamazaki K, Kimoto T, et al: A large outbreak of acute gastroenteritis associated with astrovirus among students and teachers in Osaka, Japan, *J Infect Dis* 170:439, 1994.
27. Lewis DC, Lightfoot NF, Cubitt WD, Wilson SA: Outbreaks of astrovirus type 1 and rotavirus gastroenteritis in a geriatric in-patient population, *J Hosp Infect* 14:9, 1989.
28. Mitchell DK, Van R, Morrow AL, et al: Outbreaks of astrovirus gastroenteritis in day care centers, *J Pediatr* 123:725, 1993.
29. Noel J, Cubitt D: Identification of astrovirus serotypes from children treated at the Hospitals for Sick Children, London, 1981-93, *Epidemiol Infect* 113:153, 1994.
30. Willcocks MM, Kurtz JB, Lee TW, Carter MJ: Prevalence of human astrovirus serotype 4: capsid protein sequence and comparison with other strains, *Epidemiol Infect* 114:385, 1995.
31. Guerrero ML, Noel J, Mitchell DK: A prospective study of astrovirus diarrhea of infancy in Mexico City, *Pediatr Infect Dis J* 17:723, 1998.
32. Kurtz J, Lee T: Astrovirus gastroenteritis age distribution of antibody, *Med Microbiol Immunol (Berl)* 166:227, 1978.
33. Myint S, Manley R, Cubitt D: Viruses in bathing waters, *Lancet* 343:1640, 1994 (letter).
34. Midthun K, Greenberg HB, Kurtz JB, et al: Characterization and seroepidemiology of a type 5 astrovirus associated with an outbreak of gastroenteritis in Marin County, California, *J Clin Microbiol* 31:955, 1993.
35. Monroe SS, Glass RI, Noah N, et al: Electron micro-

scopic reporting of gastrointestinal viruses in the United Kingdom, 1985-1987, *J Med Virol* 33:193, 1991.

36. Lee TW, Kurtz JB: Serial propagation of astrovirus in tissue culture with the aid of trypsin, *J Gen Virol* 57:421, 1981.

37. Moe CL, Allen JR, Monroe SS, et al: Detection of astrovirus in pediatric stool samples by immunoassay and RNA probe, *J Clin Microbiol* 29:2390, 1991.

38. Mitchell DK, Monroe SS, Jiang X, et al: Virologic features of an astrovirus diarrhea outbreak in a day care center revealed by reverse transcriptase–polymerase chain reaction, *J Infect Dis* 172:1437, 1995.

39. Jonassen TO, Kjeldsberg E, Grinde B: Detection of human astrovirus serotype 1 by the polymerase chain reaction, *J Virol Methods* 44:83, 1993.

39a. Cubitt WD, Mitchell DK, Carter MJ, et al: Application of electronmicroscopy, enzyme immunoassay, and RT-PCR to monitor an outbreak of astrovirus type 1 in a paediatric bone marrow transplant unit, *J Med Virol* 57: 313, 1999.

39b. Gaggero A, O'Ryan M, Noel JS, et al: Prevalence of astrovirus infection among Chilean children with acute gastroenteritis, *J Clin Microbiol* 36:3691, 1998.

40. Kriston S, Willcocks MM, Carter MJ, Cubitt WD: Seroprevalence of astrovirus types 1 and 6 in London, determined using recombinant virus antigen, *Epidemiol Infect* 117:159, 1996.

41. Dolin R, Reichman RC, Roessner KD, et al: Detection by immune electron microscopy of the Snow Mountain agent of acute viral gastroenteritis, *J Infect Dis* 146:184, 1982.

42. Dolin R, Levy AG, Wyatt RG, et al: Viral gastroenteritis induced by the Hawaii agent: jejunal histopathology and serologic response, *Am J Med* 59:761, 1975.

43. Wyatt RG, Dolin R, Blacklow NR, et al: Comparison of three agents of acute infectious nonbacterial gastroenteritis by cross-challenge in volunteers, *J Infect Dis* 129:709, 1974.

44. Caul EO, Appleton H: The electron microscopical and physical characteristics of small round human fecal viruses: an interim scheme for classification, *J Med Virol* 9:257, 1982.

45. Lew JF, Petric M, Kapikian AZ, et al: Identification of minireovirus as a Norwalk-like virus in pediatric patients with gastroenteritis, *J Virol* 68:3391, 1994.

46. Nakata S, Chiba S, Terashima H, et al: Microtiter solid-phase radioimmunoassay for detection of human calicivirus in stools, *J Clin Microbiol* 17:198, 1983.

47. Cubitt WD, Jiang X, Wang J, Estes MK: Sequence similarity of human caliciviruses and small round structured viruses, *J Med Virol* 43:252, 1994.

48. Jiang X, Matson DO, Velazquez FR, et al: Study of Norwalk-related viruses in Mexican children, *J Med Virol* 47:309, 1995.

49. Jiang X, Matson DO, Ruiz-Palacios GM, et al: Expression, self-assembly, and antigenicity of a Snow Mountain agent–like calicivirus capsid protein, *J Clin Microbiol* 33:1452, 1995.

50. Moe CL, Gentsch J, Ando T, et al: Application of PCR to detect Norwalk virus in fecal specimens from outbreaks of gastroenteritis, *J Clin Microbiol* 32:642, 1994.

51. Lew JF, Kapikian AZ, Jiang X, et al: Molecular characterization and expression of the capsid protein of a Norwalk-like virus recovered from a Desert Shield troop with gastroenteritis, *Virology* 200:319, 1994.

52. Matson DO, Zhong WM, Nakata S, et al: Molecular characterization of a human calicivirus with sequence relationships closer to animal caliciviruses than other known human caliciviruses, *J Med Virol* 45:215, 1995.

53. Lambden PR, Caul EO, Ashley CR, Clarke IN: Sequence and genome organization of a human small round-structured (Norwalk-like) virus, *Science* 259:516, 1993.

54. Wang J, Jiang X, Madore HP, et al: Sequence diversity of small, round-structured viruses in the Norwalk virus group, *J Virol* 68:5982, 1994.

55. Jiang X, Wang M, Wang K, Estes MK: Sequence and genomic organization of Norwalk virus, *Virology* 195:51, 1993.

56. Ando T, Monroe SS, Gentsch JR, et al: Detection and differentiation of antigenically distinct small round-structured viruses (Norwalk-like viruses) by reverse transcription–PCR and southern hybridization, *J Clin Microbiol* 33:64, 1995.

57. Wolfaardt M, Taylor MB, Grabow WO, et al: Molecular characterization of small round structured viruses associated with gastroenteritis in South Africa, *J Med Virol* 47:386, 1995.

58. Berke T, Golding B, Jiang X, et al: Phylogenetic analysis of the caliciviruses, *J Med Virol* 52:19, 1997.

59. Jiang X, Cubitt DW, Berke T, et al: Sapporo-like human caliciviruses are genetically and antigenically diverse, *Arch Virol* 142:1813, 1997.

60. Kaplan JE, Gary GW, Baron RC, et al: Epidemiology of Norwalk gastroenteritis and the role of Norwalk virus in outbreaks of acute nonbacterial gastroenteritis, *Ann Intern Med* 96:756, 1982.

61. Parker SP, Cubitt WD, Jiang X, Estes MK: Seroprevalence studies using a recombinant Norwalk virus protein enzyme immunoassay, *J Med Virol* 42:146, 1994.

62. Gray JJ, Jiang X, Morgan-Capner P, et al: Prevalence of antibodies to Norwalk virus in England: detection by enzyme-linked immunosorbent assay using baculovirus-expressed Norwalk virus capsid antigen, *J Clin Microbiol* 31:1022, 1993.

63. Lew JF, Valdesuso J, Vesikari T, et al: Detection of Norwalk virus or Norwalk-like virus infections in Finnish infants and young children, *J Infect Dis* 169: 1364, 1994.

64. Jiang X, Wang J, Graham DY, Estes MK: Detection of Norwalk virus in stool by polymerase chain reaction, *J Clin Microbiol* 30:2529, 1992.

65. Jiang X, Wang M, Graham DY, Estes MK: Expression, self-assembly, and antigenicity of the Norwalk virus capsid protein, *J Virol* 66:6527, 1992.

66. Jiang X, Cubitt D, Hu J, et al: Development of an ELISA to detect MX virus, a human calicivirus in the Snow Mountain agent genogroup, *J Gen Virol* 76:2739, 1995.

67. Jiang X, Wang J, Estes MK: Characterization of SRSVs using RT-PCR and a new antigen ELISA, *Arch Virol* 140: 363, 1995.

68. Green KY, Lew JF, Jiang X, et al: Comparison of the reactivities of baculovirus-expressed recombinant

Norwalk virus capsid antigen with those of the native Norwalk virus antigen in serologic assays and some epidemiologic observations, *J Clin Microbiol* 31:2185, 1993.

69. Treanor JJ, Jiang X, Madore HP, Estes MK: Subclass-specific serum antibody responses to recombinant Norwalk virus capsid antigen (rNV) in adults infected with Norwalk, Snow Mountain, or Hawaii virus, *J Clin Microbiol* 31:1630, 1993.

70. Parker S, Cubitt D, Jiang X, Estes M: Efficacy of a recombinant Norwalk virus protein enzyme immunoassay for the diagnosis of infections with Norwalk virus and other human candidate caliciviruses, *J Med Virol* 41:179, 1993.

71. Graham DY, Jiang X, Tanaka T, et al: Norwalk virus infection of volunteers: new insights based on improved assays, *J Infect Dis* 170:34, 1994.

72. Numata K, Nakata S, Jiang X, et al: Epidemiological study of Norwalk virus infections in Japan and Southeast Asia by enzyme-linked immunosorbent assays with Norwalk virus capsid protein produced by the baculovirus expression system, *J Clin Microbiol* 32:121, 1994.

73. Monroe SS, Stine SE, Jiang X, et al: Detection of antibody to recombinant Norwalk virus antigen in specimens from outbreaks of gastroenteritis, *J Clin Microbiol* 31:2866, 1993.

74. Parker SP, Cubitt WD, Jiang X: Enzyme immunoassay using baculovirus-expressed human calicivirus (Mexico) for the measurement of IgG responses and determining its seroprevalence in London, UK, *J Med Virol* 46:194, 1995.

75. Jiang X, Turf E, Hu J, et al: Outbreaks of gastroenteritis in elderly nursing homes and retirement facilities associated with human caliciviruses, *J Med Virol* 50:335, 1996.

76. Matson DO, Estes MK, Glass RI, et al: Human calicivirus–associated diarrhea in children attending day care centers, *J Infect Dis* 159:71, 1989.

77. Kapikian AZ, Dienstag JL, Purcell RH: Immune electron microscopy as a method for the detection, identification, and characterization of agents not cultivatable in an in vitro system. In Rose NR, Friedman H, editors: *Manual of clinical immunology*, ed 2, Washington, DC, 1980, American Society for Microbiology.

78. Blacklow NR, Cukor G, Bedigian MK, et al: Immune response and prevalence of antibody to Norwalk enteritis virus as determined by radioimmunoassay, *J Clin Microbiol* 10:903, 1979.

79. Hayashi Y, Ando T, Utagawa E, et al: Western blot (immunoblot) assay of small, round-structured virus associated with an acute gastroenteritis outbreak in Tokyo, *J Clin Microbiol* 27:1728, 1989.

79a. Jiang X, Matson DO, Cubitt WD, et al: Genetic and antigenic diversity of human caliciviruses (HuCVs) using RT-PCR and new EIAs, *Arch Virol* Suppl 12:251, 1996.

80. Lew JF, Kapikian AZ, Valdesuso J, Green KY: Molecular characterization of Hawaii virus and other Norwalk-like viruses: evidence for genetic polymorphism among human caliciviruses, *J Infect Dis* 170:535, 1994.

80a. Atmar RL, Neill FH, Romalde JL, et al: Detection of Norwalk virus and hepatitis A virus in shellfish tissues with the PCR, *Appl Environ Microbiol* 61:3014, 1995.

80b. Atmar RL, Neill FH, Woodley CW, et al: Collaborative evaluation of a method for the detection of Norwalk virus in shellfish tissues by PCR, *Appl Environ Microbiol* 62:254, 1996.

80c. Le Guyader F, Neill FH, Estes MK, et al: Detection and analysis of a small round-structured virus strain in oysters implicated in an outbreak of acute gastroenteritis, *Appl Environ Microbiol* 62:4268, 1996.

80d. Payment P, Franco E, Fout GS: Incidence of Norwalk virus infections during a prospective epidemiology study of drinking water-related gastrointestinal illness, *Can J Microbiol* 40:805, 1994.

80e. Schwab KJ, De Leon R, Sobsey MD: Concentration and purification of beef extract mock eluates from water samples for the detection of enteroviruses, hepatitis A virus, and Norwalk virus by reverse transcription-PCR, *Appl Environ Microbiol* 61:531, 1995.

81. Parrino TA, Schreiber DS, Trier JS, et al: Clinical immunity in acute gastroenteritis caused by Norwalk agent, *N Engl J Med* 297:86, 1977.

82. Black RE, Greenberg HB, Kapikian AZ, et al: Acquisition of serum antibody to Norwalk Virus and rotavirus and relation to diarrhea in a longitudinal study of young children in rural Bangladesh, *J Infect Dis* 145:483, 1982.

83. Ryder RW, Singh N, Reeves WC, et al: Evidence of immunity induced by naturally acquired rotavirus and Norwalk virus infection on two remote Panamanian islands, *J Infect Dis* 151:99, 1985.

84. Nakata S, Chiba S, Terashima H, Nakao T: Prevalence of antibody to human calicivirus in Japan and Southeast Asia determined by radioimmunoassay, *J Clin Microbiol* 22:519, 1985.

85. Brandt CD, Kim HW, Rodriguez WJ, et al: Adenoviruses and pediatric gastroenteritis, *J Infect Dis* 151:437, 1985.

86. Van R, Wun CC, O'Ryan ML, et al: Outbreaks of human enteric adenovirus types 40 and 41 in Houston day care centers, *J Pediatr* 120:516, 1992.

87. Chiba S, Nakata S, Nakamura I, et al: Outbreak of infantile gastroenteritis due to type 40 adenovirus, *Lancet* 2:954, 1983.

88. Madeley CR: The emerging role of adenoviruses as inducers of gastroenteritis, *Pediatr Infect Dis J* 5:S63, 1986.

89. Shinozaki T, Araki K, Ushijima H, Fujii R: Antibody response to enteric adenovirus types 40 and 41 in sera from people in various age groups, *J Clin Microbiol* 25:1679, 1987.

90. Yolken RH, Franklin CC: Gastrointestinal adenovirus: an important cause of morbidity in patients with necrotizing enterocolitis and gastrointestinal surgery, *Pediatr Infect Dis* 4:42, 1985.

91. Grimwood K, Carzino R, Barnes GL, Bishop RF: Patients with enteric adenovirus gastroenteritis admitted to an Australian pediatric teaching hospital from 1981 to 1992, *J Clin Microbiol* 33:131, 1995.

92. Uhnoo I, Olding Stenkvist E, Kreuger A: Clinical features of acute gastroenteritis associated with rotavirus, enteric adenoviruses, and bacteria, *Arch Dis Child* 61:732, 1986.

93. Martin AL, Kudesia G: Enzyme linked immunosorbent

assay for detecting adenoviruses in stool specimens: comparison with electron microscopy and isolation, *J Clin Pathol* 43:514, 1990.

94. Perron Henry DM, Herrmann JE, Blacklow NR: Isolation and propagation of enteric adenoviruses in HEp-2 cells, *J Clin Microbiol* 26:1445, 1988.

95. Shinozaki T, Araki K, Ushijima H, et al: Use of Graham 293 cells in suspension for isolating enteric adenoviruses from the stools of patients with acute gastroenteritis, *J Infect Dis* 156:246, 1987.

96. van der Avoort HG, Wermenbol AG, Zomerdijk TP, et al: Characterization of fastidious adenovirus types 40 and 41 by DNA restriction enzyme analysis and by neutralizing monoclonal antibodies, *Virus Res* 12:139, 1989.

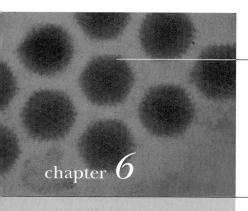

Gregory A. Storch

chapter *6*

Skin and Mucous Membrane Infections

OVERVIEW

Members of four virus families cause infection of the skin and mucous membranes (Table 6–1). *Herpesviruses*, especially herpes simplex and varicella-zoster, are common causes of vesicular skin lesions in both normal and immunocompromised individuals. *Enteroviruses*, especially the coxsackie B viruses, can also cause skin lesions from which the causative agent can be isolated. *Human papillomaviruses* cause the common wart and a variety of other cutaneous lesions. *Poxviruses* are also prominent causes of skin infections. Poxvirus diseases include smallpox, vaccinia (which can occur from smallpox vaccine), monkeypox, molluscum contagiosum, orf (contagious ecthyma) and milker's nodule (paravaccinia).

A variety of other viral diseases have cutaneous manifestations, but the causative agent is not usually isolated from the skin. These include measles; rubella; exanthem subitum; roseola (human herpesviruses 6 and 7); erythema infectiosum or fifth disease (parvovirus B19); and dengue (see Chapters 13 and 16). Infections of the genital tract are discussed in Chapter 7.

HERPES SIMPLEX VIRUS

Herpes simplex virus (HSV) is classified in the alpha virinae subfamily within the family Herpesviridae. Like all other members of the family, HSV has a large double-stranded deoxyribonucleic acid (DNA) genome. Two closely related viruses are designated HSV types 1 and 2. *HSV-1* is the usual cause of orolabial infection, whereas *HSV-2* is the major cause of genital infection. HSV-1 also accounts for some episodes of genital infection but is less likely than HSV-2 to cause recurrent genital tract disease.[1] More than 50% of the adult U.S. population has experienced infection with HSV-1, and approximately 20% has experienced infection with HSV-2.[2, 3]

As with other herpesviruses, the life cycle of HSV includes a *latent phase*. After primary infection, HSV becomes latent in neural tissue. Infected individuals may experience reactivations spontaneously or as a result of stimuli such as ultraviolet light, trauma, and fever. HSV reactivations are more common and more severe in immunocompromised individuals. Antiviral agents effective against HSV include acyclovir, famciclovir, ganciclovir, and foscarnet.

Clinical Manifestations of HSV Infection

The most common clinical manifestations of HSV infection are gingivostomatitis (herpes labialis) and herpes genitalis. In *herpetic gingivostomatitis* the lesions may involve the lips, tongue, gingiva, hard and soft palate, buccal mucosa, pharynx, and skin surrounding the mouth. The recurrent lesions often occur on the lips and are referred to as cold sores.

Herpes genitalis may involve the external genitalia, the cervix, or the skin surrounding the genital region. In any location the characteristic lesion is one or more vesicles that evolve through pustular, ulcerative, and crusted phases. Primary infection is usually much more severe than recurrent infection, although it is also frequently asymptomatic. Severe cases can be complicated by edema, localized lymphadenopathy, and fever and can last for 2 to 3 weeks. Viral shedding occurs for an average of 7 to 10 days but can persist for as long as 23 days.[4] Severe HSV reactivations can occur in immunocompromised patients, regardless of whether they have a previous history of symptomatic episodes.

Other forms of mucocutaneous HSV disease include *herpetic whitlow* (infection of the digits), *traumatic herpes* (herpes gladiatorum, wrestler's herpes), and *superinfection* of skin that is abnormal because of burn injury or skin diseases (e.g., eczema). In these cases, mucocutaneous infection can be very widespread and is referred to as *eczema herpeticum* or *Kaposi's varicelliform eruption*. HSV can also be associated with *erythema multiforme*. *Herpetic esophagitis* is recognized most often in immunocompromised hosts, especially those with acquired immunodeficiency syndrome (AIDS).

Other manifestations of HSV infection include encephalitis and meningitis (Chapter 3), conjunctivitis and keratitis (Chapter 10), pharyngitis and tracheobronchitis (Chapter 4), hepatitis (Chapter 8), and neonatal infection (Chapter 14). Many HSV infections, both primary and reactivated, are asymptomatic but still are associated with viral shedding.

Diagnosis of HSV Infections

Many HSV infections are obvious and do not require laboratory confirmation. Some lesions are atypical, however, especially in immunocompromised patients,

Table 6.1	Viruses that Infect the Skin and Mucous Membranes
Family	**Viruses**
Herpesviridae	Herpes simplex
	Varicella-zoster
	Cytomegalovirus
	Epstein-Barr
Picornaviridae	Coxsackie B
	Other enteroviruses
Papovaviridae	Human papillomaviruses
Poxviridae	Variola (smallpox)
	Vaccinia
	Monkeypox
	Molluscum contagiosum
	Orf (contagious ecthyma)
	Milker's nodule (paravaccinia)

and clinical diagnosis may not be accurate.[5] One study suggested that access to viral cultures improved accurate clinical recognition of HSV lesions.[6]

Several modalities are available for the diagnosis of HSV infections. The benchmark method is viral culture, which is widely available. Fluorescent antibody (FA) staining can provide a rapid diagnosis, as can several alternative methods of antigen detection. The polymerase chain reaction (PCR) has been used in research studies but is not in clinical use for diagnosis of cutaneous HSV infections. Serology can establish past infection with HSV but is not used for diagnosis of current infection.

Viral culture. HSV is readily cultured in diagnostic laboratories. The virus grows in a wide variety of cell culture types. Primary rabbit kidney, mink lung, guinea pig embryo, and rhabdomyosarcoma cells are particularly sensitive to HSV and allow slightly more rapid detection, although they do not greatly affect overall recovery.[7-10] HSV grows rapidly in cell culture, with approximately 50% of positive cultures producing detectable cytopathic effect (CPE) within 24 hours of inoculation of sensitive cells, 85% within 48 hours, and more than 99% within 4 days.[7] HSV-1 and HSV-2 are equally well detected. Typing of the virus can be accomplished readily by FA staining performed on a positive culture, using monoclonal antibodies that are specific for HSV-1 and HSV-2. Most laboratories hold herpes cultures for 5 to 7 days. Some laboratories perform typing of all positive cultures, whereas others perform typing only by special request.

Some laboratories have adopted shell vial culture techniques to increase the speed of detection (see Chapter 2). The specimen is centrifuged onto the cell culture monolayer, and virus is detected after 24 to 48 hours by an antigen detection technique such as FA staining or enzyme immunoassay (EIA). The sensitivity of these techniques is probably comparable to conventional culture, with individual laboratories reporting comparable,[11] decreased,[12] or increased[13] sensitivity.

An innovative genetically engineered cell line was developed by Stabell and Olivo[14] specifically for the detection of HSV (see Figure 1–5). The commercial version of the system, called ELVIS (Diagnostic Hybrids, Athens, Oh), has been adopted by a number of laboratories. The sensitivity has been shown to be comparable to that of conventional viral culture.[15] The advantage of this system compared with conventional viral culture is that detection is performed 1 day after inoculation, allowing all results to be reported within 1 to 2 days of receipt in the laboratory.

Regardless of the method used, the sensitivity of a culture for HSV depends on several factors that affect the quality of the specimen, including the stage of the lesion, the amount of material obtained, the type of swab used, and the conditions of transport. The amount

of infectious virus is higher in primary infections compared with reactivated infections. Also, the viral titer is highest in fresh vesicular lesions and decreases progressively as lesions evolve.[16-18] In one study, culture was estimated to have an overall sensitivity of 80% for patients with genital HSV. Sensitivity was higher with primary versus recurrent infections and with vesicular versus pustular or ulcerative lesions.[19] In another study, HSV culture was positive in 77% of women with first episodes of genital HSV and in 47% of women with recurrent infections.[6] Studies with PCR confirm that viral culture is not always positive when HSV is present, especially when lesions are crusted.[5, 20]

The sensitivity of culture depends greatly on how the specimen is obtained and handled. Vesicular fluid is rich in virus and should be submitted whenever possible. Unopened vesicles can be aspirated with a tuberculin syringe and the material expelled into a vial of viral transport media. To maximize the recovery of infectious material, the needle and syringe should also be rinsed by drawing up a small volume of viral transport media and expelling it back into the vial. Alternatively, the lesion to be cultured can be unroofed with a scalpel blade. A cotton, Dacron, or rayon swab is then used to soak up vesicular fluid and to rub the base of the lesion vigorously. Calcium alginate swabs should not be used because this material is inhibitory to HSV.[21] The swab should be placed in viral transport media and sent promptly to the laboratory. For ulcerative lesions, the base of the lesion should be vigorously swabbed and the swab placed in viral transport media. Extensive exudative debris should be removed by washing with sterile saline or water.

Tzanck smear. The Tzanck smear is a rapid method for establishing the presence of HSV or varicella-zoster virus (VZV). A scraping is made from the base of a lesion using a scalpel blade and placed on a glass microscope slide. The slide is stained using any of a variety of stains, including Wright's, Giemsa, Papanicolaou, or Sedi. The presence of multinucleated giant cells or intranuclear inclusions indicates HSV or VZV (see Figure 1–6, A). Intranuclear inclusions are visible only if the staining technique includes eosin.

The Tzanck smear is specific if carried out by a trained observer but is considerably less sensitive than viral culture or FA staining for the detection of HSV.[22-24] Also, it does not differentiate between HSV and VZV. Its main advantage is convenience; it can be performed rapidly with only a microscope.

Fluorescent antibody staining. Rapid diagnosis and typing of HSV infection can be achieved using FA staining of material prepared from clinical specimens. Preparation of specimens for FA staining varies among laboratories. Some laboratories request that clinicians prepare a slide by scraping or swabbing material from the base of a lesion and placing it on a glass microscope slide, which is then air-dried and fixed with acetone. Other laboratories prefer to prepare slides themselves from material submitted in viral transport media. The inoculated material is centrifuged, and the pellet is used to prepare slides for staining.

The performance of FA staining compared with culture depends greatly on the quality of the specimen submitted. The method detects cell-associated viral antigens, and therefore adequate cellular material must be present to achieve high sensitivity. Reported sensitivity has ranged from 70% to 100%.[18, 19, 25-31] The use of cytocentrifugation to prepare slides in the laboratory from swab specimens submitted in viral transport media was recently reported to increase sensitivity.[32] As with viral culture, the sensitivity is affected by the quality of the specimen and by the stage of the lesion, with progressively lower sensitivity with increasing stage and age of the lesion.[18]

A disadvantage of FA staining for HSV is that 10% to 30% of specimens tend to have an inadequate number of cells for adequate examination. Obtaining an adequate specimen may be particularly difficult from mouth lesions in children and from cervical specimens.

The specificity of FA staining can be very high with experienced laboratory personnel.[18, 19, 26-29, 32-34] Inexperienced personnel can be confused by nonspecific staining of cellular debris that may be present in skin specimens.

Other antigen detection methods. EIA can be used to detect HSV in clinical specimens. Most EIAs have been less sensitive than culture. One commercially available EIA called *HerpChek* (Dupont Medical Products, Boston) is licensed by the Food and Drug Administration (FDA) for the detection of HSV antigen in clinical specimens without the need for culture backup. The assay is a sandwich EIA performed in a 96-well microtiter tray (see Figure 1–8). It uses a polyclonal rabbit capture antibody, a biotinylated mouse monoclonal detector antibody, streptavidin–horseradish peroxidase, and a chromogenic substrate to detect HSV antigen. The assay detects both HSV-1 and HSV-2. The manufacturer claims a sensitivity of 95.6% and a specificity of 100% for HerpChek compared with culture. The assay requires approximately 5 hours to perform.

The HerpChek specimen should be collected using the manufacturer's collection and transport pack (Herptran). Specimens collected in certain other transport media certified by the manufacturer can also be tested provided they were collected using cotton- or dacron-tipped swabs with plastic shafts. The viral transport media is treated with a concentrated lysis solution (Herptran Concentrate) before performance of the assay.[35]

Independent evaluations of the HerpChek assay suggest that its sensitivity compared with viral culture depends on the stage of disease. For symptomatic lesions, HerpChek's sensitivity appears to be comparable to that of culture.[25, 36, 37] For crusted lesions, its sensitivity exceeds that of culture, most likely because viral antigen persists after infectious viral particles have disappeared.[37] For asymptomatic individuals, however, HerpChek is less sensitive than culture, consistent with the finding that it is 10- to 100-fold less sensitive in detecting dilutions of a stock virus.[36]

Nucleic acid detection. PCR assays for HSV DNA have been used to detect mucocutaneous HSV, with sensitivity exceeding that of culture.[5, 20, 38, 39] In patients with recurrent HSV who were followed with serial culture and PCR, specimens positive for PCR tended to occur in temporal clusters, suggesting that episodes of reactivation were being detected and that detection of HSV DNA on a mucosal swab indicates recent replication and release of HSV DNA from mucosal epithelial cells.[20] The relationship between PCR positivity and infectivity, however, is not yet known. A multiplex PCR that simultaneously detects the DNAs of HSV, *Treponema pallidum*, and *Haemophilus ducreyi* has been developed for the evaluation of patients with genital ulcer disease.[39] Currently, PCR assays for the detection of HSV from cutaneous lesions are developmental and are not in routine use in diagnostic virology laboratories.

The *hybrid capture assay* (Digene Corporation, Beltsville, Md) does not amplify the target DNA but amplifies the detection signal (see Chapter 1). In one preliminary study this assay was used to detect HSV DNA and was more sensitive than viral culture.[40] The analytic limit of detection was 5×10^3 to 1×10^4 virions per assay. Nonamplification assays for direct detection of HSV DNA in clinical specimens have been evaluated[41] but are not in widespread use.

Serology. Serology has little use in the diagnosis of currently active HSV infection because culture and antigen detection methods provide rapid direct evidence of infection. Serologic tests have been used in research studies of the epidemiology of HSV and are occasionally useful in unusual clinical situations.

Methods that have been used to measure HSV antibodies (anti-HSV) include complement fixation, neutralization, EIA, and Western blot. Individuals with primary infection are negative for anti-HSV at the time that lesions develop, and they subsequently develop HSV-specific immunoglobulin G (IgG) and immunoglobulin M (IgM) during the next 1 to 2 weeks. Individuals with reactivated infection have HSV-specific IgG at the time of onset and may or may not experience an increase in antibody level as the infection evolves. HSV-specific IgM is detectable in some episodes of reactivation.[16, 17, 42] Thus the presence of HSV-specific IgM is not a reliable indicator of primary infection. Increases in HSV antibodies can also occur as a result of infection with other herpesviruses, especially VZV.[43]

Extensive antigenic cross-reactivity exists between

HSV-1 and HSV-2. Until recently, serologic tests did not provide accurate information about whether a seropositive individual had been infected with HSV-1, HSV-2, or both viruses.[44] Western blot assays have been developed that can provide this information.[45] In addition, EIAs using the HSV glycoprotein G (gG) are under development. The antibody response to gG is highly specific, and gG-based assays can accurately determine whether individuals have past infection with HSV-1 and/or HSV-2[45-47] (see Chapter 7).

VARICELLA-ZOSTER VIRUS

As with HSV, VZV is a member of the alphavirinae subfamily within the family Herpesviridae. Also like HSV, the VZV life cycle includes acute primary infection, latent infection, and reactivation. The primary infection is known as *chickenpox* or *varicella*, and the reactivated form is known as *shingles* or *zoster*. More than 90% of individuals in the United States and other countries in temperate zones become infected with VZV during childhood. Most of these infections are evident as chickenpox, but some are unrecognized or asymptomatic. After primary infection the virus becomes latent in dorsal root ganglia. Approximately 15% of individuals subsequently experience one or more episodes of zoster, often later in adult life. The virus spreads through the respiratory route and is highly contagious.

Clinical Manifestations of VZV Infection

Primary infection, or chickenpox, occurs most often in children 1 to 10 years old. Infection in adolescents and adults is more serious, with higher rates of complications, hospitalization, and death.

The most important findings in uncomplicated infection include low to moderate fever and malaise. Characteristic vesicular lesions typically begin on the face and scalp and spread to involve the body and extremities. Lesions can be maculopapular or vesicular at onset and evolve through pustular and crusted ulcerative phases. The uncomplicated illness lasts 3 to 7 days. Important complications include secondary bacterial skin infection, pneumonia, and encephalitis. Reye's syndrome was a feared sequela of varicella in the past but has become rare since its association with salicylates was recognized.

Zoster occurs years after an episode of chickenpox and typically involves a single dermatome. Lesions persist for 1 to 2 weeks and may be accompanied by pain, which can persist after the skin lesions are healed (*postherpetic neuralgia*). Both varicella and zoster can be much more severe in immunocompromised individuals.

Licensed treatments for zoster include acyclovir, famciclovir, and valacyclovir. Acyclovir is also licensed for treatment of varicella. The American Academy of Pediatrics recommends acyclovir for individuals at increased risk of moderate to severe varicella, including those older than 12 years. A live attenuated vaccine is also licensed for prevention of VZV infection. It is recommended for all children at 12 to 15 months of age and for all older children, adolescents, and adults who are susceptible to VZV infection. Varicella-zoster immune globulin (VZIG) is a preparation of immunoglobulins used to prevent varicella in susceptible individuals at high risk for exposure. VZIG must be given within 96 hours of exposure.

Diagnosis of VZV Infections

No need exists for laboratory confirmation of routine varicella or typical zoster. Specific testing can be useful for atypical cases that may be confused with HSV infection or other cutaneous diseases. Techniques available for diagnosis include viral culture, FA staining, PCR, and serology. FA staining is preferred for the diagnosis of active infection because of its increased sensitivity and speed. Serology is used for the definition of VZV immune status.

Viral culture. VZV is much more difficult to grow in cell culture than HSV. It grows only in human fibroblast and monkey kidney cell cultures and typically requires 5 to 7 days before a positive culture can be recognized by the development of CPE. The virus is labile and may not grow in cell culture even when inoculated immediately into culture. Delay in transport further compromises sensitivity. The sensitivity of detection can be increased through the use of the shell vial technique, which also decreases the time to detection.[48]

The best specimen is a fresh lesion, which should be unroofed using a scalpel. Vesicular fluid can be aspirated using a syringe and inoculated directly into a cell culture tube, if possible, or into viral transport media. Alternatively, a cotton-, Dacron-, or rayon-tipped swab can be used to soak up the fluid. The swab should also be rubbed vigorously along the base of the lesion to obtain virally infected epithelial cells. The swab should be placed immediately into viral transport media and transported to the laboratory. A scalpel blade or additional swab can be used to obtain material from the base of the lesion for FA staining.

Fluorescent antibody staining. FA staining is much more sensitive than culture for detecting VZV and also provides an answer within several hours after the specimen arrives in the laboratory.[26, 48, 49] Successful detection of VZV by FA staining depends on preparation of an adequate specimen containing cellular material from the base of a lesion. This material can be obtained by scraping with a scalpel blade or by vigorous rubbing of the base of the lesion with a cotton-, Dacron-, or rayon-tipped swab. The material is then placed directly on microscope slides or in viral transport media according to instructions from the laboratory. The slides are air-dried, fixed with acetone, and stained using monoclonal antibodies specific for VZV.

In one study the sensitivity of FA staining was 86% compared with 36% for culture.[49] The specificity can be as high as 100% but depends on the skill of laboratory personnel. Staining of the same specimen for both VZV and HSV is often helpful in determining the viral etiology of confusing vesicular or pustular skin lesions.

Tzanck smear. The Tzanck smear described earlier for detection of HSV does not discriminate between HSV and VZV. Although the Tzanck smear is less sensitive than cell culture for HSV, it is more sensitive than cell culture for VZV and nearly as sensitive as FA staining.[24, 48, 50]

Polymerase chain reaction. PCR assays are available for detection of VZV DNA. They are used mainly for detection of VZV in cerebrospinal fluid (CSF) or ocular fluid of patients with central nervous system (CNS) or ocular complications (see Chapters 3 and 10). They have also been used to detect VZV DNA in air samples to study the nosocomial transmission of VZV.[51] Another important feature of PCR is that it can distinguish between wild-type varicella and the varicella vaccine strain.[52] This can be very useful in determining whether lesions occurring in patients who received the varicella vaccine represent breakthrough infection with wild-type virus or infection with the vaccine strain itself.

Serologic assays. Serologic assays for VZV are rarely used for diagnosis of VZV infection but are used frequently for determination of VZV immune status. Many assay formats have been used to measure antibodies to VZV (anti-VZV), including complement fixation, neutralization, indirect fluorescent antibody (IFA), anticomplement immunofluorescence, immune adherence hemagglutination, latex agglutination (LA), EIA, radioimmunoassay (RIA), and *fluorescent antibody to membrane antigen* (FAMA). Complement fixation is less sensitive than the other methods, often failing to detect VZV antibodies in individuals with past histories of varicella.[53, 54]

The FAMA assay has been widely accepted as the reference method. This assay uses live, VZV-infected fibroblasts as the antigenic substrate for the assay, and can test dilutions of serum as low as 1:2 without background interference. This allows very low levels of VZV antibody to be detected.

Of the other assays, IFA, LA, and EIA are currently in widespread use. IFA and EIA are slightly less sensitive than FAMA.[55] LA has been found to be less sensitive than FAMA in one study, but comparable in another.[56, 57] Lot-to-lot variation in the LA reagents was suggested as the possible explanation for the discrepant findings. The advantage of LA is that it can

be performed in approximately 15 minutes and thus can be used for emergency VZV immune status testing. A special consideration with the LA assay is the occurrence of *prozone phenomena* in serum from some individuals with high levels of VZV antibodies, causing a negative reaction even though VZV antibodies are present. To avoid this, the manufacturer recommends testing serum at dilutions of 1:2 and 1:20. Some authorities have suggested testing sera at a starting dilution of 1:4 (to avoid false-positive reactions that may occur at the 1:2 dilution) and increasing to 1:64 to avoid all prozone reactions.[57]

Serologic response to VZV infection. VZV-specific IgG and IgM antibodies appear within a few days of onset of varicella and reach peak levels within 2 to 3 weeks. VZV-specific IgM antibodies persist for several months, whereas VZV-specific IgG antibodies persist for life. During zoster, VZV-specific IgG antibodies are present at onset and increase rapidly in titer. VZV-specific IgM antibodies also appear in some cases shortly after the onset of zoster.[58] Serologic diagnosis of zoster is particularly problematic, because HSV infection can cause an increase in VZV-specific IgG antibodies. HSV does not stimulate the production of VZV-specific IgM antibodies.[58] Controversy exists about whether the VZV antibody response stimulated by HSV infection is restricted to those who were initially VZV seropositive.[58-60] Cross-reaction with other herpesviruses has not been reported.

Determination of VZV immune status. A reliable history of varicella is considered valid evidence of VZV immunity. Because 75% to 90% of individuals without a history of varicella are immune on the basis of subclinical infection, however, it is often worthwhile to perform serologic testing to define the VZV immune status of adults who do not remember having had varicella. The benchmark assay for VZV immune status determination is the FAMA. The FAMA has the advantages of high sensitivity and documented correlation with VZV immunity, but it is cumbersome and not widely available. Commercial assays are available using IFA, EIA, and LA formats, and detection of VZV antibodies by any of these methods is considered evidence of past VZV infection. IFA and EIA may fail to detect VZV antibodies in a small percentage of individuals who have VZV antibodies detectable by FAMA.[55]

Cases of varicella have occurred in individuals with low levels of VZV antibodies, especially immunocompromised patients.[60] Some authorities suggest accepting only a reliable history of clinical varicella as an indication of VZV immunity in immunocompromised individuals when deciding if VGIG should be administered after exposure to VZV.[61]

Special considerations are involved in the determination of serologic response to VZV immunization.

Serologic testing after immunization is not routinely recommended but may be indicated in special circumstances, such as evaluation of immunized health care personnel after VZV exposure. LA is more sensitive than commercially available EIAs for detecting anti-VZV after immunization.[56] The most sensitive assay for detecting antibodies after immunization is an EIA that uses membrane glycoproteins (gpELISA) as the antigenic substrate.[62] This assay is currently available only through Merck & Co., the manufacturer of varicella vaccine.

ENTEROVIRUSES

Involvement of the skin and mucous membranes is not unusual in enteroviral infection. *Herpangina* is a syndrome associated with coxsackie A viruses in which painful vesicular lesions are present on the soft palate, uvula, tonsils, and posterior pharynx. *Hand-foot-and-mouth disease* is caused by coxsackie A16 and other coxsackie A and B viruses. A recent outbreak in Taiwan was caused by enterovirus 71.[63] The hallmark of the disease is vesiculoulcerative oral lesions and papular or vesicular lesions of the hands, feet, and buttocks. The mouth lesions most often involve the tongue, hard palate, and buccal mucosa. A variety of exanthems (maculopapular, vesicular, petechial, urticarial) occur with many of the enterovirus serotypes.[64] CNS complications can occur.

Viral culture is the preferred method for diagnosis of enteroviral infections (see Chapters 3 and 13). Because these infections are systemic, specimens of the throat or nasopharynx, stool, and CSF are generally used. The causative virus can also be isolated from vesicular fluid.[65]

POXVIRUSES

The poxviruses are large DNA viruses that are members of the family Poxviridae. The family is divided into four genera (Table 6–2). The more important infections caused by these viruses are discussed in a following section. Although many of the poxviruses can grow in cell cultures, routine diagnostic virology laboratories are not accustomed to working with these viruses. Accordingly, whenever poxvirus disease is suspected, the laboratory should be informed before specimens arrive. In addition, consultation from state health department laboratories and the Poxvirus Section at the Centers for Disease Control and Prevention (CDC) is usually indicated when these infections are under consideration.

Diagnosis of Poxvirus Infections

Electron microscopy. Viral particles can be seen in material from lesions after negative staining and can

Table 6.2	Poxviruses that Infect Humans
Genus	**Viruses/infections**
Orthopoxvirus	Variola (smallpox)
	Monkeypox
	Vaccinia (smallpox vaccine)
	Cowpox
	Buffalopox
	Camelpox
Parapoxvirus	Orf (contagious ecthyma)
	Milker's nodule (paravaccinia)
	Bovine papular stomatitis
	Sealpox
Yatapoxvirus	Yabapox
	Tanapox
Molluscipoxvirus	Molluscum contagiosum

provide a rapid diagnosis. The electron microscopic appearance can be used to separate poxviruses from herpesviruses and can identify the poxvirus to the genus level. Identification of individual species cannot be made based on only the electron microscopic appearance.

Cell culture. The orthopoxviruses grow both in cell culture and on the chorioallantoic membrane of 12-day-old chick embryos. Viral growth produces characteristic "pocks" that allow identification of the individual virus species. A number of cell culture types are susceptible to orthopoxviruses, including human embryonic lung and infant foreskin fibroblasts, primary monkey kidney cells, Vero cells, and LLC-MK2 cells.[66] CPE indicative of viral growth is often apparent within 3 days. Parapoxviruses and yatapoxviruses grow in cell culture but not in chick embryos. Molluscum contagiosum virus does not grow in either cell culture or chick embryos.

Polymerase chain reaction. A PCR assay has been described that amplifies a segment of the poxvirus hemagglutinin gene and can differentiate among the 11 species of orthopoxviruses.[67] PCR can be performed directly on a specimen or on cell culture to identify a virus that is producing CPE.

Serology. Several different serologic assays are available, including neutralization, hemagglutination inhibition, EIA, and Western blot.[68] These tests can reveal evidence of past orthopoxvirus infection but cannot differentiate among the different members of the genus. The correlation of serologic tests with immunity is not fully validated. Serologic tests have also been performed for yatapoxvirus infection, but not for parapoxvirus or molluscum contagiosum. These tests are available only through poxvirus research laboratories (e.g., CDC), and require specialized interpretation.

Smallpox

The last case of smallpox was recorded in Somalia in 1979. The characteristic skin lesions have a centrifugal distribution and progress through macular, papular, vesicular, and pustular stages. Any suspected case should be reported immediately to the state health department and then to the World Health Organization (WHO) Collaborating Center for Smallpox and Other Poxvirus Infections at the CDC in Atlanta. Appropriate specimens for diagnosis include biopsy tissue, vesicular fluid, scab material, and cells scraped from the base of lesions. Specimens should be placed in a Parafilm-sealed container without transport media and sent immediately to the state health department laboratory or directly to the CDC according to instructions from the state health department. Testing methods in use include electron microscopy, inoculation of cell cultures and chick chorioallantoic membranes, DNA restriction enzyme assays, and PCR.[68] Histopathology reveals characteristic eosinophilic inclusion bodies called *Guarnieri bodies*. PCR assays are now available to identify individual orthopoxviruses.[67]

Vaccinia

Although no longer recommended for general use, smallpox vaccination with vaccinia virus is still recommended for those at risk, mainly certain laboratory workers. Side effects of vaccination include eczema vaccinatum, progressive or generalized vaccinia, conjunctivitis, and encephalitis. The approach to diagnosis is similar to that described for smallpox. Specimens from the site of disease are appropriate. Vaccinia virus grows well in a number of cell culture types used in routine diagnostic virology laboratories.[69] The laboratory should be notified in advance if vaccinia is suspected, because many laboratories may not be familiar with the CPE produced in cell culture and may not have reagents available for identifying the virus after it grows.

Monkeypox

Monkeypox is a vesicular disease of monkeys that occurs in the tropical rainforests of the Republic of Congo (formerly Zaire) and West Africa. The virus is enzootic in monkeys and squirrels in the rainforests. Human cases occur in individuals who have contact with monkeys, but human-to-human transmission can occur as well.[70, 71] During a large outbreak that occurred in the Republic of Congo in 1996-97, nearly 80% of cases were believed to result from human transmission.[72] The clinical manifestations are similar to those of smallpox, with more prominent lymphadenopathy in monkey-

pox.[68] The disease can also be confused with varicella. Smallpox vaccine is protective. The approach to diagnosis is the same as that described for smallpox. In addition, serologic testing is available through the CDC.

Tanapox

Tanapox viruses are endemic zoonoses in equatorial Africa. Human cases have occurred in animal handlers and may occur through an insect bite as well. The skin lesions are described as firm, elevated, round, maculopapular nodules.[68] The appropriate diagnostic specimen is a skin biopsy that can be examined by light and electron microscopy and inoculated into appropriate culture systems. Tanapox viruses tend to grow in cells of monkey origin, such as primary monkey kidney, Vero, and LLC-MK2.

Orf and Other Parapoxviruses

Orf is a disease of sheep and goats that can occur as a self-limited disease (*contagious ecthyma*) in humans exposed to these animals.[73] Nodular lesions that can vesiculate and ulcerate occur typically on the hands and arms as a result of direct exposure to infected animals. The lesions can be painful, and regional lymphadenopathy may be present. The lesion of *milker's nodule*, (*paravaccinia*) is similar but is acquired from contact with the teat of an infected cow.

Diagnosis of these infections is often clinical. Laboratory diagnosis can be made by visualizing poxvirus particles by electron microscopy of lesional material or by culture.[74] Orf virus grows in bovine or ovine embryo kidney or testis cells and in human amnion cells. Biopsy of the lesion reveals distinctive large, intracytoplasmic inclusions that contain viral particles visible by electron microscopy.

Molluscum Contagiosum

Molluscum contagiosum is a common disease characterized by multiple small, firm umbilicated nodules often occurring on the trunk and face of children infected by direct or indirect contact. The disease may also be transmitted by sexual contact with lesions in the genital area. Severe disseminated cases have occurred in patients with human immunodeficiency virus (HIV) infection. The diagnosis is usually clinical. Biopsy of lesions reveals minimal inflammation and enlarged epithelial cells with pathognomonic Feulgen-positive intracytoplasmic inclusions called *molluscum* (*Henderson-Paterson*) *bodies*.

PAPILLOMAVIRUSES

The human papillomaviruses (HPVs) are DNA viruses that are classified along with the polyomaviruses as members of the family Papovaviridae. The papillomaviruses are divided into numerous genotypes with different disease. Common and plantar warts are associated with types 1 and 2. Genital warts, also known as condylomata acuminata, are associated with types 6 and 11, which are also associated with recurrent laryngeal papillomatosis. Types 16 and 18 as well as higher-number genotypes are associated with cervical neoplasia. Genital papillomavirus disease is discussed in Chapter 7.

The laboratory diagnosis of cutaneous warts or respiratory papillomatosis is limited. HPVs cannot be grown in cell culture. Biopsy of a lesion with light microscopic examination can reveal characteristic histologic findings, including hyperkeratosis, papilloma formation, and characteristic pyknotic nuclei with a surrounding vacuolated cytoplasmic halo. These characteristic cells are called *koilocytes*. Immunohistochemistry can be performed but is of low sensitivity.[75] In situ hybridization can be used to detect HPV DNA or RNA in formalin-fixed, paraffin-embedded tissue; its advantage is that it can be used to determine the HPV type. Southern blotting has also been used to detect HPV DNA in tissues and can provide information about HPV type. Southern blotting has been largely replaced by the hybrid capture assay (see Chapters 1 and 7) and by PCR.[76, 77] PCR has the greatest sensitivity of any of the methods and can provide type identification.[78] Serologic assays are currently investigational and not routinely used.

References

1. Corey L, Adams HG, Brown ZA, Homes KK: Genital herpes simplex virus infections: clinical manifestations, course, and complications, *Ann Intern Med* 98:958, 1983.
2. Nahmias AJ, Lee FK, Beckman-Nahmias S: Seroepidemiological and sociological patterns of herpes simplex virus infection in the world, *Scand J Infect Dis* 69 (suppl):19, 1990.
3. Fleming DT, McQuillan GM, Johnson RF, et al: Herpes simplex virus type 2 in the United States, 1976 to 1994, *N Engl J Med* 337:1105, 1997.
4. Whitley RJ, Roizman B: Herpes simplex viruses, In Richman DD, Whitley RJ, Hayden FG, editors: *Clinical virology*, New York, 1997, Churchill Livingstone.
5. Safrin S, Shaw H, Bolan G, et al: Comparison of virus culture and the polymerase chain reaction for diagnosis of mucocutaneous herpes simples virus infection, *Sex Transm Dis* 24:176, 1997.
6. Koutsky LA, Stevens CE, Holmes KK, et al: Underdiagnosis of genital herpes by current clinical and viral-isolation procedures, *N Engl J Med* 326:1533, 1992.
7. Callihan DR, Menegus MA: Rapid detection of herpes simplex virus in clinical specimens with human embryonic lung fibroblast and primary rabbit kidney cell cultures, *J Clin Microbiol* 19:563, 1984.
8. Chang RS, Arnold D, Chang YY, et al: Relative sensitivity of cell culture systems in the detection of herpes simplex viruses, *Diagn Microbiol Infect Dis* 5:135, 1986.
9. Zhao L, Landry ML, Balkovic ES, Hsiung GD: Impact of cell culture sensitivity and virus concentration on rapid detection of herpes simplex virus by cytopathic effects and immunoperoxidase staining, *J Clin Microbiol* 25:1401, 1987.
10. Landry ML, Mayo DR, Hsiung GD: Comparison of guinea pig embryo cells, rabbit kidney cells, and human embryonic lung fibroblast cell strains for isolation of herpes simplex virus, *J Clin Microbiol* 15:842, 1982.
11. Gleaves CA, Wilson DJ, Wold AD, Smith TF: Detection and serotyping of herpes simplex virus in MRC-5 cells by use of centrifugation and monoclonal antibodies 16 h postinoculation, *J Clin Microbiol* 21:29, 1985.
12. Peterson EM, Hughes BL, Aarnaes SL, de la Maza L: Comparison of primary rabbit kidney and MRC-5 cells and two stain procedures for herpes simplex virus detection by a shell vial centrifugation method, *J Clin Microbiol* 26:222, 1988.
13. Salmon VC, Turner RB, Speranza MJ, Overall JC Jr: Rapid detection of herpes simplex virus in clinical specimens by centrifugation and immunoperoxidase staining, *J Clin Microbiol* 23:683, 1986.
14. Stabell EC, Olivo EC: Isolation of a cell line for rapid and sensitive histochemical assay for the detection of herpes simplex virus, *J Virol Methods* 38:195, 1992.
15. Stabell EC, O'Rourke SR, Storch GA, Olivo PD: Evaluation of a genetically engineered cell line and a histochemical beta-galactosidase assay to detect herpes simplex virus in clinical specimens, *J Clin Microbiol* 31:2796, 1993.
16. Spruance S, Overall JC Jr, Kern ER, et al: The natural history of recurrent herpes simplex labialis: implications for antiviral therapy, *N Engl J Med* 297:69, 1977.
17. Bader C, Crumpacker CS, Schnipper LE, et al: The natural history of recurrent facial-oral infection with herpes simplex virus, *J Infect Dis* 138:897, 1978.
18. Lafferty WE, Krofft S, Remington M, et al: Diagnosis of herpes simplex virus by direct immunofluorescence and viral isolation from samples of external genital lesions in a high-prevalence population, *J Clin Microbiol* 25:323, 1987.
19. Moseley RC, Corey L, Benjamin D, et al: Comparison of viral isolation, direct immunofluorescence, and indirect immunoperoxidase techniques for detection of genital herpes simplex virus infection, *J Clin Microbiol* 13:913, 1981.
20. Wald A, Corey L, Cone R, et al: Frequent genital herpes simplex virus 2 shedding in immunocompetent women: effect of acyclovir treatment, *J Clin Invest* 99:1092, 1997.
21. Crane LR, Gutterman PA, Chapel T, Lerner AM: Incubation of swab materials with herpes simplex virus, *J Infect Dis* 141:531, 1980.
22. Solomon AR, Rasmussen JE, Varani J, Pierson CL: The Tzanck smear in the diagnosis of cutaneous herpes simplex, *JAMA* 251:633, 1984.
23. Nahass GT, Goldstein BA, Zhu WY, et al: Comparison of Tzanck smear, viral culture, and DNA diagnostic methods in detection of herpes simplex and varicella-zoster infection, *JAMA* 268:2541, 1992.

24. Zirn JR, Tompkins SD, Huie C, Shea CR: Rapid detection and distinction of cutaneous herpesvirus infections by direct immunofluorescence, *J Am Acad Dermatol* 33:724, 1995.

25. Lee SF, Storch GA, Reed CA, et al: Comparative laboratory diagnosis of experimental herpes simplex keratitis, *Am J Ophthalmol* 109:8, 1990.

26. Schmidt NJ, Gallo D, Devlin V, et al: Direct immunofluorescence staining for detection of herpes simplex and varicella-zoster virus antigens in vesicular lesions and certain tissue specimens, *J Clin Microbiol* 12:651, 1980.

27. Goldstein LC, Corey L, McDougall JK, et al: Monoclonal antibodies to herpes simplex viruses: use in antigenic typing and rapid diagnosis, *J Infect Dis* 147:829, 1983.

28. Schmidt HJ, Dennis J, Devlin V, et al: Comparison of direct immunofluorescence and direct immunoperoxidase procedures for detection of herpes simplex virus antigen in lesion specimens, *J Clin Microbiol* 18:445, 1983.

29. Fung JC, Shanley J, Tilton RC: Comparison of the detection of herpes simplex virus in direct clinical specimens with herpes simplex virus-specific DNA probes and monoclonal antibodies, *J Clin Microbiol* 22:748, 1985.

30. Pouletty P, Chomel JJ, Thouvenot D, et al: Detection of herpes simplex virus in direct specimens by immunofluorescence assay using a monoclonal antibody, *J Clin Microbiol* 25:958, 1987.

31. Goodyear HM, Wilson P, Cropper L, et al: Rapid diagnosis of cutaneous herpes simplex infections using specific monoclonal antibodies, *Clin Exp Dermatol* 19:294, 1994.

32. Landry ML, Ferguson D, Wlochowski J: Detection of herpes simplex virus in clinical specimens by cytospin-enhanced direct immunofluorescence, *J Clin Microbiol* 35:302, 1997.

33. Taber LH, Brasier F, Couch RB, et al: Diagnosis of herpes simplex virus infection by immunofluorescence, *J Clin Microbiol* 3:309, 1976.

34. Gardner PS, McQuillin J: *Rapid virus diagnosis: application of immunofluorescence*, ed 2, London, 1980, Butterworths.

35. Dascal AJ, Chan-Thim, Morahan M, et al: Replacement of special enzyme immunoassay transport medium by a direct antigen detection enzyme immunoassay kit, *Diagn Microbiol Infect Dis* 12:473, 1989.

36. Verano L, Michalski FJ: Herpes simplex virus antigen direct detection in standard virus transport medium by Du Pont HerpChek enzyme-linked immunosorbent assay, *J Clin Microbiol* 28:2555, 1990.

37. Cone RW, Swenson PD, Hobson AC, et al: Herpes simplex virus detection from genital lesions: a comparative study using antigen detection (HerpChek) and culture, *J Clin Microbiol* 31:1774, 1993.

38. Hardy DA, Arvin AM, Yasukawa LL, et al: Use of polymerase chain reaction for successful identification of asymptomatic genital infection with herpes simplex virus in pregnant women at delivery, *J Infect Dis* 162:1031, 1990.

39. Orle KA, Gates CA, Martin DH, et al: Simultaneous PCR detection of *Haemophilus ducreyi, Treponema pallidum,* and herpes simplex virus types 1 and 2 from genital ulcers, *J Clin Microbiol* 34:49, 1996.

40. Cullen AP, Long CD, Lörincz AT: Rapid detection and typing of herpes simplex virus DNA in clinical specimens by the Hybrid Capture II signal amplification probe test, *J Clin Microbiol* 35:2275, 1997.

41. Langenberg A, Smith D, Brakel CL, et al: Detection of herpes simplex virus DNA from genital lesions by in situ hybridization, *J Clin Microbiol* 26:933, 1988.

42. Kurtz JB: Specific IgG and IgM antibody responses in herpes-simplex virus infections, *Med Microbiol* 7:333, 1974.

43. Arvin AM, Prober CG: Herpes simplex viruses. In Murray PM, Baron EJ, Pfaller MA, et al, editors: *Manual of clinical microbiology,* ed 7, Washington, DC, 1999, ASM Press.

44. Ashley R, Cent A, Maggs V, et al: Inability of enzyme immunoassays to discriminate between infections with herpes simplex virus types 1 and 2, *Ann Intern Med* 115:520, 1991.

45. Ashley RL, Militoni J, Lee F, et al: Comparison of Western blot (immunoblot) and glycoprotein G–specific immunodot enzyme assay for detecting antibodies to herpes simplex virus types 1 and 2 in human sera, *J Clin Microbiol* 26:662, 1988.

46. Lee FK, Coleman RM, Pereira L, et al: Detection of herpes simplex virus type 2–specific antibody with glycoprotein G, *J Clin Microbiol* 22:641, 1985.

47. Ashley RL, Wu L, Pickering JW, et al: Premarket evaluation of a commercial glycoprotein G–based enzyme immunoassay for herpes simplex virus type–specific antibodies, *J Clin Microbiol* 36:294, 1998.

48. Schirm J, Janneke JM, Meulenberg J, et al: Rapid detection of varicella-zoster virus in clinical specimens using monoclonal antibodies on shell vials and smears, *J Med Virol* 28:1, 1989.

49. Drew WL, Mintz L: Rapid diagnosis of varicella-zoster virus infection by direct immunofluorescence, *Am J Clin Pathol* 73:699, 1980.

50. Sadick NS, Swenson PD, Kaufman RL, Kaplan MH: Comparison of detection of varicella-zoster virus by the Tzanck smear, direct immunofluorescence with a monoclonal antibody, and virus isolation, *J Am Acad Dermatol* 17:64, 1987.

51. Sawyer MH, Chamberlin CJ, Wu YN, et al: Detection of varicella-zoster virus DNA in air samples from hospital rooms, *J Infect Dis* 169:91, 1994.

52. LaRussa P, Lungu O, Hardy I, et al: Restriction fragment length polymorphism of polymerase chain reaction products from vaccine and wild-type varicella-zoster virus isolates, *J Virol* 66:1016, 1992.

53. Williams V, Gershon A, Brunnell PA: Serologic response to varicella-zoster membrane antigens measured by indirect immunofluorescence, *J Infect Dis* 130:669, 1974.

54. Zaia JA, Oxman MN: Antibody to varicella-zoster virus–induced membrane antigen: immunofluorescence assay using monodisperse glutaraldehyde–fixed target cells, *J Infect Dis* 136:519, 1977.

55. LaRussa P, Steinberg S, Waithe E, et al: Comparison of

five assays for antibody to varicella-zoster virus and the fluorescent -antibody-to-membrane-antigen test, *J Clin Microbiol* 25:2059, 1987.

56. Steinberg SP, Gershon AA: Measurement of antibodies to varicella-zoster virus by using a latex agglutination test, *J Clin Microbiol* 29:1527, 1991.

57. Gershon AA, LaRussa P, Steinberg S: Detection of antibodies to varicella-zoster virus using a latex agglutination assay, *Clin Diagn Virol* 2:271, 1994.

57a. Arvin AH, Koropehak CM: Immunoglobulins M and G to varicella-zoster virus measured by solid-phase radioimmunoassay: antibody responses to varicella and herpes zoster infections, *J Clin Microbiol* 12:367, 1980.

58. Cradock-Watson JE, Ridehalgh MKS: Specific immunoglobulin responses after varicella and herpes zoster, *J Hyg (Camb)* 82:319, 1979.

59. Gallo D, Schmidt NJ: Comparison of anticomplement immunofluorescence and fluorescent antibody–to–membrane antigen tests for determination of immunity status to varicella-zoster virus and for serodifferentiation of varicella-zoster and herpes simplex infections, *J Clin Microbiol* 14:539, 1981.

60. Gershon AA, LaRussa P, Steinberg SP: Varicella-zoster virus. In Murray PR, Baron EJ, Pfaller MA, et al, editors: *Manual of clinical microbiology*, ed 7, Washington, DC, 1999, ASM Press.

61. Committee on Infectious Diseases: *1997 Red Book: report of the Committee on Infectious Diseases*, ed 24, Elk Grove Village, Ill, 1997, American Academy of Pediatrics.

62. Provost PJ, Krah DL, Kuter BJ, et al: Antibody assays suitable for assessing immune response to live varicella vaccine, *Vaccine* 9:111, 1991.

63. Centers for Disease Control and Prevention: Deaths among children during an outbreak of hand, foot, and mouth disease—Taiwan, Republic of China, April-July 1998, *MMWR* 47:629, 1998.

64. Cherry JD: Enteroviruses: coxsackieviruses, echoviruses, and polioviruses. In Feigin RD, Cherry JD, editors: *Textbook of pediatric infectious diseases*, Philadelphia, 1998, WB Saunders.

65. Adler JL, Mostow RS, Mellin H, et al: Epidemiologic investigation of hand, foot, and mouth disease, *Am J Dis Child* 120:309, 1970.

66. Behbehani AM: Poxviruses. In Lennette EH, Lennette DA, Lennette ET, editors: *Diagnostic procedures for viral, rickettsial, and chlamydial infections*, ed 7, Washington, DC, 1995, American Public Health Association.

67. Ropp SL, Jin Q, Knight JC, et al: PCR strategy for identification and differentiation of small pox and other orthopoxviruses, *J Clin Microbiol* 33:2069, 1995.

68. Ropp SL, Esposito JJ, Loparev VN, Palumbo GJ: Poxviruses infecting humans. In Murray PM, Baron EJ, Pfaller MA, et al, editors: *Manual of clinical microbiology*, ed 7, Washington, DC, 1999, ASM Press.

69. Lee SF, Buller R, Chansue E, et al: Vaccinia keratouveitis manifesting as a masquerade syndrome, *Am J Ophthalmol* 117:480, 1994.

70. Arita I, Jezek Z, Khodakevich L, Ruti K: Human monkeypox: a newly emerged orthopoxvirus zoonosis in the tropical rain forests of Africa, *Am J Trop Med Hyg* 34:781, 1985.

71. Jezek Z, Arita I, Mutumbo M, et al: Four generations of probable person-to-person transmission of human monkeypox, *Am J Epidemiol* 123:1004, 1986.

72. Mukinda VB, Mwema G, Kilundu M, et al: Re-emergence of human monkeypox in Zaire in 1996, *Lancet* 349:1449, 1997.

73. Leavell UWJ, NcNamara MJ, Muelling R, et al: Orf: report of 19 human cases with clinical and pathologic observations, *JAMA* 204:657, 1968.

74. Fenner F: Poxviruses. In Richman DD, Whitley RJ, Hayden FG, editors: *Clinical virology*, New York, 1997, Churchill Livingstone.

75. Bonnez W: Papillomavirus. In Richman DD, Whitley RJ, Hayden FG, editors: *Clinical virology*, New York, 1997, Churchill Livingstone.

76. Bauer HM, Ting Y, Greer CE, et al: Genital human papillomavirus infection in female university students as determined by a PCR-based method, *JAMA* 265:472, 1991.

77. Schiffman MH, Bauer HM, Lorincz AT, et al: Comparison of Southern blot hybridization and polymerase chain reaction methods for the detection of human papillomavirus DNA, *J Clin Microbiol* 29:573, 1991.

78. Cope JU, Hildesheim A, Schiffman MH, et al: Comparison of the hybrid capture tube test and PCR for detection of human papillomavirus DNA in cervical specimens, *J Clin Microbiol* 35:2262, 1997.

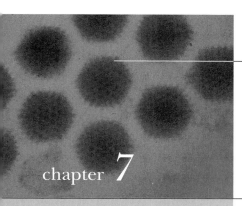

chapter *7*

Kenneth H. Fife

Genital Tract Infections

OVERVIEW

Viral sexually transmitted diseases (STDs) constitute a large proportion of all STDs. Several viruses are typically transmitted by sexual contact. Hepatitis B virus (Chapter 8) and human immunodeficiency virus (Chapter 17) cause primarily systemic illness and are not usually included with the viral STDs. This chapter considers the diagnosis of viral infections that cause symptoms in the genital area: herpes simplex virus, human papillomavirus, and molluscum contagiosum virus. Diagnosis of these common infections is often made by the clinical appearance of lesions. For some patients, laboratory confirmation of the diagnosis is important for appropriate management or counseling.

HERPES SIMPLEX VIRUS

Genital tract infections with herpes simplex virus (HSV) are quite common. Infection typically leads to the development of painful lesions on the genitals, perineum, perianal area, buttocks, or thighs. The lesions may be red papules, vesicles (blisters), small shallow ulcers, or dried crusted lesions. With the first episode of *genital herpes*, systemic symptoms such as fever, headache, and muscle aches are sometimes present along with the genital lesions. Some genital herpes infections are asymptomatic or minimally symptomatic, however, and may go unrecognized.

Recurrences of the lesions after the initial infection are a hallmark of genital herpes. Most patients with symptomatic first episodes of genital herpes will have recurrences, although the frequency of recurrences varies greatly.

The two HSV serotypes are HSV types 1 and 2. *HSV-1* is generally associated with infections of the face (fever blisters or cold sores), whereas *HSV-2* usually causes genital infections. Either virus can infect either location, however, and produce disease that cannot be distinguished on clinical grounds from that caused by the other type. Between 10% and 30% of first episodes of genital herpes are caused by HSV-1 in most series.[1]

When a patient presents with a classic history and has characteristic lesions, clinical diagnosis alone may be adequate. Many clinicians prefer to obtain laboratory documentation of the diagnosis, however, especially if antiviral therapy is being contemplated. If the diagnosis is in question, laboratory confirmation is essential. Genital herpes is underdiagnosed, and more frequent use of laboratory diagnostic methods is appropriate.[2] The clinician should suspect HSV infection in any patient with any type of genital ulcer, no matter how atypical, and consider diagnostic testing.

For the acute diagnosis of HSV, diagnostic methods can be divided into culture and nonculture techniques. Viral culture has been considered the gold standard of diagnostic techniques because it has a relatively high sensitivity and very high specificity. Most other diagnostic tests have been compared with culture to determine their merit.

Specimen Collection and Transport

One of the most critical factors determining the sensitivity of viral culture is how cultures are obtained and subsequently handled. When dealing with STDs, it is likely that a genital lesion is being evaluated. Viral cultures are usually collected on cotton or dacron swabs; swabs impregnated with calcium alginate *never* should be used for HSV cultures because the chemical inactivates HSV and will lead to false-negative cultures. If the lesion is vesicular (blisterlike), the lesion should be unroofed using the swab or a small (25- to 30-gauge) needle and the vesicular fluid collected on the swab. This fluid contains millions of viral particles and is the best source of material for culture.

If the lesions are ulcers, the base of the ulcer should be rubbed vigorously. Because such ulcers are usually tender, this procedure is often uncomfortable for the patient. Most of the virus in ulcerative lesions is contained in cells, however, so the swab must remove cells from the base of the ulcer to achieve a high probability of yielding a positive result. Dry and crusted lesions are less likely to be positive. Actively removing crusts from such lesions is not generally recommended, but the clinician should seek the area(s) still somewhat moist for culture at this stage of disease. Moistening the swab with transport medium before swabbing dry lesions may be helpful, but this has not been established.

Many diagnostic laboratories will supply viral transport medium in small tubes into which swabs can be placed. Self-contained systems contain a swab and transport medium that can also be used. It is best to check with the laboratory if uncertain. Most transport media contain buffers to maintain a near-neutral pH, and many contain antibiotics to inhibit bacterial growth. Although HSV is relatively stable in most transport media under a variety of conditions, it is best to place specimens for HSV culture on ice (or in a standard refrigerator) as soon as possible while awaiting transport to the laboratory. Specimens for HSV culture should never be frozen in a standard freezer ($-20°C$) because HSV is rapidly inactivated at this temperature.

Viral Culture

Most laboratories should be able to report positive HSV cultures within a few days of receipt. On arrival the swab is removed from the transport medium, and an aliquot of the medium is inoculated onto a monolayer culture of animal cells susceptible to HSV infection. The cell line used varies among laboratories. Some laboratories

Figure 7.1 Effect of herpes simplex virus (HSV) on cells in culture. Monkey kidney (Vero) cells were grown in culture and infected with three different quantities of HSV-2. These photomicrographs were taken 24 hours after infection. **A,** Mostly normal, cuboidal cells, with small area in center where some cells have been lost and some surrounding cells are rounded and more refractile. **B,** Larger area of monolayer is affected, with more extensive cell loss and many rounded cells and one giant cell. **C,** Most of area shown is infected, with extensive cell loss and almost universal rounding of remaining cells.

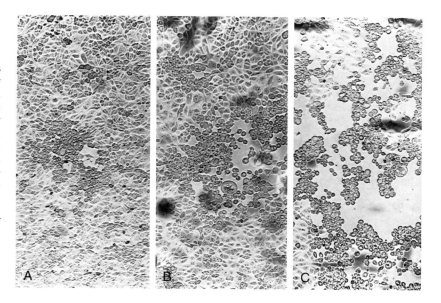

use monkey kidney cells, and others use one of several types of human epithelial or fibroblast cells. Because HSV will grow in a variety of mammalian cells, several different cell types are appropriate. Although small differences may exist in sensitivity of different cell types to detection of HSV growth, most laboratories have systems in place to optimize the detection of HSV in their particular culture setup.

HSV cultures are frequently observed for microscopic evidence of viral growth, often daily. Typical cytopathic changes consistent with HSV infection are easily recognized under the microscope (Figure 7–1). When cytopathic changes suggestive of HSV are detected, a portion of the culture may be stained with antibodies to HSV to confirm the identification, although this step is omitted in some laboratories when the cytopathic effect is very clear cut. In most laboratories, type-specific monoclonal antibodies are used to provide information about HSV type as well. In some laboratories, typing is not performed routinely and must be specifically requested. When observed daily, many HSV cultures become positive within 48 to 72 hours. Some laboratories do not observe the cultures as frequently but routinely stain cultures at fixed times (e.g., at 3 and 5 days) for evidence of HSV. Most laboratories observe HSV cultures for 5 to 10 days before signing them out as negative.

Modified culture procedures for HSV are also widely used (see Chapters 1 and 6). These procedures (e.g., shell vial culture) involve inoculation of the specimen into cell culture followed by a procedure to detect the production of a HSV-specific antigen using fluorescent antibody (FA) staining or enzyme immunoassay (EIA). The antigen detection is done at a fixed time after inoculation, most often 1 or 2 days. The ELVIS system (Diagnostic Hybrids, Athens, Oh) consists of a geneti-

cally engineered cell line that detects a specific HSV protein in the specimen. The advantage of all these systems is that they provide a final answer as the procedure is carried out, usually in 1 or 2 days.

Cytologic and Immunologic Methods

One of the most rapid and direct methods for diagnosing HSV infections is microscopic examination of lesion material. Cells are removed from the base of a lesion (usually an ulcer) with either a swab or a scalpel blade and placed on a microscope slide. The slide is stained (Wright's, Giemsa) and examined for typical cytologic changes (Tzanck smear).[3, 4] Alternatively, the slide can be stained with fluorescein-conjugated antibody to HSV and examined by immunofluorescent microscopy. Both methods are rapid, but both require some equipment and a significant amount of experience in interpreting the tests.

The sensitivity of these tests ranges from 60% to 80% compared with viral culture, with FA staining generally considered more sensitive than the Tzanck smear[5] (see also Chapters 1 and 6).

DNA Amplification Methods

The development of the polymerase chain reaction (PCR) method[6] has led to PCR-based tests for many different infectious agents, including HSV. As with many infectious agents, however, currently no standardized, quality-controlled PCR assay for HSV exists that can be run by different laboratories to obtain consistent results. Several groups have reported taking advantage of the high sensitivity of PCR to detect HSV deoxyribonucleic acid (DNA) in a variety of clinical settings. Examples include detection of HSV in the genital tract of pregnant women[7, 8] or in the spinal fluid of patients with herpes encephalitis.[9] Others study the dynamics of asymptomatic HSV shedding in patients with a history of recurrent genital herpes.[10, 11] PCR-based assays for HSV are more sensitive than culture.[10, 12] The specificity is very high provided laboratory conditions are carefully controlled to avoid contamination of specimens with previously amplified DNA. The PCR assay can be done relatively quickly, with turnaround times similar to or faster than viral culture.

As PCR-based assays become more common in routine diagnostic laboratories, standardized PCR assays for HSV likely will be developed and used more often. Specimens similar to those collected for HSV culture are usually sufficient for PCR assays, although the transport medium may be different. Some PCR systems are inhibited by the presence of red blood cells in the assay, so care should be taken to avoid induction of bleeding during specimen collection.

Serology

Serologic diagnosis is a mainstay for many viral infections, but serology for HSV has not been helpful in most clinical settings. Substantial serologic cross-reactivity occurs between HSV-1 and HSV-2, and none of the tests commercially available reliably distinguishes between reactivity to the two HSV types (even though many laboratories report type-specific results).[13] The clinician must know the exact method used by their usual laboratory to determine if adequate HSV serologic testing is available to them.

The most extensively evaluated test available for measuring type-specific HSV antibodies is the *Western blot assay*,[14] which has been neither commercialized nor widely distributed. A few reference laboratories perform this assay, but most do not. Western blot has not been approved by the U.S. Food and Drug Administration (FDA) for sale as a diagnostic test.

Newer assays using recombinant HSV proteins have been developed, and some may become commercialized and widely available in the future.[14, 15] Figure 7–2 shows an immunoassay that is easily performed, is easily interpreted, and compares favorably with Western blot.[16]

When reliable, type-specific HSV serologic testing becomes available, it will have limited usefulness. Serologic assays for HSV are rarely helpful in the setting of an acute illness. Because antibodies to HSV develop slowly (over weeks to months) after acquisition of genital herpes,[17] patients are usually antibody negative for the infecting HSV type during their first episode of genital herpes. Antibody testing is only helpful if conversion from negative to positive can be docu-

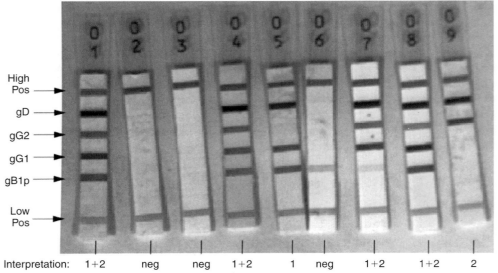

Figure 7.2   Strip HSV immunoassay (RIBA, Bayer Diagnostics, Emeryville, Calif). Premade strips are supplied with several recombinant HSV proteins: glycoprotein D (*gD*), which is broadly cross-reactive between HSV types, and glycoprotein G of HSV-2 (*gG2*), glycoprotein G of HSV-1 (*gG1*), and a peptide fragment of glycoprotein B of HSV-1 (*gB1p*), all of which contain type-specific epitopes. Two quantities of antibody to human IgG are also placed on the strip as positive controls and must react for test to be interpretable. To be considered positive for HSV antibody, gD band must react at least as strongly as low-positive control. Type-specificity is determined by type-specific bands that also react. Because some individuals do not form antibody to gG1 after HSV-1 infection, gB1p band is also included. Reaction to either (or both) bands is considered reactive for HSV-1. Occasional samples (<2%, author's observations) will react to gD but not to any type-specific band. These sera are considered positive but untypable.

mented between serum collected at the time of the acute illness and one obtained 3 to 6 weeks later. This type of evidence may be helpful if cultures are negative or cannot be obtained.

HSV antibody testing also may be helpful in a patient with a clinical history suggestive of recurrent genital herpes who has never had a positive HSV culture during a clinical episode. Because genital HSV-2 infection is much more likely to recur than genital HSV-1 infection,[18] the presence of antibody to HSV-2 and a compatible clinical history would be strong presumptive evidence that the disease was recurrent genital herpes, whereas the absence of any HSV antibody would argue strongly against that diagnosis. The presence of only HSV-1 antibody would be inconclusive.

Serologic testing is also useful in couples, one of whom has a history of genital herpes and the other who does not. Testing the "uninfected" partner often reveals that this individual has antibody to the relevant HSV type already and is thus immune to new infection from the partner with active disease.[19, 20] Conversely, if the uninfected partner is HSV antibody negative, appropriate precautions need to be taken to reduce the risk of transmission.

Finally, testing of pregnant women for HSV-2 antibody may be done with a type-specific assay for HSV antibodies. Studies of neonatal HSV infections have generally shown that most infected infants are born to women who have no clinical history of recurrent genital herpes but who are HSV-2 antibody positive at term.[21-23] Early identification of these women by serologic testing might be used as part of a strategy to prevent some perinatal transmission of HSV. Some studies have suggested, however, that women who are HSV seronegative but in danger of acquisition of HSV late in pregnancy have the greatest risk of having infants who may acquire life-threatening infection.[22, 24, 25]

Currently no consensus exists on how to use type-specific HSV antibody testing optimally in pregnancy. One approach might seek to identify the HSV-seronegative pregnant woman with an HSV-2–seropositive partner. This situation would present a risk of primary infection with high risk of peripartum transmission. Such couples might choose to take precautions to avoid transmission during the pregnancy. Thus good arguments can be made for identifying both unrecognized HSV-2–positive women and women who are HSV antibody negative but in danger of becoming infected.

HUMAN PAPILLOMAVIRUS

Human papillomaviruses (HPVs) are the most prevalent sexually transmitted viruses. The spectrum of clinical manifestations is broad and includes genital warts (condylomata acuminata), flat warts, cervical dysplasia, and cervical carcinoma. Subclinical infections with no overt clinical manifestations are also common. Visible lesions such as genital warts can appear anywhere on the external genitalia, thighs, perineum, or perianal area. They can also occur in the vagina, cervix, or urethra and rectum (either gender). Solitary lesions are occasionally seen, but most patients have multiple lesions, sometimes at multiple locations.

More than 75 types of HPVs have been characterized, and new types continue to be identified. Almost half of those described have been found in specimens from the genital tract. Among the genital HPVs, some (e.g., HPV-16) are often associated with dysplastic or malignant lesions, whereas others (e.g., HPV-6) are seldom found in dysplastic or malignant tissue. This has led to an informal grouping of HPV types as "low risk" (those rarely associated with dysplasia or cancer) and "high risk" (those more often associated with dysplasia or cancer). Grouping the HPV types in this manner is often helpful but can occasionally be misleading. For example, well-documented cases of cancers are associated with "low-risk" HPV types, and many infections with "high-risk" HPV types resolve spontaneously and never become dysplastic.

No reproducible culture system exist for HPVs, so only nonculture methods of diagnosis are available.

Testing Considerations

Currently, most therapeutic decisions regarding HPV testing are made based on the lesion's clinical appearance and cytology or histology. It can be argued that detection and typing of HPV add little to the decision-making process.[26] Typical condylomata acuminata are usually treated based on appearance alone. Lesions of the cervix or atypical lesions of the skin are usually biopsied before a final treatment strategy is determined. High-grade dysplastic lesions are treated more aggressively than are low-grade lesions. Clinicians assume that the condyloma will contain a low-risk HPV type and that the high-grade dysplastic lesion of the cervix will contain a high-risk HPV type.

HPV testing may be helpful in the patient with a cervical lesion that is mildly atypical or shows low-grade dysplasia.[27] Women with large quantities of a high-risk HPV type may deserve more aggressive management than those with a low-risk type.[28-30] As more studies that apply HPV testing to large populations of women in cervical cancer screening programs are completed, more specific recommendations may be made. HPV testing also could be used as an adjunct to cervical cytology screening. One study showed that adding HPV testing to cytology identified a number of women with high-grade lesions on cervical biopsy who had normal or minimally abnormal screening cervical cytology.[31]

Thus a role for HPV testing is emerging in the management of cervical disease, although specific guidelines cannot yet be formulated. HPV testing of other types of specimens occasionally provides useful information, but its role in the routine evaluation of noncervical specimens remains to be established.

Southern Blot

With no reliable culture system and thus no gold standard for the diagnosis of HPV, Southern blot is the method of choice. Deoxyribonucleic acid (DNA) is extracted from a clinical specimen and digested with a site-specific restriction endonuclease. The fragments are separated by electrophoresis, transferred to a membrane, and hybridized with labeled HPV DNA. This method detects specific HPV types based on the fragment pattern and reaction with individual probes. Using low-stringency hybridization conditions, HPV types other than those in the probe mixture also can be detected because some regions of DNA sequence homology exist among all papillomaviruses.

Despite the reliability of Southern blot, it has significant limitations. A relatively large amount of DNA is required, making it difficult to do a Southern blot on any specimen other than tissue. Exfoliated cells of the cervix (or other sites) sometimes yield enough DNA for Southern blot analysis but often do not. In addition, the method is relatively insensitive, detecting only about 0.1 to 0.5 copies of HPV DNA per cell.[26] It is even less sensitive at detecting heterologous HPV types under low-stringency conditions. Finally, the method is cumbersome and expensive and thus impractical for large screening studies or in clinical diagnosis. Southern blot is neither fully standardized nor FDA approved as a commercial diagnostic test.

DNA Amplification Methods

Because of the large number of HPV types, a relatively nonselective method of HPV identification is most useful. Despite the many types, all HPVs have regions of DNA that show significant nucleotide sequence homology.[32] One of these conserved regions is in the L1 major capsid protein gene. It has been possible to design consensus PCR primers containing a variety of sequences that permit amplification of any genital HPV type (including previously uncharacterized types) with high efficiency.[33]

Although other consensus primer systems have been developed,[34-36] the *L1 system* has received the widest use. Because of its high sensitivity and ability to detect a broad range of HPV types, this method has become widely used. Although not a true gold standard, many investigators consider the L1 consensus primer PCR assay the most sensitive test for HPV available, far exceeding the sensitivity of the Southern blot method.[37] In addition to detecting the presence of HPV DNA, this assay can also provide typing information using a battery of type-specific DNA probes that bind to unique regions between the common primers. Most series using this assay, however, still report a number of specimens that are positive but cannot be typed. These untypable specimens may represent novel HPV types or uncharacterized DNA sequence variability among known types. The L1 method has not been fully standardized and has not received FDA approval for sale as a diagnostic test.

A recent attempt has been made to provide better standardization and reproducibility of the consensus primer PCR assay.[38] In this format the primers are biotinylated, and the product from the PCR reaction is used as a probe for a membrane that contains type-specific sequences for 27 commonly identified genital HPV types. Subsequent reaction of the membrane with avidin-peroxidase and a peroxidase substrate permits easy identification of areas that bind the biotinylated DNA. By carefully manufacturing these membrane strips so that the probes are immobilized in exactly the same positions, it is relatively easy to align the strip with a reading template and identify the HPV types amplified (Figure 7-3).

Current versions of consensus primer PCR are not quantitative and provide only a crude estimate of the amount of HPV DNA in a sample. Developing a quantitative PCR assay for a specific HPV type should be possible, but the consensus primers are mixtures of different sequences and clinical specimens may contain more than one HPV type.[39] Despite these technical barriers to quantitation, progress is being made toward quantitative PCR assays that eventually may be available.[40]

PCR can analyze a variety of clinical specimens for HPV DNA. Because the cervix is the usual target organ for diagnosis, cervical scrapes, cervical swabs, or cervicovaginal lavage specimens are often used. The cells are concentrated and DNA is extracted for the PCR assay. DNA from biopsy material can also be extracted for PCR analysis. The PCR assay is so sensitive that a section from a fixed and embedded tissue specimen can also be used for HPV analysis.

Hybrid Capture Assay

The only FDA-approved diagnostic test for HPV identification is the Hybrid Capture assay (Digene Corporation, Beltsville, Md)[41-43] (see Figure 1-13). Specimens (usually from the cervix) are collected on a Dacron swab and placed in a solution that lyses the cells and preserves DNA. Purified DNA (e.g., from a biopsy specimen) can also be used. The key components of the assay are ribonucleic acid (RNA) probes for 14 commonly identified genital HPV types and a monoclonal antibody that recognizes molecular hybrids formed between RNA (the supplied probes) and DNA (viral DNA in the specimen). The test is configured to detect HPV DNA according to associated risk of dysplasia. The

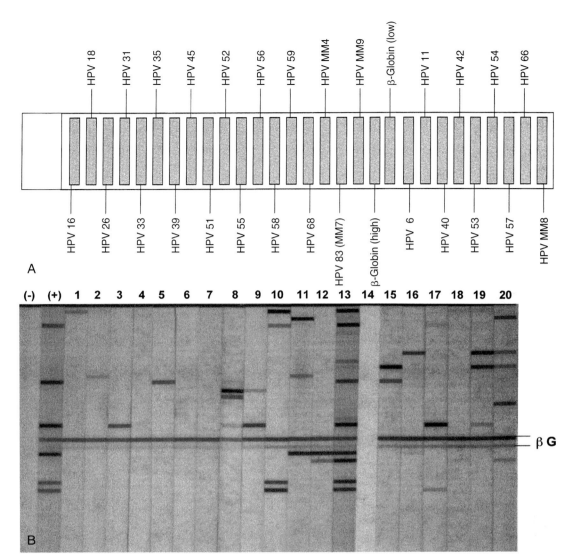

Figure 7.3   Type-specific polymerase chain reaction (PCR) strip assay for human papillomavirus (HPV). Biotin-labeled PCR products are hybridized to a membrane containing 27 type-specific probes and two control probes. **A,** Organization of probe strip. High-concentration and low-concentration probes for β-globin gene are present on strip as amplification controls. β-globin sequence is coamplified with HPV sequences in specimen. Cancer-associated HPV types are located above (to left in figure) β-globin controls, and HPV types usually associated with benign lesions are below controls. **B,** Results from assay of 20 clinical specimens for HPV. Negative control reaction (no DNA template) is shown on left (−) next to known positive control (+) that contains similar quantities of HPV types 26, 55, 83, 6, 53, and 54 DNA. Location of β-globin control bands (βG) is shown on right. Lanes 4, 6, 7, and 18 contain no detectable HPV DNA; lane 14 is invalid because no control bands are present, suggesting that no amplification occurred. DNA template for lane 13 is a mixture of DNA from 33 different HPV-associated lesions and contains strong bands for HPV types 16, 26, 55, 83, 6, 11, 53, and 54 and fainter bands for at least five additional types. Each of the other lanes is derived from different individual patients.

RNA probes are used in two pools, a low-risk group (currently containing HPV types 6, 11, 42, 43, and 44) and a high-risk group (currently containing HPV types 16, 18, 31, 33, 35, 45, 51, 52, and 56). The results are easily interpreted and provide quantitative information, permitting an estimate of the amount of HPV DNA present in the specimen. Evidence suggests that quantity of HPV may have important prognostic implications.[28-30] Because it is standardized, the assay also is reproducible between laboratories.[27, 44] The sensitivity of the Hybrid Capture assay, about 0.05 copies per cell, is intermediate between PCR and Southern blot.

The Hybrid Capture assay has significant limitations. First, the range of HPV types is limited to the 14 types contained in the assay. Although these types are among the most prevalent types found in the human genital tract, many genital types are not represented in the probe pools used. Some of these other types, including uncharacterized types, are relatively common in some series.[45] This aspect gives PCR a distinct advantage. Second, the Hybrid Capture assay is less sensitive than PCR for the types contained in the probe pools.[45] Although this is a relative disadvantage of the Hybrid Capture assay, the significance of detecting minute quantities of HPV DNA in clinical samples is uncertain. Third, the hybrid capture assay requires more DNA for optimal performance than does PCR. Most clinical specimens yield sufficient DNA for analysis by either method, but specimen adequacy is occasionally a problem with the Hybrid Capture assay.

Other DNA Detection Methods

Dot blot assays,[46] reverse blot assays,[47, 48] and tissue in situ[49-51] and filter in situ[52-54] hybridization assays may be helpful under certain circumstances, but none has sufficient sensitivity, specificity, or ability to detect novel HPV types to make them generally useful in a clinical setting. They cannot be recommended for diagnostic applications.

Serology

Attempt to establish serologic assays for HPV have met with limited success. Early studies using recombinant protein antigens were disappointing, but more recent efforts using viruslike particles that preserve conformational epitopes have been more promising.[55-57] These assays have demonstrated type-specific antibodies in study subjects. In most reports, not all persons with clinical disease or detectable HPV DNA were antibody positive, so the sensitivity of these tests may still be inadequate.

One study correlated acquisition of HPV-16 DNA in genital tract specimens with development of HPV-16 antibody and found a significant delay between the two events.[56] More than 90% of women who had HPV-16 DNA detected on entry into the study had or developed HPV-16 antibody over the 16 months they were followed. This suggests that most women may eventually develop antibody, but the timing may be highly variable.

Serologic assays are being more thoroughly characterized and could have a more clearly defined role in HPV diagnosis in the future.

MOLLUSCUM CONTAGIOSUM VIRUS

Molluscum contagiosum virus (MCV) is a member of the poxvirus family that causes small papular lesions of the genital area that are sometimes mistaken for genital warts (see Chapter 6). Although MCV is not exclusively transmitted by sexual contact, lesions on the genital skin usually are the result of sexual interaction with an infected individual. MCV infections in children usually occur on the trunk, extremities, or face and are not acquired by sexual contact.

The epidemiology of MCV infection is incompletely characterized, in part because the virus cannot be grown in cell culture. At least two genotypes of MCV exist,[58-60] but both types have been described in genital lesions, and data are conflicting on whether one type predominates in any age group or anatomic location. MCV infections are usually diagnosed clinically. The umbilicated center of the MCV lesion usually distinguishes it from a genital wart, although some lesions may be less typical and may engender more confusion. Because genital warts and MCV lesions are both often treated with cryotherapy, distinguishing between the two possible causes is not always critical.

Currently, histologic examination of a biopsy is the only way to diagnose MCV infection other than by clinical appearance. MCV-infected tissue shows characteristic inclusions that are diagnostic.[61] Molecular diagnosis of MCV will be facilitated by the recent sequencing of the MCV genome.[62] PCR assays to detect and type MCV have been described[63, 64] but are not in routine use. Serologic assays for MCV have been attempted[65] but not subjected to widespread testing. Serology currently has no role in the diagnosis of MCV infections.

References

1. Corey L, Adams HG, Brown ZA, Holmes KK: Genital herpes simplex virus infections: clinical manifestations, course, and complications, *Ann Intern Med* 98:958, 1983.
2. Koutsky LA, Stevens CE, Holmes KK, et al: Underdiagnosis of genital herpes by current clinical and viral-isolation procedures, *N Engl J Med* 326:1533, 1992.
3. Blank H, Burgoon CF, Baldridge GD, et al: Cytologic smears in the diagnosis of herpes simplex, herpes zoster, and varicella, *JAMA* 146:1410, 1951.
4. Tzanck A, Melki GR: Cytodiagnosis in dermatology. In MacKenna RMB, editor: *Modern trends in dermatology*, New York, 1954, Hoeber.
5. Nahass GT, Goldstein BA, Zhu WY, et al: Comparison of Tzanck smear, viral culture, and DNA diagnostic methods in detection of herpes simplex and varicella-zoster infection, *JAMA* 268:2541, 1992.
6. Saiki RK, Scharf S, Faloona F, et al: Enzymatic amplification of β-globin genomic sequences and restriction site analysis for diagnosis of sickle cell anemia, *Science* 230:1350, 1985.
7. Hardy DA, Arvin AM, Yasukawa LL, et al: Use of polymerase chain reaction for successful identification of asymptomatic genital infection with herpes simplex virus in pregnant women at delivery, *J Infect Dis* 162: 1031, 1990.

8. Cone RW, Hobson AC, Brown Z, et al: Frequent detection of genital herpes simplex virus DNA by polymerase chain reaction among pregnant women, *JAMA* 272: 792, 1994.

9. Lakeman FD, Whitley RJ, Alford C, et al: Diagnosis of herpes simplex encephalitis: application of polymerase chain reaction to cerebrospinal fluid from brain-biopsied patients and correlation with disease, *J Infect Dis* 171:857, 1995.

10. Cone RW, Hobson AC, Palmer J, et al: Extended duration of herpes simplex virus DNA in genital lesions detected by the polymerase chain reaction, *J Infect Dis* 164:757, 1991.

11. Wald A, Corey L, Cone R, et al: Frequent genital herpes simplex virus 2 shedding in immunocompetent women: effect of acyclovir treatment, *J Clin Invest* 99:1092, 1997.

12. Cone RW, Swenson PD, Hobson AC, et al: Herpes simplex virus detection from genital lesions: a comparative study using antigen detection (HerpChek) and culture, *J Clin Microbiol* 31:1774, 1993.

13. Ashley R, Cent A, Maggs V, et al: Inability of enzyme immunoassays to discriminate between infections with herpes simplex virus types 1 and 2, *Ann Intern Med* 115:520, 1991.

14. Ashley RL, Militoni J, Lee F, et al: Comparison of Western blot (immunoblot) and glycoprotein G–specific immunodot enzyme assay for detecting antibodies to herpes simplex virus types 1 and 2 in human sera, *J Clin Microbiol* 26:662, 1988.

15. Johnson RE, Nahmias AJ, Magder LS, et al: A seroepidemiologic survey of the prevalence of herpes simplex virus type 2 infection in the United States, *N Engl J Med* 321:7, 1989.

16. Ashley R, Alexander D, Burke, RL: Personal communication, 1997.

17. Ashley R, Benedetti J, Corey L: Humoral immune response to HSV-1 and HSV-2 viral proteins in patients with primary genital herpes, *J Med Virol* 17:153, 1985.

18. Reeves WC, Corey L, Adams HG, et al: Risk of recurrence after first episodes of genital herpes: relation to HSV type and antibody response, *N Engl J Med* 305:315, 1981.

19. Mertz GJ, Benedetti J, Ashley R, et al: Risk factors for the sexual transmission of genital herpes, *Ann Intern Med* 116:197, 1992.

20. Bryson Y, Dillon M, Bernstein DI, et al: Risk of acquisition of genital herpes simplex virus type 2 in sex partners of persons with genital herpes: a prospective couple study, *J Infect Dis* 167:942, 1993.

21. Prober CG, Hensleigh PA, Boucher FD, et al: Use of routine viral cultures at delivery to identify neonates exposed to herpes simplex virus, *N Engl J Med* 318:887, 1988.

22. Kulhanjian JA, Soroush V, Au DS, et al: Identification of women at unsuspected risk of primary infection with herpes simplex virus type 2 during pregnancy, *N Engl J Med* 326:916, 1992.

23. Frenkel LM, Garratty EM, Shen JP, et al: Clinical reactivation of herpes simplex virus type 2 infection in seropositive pregnant women with no history of genital herpes, *Ann Intern Med* 118:414, 1993.

24. Brown ZA, Benedetti J, Ashley R, et al: Neonatal herpes simplex virus infection in relation to asymptomatic maternal infection at the time of labor, *N Engl J Med* 324:1247, 1991.

25. Brown ZA, Selke S, Zeh J, et al: The acquisition of herpes simplex virus during pregnancy, *N Engl J Med* 337:509, 1997.

26. Roman A, Fife KH: Human papillomaviruses: are we ready to type? *Clin Microbiol Rev* 2:166, 1989.

27. Cox JT, Lorincz AT, Schiffman MH, et al: Human papillomavirus testing by hybrid capture appears to be useful in triaging women with a cytologic diagnosis of atypical squamous cells of undetermined significance, *Am J Obstet Gynecol* 172:946, 1995.

28. Morrison EA, Ho GY, Vermund SH, et al: Human papillomavirus infection and other risk factors for cervical neoplasia: a case-control study, *Int J Cancer* 49:6, 1991.

29. Cuzick J, Terry G, Ho L, et al: Human papillomavirus type 16 DNA in cervical smears as predictor of high-grade cervical cancer, *Lancet* 339: 959, 1992.

30. Schiffman MH, Brinton LA: The epidemiology of cervical carcinogenesis, *Cancer* 76:1888, 1995.

31. Cuzick J, Szarewski A, Terry G, et al: Human papillomavirus testing in primary cervical screening, *Lancet* 345:1533, 1995.

32. Danos O, Engel LW, Chen EY, et al: A comparative analysis of the human type 1a and bovine type 1 papillomavirus genomes, *J Virol* 46:557, 1983.

33. Manos MM, Ting Y, Wright DK, et al: Use of polymerase chain reaction amplification for the detection of genital human papillomaviruses, *Cancer Cells* 7:209, 1989.

34. Lucotte G, François MH, Petit MC, et al: A multiple primer pairs polymerase chain reaction for the detection of human genital papillomavirus types, *Mol Cell Probes* 7:339, 1993.

35. de Roda Husman AM, Walboomers JMM, van den Brule AJC, et al: The use of general primers GP5 and GP6 elongated at their 3′ ends with adjacent highly conserved sequences improves human papillomavirus detection by PCR, *J Gen Virol* 76:1057, 1995.

36. Baay MFD, Quint WGV, Koudstaal J, et al: Comprehensive study of several general and type-specific primer pairs for detection of human papillomavirus DNA by PCR in paraffin-embedded cervical carcinomas, *J Clin Microbiol* 34:745, 1996.

37. Schiffman MH, Bauer HM, Lorincz AT, et al: Comparison of Southern blot hybridization and polymerase chain reaction methods for the detection of human papillomavirus DNA, *J Clin Microbiol* 29:573, 1991.

38. Gravitt PE, Peyton CL, Apple RJ, Wheeler CM: Genotyping of 27 HPV types from L1 consensus PCR products using a single hybridization, reverse line-blot detection method, *J Clin Microbiol* 36:3020, 1998.

39. Brown DR, Bryan JT, Cramer H, et al: Detection of multiple human papillomavirus types in condylomata acuminata from immunosuppressed patients, *J Infect Dis* 170:759, 1994.

40. Swan DC, Tucker RA, Tortolero-Luna G et al: Human papillomavirus (HPV) DNA copy number is dependent on grade of cervical disease and HPV type, *J Clin Microbiol* 37:1030; 1999.

41. Lörincz A: Diagnosis of human papillomavirus infection by the newer generation of molecular DNA assays, *Clin Immunol Newslett* 12:123, 1992.

42. Brown DR, Bryan JT, Cramer H, Fife KH: Analysis of human papillomavirus types in exophytic condylomata acuminata by hybrid capture and Southern blot techniques, *J Clin Microbiol* 31:2667, 1993.

43. Lörincz A: Hybrid Capture method for detection of human papillomavirus DNA in clinical specimens, *Papillomavirus Rep* 7:1, 1996.

44. Schiffman MH, Kiviat NB, Burk RD, et al.: Accuracy and interlaboratory reliability of human papillomavirus DNA testing by hybrid capture, *J Clin Microbiol* 33:545, 1995.

45. Shah KV, Solomon L, Daniel R, et al: Comparison of PCR and hybrid capture methods for detection of human papillomavirus in injection drug-using women at high risk of human immunodeficiency virus infection, *J Clin Microbiol* 35:517, 1997.

46. Weintraub J, Redard M, Seydoux J: The comparative test performance of dot filter hybridization (Viratype) and conventional morphologic analysis to detect human papillomavirus, *Am J Clin Pathol* 97:46, 1992.

47. de Villiers E-M, Schneider A, Gross G, zur Hausen H: Analysis of benign and malignant urogenital tumors for human papillomavirus infection by labelling cellular DNA, *Med Microbiol Immunol* 174:281, 1986.

48. Webb DH, Rogers RE, Fife KH: A one-step method for detecting and typing human papillomavirus DNA in cervical scrape specimens from women with cervical dysplasia, *J Infect Dis* 156:912, 1987.

49. Beckmann AM, Myerson D, Daling JR, et al: Detection and localization of human papillomavirus DNA in human genital condylomas by in situ hybridization with biotinylated probes, *J Med Virol* 16:265, 1985.

50. Gupta J, Gendelman HE, Naghashfar Z, et al: Specific identification of human papillomavirus type in cervical smears and paraffin sections by in situ hybridization with radioactive probes: a preliminary communication, *Int J Gynecol Pathol* 4:211, 1985.

51. Gupta JW, Gupta P, Rosenshein N, Shah KV: Detection of human papillomavirus in cervical smears: a comparison of in situ hybridization, immunocytochemistry and cytopathology, *Acta Cytol* 31:387, 1987.

52. Wagner D, Ikenberg H, Boehm N, Gissmann L: Identification of human papillomavirus in cervical swabs by deoxyribonucleic acid in situ hybridization, *Obstet Gynecol* 64:767, 1984.

53. McCance DJ, Campion MJ, Singer A: Non-invasive detection of cervical papillomavirus DNA, *Lancet* i:558, 1986.

54. de Villiers E-M, Wagner D, Schneider A, et al: Human papillomavirus infections in women with and without abnormal cervical cytology, *Lancet* ii:703, 1987.

55. Carter JJ, Wipf GC, Hagensee ME, et al: Use of human papillomavirus type 6 capsids to detect antibodies in people with genital warts, *J Infect Dis* 172:11, 1995.

56. Carter JJ, Koutsky LA, Wipf GC, et al: The natural history of human papillomavirus type 16 capsid antibodies among a cohort of university women, *J Infect Dis* 174:927, 1996.

57. Wideroff L, Schiffman MH, Hoover R, et al: Epidemiologic determinants of seroreactivity to human papillomavirus (HPV) type 16 virus–like particles in cervical HPV-16 DNA-positive and -negative women, *J Infect Dis* 174:937, 1996.

58. Darai G, Reisner H, Scholz J, et al: Analysis of the genome of molluscum contagiosum virus by restriction endonuclease analysis and molecular cloning, *J Med Virol* 18:29, 1986.

59. Porter CD, Blake NW, Archard LC, et al: Molluscum contagiosum virus types in genital and non-genital lesions, *Br J Dermatol* 120:37, 1989.

60. Thompson CH, De Zwart-Steffe RT, Biggs IM: Molecular epidemiology of Australian isolates of molluscum contagiosum, *J Med Virol* 32:1, 1990.

61. Reed RJ, Parkinson RP: The histogenesis of molluscum contagiosum, *Am J Surg Pathol* 1:161, 1977.

62. Senkevich TG, Bugert JJ, Sisler JR, et al: Genome sequence of a human tumorigenic poxvirus: prediction of specific host response–evasion genes, *Science* 273:813, 1996.

63. Thompson CH: Identification and typing of molluscum contagiosum virus in clinical specimens by polymerase chain reaction, *J Med Virol* 53:205, 1997.

64. Nunez A, Funes JM, Agromayor M, et al: Detection and typing of molluscum contagiosum virus in skin lesions by using a simple lysis method and polymerase chain reaction, *J Med Virol* 50:342, 1996.

65. Konya J, Thompson CH, De Zwart-Steffe RT: Enzyme-linked immunosorbent assay for measurement of IgG antibody to molluscum contagiosum virus and investigation of the serological relationship of the molecular types, *J Virol Methods* 40:183, 1992.

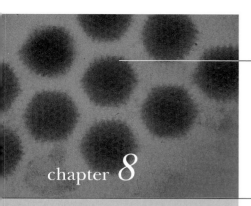

Teddy F. Bader

chapter *8*

Viral Hepatitis

OVERVIEW

Many different viruses can infect the liver and produce hepatitis (Box 8–1). Five viruses, designated *hepatitis A, B, C, D,* and *E,* have been identified as causes of acute viral hepatitis. The role of a sixth possible hepatitis virus, designated *GB* or *hepatitis G,* is still being defined. Other viruses can involve the liver, but extrahepatic clinical manifestations are usually predominant. Except for the viruses that cause common viral respiratory illnesses, the hepatitis viruses are the most common viral infectious agents in the world. In many areas, virtually the entire population has been infected with hepatitis A virus (HAV). More than 300 million people worldwide are chronically infected with hepatitis B virus (HBV), and probably as many are chronic carriers of hepatitis C virus (HCV).

The principal focus of this chapter is the diagnosis of infection with each of the five well-established hepatitis viruses, with limited discussion of clinical manifestations and treatment. (For a comprehensive clinical approach and other references, see Bader.[1])

The diagnosis of infection with the hepatitis viruses differs from the diagnosis of most other infections in that viral culture has virtually no role. All diagnostic tests are either serologic tests for hepatitis virus–associated antibodies or antigens or tests for hepatitis virus nucleic acids. Therefore hepatitis diagnostic tests are often performed outside of diagnostic virology laboratories, frequently in blood bank laboratories. Diagnosis of infection with HAV or HBV is relatively straightforward and reliable. Diagnosis of infections with HCV, the delta agent (hepatitis D virus [HDV]), and hepatitis E virus (HEV) is more challenging, and diagnostic tests for these agents are still evolving.

HEPATITIS A

Hepatitis A is an acute, self-limited disease caused by a ribonucleic acid (RNA) virus in the family Picornaviridae. HAV is closely related to the enteroviruses. It is fairly homogeneous, and only one serotype has been recognized. As with the enteroviruses, HAV is believed to replicate in the gastrointestinal tract and is spread by the fecal-oral route. Infection occurs either as sporadic cases or in association with outbreaks. Older children and young adults are at highest risk for symptomatic hepatitis A.

The clinical course of HAV infection is variable and age dependent. The incubation period is approximately 4 weeks, with a range of 2 to 6 weeks. When infected with HAV, most preschool-age children have minimal symptoms without jaundice, whereas a majority of adults experience full-blown hepatitis. The illness is self-limited, although periodic relapses may occur during the recovery period. Rarely, fulminant hepatitis can occur, but the overall fatality rate is substantially less than 1%. Older age and preexisting liver disease are risk factors for severe hepatitis A.

Diagnosis of Acute Infection

Figure 8–1 shows the temporal course of HAV infection. Viremia and viral shedding in feces occur before and during the symptomatic period but are not relevant for diagnosis because HAV is not readily cultured in clinical laboratories. The test of choice for diagnosis of acute HAV infection is an assay for immunoglobulin M antibodies to HAV (*IgM anti-HAV*). Commercial enzyme immunoassays (EIAs) and radioimmunoassays (RIAs) are widely available.

IgM anti-HAV is virtually always detectable at the onset of symptoms. Occasional results are reported as "gray zone" or indeterminate. In these patients it may be helpful to repeat the test at about 1-week intervals to distinguish between an increasing level associated with acute infection and a stable or declining level associated with recovery. In my experience, gray zone results are usually negative on repeat testing. Because false-positive tests are unusual, a positive test is considered diagnostic of hepatitis A. This test has such high predictive value

---

Box 8.1 Viruses that Infect the Liver

Hepatitis viruses

Hepatitis A (HAV)
Hepatitis B (HBV)
Hepatitis C (HCV)
Hepatitis D (HDV, delta agent)
Hepatitis E (HEV)
Hepatitis G (GB virus C)

Other viruses: encountered in United States

Cytomegalovirus (CMV)
Epstein-Barr (EBV)
Herpes simplex (HSV)
Varicella-zoster (VZV)
Human herpesvirus type 6 (HHV-6)
Measles
Rubella
Enteroviruses

Other viruses: not endemic in United States

Yellow fever
Junin (Argentinian hemorrhagic fever)
Machupo (Bolivian hemorrhagic fever)
Lassa fever
Rift Valley fever
Congo-Crimean hemorrhagic fever
Marburg
Ebola

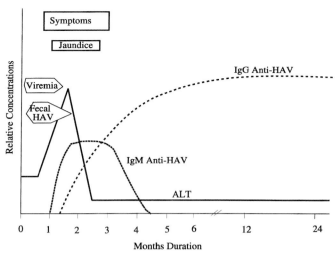

Figure 8.1 Sequence of events and serologic markers in hepatitis A virus (HAV) infection. *IgG, IgM,* Immunoglobulin G, M; *Anti-HAV,* antibodies to HAV; *ALT,* alanine transaminase. (From Bader TF: *Viral hepatitis: practical evaluation and treatments,* ed 3, Seattle, 1999, Hogrefe and Huber.)

that experienced clinicians suggest no further diagnostic testing looking for other causes of jaundice, particularly in the syndrome of prolonged *cholestasis* (defined as jaundice persisting for more than 2 months), which can occur as a complication of acute hepatitis A.[2]

IgM anti-HAV levels gradually decline after acute infection. The cutoff value used in the HAVAB-M assay (Abbott Laboratories, Abbott Park, Ill) is designed to have the test become negative 3 months after the onset of illness. IgM anti-HAV can rarely be detected for as long as 18 months; persistence beyond this time should raise suspicion for a false-positive test.

Polymerase chain reaction (PCR) assays for HAV have been developed but are of interest mainly for research and in studies of the extent and distribution of HAV in environmental water supplies.

Immunity

Immunoglobulin G (IgG) antibodies to HAV develop during the acute illness and persist for life. No IgG-specific anti-HAV assay is available in the United States; the commercially available tests (EIA, RIA) measure total antibody to HAV, including both IgM and IgG anti-HAV. A positive test is evidence of current or past infection with HAV and indicates immunity to new infection. This test has been very valuable in epidemiologic studies defining the prevalence of past infection with HAV. In the United States, seroprevalence rates are age dependent, with much higher rates in adults over age 40 than in children.

The main clinical uses for total anti-HAV testing are in travel clinics and for determining the need for HAV vaccine. Such testing is only cost-effective if the likelihood of an individual being positive is high.[3] This

applies to individuals born in underdeveloped countries and to U.S. natives over age 40 or from lower socioeconomic backgrounds. False-positive tests can occur after receipt of immunoglobulin or blood products. IgG, but not IgM, anti-HAV can be transmitted across the placenta. Thus a positive test for total anti-HAV in an infant during the first 6 months of life more likely indicates past HAV infection in the mother rather than current HAV infection in the infant.

HEPATITIS B

HBV is a member of the family Hepadnaviridae. The members of this unusual viral family contain a unique deoxyribonucleic acid (DNA) genome that is partially double stranded and partially single stranded. A reverse transcriptase step is included in viral replication. Four subtypes of HBV are recognized: *adw, ayw, adr,* and *ayr.* The subtypes do not have clinical significance but can be useful as epidemiologic markers. Although HBV has been grown in certain specialized cell types, isolation of the virus plays no role in clinical diagnosis.

HBV is worldwide in distribution and is highly endemic in the Far East, sub-Saharan Africa, the Middle East, and parts of South America. The routes of transmission are parenteral, sexual, and vertical. The incubation period is typically about 100 days, although it ranges from 2 to 6 months. The clinical manifestations of HBV infection vary from asymptomatic to fatal fulminant hepatitis. Many cases consist of an acute hepatitis that resolves without sequelae. The likelihood of chronic carriage after acute infection is greatly affected by age. Approximately 5% to 10% of acutely infected adults become carriers, compared with more than 90% of infected newborns. Less than 1 in 1000 cases of hepatitis B has a fulminant course that can be fatal. A serum sickness–like syndrome can occur during the prodromal phase of infection; many of these patients have urticaria and polyarticular arthralgias or arthritis. Other extrahepatic manifestations include polyarteritis nodosa, essential mixed cryoglobulinemia, membranous glomerulonephritis, and rare neurologic complications. Complications of chronic carriage may include chronic active hepatitis, cirrhosis, and hepatocellular carcinoma. Most carriers do not suffer hepatic morbidity.

Serologic Markers

The main diagnostic tests for HBV infection are serologic assays to detect several HBV-associated antigens and antibodies. Both EIA and RIA formats are available for most assays, although EIA has largely replaced RIA in most laboratories. Table 8–1 summarizes HBV markers, and Table 8–2 shows common HBV serologic profiles.

Table 8.1   Hepatits B Serologic Markers

Marker	Abbreviation	Meaning
Hepatitis B surface antigen	HBsAg	Active infection (acute or chronic carrier state)
Antibody to hepatitis B surface antigen	Anti-HBs	Past infection
		Immunity
		Positive after successful hepatitis B vaccination
Antibody to hepatitis B core antigen	Anti-HBc	Current or past infection
		Measures all antibody classes
		Not present after hepatitis B vaccination
Immunoglobulin M antibody to hepatitis B core antigen	IgM anti-HBc	Recent infection
		Occasionally present at low levels in chronic carriers
Hepatitis B e antigen	HBeAg	Active infection
		Present in some HBsAg-positive individuals
		Relatively high level of viral replication, with greater risk of progression and contagion
Antibody to hepatitis B e antigen	Anti-HBe	Lower level of viral replication, with lower risk of progression and contagion
Hepatitis B DNA	HBV DNA	Detectable in some HBsAg-positive individuals
		Quantitative information on level of viral replication

Hepatitis B surface antigen. HBsAg is a component of the viral capsid that is produced in excess quantities by the virus. As many as 10^{15} HBsAg particles may exist in the bloodstream. In some HBV carriers the weight of HBsAg in the blood exceeds that of serum albumin. A neutralization assay is used to confirm the specificity of a reactive assay. According to the manufacturer of Auszyme Monoclonal (Abbott Laboratories), a widely used EIA for HBsAg, all reactive EIAs should be confirmed with a neutralization assay to confirm specificity; this is desirable but not mandatory with RIAs. The laboratory should perform the assay before a patient is informed about having a positive test.

Antibody to HBsAg. Anti-HBs is evidence of immunity to HBV. Except for a small percentage of those with acute or chronic HBV infection, HBsAg and anti-HBs are not present simultaneously in serum. The EIA used to measure anti-HBs is a semiquantitative assay. The RIA is also semiquantitative and provides an estimate of the

anti-HBs level in RIA units. A more standardized quantitative result, expressed in milli-International Units per milliliter of serum (mIU/ml), can be obtained using either EIA or RIA with a commercially available quantitation panel. For some purposes (e.g., reimmunization of dialysis patients) a level less than 10 mIU/ml indicates the need for a booster dose of hepatitis B vaccine.

Dane particle. The Dane particle refers to the complete HBV virion and is present in serum at much lower levels of serum than HBsAg.

Hepatitis B core antigen. HBcAg is an interior antigen that is detected in liver tissue but not in blood. Therefore no serologic assay exists for HBcAg.

Antibody to HBcAg. Anti-HBc is detected earlier in infection than anti-HBs. Commercial assays exist for both IgM anti-HBc and total anti-HBc. IgM anti-HBc is present with acute infection and occasionally is present

Table 8.2   HBV Marker Profiles

HBsAg	Anti-HBs	IgM anti-HBc	Total anti-HBc	Meaning
+	−	+	+	Acute HBV infection
−	−	+	+	Acute HBV infection (window period)
+	+	+	+	Acute HBV infection
+	−	−	+	Chronic HBV infection (carrier)
−	+	−	+	Past HBV infection
−	−	−	+	Past HBV infection, or chronic HBV infection with undetectable HBsAg, or false-positive test
−	+	−	−	Successful HBV vaccination

See Table 8-1 for abbreviations.

at low levels in chronic carriers, especially during periods of disease activity. Anti-HBc becomes detectable at about the same time as IgM anti-HBc but persists indefinitely. Anti-HBc may be present simultaneously with either HBsAg or anti-HBs. The presence of anti-HBc does not signify immunity to HBV.

Hepatitis B e antigen and antibody to HBeAg. HBeAg, a component of the core antigen, can be detected in serum during acute infection, first appearing at about the same time as HBsAg. The presence of HBeAg indicates active viral replication and correlates with infectivity. The presence of anti-HBe usually denotes that viral replication has diminished or stopped. The e antigen and antibody markers are not needed for the diagnosis of acute or chronic HBV infection but can be useful for assessing disease activity.

Recent attention has focused on a group of patients with progressive, chronic HBV infection who lack detectable HBeAg, even though other evidence of active viral replication is present. These patients have a mutation at position 28 in the precore region of the viral genome. The mutation's effect is to change a codon coding for tryptophan to a stop codon, leading to failure to synthesize and secrete HBeAg. Detection of the precore mutation requires amplification of HBV DNA from serum by PCR, followed by nucleotide sequencing. This procedure is currently available only in research or reference laboratories.

Hepatitis B DNA. HBV DNA can be detected in serum by several means. The original method is the *liquid hybridization* assay (Abbott Laboratories). This assay is quantitative and provides a measure of the level of HBV replication. The quantitative result is expressed in picograms of HBV DNA per milliliter of serum. HBV DNA testing is not needed for the diagnosis of acute or chronic HBV infection but can be used to measure viral load. Compared with the HBeAg system, the HBV DNA assay is quantitative and is positive in some HBeAg-negative patients. It also provides a measure of infectivity in patients with precore mutations who may not have detectable HBeAg despite highly replicative HBV infection.

Other molecular techniques are also becoming available for the measurement of HBV DNA. The *branched-chain DNA* (bDNA) assay (Quantiplex HBV DNA, Bayer Corporation, Emeryville, Calif) and the hybrid capture assay (Digene Corporation, Beltsville, Maryland) are non-amplification methods that provide a quantitative measure of HBV DNA in serum (see Chapter One). PCR can also be used to detect HBV DNA in serum or in mononuclear cells. This assay is typically qualitative but can be made quantitative. PCR is much more sensitive than the other assays; in one recent study its limit of detection was 2.5×10^2 genomes/ml of serum, compared with 2.5×10^6 for bDNA and 2.5×10^7 for liquid hybridization.[4] In the same study HBV DNA was assayed in specimens that were positive or negative for HBeAg. In the HBeAg-positive samples, 100%, 73%, and 67% were positive for HBV DNA by PCR, bDNA, and liquid hybridization, respectively. In the HBeAg-negative samples the three assays detected HBV DNA in 90%, 25%, and 13%. Levels of HBV DNA measured by the different assays are not necessarily comparable. For example, levels measured by liquid hybridization were 31 times lower than levels measured by bDNA.[4] Although the U.S. Food and Drug Administration (FDA) has not yet approved a PCR assay for HBV DNA, testing is available in some reference laboratories. Recent studies show that PCR can detect HBA DNA in the serum of some patients who are negative for all other HBV markers.[4a]

Diagnosis of Acute Infection

Figure 8–2, *A*, shows the temporal course of acute HBV infection. HBsAg is first detectable in serum during the incubation period, 2 to 12 weeks after exposure. The median time for clearance of HBsAg is 7 weeks after onset of symptoms. Anti-HBs usually becomes detectable 1 to 3 months after the disappearance of HBsAg, although in some patients, HBsAg and anti-HBs may be present simultaneously for a time. The prodromal symptoms of arthralgias or arthritis and rash that occur in some patients are thought to be caused by immune complex formation between HBsAg and anti-HBs, although the syndrome does not occur in all patients who have both markers.

The titer of anti-HBs rises slowly during recovery for up to 12 months and often remains detectable indefinitely. Total anti-HBc and IgM anti-HBc can be detected about 4 weeks after the appearance of HBsAg and are always present before the onset of symptoms. IgM anti-HBc declines much more rapidly than total anti-HBc, but may be detectable for 2 years in 20% of patients. Because of the persistence of IgG anti-HBc, the total anti-HBc assay remains positive for many years and is generally more persistent than anti-HBs. Approximately 10% of patients never form measurable anti-HBs and have only anti-HBc as evidence of exposure to HBV. Why these individuals fail to produce anti-HBs is unknown, but they appear to be immune from subsequent HBV infection.[5]

The most important marker for the diagnosis of acute hepatitis B is HBsAg. The presence of HBsAg in serum is evidence of active HBV infection, which may be either acute or chronic. IgM anti-HBc is useful in resolving this distinction; a positive test suggests acute infection, but IgM anti-HBc is also occasionally detected during chronic carriage. Knowing the strength of positivity can be helpful, since the test is usually strongly positive in acute infection but only weakly positive in chronic infection.

A negative test for HBsAg does not rule out the diagnosis of acute hepatitis B, since 12% to 46% of

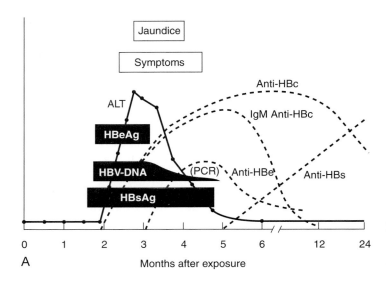

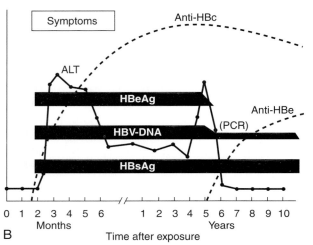

Figure 8.2 Sequence of events and serologic markers in acute hepatitis B virus (HBV) infection. **A,** Acute HBV infection with resolution. **B,** Acute HBV infection progressing to chronicity. *ALT,* Alanine transaminase; *PCR,* polymerase chain reaction; see Table 8–1 for serologic markers. (From Wright TL, Terrault NA, Ganem D: In Richman DD, Whitley RJ, Hayden FG, editors: *Clinical virology,* New York, 1997, Churchill Livingstone.)

patients may be negative for HBsAg when tested during acute HBV infection.[5, 6] In rare cases the HBsAg level never exceeded the assay's threshold of detection. More often the test was performed during the *window period,* the interval between the disappearance of HBsAg and the appearance of anti-HBs. The test for IgM anti-HBc is useful for making the diagnosis of acute hepatitis B in these patients, since it is positive during the window period in virtually all cases. Therefore the assay for IgM anti-HBc is a useful adjunct to the HBsAg assay for the diagnosis of acute HBV infection and is frequently included in acute hepatitis panels.

Chronic Infection

The chronic carrier state, defined as HBsAg positivity for more than 6 months, occurs in 1% to 95% of patients depending on (1) age when infected, (2) gender, (3) form of expression of the acute disease, and (4) immune status of the infected host.[7] Age is the most important factor in chronic infection: 90% of neonates, 20% of children, and 1% to 5% of adults with acute

HBV infection become chronic carriers. Males have a greater likelihood of becoming carriers than females. The mean annual clearance rate of HBsAg in female carriers is 1.9%, compared with 0.4% for males.[8]

The effect of immune status is illustrated by the behavior of HBV in renal dialysis units. Dialysis patients have a mild illness and a chronic carrier rate of 40% to 90%. In contrast, dialysis staff typically develop icteric hepatitis that resolves completely. Other immunodeficiency states with an increased rate of chronic HBV carriage are hemophilia, human immunodeficiency virus (HIV) disease, and Down syndrome.

Figure 8–2, *B,* shows the sequence of events involving HBV markers in the individual who becomes a chronic carrier. Initially the patient is positive for HBsAg and HBeAg and has high levels of serum HBV DNA, indicating intensive viral replication. Significant liver damage may or may not occur during this phase. The phase of active replication may last 1 to 20 years or longer.

The first step in HBV clearance involves the loss of detectable HBeAg and the appearance of anti-HBe.

This may occur at any time during chronic HBV infection. An exacerbation of clinical hepatitis can occur during HBeAg clearance and mimic an attack of acute hepatitis B, except for the presence of anti-HBe. The annual rate of conversion from HBeAg positivity to anti-HBe positivity is 2.7% to 25%.[7] Coincident with HBeAg seroconversion, HBV DNA and alanine aminotransferase (ALT) levels fall. HBV replicates at low levels during the phase of positivity for HBsAg and anti-HBe. Low levels of replication predict diminished infectivity, mild liver injury, and a decreased likelihood of progression to cirrhosis.

Unfortunately, this phase is not always stable, and reactivation of HBeAg positivity can mimic acute viral hepatitis. Chemotherapeutic agents, other immunosuppressive agents, and withdrawal of short-term corticosteroids have also caused HBeAg reactivation. Unless the clinician knows that a patient has previously been an HBV carrier, it is difficult to distinguish between HBeAg reactivation and acute HBV infection. A negative test for IgM anti-HBc is consistent with HBeAg reactivation rather than acute hepatitis B, although IgM is present in some cases of HBeAg reactivation.

The final phase of the HBV carrier state is the disappearance of HBsAg. HBsAg seroreversion occurs at the rate of 1% to 2% per year. Liver function tests and histology become normal unless irreversible damage had already occurred. The patient is considered noninfectious when anti-HBs is present.

Unusual Serologic Profiles

Isolated anti-HBc. One of the most common confusing serologic profiles in HBV infection is the presence of anti-HBc in the absence of any other HBV markers. In a series of 700 asymptomatic federal prisoners tested by RIA, 3% were found to have isolated anti-HBc.[9] Smaller studies have noted this finding in 0.5% to 20% of cases using RIA. In acute hepatitis B, isolated anti-HBc can occur during the window phase after disappearance of HBsAg and before the appearance of anti-HBs. In these patients, IgM anti-HBc is usually present.

The pattern of isolated positive total anti-HBc with negative IgM anti-HBc has several possible explanations. The usual explanation is a false-positive test for total anti-HBc. This problem has become more common since RIA has been largely replaced by EIA to test for total anti-HBc. In one study, 60% of patients with isolated total anti-HBc given hepatitis B vaccine had a low-level anti-HBs response consistent with lack of prior exposure to HBV, suggesting that the positive total anti-HBc assay was a false positive.[10] A second explanation is past HBV infection, since anti-HBs is shorter lived than anti-HBc. A third explanation is chronic HBV infection with undetectable HBsAg. This pattern occurs because up to 10% of individuals infected with HBV never form anti-HBs. This phenomenon is well recognized but accounts for a small proportion of all patients with isolated anti-HBc. For example, one study found HBV DNA in only 1 of 109 patients with isolated anti-HBc detected by EIA.[11]

Isolated total anti-HBc positivity becomes a greater concern when discovered during a workup for asymptomatic ALT elevation. For practical purposes the finding can be ignored in this situation. The possibility that the isolated anti-HBc represents low-level infection is unlikely because hepatic injury does not occur when levels are this low. For this reason the assay for total anti-HBc should not be a component of hepatitis panels used to evaluate patients with occult liver disease. The total anti-HBc assay is useful primarily for screening blood donors to help identify recently infected donors who may not be positive for HBsAg because they are in the window phase.

Isolated anti-HBs. Anti-HBs is the only HBV marker that is positive after HBV vaccine. In other settings this finding is unusual. None of the 700 prisoners described earlier had this finding.[9] Smaller studies in which testing was performed by RIA have shown rates of 0% to 7%. Isolated anti-HBs has occasionally been detected in health care workers with no history of vaccination. Personnel with this profile may not be immune to HBV. In one study, HBV vaccine given to patients with isolated anti-HBs produced an anamnestic response indicative of immunity in only 25%.[12]

Coexisting HBsAg and anti-HBs. Occasionally, HBsAg and anti-HBs are positive simultaneously. This pattern is present in some patients with the HBV *arthritis-dermatitis syndrome*, which is thought to be related to the presence of immune complexes. Anti-HBs is not always detected in these patients' serum because it is bound to circulating HBsAg. Arthritis-dermatitis syndrome is not present in all patients who have both HBsAg and anti-HBs positivity.

Response to Treatment

Interferon-α (IFN-α) is FDA approved for treatment of chronic HBV infection, with a response rate of approximately 35%.[13] The HBV DNA level has been useful in assessing the likelihood that HBsAg carriers will respond, and in following the response of HBsAg carriers to IFN-α treatment. The U.S. trial of IFN-α demonstrated that patients with lower pretreatment HBV DNA levels (e.g., less than 100 pg/ml) were much more likely to have a sustained response (defined as absence of HBV DNA from serum for more than 6 months after treatment) than patients with higher levels.[8] Measurement of HBeAg at the end of therapy is recommended, since in patients with a sustained response, HBeAg often becomes undetectable after 6 to 12 months, followed 1 to 2 years later by disappearance of HBsAg.

Quantitative tests for HBV DNA can also be used to monitor the effect of therapy, although the necessity for this is not firmly established.

Other agents. Other agents, including lamivudine, famciclovir, and adefovir are active against HBV. Monitoring of therapy with these agents when used for the treatment of chronic HBV infection has included measurements of HBsAg, HBeAg, and HBV DNA. Emergence of viral mutants resistant to lamivudine is common.[13a] A mutation at position 552 within the YMDD motif of the HBV DNA polymerase is detected most frequently. Nucleotide sequencing of portions of the HBV genome after amplification by PCR can detect this and other mutations. This testing is currently performed only in selected research and reference laboratories.

HEPATITIS C

When serology for hepatitis A and B became available in 1974, the existence of one or more additional hepatitis viruses was apparent, and hepatitis caused by this agent(s) was given the awkward name of "non-A, non-B hepatitis." In 1989, molecular biologic techniques were used to clone a new virus, hepatitis C virus (HCV).[14] HCV is common worldwide and responsible for 80% to 90% of non-A, non-B hepatitis. An estimated 4 million people in the United States are infected.[15]

Although HCV has still not been cultured, it has been classified as a member of the Flaviviridae family on the basis of nucleotide sequence analysis. This family also includes yellow fever virus, dengue virus, St. Louis encephalitis virus, and numerous other viruses that cause encephalitis. HCV is divided into six major genotypes and 11 or more subtypes, based on nucleotide sequence differences.[16] The genotypes are designated 1 to 6, and subtypes are designated by letter suffixes (e.g., 1a, 1b). The prevalence of different genotypes varies greatly in different geographic regions, and evidence suggests that the genotype affects response to therapy with IFN-α.

HCV is transmitted almost exclusively by parenteral means. Major risk factors for infection include blood transfusion and intravenous drug abuse. The incubation period varies from 2 weeks to 6 months but is usually 7 to 8 weeks. *Acute* HCV infection can present as acute hepatitis indistinguishable from hepatitis A or B, but about two thirds of patients are asymptomatic. Extrahepatic complications include essential mixed cryoglobulinemia, membranoproliferative glomerulonephritis, and nonfamilial porphyria cutanea tarda.

HCV is not easily cleared, and *chronic* infection develops in as many as 85% of infected patients. Patients with chronic infection have detectable levels of HCV RNA present in serum. ALT levels may be normal or intermittently or persistently elevated. Chronic infection may lead to cirrhosis and hepatocellular carcinoma. The rate of progression is slow in most patients, but HCV is currently the most common indication for liver transplantation in the United States.[17]

Diagnosis

Figure 8–3 shows the temporal course of acute HCV infection. Diagnostic tests for HCV can be divided into serologic assays for HCV antibodies (anti-HCV) and molecular assays that measure HCV RNA in serum or plasma. The virus cannot be cultured, and thus no gold standard exists for HCV detection. Serologic assays detect current or past infection with HCV. Molecular tests for HCV RNA detect currently active infection. Clinical judgment is still needed to combine the results of testing with the patient's history.

Serologic assays. Although HCV has not been cultured, individual viral proteins have been expressed using genetic engineering techniques. These proteins have been used as antigens in tests for HCV antibodies. The current standard for HCV screening in the United States is the *second-generation EIA* (EIA-2), which tests for antibodies to multiple recombinant HCV antigens, including c22-3, c33c, c100-3, and 5-1-1 (Figure 8–4). The two FDA-approved EIAs are sold by Ortho Diagnostic Systems (Raritan, NJ) and Abbott Laboratories (North Chicago, Ill.). Both tests are produced under licensure from Bayer Diagnostics, which first developed the HCV antibody test. Advantages of the EIA method include relatively low cost, possibility for automation, and reproducibility. Using the presence of HCV RNA as a refer-

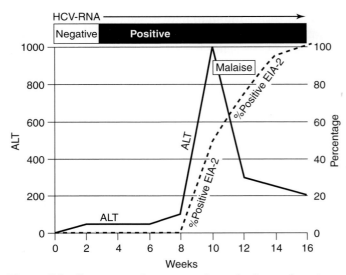

Figure 8.3 Sequence of events and serologic markers in hepatitis C virus (HCV) infection. *ALT,* Alanine transaminase; *EIA-2,* second-generation enzyme immunoassay. (From Bader TF: *Viral hepatitis: practical evaluation and treatments,* ed 3, Seattle, 1999, Hogrefe and Huber.)

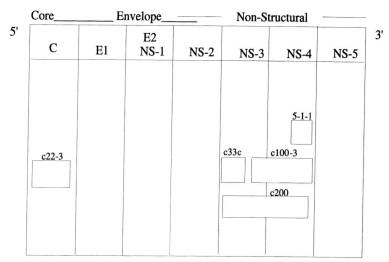

Figure 8.4   Structure of HCV genome and associated proteins. (From Bader TF: *Viral hepatitis: practical evaluation and treatments,* ed 3, Seattle, 1999, Hogrefe and Huber.)

ence standard, the sensitivity of EIA-2 is an estimated 92% to 95%.[15] The specificity is not well defined.

A *third-generation EIA* (EIA-3) test detects an additional antibody to the viral protein NS-5 that is not detected by EIA-2. U.S. blood banks recently began using EIA-3. Although preliminary studies suggest a small improvement in sensitivity over EIA-2, the specificity of the EIA-3 test has not been adequately defined in the routine diagnostic setting to justify the additional cost.[17] Most clinical laboratories still use EIA-2.

Because some positive EIA results are false positives, a method for confirming (supplementing) positive EIA screening tests is desirable. The assay most widely used for this purpose is a *second-generation radioimmunobinding assay* (RIBA). Several HCV antigens produced as recombinant antigens or synthetic peptides are bound on a membrane strip that is incubated with the patient's serum. A recently approved version called RIBA HCV 3.0 (Ortho Diagnostic Systems, Raritan, New Jersey) includes an additional antigen(NS-5) besides the four included in the previous version. Antibodies to these

antigens that are present in the serum bind to the antigens and are detected using an enzyme-labeled antiimmunoglobulin and a colorimetric substrate (Figure 8–5). The RIBA is considered positive when antibodies to at least two HCV antigens are detected. RIBA assays in which antibodies to only one HCV antigen are detected are considered indeterminate. The RIBA is not more sensitive than EIA-2 but is more specific because RIBA can determine whether reactivity is related to the presence of antibodies to specific antigens. Because RIBA uses the same antigens used in HCV EIA, it is considered a supplemental test rather than a confirmatory test.

In testing blood donor populations, the rate of EIA-2–positive results that are considered false positives because they are not positive by RIBA is 30%. Therefore a supplemental test is required in this setting. Among blood donors, few specimens with indeterminate RIBA results are found to be positive for HCV RNA. In contrast, in a high-prevalence population such as patients with hepatitis, approximately 90% of EIA-2–

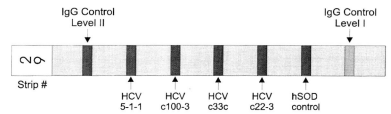

Figure 8.5   Second-generation radioimmunobinding assay (RIBA-2) for hepatitis C. A newer version also contains antigen NS-5. *hSOD,* Human superoxide dismutase, used as a control. The c33c and NS-5 recombinant antigens are produced as fusion proteins with hSOD. Accordingly, hSOD is included as a separate antigen on the strip to detect antibodies to hSOD that could account for nonspecific reactivity. To be valid, a test strip must show visible bands for IgG level I and level II controls. HCV bands are considered reactive only if the intensity of the band is equal to or greater than that of the level I IgG control. A positive test is defined as a strip showing at least two reactive HCV bands. A test is considered indeterminate if there is only one reactive HCV band or if there is a reactive hSOD band plus one or more reactive HCV bands. A negative test is a strip with no reactive HCV bands. (Figure courtesy of Bayer Diagnostics, Emeryville, Calif.)

positive specimens are positive by RIBA, and supplemental testing may not be necessary.

HCV antibodies can be delayed in appearance and are often not detectable at the time the patient presents with acute hepatitis (see Figure 8–3). In one study, only 68% of patients with acute hepatitis C were EIA-2 positive 6 weeks after onset, 13% did not have positive tests until 6 months after onset, and 2% were not positive until 9 months after onset.[18] In all, EIA-2 was positive in only 86% of patients found to have hepatitis C by research test methods.

Molecular tests. Molecular testing for HCV is directed at the detection, quantitation, and typing of HCV RNA in serum. The most widely used molecular method is *reverse-transcription PCR* (RT-PCR), but other methods (e.g., bDNA) are also used. HCV RNA becomes detectable in serum 1 to 3 weeks after infection, and levels increase rapidly to 10^6 through 10^8 genomes/ml of serum. Up to 85% of infected individuals become chronically infected and continue to have HCV RNA detectable in serum for many years.

Qualitative HCV RNA. Amplicor (Roche Diagnostic Systems, Indianapolis, In.) is a commercial RT-PCR assay for HCV RNA, currently available for "research use only" in the United States. A number of laboratories also use "home brew" versions. The limit of detection of qualitative RT-PCR assays can be as low as 100 copies/ml. Currently, testing is nonstandardized, and results may vary between laboratories. Numerous factors contribute to PCR variability, including specimen handling, assay differences, and detection method.[19] The College of American Pathologists recently began a proficiency testing program.

Qualitative HCV RNA testing may be useful in diagnosing acute hepatitis C, since HCV RNA is detectable much earlier after infection than anti-HCV (see Figure 8–3). It also may be useful as an alternative to RIBA to confirm positive EIA results. This approach is most appropriate in high-risk populations, and the HCV RNA result may also assist in determining the need and suitability of IFN-α therapy (see later discussion). HCV RNA testing may also help to clarify ambiguous serologic results, especially indeterminate RIBA assays. When used for this purpose, a positive HCV RNA test confirms active HCV infection. A negative HCV RNA test is consistent with a false-positive serologic test or with past infection in which virus has been cleared from the bloodstream.

Quantitative HCV RNA testing. Possible uses of quantitative HCV RNA testing include assessing disease activity and response to treatment. The methods used for quantitation of HCV RNA are similar to those used for HIV (see Chapter 17). A commercial RT-PCR assay (Roche Monitor) and a bDNA assay (*Quantiplex HCV RNA*) have been developed but are not yet FDA approved. Although both assays measure the level of HCV RNA in serum, they differ fundamentally in methodolgy. RT-PCR involves amplification of the HCV RNA itself. In contrast, bDNA amplifies the detection signal, not the HCV RNA. The detection limit of the Roche Monitor assay is 1000 copies/ml. The Quantiplex version 2.0 bDNA assay is much less sensitive, with a detection limit of 250,000 copies/ml.[20, 21] The Quantiplex assay may be more reproducible, with a between-run coefficient of variation of 23% in one study.[20] Serum HCV RNA levels are fairly stable over time in untreated patients with chronic HCV infection.[22]

The accuracy of the quantitative HCV assays for measuring the level of HCV RNA in infection caused by different HCV genotypes is an important question that is still under investigation. Quantiplex 2.0 has been shown to be less affected by the genotype than Quantiplex 1.0 or Roche Monitor.[23]

Diagnostic Algorithm. Because of its simplicity, the first test used to test for HCV infection is EIA. An exception to this is during the early period after exposure when HCV RNA may be detectable in the absence of anti-HCV. The approach to the patient with a positive EIA depends on the risk of the patient for HCV.

In a *low-risk patient* such as a blood donor, a positive EIA should be followed by RIBA to confirm the presence of HCV antibodies. Additional workup may include ALT and a quantitative HCV RNA test to assess disease activity. A positive RIBA confirms that the individual has antibodies to HCV. A negative RIBA indicates that the positive EIA was a false positive, and rules out HCV. If the RIBA is indeterminate, qualitative HCV RT-PCR should be performed. A positive RT-PCR confirms HCV infection. A negative RT-PCR is consistent with a false-positive test but should be interpreted cautiously because PCR can be intermittently positive. Depending on the level of clinical concern, it may be worthwhile to repeat all tests after several months.

In a *high-risk patient* with a positive EIA, RIBA may be unnecessary. Some experts perform RT-PCR instead, since it can both confirm the diagnosis and provide information about viral activity. Quantitative RT-PCR may provide further information about disease status and likelihood of response to treatment.

Response to Treatment

Treatment recommendations for HCV have been developed by an NIH Consensus Developmental Panel (Box 8–2). Interferon-α is FDA-approved for treatment of chronic HCV infection. With 12 months of monotherapy, approximately 10% to 20% of treated patients have a long-term response with clearance of HCV. Absence of cirrhosis, low levels of pretreatment HCV RNA, and infection with HCV genotype 2 or 3 predict a higher likelihood of response.[17] When pretreatment

HCV RNA levels are less than 10^6 genome equivalents/ml, the response rate is 50%, compared with a much lower rate with higher pretreatment levels.[24] Thus quantitative HCV RNA testing may be useful in evaluating the likelihood of response.

Rebetron (combined therapy of oral ribavirin and IFN-α by injection) is FDA approved for hepatitis C patients who respond either by ALT normalization or viral negativity during IFN monotherapy and then relapse after withdrawal of therapy. It is also indicated for HCV-infected patients who have not received prior interferon therapy. As in monotherapy, the viral genotype influences the likelihood of *sustained remission* (SR). Non–type 1 genotypes have a 70% to 80% SR, compared with 20% to 40% for type 1.[25]

Combination therapy appears to have little efficacy in patients who do not respond to IFN monotherapy, but more research is needed in this group. Based on limited data, SR in patients who have never received IFN appears to be similar to SR in patients experiencing relapse.

The response to treatment is evaluated using qualitative HCV RNA testing. Patients who are still positive by RT-PCR after 6 months of combination therapy should not receive further treatment. The bDNA assay should not be used for this purpose because of its lack of sensitivity. Long-term response to IFN-α treatment should be based on ALT level and presence of serum HCV-RNA measured 6 months posttreatment to evaluate SR. Patients with undetectable HCV RNA at 6 months after treatment are usually negative at 2- and 4-year follow-up and may be considered cured if HCV RNA remains undetectable for an extended time.[26]

Genotyping

HCV is a heterogeneous family of viruses with at least six distinct genotypes and numerous subtypes found worldwide. *Genotype 1* is the most common genotype both worldwide and in the United States. Unfortunately, patients with type 1 have a poor response to IFN-α therapy. Types 2 and 3 are much more responsive to IFN-α therapy. Methods for performing genotyping include the line probe assay, RT-PCR combined with enzyme immunoassay, and nucleotide sequencing (see Chapter 19).

Box 8.2   Treatment Recommendations for Hepatitis C Patients

1. EIA-2* should be the initial test for the diagnosis of hepatitis C. In low-risk populations, supplemental RIBA-2 and/or HCV RNA testing should be performed. In patients with clinical findings of liver disease, qualitative HCV RNA PCR can be used for confirmation.
2. Liver biopsy is indicated when histologic findings will assist decision making regarding patient management. In patients who are not treated with antiviral therapy initially, liver biopsy can be repeated to assess disease progression.
3. Because of assay variability, HCV RNA PCR testing must be interpreted cautiously. Rigorous proficiency testing of clinical laboratories performing the assay is recommended.
4. HCV genotyping may provide useful prognostic information but at present must be considered a research tool (see Genotyping above box for update).
5. Currently available therapy for chronic hepatitis is clearly indicated for patients who have persistently elevated abnormal ALT (>6 months), a positive HCV RNA, and liver biopsy evidence of septal fibrosis and/or moderate to severe necroinflammatory changes. Patients with milder histologic disease, compensated cirrhosis, or age under 18 or over 60 should be managed on an individual basis or in the context of clinical trials. Patients with decompensated cirrhosis should not be treated with interferon but should be considered for liver transplantation. Patients with persistently normal ALT should not be treated outside of clinical trials. Treatment with interferon is contraindicated in patients with a history of major depressive illness, cytopenias, active alcohol use or illicit drug use, hyperthyroidism, renal transplantation, or autoimmune disease. Therapy should not be limited by mode of acquisition, risk group, HIV status, HCV RNA levels, or genotype.
6. Since 12-month regimens with interferon are more successful in achieving sustained responses, initial therapy with interferon alpha (or its equivalent) should be 3 million units thrice weekly subcutaneously for 12 months. (Preferred initial treatment is now alfa 2b interferon plus ribavirin.)
7. Nonresponders to interferon therapy can be identified early by assessing the serum ALT levels and presence of serum HCV RNA after 3 months of therapy. If the ALT level remains abnormal and the serum HCV RNA remains detectable, interferon therapy should be stopped, as further treatment is unlikely to produce a response. Nonresponders should not receive further therapy with interferon alone but should be considered for combination therapy or enrollment in investigational protocols.
8. Patients who relapse should receive retreatment with their original therapy or combination interferon-ribavirin therapy, preferably in a clinical trial.

From National Institutes of Health Consensus Development Conference Statement: *Management of hepatitis C,* Bethesda, Md, 1997, The Institutes. Updated by the author where indicated by parentheses.
*See text for abbreviations.

Genotyping is important for determining duration of treatment in patients receiving combination therapy. Genotype 1 patients who are negative by RT-PCR after 6 months should receive an additional 6 months of consolidation therapy to help prevent relapse. Treatment longer than 6 months has not been shown helpful for genotypes 2 and 3.

HEPATITIS D (DELTA HEPATITIS)

Studies by Mario Rizzetto in 1977 led to the identification of a small (1700-nucleotide), single-stranded RNA virus in patients also infected with HBV. The agent was called the *delta agent* or *hepatitis D virus* (HDV). It resembles small RNA viruses found in plants called *viroids* or *satellite RNAs*. HDV is defective and requires the simultaneous presence of HBV for its replication. The HDV genome encodes only a single protein. The HDV virion consists of the HDV RNA genome and the HDV antigen (HDAg), both surrounded by HBsAg. The transmission of HDV is primarily parenteral, similar to HBV. HDV is distributed unevenly throughout the world, with endemic foci in sub-Saharan Africa, certain regions of South America, and southern Europe.

Two modes of HDV infection can occur: *coinfection*, in which HDV and HBV are acquired at the same time, and *superinfection*, in which HDV infection is superimposed on chronic HBV carriage. Clinical manifestations, incidence of fulminant hepatitis, and progression to chronic carriage differ between coinfection and superinfection, with superinfection generally being more severe. In coinfection, HBsAg and HDAg appear in the serum several weeks apart, causing two peaks of ALT, known as *biphasic* (or *relapsing*) *illness*. Biphasic illness has been reported in 14% to 80% of patients with acute HDV coinfections. The first ALT peak results from the immune response to HBsAg and the second peak from response to HDAg (Figure 8–6). Superinfection of an HBV carrier causes acute hepatitis in 50% to 70% of patients.

An Italian study compared the clinical courses of coinfection and superinfection.[27] The diseases did not differ in average height of serum ALT elevations, bilirubin, or prothrombin time (PT); however, superinfection was more severe, as measured by increased hospital time, more prolonged illness, and higher frequency of greatly elevated PT. Fulminant hepatitis is not common with coinfection but is a serious complication of superinfection that does occur. The reported rate of chronic HDV carriage after coinfection is 2.4% to 4.7%. In contrast, superinfection leads to chronic carriage in more than 90% of cases.

The only commercially available diagnostic test available in the United States for the diagnosis of HDV infection is a *blocking radioimmunoassay for total HDV antibody* (anti-HD). Anti-HD measures both IgG and

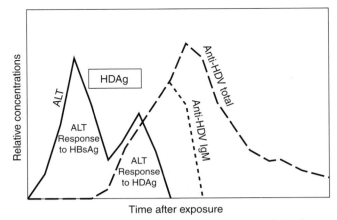

Figure 8.6 Typical serologic course of acute resolving hepatitis D virus (HDV, delta agent) coinfection. HDV antigen (*HDAg*) is detected for only 7 to 21 days. IgM antibody to HDV (*anti-HDV*) persists for 2 months. Total anti-HDV lasts 1 to 2 years. *ALT,* Alanine transaminase; *HBsAg,* hepatitis B surface antigen. (From Bader TF: *Viral hepatitis: practical evaluation and treatments,* ed 3, Seattle, 1999, Hogrefe and Huber.)

IgM antibodies, although in practice the principal antibody class is IgG. A disadvantage of the anti-HD assay is that it may not be positive in either coinfection or superinfection at the onset of symptomatic illness. In one study of acute coinfection, 15% of cases were positive at admission, whereas 92% were positive after 30 days.[28]

In theory, assays for HDAg, IgM anti-HD, and HDV RNA could be positive earlier than total anti-HD. HDAg occurs in low titer, may be difficult to detect because it is complexed with anti-HD, and may be short-lived (less than 1 week) after acute infection. Only 35% of patients with acute HDV infection have this marker on admission. IgM anti-HD can also appear late and be present only transiently. It persists for about 2 weeks, then disappears in resolving infections after 21 to 43 days.[29] Little information is available on HDV RNA. These assays are currently available only in research laboratories.

If all markers of HDV are used, only 69% of patients can be correctly diagnosed at the time of onset of illness. Thus the most cost-effective approach of testing for acute HDV infection during an episode of acute hepatitis B is to measure total anti-HD 30 to 40 days after the onset of illness.[28] Chronic HDV infection can be diagnosed simply by testing for anti-HD, since anti-HD levels in this disease are persistently high. After acute HDV infection, anti-HD persists for 1 to 2 years. Therefore the finding of anti-HD in a carrier of HBsAg is much more likely to reflect active infection than past exposure to HDV.

Testing for HDV should be performed in patients with reactivated hepatitis B and in unusually severe cases of hepatitis B. HDV testing should also be performed before treatment of HBV infection with IFN-α.

HEPATITIS E

After the development of specific tests for hepatitis A, it became apparent that another form of viral hepatitis could be transmitted by contaminated water. The causative agent was molecularly cloned in 1990[30] and termed *hepatitis E virus* (HEV). Analysis of the nucleotide sequence revealed that the virus has similarities to the Caliciviridae family of single-stranded RNA viruses, quite distinct from HAV. Nevertheless, the clinical picture is indistinguishable from hepatitis A. A noteworthy aspect is a high incidence of fulminant hepatitis in pregnant women with acute infection. Chronic HEV infection does not occur.

HEV is endemic in much of the underdeveloped world, with reports predominantly from the Indian subcontinent, the South Asian republics of the former U.S.S.R., Southeast Asia, North Africa, and Mexico. Thus the greatest relevance of HEV for U.S. physicians is the possibility of its occurrence in travelers or immigrants. In 1998, HEV was also detected in the United States,[31] but the frequency is low.

Limited propagation of HEV in cell culture has been achieved, but the diagnostic approach to date is mainly serologic. Recombinant proteins have been used as antigens in EIAs to detect IgG and IgM antibodies to HEV. Figure 8–7 shows the temporal course of HEV infection. In one study, IgG antibody to HEV was detected by Western blot in 93% of patients with acute hepatitis thought to be caused by HEV. IgG anti-HEV was continuously present in 90% of patients over a 24-month observation period. IgM anti-HEV was detected in 73% of patients within 26 days after onset of jaundice, in 50% 1 to 4 months after onset, in 6% after 6 to 7 months and in none after 8 months.[32] RT-PCR assays have been used to detect HEV RNA in stool and serum. They are currently research tools, however, and unavailable for clinical diagnosis.

Testing for HEV in the United States is currently available only through the Centers for Disease Control and Prevention in Atlanta (404-639-2709). Physicians should note that attempts to order tests for HEV from a local laboratory often result in testing for HBeAg or anti-HBe.

FINAL DIAGNOSTIC CONSIDERATIONS

In an era of "cost awareness," a parsimonious approach to ordering tests is appropriate. Testing for acute hepatitis should include IgM anti-HAV, HBsAg, IgM anti-HBc, and anti-HCV. A caution is given that only 50% of patients with acute hepatitis C will be positive for anti-HCV at the time of presentation, and repeat testing by EIA should be done in 1 to 2 months if suspicion for hepatitis C remains. Alternatively, HCV RT-PCR can be ordered if clinical suspicion is high. Testing for *chronic hepatitis* should include HBsAg and anti-HCV.

Table 8–3 summarizes the diagnostic approach to acute viral hepatitis.

Table 8.3	Approach to Patients with Acute Viral Hepatitis	
Agent	**Clinical/epidemiologic clues**	**Diagnostic test**
A	Child or young adult Contact with another case Occurrence as part of outbreak	IgM anti-HAV*
B	Parenteral or sexual exposure Arthralgias/arthritis and urticaria before onset of jaundice	HBsAg† IgM anti-HBc†
C	Parenteral exposure	Anti-HCV‡ HCV RT-PCR‡
D	Parenteral or sexual exposure Concomitant HBV infection	Anti-HD
E	Exposure in underdeveloped country Occurrence as part of outbreak	Anti-HEV§

*Rarely negative at presentation; will always be positive if repeated within 4 to 7 days.
†Presence of HBsAg occurs in acute hepatitis B and in chronic carriers. Strongly positive test for IgM anti-HBc is compatible with acute infection. Weakly positive tests for IgM anti-HBc can occur in chronic carriers.
‡Anti-HCV is positive at presentation in only about 50% of patients. Repeat in 1 to 2 months or perform HCV RT-PCR if suspicion is high.
§Available through Centers for Disease Control (see text).

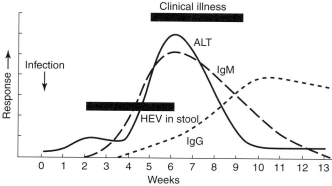

Figure 8.7 Sequence of events and serologic markers in hepatitis E virus (HEV) infection. (From Robertson BH, Bradley DW: In Lennette EH, Lennette DA, Lennette ET, editors: *Diagnostic procedures for viral, rickettsial, and chlamydial infections*, ed 7, Washington, DC, 1995, American Public Health Association).

References

1. Bader TF: *Viral hepatitis: practical evaluation and treatments,* ed 3, Seattle, 1999, Hogrefe and Huber.

2. Gordon SC, Reddy KR, Schiff L, Schiff ER: Prolonged intrahepatic cholestasis secondary to acute hepatitis A, *Ann Intern Med* 101:635, 1984.

3. Bader TF: Hepatitis A vaccine, *Am J Gastroenterol* 91: 217, 1996.

4. Zaaijer HL, ter Borg F, Cuypers HTM, et al: Comparison of methods for detection of hepatitis B virus DNA, *J Clin Microbiol* 32:2088, 1994.

4a. Cacciola I, Pollicino T, Squdrito g, et al: Occult hepatitis B virus infection in patients with chronic hepatitis C liver disease, *N Eng J Med* 341:22, 1999.

5. Hoofnagle JH, Seeff LB, Boles AB, et al: Serologic response in hepatitis B, In Vyas GN, Cohen SN, Schmid R, editors: *Viral hepatitis,* Philadelphia, 1978, Franklin Institute.

6. Gitnick G: Immunoglobulin M hepatitis B core antibody: to titer or not to titer? *Gastroenterology* 84:653, 1983.

7. Seeff LB, Koff RS: Evolving concepts of the clinical and serologic consequences of hepatitis B virus infection, *Semin Liver Dis* 6:11, 1986.

8. Alward WL, McMahon BJ, Hall DB, et al: The long-term serological course of asymptomatic hepatitis B virus carriers and the development of primary hepatocellular carcinoma, *J Infect Dis* 151:604, 1985.

9. Bader TF, T Kibby: Unpublished data, 1984.

10. McIntyre A, Nimmo GR, Wood GM, et al: Isolated hepatitis B core antibody: can response to hepatitis B vaccine help elucidate the cause? *Aust NZ J Med* 22:19, 1992.

11. Silva AEB, McMahon BJ, Parkinson AJ, et al: HBV DNA by PCR in individuals with anti-HBc as the only marker of hepatitis B virus infection, *Hepatology* 16(suppl): 65A, 1992.

12. Kessler HA, Harris AA, Payne JA, et al: Antibodies to hepatitis B surface antigen as the sole hepatitis B marker in hospital personnel, *Ann Intern Med* 103:21, 1985.

13. Perrillo RP, Schiff ER, Davis GL, et al: A randomized, controlled trial of interferon alfa-2b alone and after prednisone withdrawal for the treatment of chronic hepatitis B: the Hepatitis Interventional Therapy Group, *N Engl J Med* 323:295, 1990.

13a. Dusheiko G: Lamivudine treatment of chronic hepatitis B, *Rev Med Virol* 8:153, 1998.

14. Choo QL, Kuo G, Weiner AJ, et al: Isolation of a cDNA clone derived from a blood-borne non-A, non-B viral hepatitis genome, *Science* 244:359, 1989.

15. National Institutes of Health Consensus Development Conference Statement: *Management of hepatitis C,* http://consensus.nih.com, Bethesda, Md, 1997, The Institutes.

16. McOmish F, Yap PL, Dow BC, et al: Geographical distribution of hepatitis C virus genotypes in blood donors: an international collaborative survey, *J Clin Microbiol* 32:884, 1994.

17. Hoofnagle JH: Hepatitis C: the clinical spectrum of disease. In National Institutes of Health Consensus Development Conference Statement: *Management of hepatitis C,* http://consensus.nih.com, Bethesda, Md, 1997, The Institutes.

18. Alter MJ, Margolis HS, Krawczynski K, et al: The natural history of community-acquired hepatitis C in the United States: the Sentinel Counties Chronic Non-A, Non-B Hepatitis Study Team, *N Engl J Med* 327: 1899, 1992.

19. Gretch D: Diagnostic assays for hepatitis C. In National Institutes of Health Consensus Development Conference: *Management of hepatitis C,* http://consensus.nih.com, Bethesda, Md, 1997, The Institutes.

20. Gretch DR, dela Rosa C, Carithers RL Jr, et al: Assessment of hepatitis C viremia using molecular amplification technologies: correlations and clinical implications, *Ann Intern Med* 123:321, 1995.

21. Hayashi J, Yoshimura E, Kishihara Y, et al: Hepatitis C virus RNA levels determined by branched DNA probe assay correlated with levels assessed using competitive PCR, *Am J Gastroenterol* 91:314, 1996.

22. Nguyen TT, Sedghi-Vaziri A, Wilkes LB, et al: Fluctuations in viral load (HCV RNA) are relatively insignificant in untreated patients with chronic HCV infection, *J Viral Hepat* 3:75, 1996.

23. Hawkins A, Davidson F, Simmonds P: Comparison of plasma virus loads among individuals infected with hepatitis C virus (HCV) genotypes 1, 2, and 3 by quantiplex HCV RNA assay versions 1 and 2, Roche Monitor assay, and an in-house limiting dilution method, *J Clin Microbiol* 35:187, 1997.

24. Hagiwara W, Hayashi N, Fusamoto H, Kamada T: Quantitative analysis of hepatitis C virus RNA: relationship between the replicative level and the various stages of the carrier states or the response to interferon therapy, *Gastroenterol Jpn* 28 (suppl 5):48, 1993.

25. McHutchison JG, Gordon SC, Schiff ER, et al: Interferon alfa-2b alone or in combination with ribavirin as initial treatment for chronic hepatitis C, *N Eng J Med* 339:1485, 1998.

26. Hoofnagle JH, di Bisceglie AM: The treatment of chronic viral hepatitis, *N Engl J Med* 336:347, 1997.

27. Hoofnagle JH: Delta hepatitis and the hepatitis delta virus. In Seeff LB, Lewis JH, editors: *Current perspectives in hepatology,* New York, 1989, Plenum.

28. Salassa B, Daziano E, Bonino F, et al: Serological diagnosis of hepatitis B and delta virus (HBV/HDV) coinfection, *J Hepatol* 12:10, 1991.

29. Aragona M, Macagno S, Caredda F, et al: Serological response to the hepatitis delta virus in hepatitis D, *Lancet* 1:478, 1987.

30. Reyes GR, Purdy MA, Kim JP, et al: Isolation of a cDNA from the virus responsible for enterically transmitted non-A, non-B hepatitis, *Science* 247:1335, 1990.

31. Schlauder GG, Dawson GJ, Erker JC, et al: The sequence and phylogenetic analysis of a novel hepatitis E virus isolated from a patient with acute hepatitis reported in the United States, *J Gen Virol* 79:447, 1998.

32. Favorov MO, Fields HA, Purdy MA, et al: Serologic identification of hepatitis E virus infections in epidemic and endemic settings, *J Med Virol* 36:246, 1992.

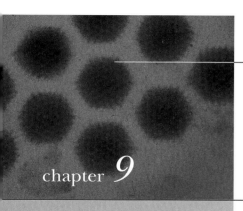

chapter *9*

Gail J. Demmler

Cardiac Infections (Viral Myocarditis and Pericarditis)

OVERVIEW

Although viruses are a well-recognized cause of cardiac infection, making a specific viral diagnosis in patients with myocarditis or pericarditis is difficult. The traditional methods include viral cultures and serology, but these methods lead to diagnosis in a relatively small number of cases. The increasing use of endomyocardial biopsy and the availability of molecular techniques may improve the ability to assess the role of viruses in cardiac infection.

This chapter reviews clinical aspects of viral infections of the heart, then discusses the laboratory techniques used to make a specific viral diagnosis.

CLINICAL SYNDROMES AND ETIOLOGIC AGENTS

Myocarditis is a clinical condition characterized by inflammation of the heart tissue. The inflammation is predominantly mononuclear in viral myocarditis, and it may be diffuse or focal. In severe cases, myocardial necrosis may occur. Myocarditis also may occur with *pericarditis*, which is inflammation of the pericardium surrounding the heart. In my experience, viral pericarditis almost always occurs in association with viral myocarditis, but viral myocarditis may not always have a significant, accompanying pericarditis. Furthermore, in patients with *myopericarditis* in whom viral isolation has been performed on both myocardium and pericardial fluid, the same virus is detected in both samples. Therefore, in a patient with suspected viral pericarditis, the clinician should also consider myocarditis. Similarly, in a patient with suspected myocarditis, the clinician should determine whether significant pericardial fluid is present.

Myocarditis and pericarditis have many infectious (both viral and nonviral) and noninfectious causes. *Enteroviruses,* especially Coxsackie B viruses, but also Coxsackie A viruses, echoviruses, and polioviruses, have been associated most often with viral myocarditis.[1, 2] Other ribonucleic acid (RNA) viruses implicated as causes of myocarditis include influenza viruses types A and B, parainfluenza virus type 3, measles virus, mumps virus, lymphocytic choriomeningitis (LCM) virus, arboviruses, and human immunodeficiency virus (HIV). The deoxyribonucleic acid (DNA) viruses also have been associated with myocarditis, including smallpox, cytomegalovirus (CMV), herpes simplex virus (HSV), varicella-zoster virus (VZV), Epstein-Barr virus (EBV), and adenovirus. In the fetus and newborn, parvovirus and rubella virus also may cause cardiac disease. This chapter discusses the diagnostic consideration of each of these agents as the cause of myocarditis or pericarditis, as well as the approach to establishing an etiologic role using a variety of laboratory methods.

CLINICAL MANIFESTATIONS

The clinical presentation of the patient with myocarditis varies from subclinical to fulminant and rapidly fatal. Disease may be confined to the heart or may be part of a disseminated, multisystem viral illness, often with hepatitis and encephalitis. Patients of all ages may have myocarditis, but it is usually most severe in newborns and younger infants and less fulminant in older infants and children. In adults, myocarditis often is subclinical and self-limited.

Acute Myocarditis

Acute myocarditis may be preceded by a nonspecific viral illness, with fever, nausea, vomiting, diarrhea, cough, sore throat, or rash that occurs 1 to 3 weeks before onset of symptoms. With the onset of myocarditis, fever, chest pain, palpitations, dyspnea, and fatigue may occur. Infants may exhibit irritability or pallor. Tachycardia, dysrhythmias, pericardial rubs, heart block, signs of congestive heart failure, and even circulatory collapse, clinical shock, or sudden death may occur.

Since acute myocarditis often is part of a multisystem illness, specific clues may indicate a viral etiology. For example, a patient who is immunocompromised by organ or marrow transplantation is likely to have CMV myocarditis, whereas previously healthy individuals are more likely to have myocarditis caused by enteroviruses or adenoviruses. An acute myocarditis occurring in late summer or early fall also is more likely to be caused by an enterovirus, especially if these viruses are known to be circulating in the community. On the other hand, acute myocarditis associated with a respiratory illness in late winter is more likely caused by influenza virus. In infants with other manifestations of congenital infection (e.g., hepatosplenomegaly, petechiae), CMV, rubella virus, parvovirus, and adenovirus are probable causes. Myocarditis also should be suspected in all patients, whether immunocompromised or apparently healthy, who have disseminated viral disease, especially when VZV, adenovirus, enterovirus, CMV, or EBV is the suspected etiologic agent.

Recurrent and Chronic Myocarditis

Some patients with myocarditis may have subacute, recurrent, or chronic courses. Others may develop *dilated cardiomyopathy*, with enlargement of the heart, severely impaired cardiac function, and heart failure, long after the original viral infection.[1, 3-5] Other late sequelae include constrictive pericarditis and aortic or mitral valve incompetence. These chronic phases of myocarditis most likely are caused by T lymphocytes, which infiltrate the myocardium in response to virus-containing myofibers. The continued presence of viral components may contribute to the ongoing inflammatory responses.[1]

The often biphasic presentation of acute myocarditis, as well as the immunopathogenic and insidious nature of its late sequelae, are critical to making a definitive viral diagnosis in most patients. In contrast to acute myocarditis, in which the etiology often is evident from clinical clues, the etiology of myocarditis that presents in the subacute or chronic phases often remains elusive.

Supportive Evidence of Myocarditis

In addition to the clinical presentation, noninvasive laboratory and imaging tests support the diagnosis of myocarditis.[6] None of these tests, however, is specific for myocardial damage secondary to viral myocarditis. Blood tests may reveal an elevated erythrocyte sedimentation rate or elevated cardiac enzyme levels. Electrocardiographic changes that support the diagnosis of acute myocarditis include ST-segment elevations and T-wave inversions. Echocardiography may show ventricular dilation, thickening of the myocardium from edema, a lowered ejection fraction, or a pericardial effusion. A chest radiograph may reveal cardiac enlargement. Noninvasive nuclear imaging using a variety of radioisotopes, including technetium-99m pyrophosphate, gallium-97, and indium-111 antimyosin antibody, may detect myocardial necrosis or inflammation. Magnetic resonance imaging also may be useful in detecting tissue alterations caused by myocardial inflammation. Hemodynamic studies using cardiac catheterization rarely are performed in patients with myocarditis, unless a structural anomaly or infarction is strongly suspected.

Endomyocardial biopsy performed by a cardiologist is an invasive but relatively safe diagnostic modality that currently is the established, reference standard for the pathologic diagnosis of myocarditis. It also may be appropriate for some patients with suspected myocarditis.[6] The histology may suggest a viral etiology of the myocarditis, especially if the cellular infiltrate is mononuclear, but it does not definitively establish a viral etiology for the inflammation. Biopsies often are taken through the right ventricle and obtained from the interventricular septum. Because of the often-focal nature of myocarditis and the small size of the tissue samples, several specimens should be obtained.

Dallas Criteria

In 1987 the *Dallas criteria* were established to provide a set of standardized pathologic definitions for the histologic diagnosis of myocarditis[7, 8] (Table 9–1). The categories of myocarditis include the following:

1. No myocarditis, with no evidence of inflammatory cell infiltrate and no myocardial damage or necrosis

Table 9.1	Dallas Criteria for Histopathologic Diagnosis of Myocarditis
Category	**Histopathologic findings**
1. No myocarditis	No evidence of inflammatory cell infiltrate No myocardial damage or necrosis
2. Borderline myocarditis	Sparse inflammatory cell infiltrate No myocardial damage or necrosis
3. Active/acute myocarditis	Intense inflammatory cell infiltrate Widespread or focal myocardial degeneration and necrosis
4. Ongoing/persistent myocarditis (second endomyocardial biopsy required for diagnosis)	Same or more severe inflammatory cell infiltrate and myocardial damage
5. Resolving/healing myocarditis (second endomyocardial biopsy required for diagnosis)	Less severe inflammatory cell infiltrate Occasional myocardial lesions
6. Resolved/healed myocarditis	Some or no inflammatory cells Fibrosis and connective tissue healing

Modified from Aretz HT: *Hum Pathol* 18:619, 1987, and Aretz HT, Billingham ME, Edwards WD, et al: *Am J Cardiovasc Pathol* 1:3, 1987.

2. Borderline myocarditis, with sparse inflammation and no myocardial damage or necrosis

3. Active or acute myocarditis with intense inflammatory cell infiltration, usually in the interstitium, and associated with widespread myocardial degeneration or necrosis

4. Ongoing or persistent myocarditis, with the same or more severe inflammation and myocardial damage present on repeat endomyocardial biopsy

5. Resolving or healing myocarditis, with less severe inflammation and occasional myocardial lesions present on repeat myocardial biopsy

6. Resolved or healed myocarditis, with some or no inflammatory cells detectable within regions of fibrosis, with evidence of connective tissue healing

Criteria for Specific Diagnosis

The diagnosis of viral myocarditis can be made by adapting the criteria for enterovirus-associated myocarditis[9] (Box 9–1).

A definitive diagnosis of viral myocarditis can be established only by isolation of the virus from the myocardium, endocardium, or pericardial fluid obtained by myocardial biopsy, pericardiocentesis, or

Definitive diagnosis: high-order association

Isolation of virus from myocardium, endocardium, or pericardial fluid

or

Detection of viral component (antigen or nucleic acid) in myocardial, endocardial, or pericardial tissue, preferably at sites of histopathologic change (Dallas criteria)

Probable diagnosis: moderate-order association

Isolation of virus from blood, serum, buffy coat, pharynx/throat, feces, or urine

and

Demonstration of significant, viral type-specific serologic response (seroconversion, fourfold rise, or IgM antibody response)

Possible diagnosis: low-order association

Isolation of virus or detection of viral components from pharynx/throat, feces, or urine

or

Demonstration of significant, viral type-specific serologic response (seroconversion, fourfold rise, or IgM antibody response)

Modified from Lerner AM, Wilsom FM, Reyes MP: *Mod Concepts Cardiovasc Dis* 64:11, 1975.

autopsy. The diagnosis also can be made by detecting components of the virus at sites of pathologic change in these tissues. For example, viral type-specific viral antigen may be detected by immunofluorescent or peroxidase-labeled antibodies, and viral nucleic acid may be detected by hybridization or nucleic acid amplification techniques performed on cardiac tissue. This degree of circumstantial evidence implicates the virus in a *high-order association* with the patient's myocarditis. This approach is therefore recommended, whenever possible, to establish the diagnosis of acute viral myocarditis and pericarditis.

A *moderate-order association* for virus-induced myocarditis can be established by isolation and typing of the virus from the blood, serum, buffy coat, pharynx, feces, or urine. This is done *in conjunction with* demonstration of a significant, viral type-specific serologic response that indicates the virus isolated was an acute infection rather than an infection weeks or months old. Often this moderate-order association is the only practical way to diagnose viral myocarditis, since direct myocardial biopsy may be inappropriate for some patients or beyond the technical expertise of many hospitals. It is therefore recommended for patients who do not undergo direct myocardial biopsy.

This approach has limitations. Isolation of a virus from a site peripheral to the end organ involved (e.g., heart) only provides circumstantial evidence that the patient is acutely infected with a virus. It does not definitively prove the virus was present in the heart. For example, some viruses (e.g., enteroviruses, adenoviruses) may be shed for several weeks to months from peripheral sites (e.g., throat, urine, feces), whereas others (e.g., CMV) may produce a chronic viremia, particularly in immunocompromised patients. Therefore serologic evidence that the viral infection is acute supports a viral etiology for the patient's myocarditis. Examples of significant serologic responses include (1) a temporally associated seroconversion from viral type-specific immunoglobulin G (IgG) antibody–negative status to IgG antibody–positive status on paired acute and convalescent sera, (2) concomitant fourfold rise in viral type-specific neutralizing or other antibodies from paired acute and convalescent sera, and (3) significant, viral type-specific immunoglobulin M (IgM) response on one acute serum specimen.

A *low-order association* for virus-induced myocarditis provides circumstantial evidence that is less convincing than the high-order and moderate-order associations. Low-order associations include isolation or detection of a virus from pharynx, feces, or urine; a fourfold rise in viral type-specific antibody on acute and convalescent serum specimen; or a significantly positive, viral type-specific IgM titer on a single serum specimen. Clinicians should consider this approach a minimal evaluation for patients with suspected viral myocarditis or pericarditis, but it is better than no attempt to implicate a virus.

DETECTION OF VIRUSES CAUSING MYOCARDITIS AND PERICARDITIS

Sample Selection and Transport

Obtaining the appropriate specimen and transporting it under the proper conditions is the first step in establishing a viral etiology for myocarditis or pericarditis and ensuring optimal results from the virology laboratory (see Chapter 2).

Samples obtained from endomyocardial biopsy should be 2 to 3 mm in size and preferably at least three to five in number to minimize sampling differences.[7, 8, 10] They should be placed in viral transport media or phosphate-buffered saline, kept cool on ice, and transported to the virology laboratory immediately. The tissue is then minced, ground, and processed before inoculation into cell culture. Samples of pericardial fluid should be placed in a sterile container and kept cool on ice during transport to the virology laboratory. The addition of viral transport media is not necessary.

If urine or samples of feces are collected, they also may be placed directly in a sterile container. Samples collected by swabbing the throat, nose, or rectum, however, should be placed in viral transport media and transported promptly while being kept cool on ice.

If blood samples are obtained, they should be 3 to 10 ml, collected in a green-top heparinized tube, and transported at room temperature. If polymerase chain reaction (PCR) is to be performed, a purple-top (EDTA) or yellow-top (acid citrate dextrose, ACD) tube may be preferred because heparin can be inhibitory to PCR. Transport media and ice should not be used when transporting blood samples for virus isolation.

The clinician should consult with the virology laboratory if questions or concerns arise about the proper specimens appropriate for an individual patient.

Virus Isolation

The viruses most often associated with myocarditis in humans include enteroviruses, adenoviruses, CMV, influenza virus, parainfluenza virus (especially type 3), and mumps virus (Box 9–2). These viruses can be identified on the cell culture monolayers routinely used in most clinical and diagnostic virology laboratories. Even though viral isolation is the reference standard for the definitive diagnosis of myocarditis, it is unusual to isolate a virus from heart tissue or pericardial tissue or fluid.

Box 9.2   Viruses Most Often Associated with Myocarditis

DNA viruses

Cytomegalovirus (CMV)
Epstein-Barr (EBV)
Herpes simplex (HSV)
Varicella-zoster (VZV)
Adenovirus
Parvovirus
Smallpox

RNA viruses

Enteroviruses
   Coxsackieviruses
   Echoviruses
   Untyped enteroviruses
Influenza types A and B
Parainfluenza type 3
Measles
Mumps
Rubella
Arboviruses
Lymphocytic choriomeningitis (LCM)
Human immunodeficiency (HIV)

A review of viral cultures of heart tissue and pericardial tissue or fluid submitted from 1990 to 1997 to the Diagnostic Virology Laboratory at Texas Children's Hospital revealed 299 cardiac specimens from 260 patient encounters.[11] Only 12 specimens (4%) from nine patients (3.5%) grew a virus: CMV from three patients, adenovirus from two, echovirus type 7 from two, Coxsackie B2 from one, and parainfluenza type 3 from one patient. In three patients the same virus was isolated from both the heart tissue and pericardial fluid (two CMV and one adenovirus).

Enteroviruses. The enteroviruses are most often associated with myocarditis. No single cell culture system will support the growth of all enteroviruses, and a combination of at least two cell culture systems is recommended. The enteroviruses, especially Coxsackie B virus and echoviruses, may produce cytopathic effect (CPE) in human cell culture systems such as foreskin fibroblasts (HFF), embryonic lung fibroblasts (HEL), embryonic kidney (HEK), MRC-5, WI-38, HeLa, or HEp-2 cell lines.[12] They also produce CPE on primary monkey kidney (PMK) cell cultures, including rhesus monkey (RhMK), buffalo monkey (BMK), and cynomologus monkey (CMK). Rhabdomyosarcoma (RD) cell cultures also support the growth of many enteroviruses.[13] Coxsackie A viruses usually do not grow in cell culture monolayer systems and require inoculation into suckling mice for cultivation and identification.

Presumptive identification of enteroviruses can be made by detection of the typical teardrop-shaped CPE, which is detectable within 2 to 5 days of incubation. Enteroviruses grow best at 35° to 37°C, and are acid stable (Figure 9–1). Both rhinoviruses and enteroviruses are members of the Picornaviridae family and have similar growth characteristics, but rhinoviruses

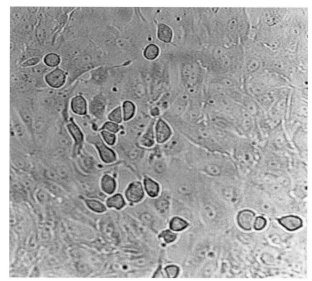

Figure 9.1 Typical, teardrop-shaped cytopathic effect of enterovirus on rhesus monkey kidney cell culture.

prefer cooler temperatures of 33°C and are inactivated by an acid pH. Therefore a virus isolated from a nose or throat swab that produces a teardrop-shaped CPE should undergo temperature preference and pH testing to determine if it is an enterovirus or rhinovirus. Similarly, if an enterovirus is isolated from feces, especially from an infant or toddler, the clinician should determine if it is in the polio or nonpolio group of enteroviruses, since this age group may receive live poliovirus vaccines that are shed in the feces for extended periods.

Differential appearance of CPE on different cell lines may allow presumptive identification of different enterovirus groups.[13] For example, echoviruses and group A coxsackieviruses usually are isolated in RD and RhMK cells but not HEp-2 cells, whereas group B coxsackieviruses can be isolated in RhMK and HEp-2 cell lines but not RD cells. Poliovirus, usually grows in all three cell lines.

The definitive typing of enteroviruses, however, can be achieved only by performing a neutralization test with the World Health Organization Lim–Benyesh–Melnick antiserum pools.[14] These antiserum pools are in limited supply, and generally their use is restricted to identification of outbreaks or serious infection. Antibodies are commercially available for typing enteroviruses using fluorescent antibody (FA) staining. These reagents may allow more widespread typing of enterovirus isolates.

Adenoviruses. Adenoviruses are best isolated in human cell culture systems (e.g., HFF, HEK, HEp-2, HeLa, A549).[15] They also may grow in PMK cell lines (e.g., RhMK). Adenoviruses produce large, round, grapelike clusters of CPE, usually detected first at the periphery of the cell culture monolayer within three to five days of incubation. Confirmation that the virus is an adenovirus usually is performed by FA staining using antisera containing antibodies directed against the hexon subunit that recognize all human adenoviruses. Specific adenovirus serotyping of the more than 40 different serotypes can be performed in research or reference laboratories using type-specific antibodies.

Cytomegalovirus. CMV grows in human fibroblast cell lines (e.g., HFF, WI-38, MRC-5).[16] It produces a focal, refractile CPE that often grows slowly and may require up to 21 days or longer to detect. Confirmation that the virus isolated is CMV can be achieved by FA staining using one of the many antibodies to CMV early or late antigens available in most clinical virology laboratories.

Parainfluenza, influenza, and mumps viruses. These viruses are best isolated in RhMK cell lines and usually are detected within 2 to 5 days of incubation.[17] Influenza viruses also may be detected in MRC-5, RD, or MDCK (canine kidney) cell culture systems. Parainfluenza, influenza, and mumps viruses may produce a nonspecific CPE or toxic effect; accordingly their presence is best identified by detection of hemadsorption using guinea pig red blood cell suspensions (see Chapters 1 and 4). Influenza viruses also may be identified using hemagglutination testing.[17] Confirmation of the specific hemadsorbing virus type usually is performed by FA staining using type-specific antibodies. Influenza A virus also may be identified by enzyme immunoassays (EIAs) in research and reference laboratories.

Unusual viral causes. Routine cell culture also will detect unusual causes of myocarditis, such as HSV types 1 and 2 and VZV. Special culture methods are necessary, however, to identify HIV or rubella virus (see Chapters 1, 13, and 17). Parvovirus is not detectable in routine cell culture and usually requires serology to detect virus-specific antibodies or molecular techniques to detect viral DNA in tissue or blood for detection and identification (see Chapter 13).

Serology

IgM antibody. Detection of a specific IgM antibody response indicates that the patient is acutely infected with a particular virus. Detection of IgM antibodies using neutralization tests or EIAs has been used in research and reference laboratories to diagnose acute infections with Coxsackie B virus.[18-22] In one study, IgM antibody to Coxsackie B virus was detected in 52% of patients with acute myocarditis and pericarditis and in only 8% of control patients.[22] This response often is detectable within 3 days of onset of myocarditis symptoms but usually resolves within 4 to 6 weeks. In some patients the IgM antibody response may last 6 months or longer.[20] Cross-reactivity with the other nonpolio enterovirus groups (echoviruses, Coxsackie A virus) also occurs.[21]

Assays for enterovirus IgM antibodies are not widely available, even in reference laboratories. In contrast, many laboratories perform assays for CMV-specific IgM antibodies. This response usually lasts 8 to 12 weeks, but individual variation occurs, and IgM antibody may be detectable in as short as 2 weeks and as long as 9 months after a primary infection with CMV.[23] Tests for parvovirus-specific and rubella virus–specific IgM antibodies also are available. These tests may be particularly helpful in newborns with suspected congenital infections caused by these viruses. Tests for specific IgM responses to adenoviruses, influenza virus, and parainfluenza virus are not readily available to the clinician.

IgG antibody. Detection of a significant, fourfold rise in virus-specific IgG antibody on acute and convalescent serum samples may be helpful in providing retrospective evidence of a recent viral infection. This approach is not the diagnostic test of choice, however, and has the following limitations:

1. Because at least 2 weeks are usually needed between acute and convalescent sera samples, the diagnosis is delayed.

2. IgG antibody levels to certain viruses (e.g., CMV) may fluctuate during times of recurrent viral infection, either reactivation or reinfection, and therefore rises may not always signify a recent primary infection.

3. Patients with CMV myocarditis most often are heart transplant recipients or other immunocompromised patients who typically experience asymptomatic recurrent infections with concomitant rises in IgG antibody.[24]

Tests for detection of IgG antibody to adenovirus are available only in research or reference laboratories. Adenovirus-specific (but not serotype-specific) antibodies can be detected by complement fixation or EIA techniques. Considerable cross-reactivity occurs among different serotypes, however, and these techniques are useful primarily for seroepidemiologic studies on the prevalence of adenovirus infection in a group or population.[25] Furthermore, adenovirus is a common infection, and many people will have detectable antibody to adenovirus. Serotype-specific assays using hemagglutination inhibition or neutralization techniques are primarily research tools and not readily available to the clinician. These serotype-specific serologic assays, however, may be combined with a viral culture that identifies a specific adenovirus serotype in the throat or stool. This helps to define a recent infection and establish a moderate-order association of the virus with the patient's myocarditis.

Similarly, serotype-specific IgG responses using neutralization assays against the enteroviruses can be used in combination with a positive viral culture from the throat or stool to identify a recent enterovirus infection and establish a moderate order association.[26] IgG antibody production to enteroviruses also may be measured using complement fixation, hemagglutination inhibition, and EIA. As with adenovirus, however, cross-reactivity between enterovirus groups may occur, and anamnestic heterotypic responses may occur in the host.

Antigen Assays

Viral antigen may be detected in body fluids using EIAs developed for HSV, influenza A virus, respiratory syncytial virus (RSV), and Coxsackie B virus. An HSV antigen test is used in many clinical virology laboratories to detect HSV antigen in vesicle fluid and swabs.[27]

This test's capability to detect HSV antigen in heart tissue is unknown.

Yolken and Torsch[28, 29] developed an EIA to detect and serotype Coxsackie A and B virus antigens. This diagnostic test primarily has been applied to stool specimens, and its usefulness in heart tissue also is unknown. Furthermore, the mouse and monkey antisera used in the test are difficult to obtain, expensive, and therefore not readily available. Also, the clinical specimen must be tested against all serotypes plus controls, making it an impractical test for routine diagnostic laboratories.

Immunofluorescence and immunoperoxidase assays also may be used to detect viral antigens in tissue. They are particularly useful in enhancing the visibility of virus-infected cells, as well as in confirming the etiology of viral inclusion cells.

The clinician is encouraged to consult with the pathologist examining the tissue regarding the availability and appropriateness of these techniques in individual patients.

Nucleic Acid Probes

Viral nucleic acid in cardiac tissue can be detected using hybridization probes. Nucleic acid probes, consisting of a complementary strand of DNA (cDNA), RNA, or synthetic oligonucleotides, have been used to detect enteroviruses in cell culture, in body fluids during reconstruction experiments, and directly in clinical samples (e.g., cardiac tissue).[30, 31] These probes usually contain regions of the enterovirus genome that is conserved among all enterovirus serotypes. Therefore these may be used as "universal" probes for enterovirus nucleic acid. They also may be designed to be group or type specific to allow identification of a particular serotype.

In general, RNA probes are more sensitive but less specific than cDNA probes. Oligonucleotide probes, while convenient and easily synthesized, are less sensitive. Furthermore, the limit of detection sensitivity of all hybridization assays for enteroviruses appears lower than that of culture. Sampling differences and the low titer of virus in most clinical specimens probably contribute to the lower sensitivity of hybridization probes compared with viral culture. Hybridization assays may be performed on paraffin-embedded tissue and archived samples, however, whereas cell culture requires a fresh tissue sample. Detection of the enterovirus genome by hybridization assays is available only in selected research or reference laboratories. Enzyme-labeled nucleic acid probes that may be applied to heart tissue specimens also are available in many histology laboratories for viruses other than the enteroviruses, including CMV, EBV, HSV, and adenovirus. Because these immunohistochemical tests enhance the visibility of virus-infected cells, they can help in establishing a viral etiology for myocarditis and are recommended if available.

Again, the clinician is encouraged to consult with the pathologist handling the tissue regarding the availability and appropriateness of these tests for each patient.

Polymerase Chain Reaction

Viral nucleic acid also can be detected by newer amplification techniques, especially PCR methodology (see Chapter 1). Three general strategies have been developed by research and reference laboratories to detect enterovirus by PCR. The strategy most useful to the clinician is "universal" detection of most or all enterovirus serotypes in a clinical sample. Primers directed at a highly conserved region of the 5' non-coding region of the enterovirus genome have been designed for reverse transcription and subsequent PCR (RT-PCR).[32] These "universal" primers used in an RT-PCR assay appear almost 100% specific and more sensitive than cell culture in detecting enteroviruses in many different types of clinical samples, including cardiac tissue. Detection of enterovirus by PCR in cardiac tissue from a patient with acute myocarditis establishes a high-order association of the virus with the patient's acute myocarditis. The primers also may be used in paraffin-embedded and archived samples.[33]

PCR-based assays have been used to study the role of enteroviruses in chronic myocarditis and dilated cardiomyopathy. Enterovirus RNA has been detected in both animal models of chronic myocarditis and in patients with dilated cardiomyopathy, indicating that the ongoing inflammatory reaction that produces chronic myocarditis may depend on the persistence of viral nucleic acid in the myocardium.[5, 33-38]

Tests to detect group-specific or serotype-specific nucleic acid may be combined with "universal" primer RT-PCR to determine the group or serotype of enterovirus in the clinical sample,[38] providing a second-order strategy to further identify an enterovirus. Tests to detect strain-specific variations within a single serotype are also possible but usually limited to research laboratories studying the molecular epidemiology of enteroviruses. This third order of definitive identification is rarely needed clinically but may provide useful epidemiologic information in selected cases.

Other viruses associated with myocarditis and pericarditis may be detected using PCR-based methods, providing a high-order association of the particular virus with the patient's episode of myocarditis. For example, adenovirus has been detected by PCR using "universal" primers that amplify a highly conserved region of the hexon gene that shares sequence homology among most adenovirus serotypes. Clinical conditions in which adenovirus has been detected in cardiac tissue include acute myocarditis with dilated cardiomyopathy and intrauterine myocarditis with fetal hydrops.[32, 33, 39, 40]

CMV may be detected in cardiac tissue by using primers that amplify conserved regions of the immediate early or late regions of the viral genome.[32, 33] The clinical conditions most likely associated with CMV myocarditis include congenital CMV disease and immu-

Table 9.2 Clinical and Laboratory Clues for the Diagnosis of Viral Myocarditis and Pericarditis

Clue	Virus(es)	Supporting laboratory tests*
Febrile illness	Enteroviruses	Viral culture of stool and nasopharynx or throat
Respiratory illness	Adenovirus, influenza A and B, parainfluenza type 3	Fluorescent antibody stain and/or culture of respiratory specimens
Parotitis	Mumps	IgM serology, viral culture of saliva and urine
	Enteroviruses	Viral culture of stool and nasopharynx or throat
	Parainfluenza	Fluorescent antibody stain and/or culture of respiratory specimens
Newborn	Enterovirus	Viral culture of stool and nasopharynx
	CMV	Viral culture of urine
	Rubella (only if other signs of congenital rubella are present)	Viral culture of pharynx, conjunctiva, urine, stool, blood, and/or CSF; IgM serology
Fetus	Parvovirus B19	Amniotic fluid PCR
	Rubella	Viral culture or PCR of amniotic fluid, IgM serology on fetal blood
Immunosuppression	Cytomegalovirus	Viral culture, pp65 antigenemia assay or PCR of blood, culture of urine

*Does not include viral cultures or nucleic acid detection performed on pericardial fluid or tissue.

nosuppression, especially related to organ transplantation.[33] CMV also has been detected in the myocardium of cardiac transplant recipients with moderate to severe multifocal rejection.[41]

PCR-based methods recently demonstrated mumps virus in the myocardium of patients with endocardial fibroelastosis.[42] Parvovirus also may be detected by PCR-based methods in the cardiac tissue of immunocompromised patients, and it also may cause hydrops fetalis. The cardiac complications of HIV infection have recently been studied, and PCR-based methods may be useful in determining the role of HIV in the chronic cardiomyopathy seen in some of these patients.[43]

The detection of viral nucleic acid by PCR-based methods provides strong circumstantial evidence that a viral component is present in the heart tissue. The clinician must be cautious, however, and choose reference laboratories skilled in performing these tests. False-positive results may occur if contamination occurs or if the primers selected are not specific for the particular virus. False-negative results may occur if nucleic acid isolation techniques are not adequate, if inhibitors are present in the sample, or if the PCR amplification or product detection conditions do not optimize the sensitivity and specificity of the assay.

DIAGNOSTIC APPROACH

An approach to determining the viral etiology of myocarditis and pericarditis is shown in Table 9–2.

References

1. Woodruff JF: Viral myocarditis: a review, *Am J Pathol* 101:421, 1980.
2. Grist NR, Bell EJ: A six-year study of Coxsackie virus B infections in heart disease, *J Hyg (Camb)* 73:165, 1974.
3. Fuster V, Gersh B, Giuliani E, et al: The natural history of idiopathic dilated cardiomyopathy, *Am J Cardiol* 47:525, 1981.
4. Reyes M, Lerner M: Coxsackie virus myocarditis: with special reference to acute and chronic effects, *Prog Cardiovasc Dis* 27:373, 1985.
5. Martino T, Liu P, Sole M: Viral infection and the pathogenesis of dilated cardiomyopathy, *Circ Res* 74:182, 1994.
6. Friedman RA, Duff DF: Myocarditis. In Feigin R, Cherry J (editors): *Textbook of pediatric infectious diseases,* ed 3, Philadelphia, 1992, WB Saunders.
7. Aretz HT: Myocarditis: the Dallas criteria, *Hum Pathol* 18:619, 1987.
8. Aretz HT, Billingham ME, Edwards WD, et al: Myocarditis: a histopathologic definition and classification, *Am J Cardiovasc Pathol* 1:3, 1987.
9. Lerner AM, Wilson FM, Reyes MP: Enteroviruses in the heart (with special emphasis on the probable role of Coxsackie viruses, group B, types 1-5). II. Observations in humans, *Mod Concepts Cardiovasc Dis* 64:11, 1975.
10. Hauck AJ, Kearney DL, Edwards WD: Evaluation of postmortem endomyocardial biopsy specimens from 38 patients with lymphocytic myocarditis: implications for role of sampling error, *Mayo Clin Proc* 64:1235, 1989.
11. Demmler G: Unpublished data, 1997.
12. Chonmaitree T, Ford C, Sanders C, et al: Comparison of cell cultures for rapid isolation of enteroviruses, *J Clin Microbiol* 26:2576, 1988.
13. Johnston S, Siegel C: Presumptive identification of enteroviruses with RD, HEp-2, and RMK cell lines, *J Clin Microbiol* 28:1049, 1990.
14. Lim KA, Benyesh-Melnick M: Typing of viruses by combinations of antiserum pools: application to typing of enteroviruses (Coxsackie and Echo), *J Immunol* 84:309, 1960.
15. Wiedbrauk DL, Johnston SLG: Adenoviruses. In *Manual of clinical virology,* New York, 1993, Raven.
16. Weidbrauk DL, Johnston SLG: Cytomegaloviruses. In *Manual of clinical virology,* New York, 1993, Raven.
17. Weidbrauk DL, Johnston SLG: Influenza virus. In *Manual of clinical virology,* New York, 1993, Raven.
18. Dorries R, Meulen TR: Specificity of IgM antibodies in acute human Coxsackie B infections, analyzed by indirect phase enzyme immunoassay and immunoblot technique, *J Gen Virol* 64:159, 1983.
19. Bell EJ, McCarthey RA, Basquill D, et al: μ-antibody capture ELISA for the rapid diagnosis of enterovirus infections in patients with aseptic meningitis, *J Med Virol* 19:213, 1986.
20. McCartney RA, Banatvala JE, Bell EJ: Routine use of μ-antibody-capture ELISA for the serological diagnosis of Coxsackie B virus infections, *J Med Virol* 19: 205, 1986.
21. Pugh SF: Heterotypic reactions in a radioimmunoassay for Coxsackie B virus specific IgM, *J Clin Pathol* 37:433, 1984.
22. Schmidt NJ, Magoffin RL, Lennette EH: Association of group B Coxsackie viruses with cases of pericarditis, myocarditis, or pleurodynia by demonstration of immunoglobin M antibody, *Infect Immunol* 8:341, 1973.
23. Schaefer L, Cesario A, Demmler G, et al: Evaluation of Abbott CMV-M enzyme immunoassay for detection of cytomegalovirus immunoglobulin M antibody, *J Clin Microbiol* 26:2041, 1988.
24. Rasmussen L, Kelsall D, Nelson R, et al: Virus-specific IgG and IgM antibodies in normal and immunocompromised subjects infected with cytomegalovirus, *J Infect Dis* 145:191, 1982.
25. Hierholzer JC: Adenoviruses. In Schmidt NJ, Emmonds RW, editors: *Diagnostic procedures for viral, rickettsial and chlamydial infections,* ed 7, Washington, DC, 1995, American Public Health Association.
26. Grandien M, Forsgren M, Ehrnst A: Enteroviruses and reoviruses. In Schmidt NJ, Emmons RW, editors: *Diagnostic procedures for viral, rickettsial and chlamydial infections,* ed 6, Washington, DC, 1989, American Public Health Association.
27. Ashley RL: Herpes simplex viruses. In Schmidt NJ, Emmons RW, editors: *Diagnostic procedures for viral,*

rickettsial and chlamydial infections, ed 7, Washington, DC, 1995, American Public Health Association.

28. Yolken RH, Torsch VM: Enzyme-linked immunosorbent assay for detection and identification of Coxsackie B antigen in tissue cultures and clinical specimens, *J Med Virol* 6:45, 1980.

29. Yolken RH, Torsch VM: Enzyme-linked immunosorbent assay for detection and identification of Coxsackie virus A, *Infect Immunol* 31:742, 1981.

30. Easton AJ, Eglin RP: The detection of Coxsackie virus RNA in cardiac tissue by *in situ* hybridization, *J Gen Virol* 69:285, 1988.

31. Bowles NE, Olsen EG, Richardson PJ, et al: Detection of Coxsackie-B-virus-specific RNA sequences in myocardial biopsy samples from patients with myocarditis and dilated cardiomyopathy, *Lancet* 1:1120, 1986.

32. Martin AB, Webber S, Fricker FJ, et al: Acute myocarditis: rapid diagnosis by PCR in children, *Circulation* 90:330, 1994.

33. Griffin LD, Kearney D, Ni J, et al: Analysis of formalin-fixed and frozen myocardial autopsy samples for viral genome in childhood myocarditis and dilated cardiomyopathy with endocardial fibroelastosis using polymerase chain reaction (PCR), *Cardiovasc Pathol* 4:3, 1995.

34. Klingel K, Hohenadl C, Canu A, et al: Ongoing enterovirus-induced myocarditis is associated with persistent heart muscle infection: quantitative analysis of virus replication, tissue damage, and inflammation, *Proc Natl Acad Sci* 89:314, 1992.

35. Jin O, Sole M, Butany J, et al: Detection of enterovirus RNA in myocardial biopsies from patients with myocarditis and cardiomyopathy using gene amplification by polymerase chain reaction, *Circulation* 82:8, 1990.

36. Andreoletti L, Hober D, Decoene C, et al: Detection of enteroviral RNA by polymerase chain reaction in endomyocardial tissue of patients with chronic cardiac diseases, *J Med Virol* 48:53, 1996.

37. Weiss L, Liu Y, Chang K, et al: Detection of enteroviral RNA in idiopathic dilated cardiomyopathy and other human cardiac tissues, *J Clin Invest* 90:156, 1992.

38. Schwaiger A, Umlauft F, Weyrer K, et al: Detection of enteroviral ribonucleic acid in myocardial biopsies from patients with idiopathic dilated cardiomyopathy by polymerase chain reaction, *Am Heart J* 126:406, 1993.

39. Lozinski GM, Davis G, Krous H, et al: Adenovirus myocarditis, *Hum Pathol* 25:831, 1994.

40. Towbin J, Griffin LD, Martin AB, et al: Intrauterine adenoviral myocarditis presenting as nonimmune hydrops fetalis: diagnosis by polymerase chain reaction, *Pediatr Infect Dis J* 13:144, 1994.

41. Schowengerdt KO, Ni J, Denfield S, et al: Diagnosis, surveillance, and epidemiologic evaluation of viral infections in pediatric cardiac transplant recipients with the use of the polymerase chain reaction, *J Heart Lung Transplant* 15:111, 1996.

42. Ni J, Bowles NE, Kim Y-H, et al: Viral infection of the myocardium in endocardial fibroelastosis: molecular evidence for the role of mumps virus as an etiologic agent, *Circulation* 95:133, 1997.

43. The P^2C^2 HIV Study Group: The pediatric pulmonary and cardiovascular complications of vertically transmitted human immunodeficiency virus (P^2C^2 HIV) infection study: design and methods, *J Clin Epidemiol* 49:1285, 1996.

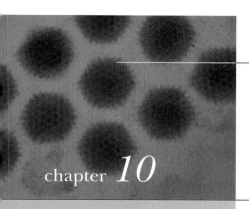

Ruben Lim-Bon-Siong, Jay S. Pepose

chapter *10*

Ocular Infections

OVERVIEW

Viral infections of the eye can be classified according to the anatomic location of the disease process and the resulting clinical syndrome. Because the clinician must establish a specific etiologic diagnosis for a patient with a particular clinical syndrome, this chapter first discusses ocular infections at three anatomic locations: conjunctiva and surrounding structures, cornea, and retina. Clinical findings are provided, emphasizing those that may be helpful in defining the etiologic agent, followed by instructions on specimen collection. Infections caused by specific viral agents are then discussed, focusing on diagnostic procedures appropriate for these viruses.

Table 10–1 lists the viruses most often associated with infection at each ocular anatomic location. Table 10–2 lists ocular infections caused by each viral agent and useful diagnostic tests.

CLINICAL SYNDROMES

Conjunctivitis and Other Surface Infections

Conjunctivitis, the most common infection of the ocular surface, is most often caused by *adenoviruses*, especially types 1 to 11, 14, 19, and 37. The most common clinical finding associated with conjunctivitis (or with infections of other portions of the ocular surface, such as the eyelid or the cornea) is redness, which may be acute or subacute in onset and is often accompanied by nonspecific symptoms such as burning, itching, foreign body sensation, and light sensitivity. Increased tearing may be present, but a thick discharge is not a prominent finding.

Other findings in some patients include lid swelling and erythema, with or without lid lesions; conjunctival congestion and edema, which may be marked; and conjunctival papillae, follicles, and membranes. Lymphoid follicles in the tarsal conjunctiva may also be prominent. Tender preauricular adenopathy ipsilateral to the involved eye suggests viral conjunctivitis but can be seen in some nonviral infections as well (e.g., cat-scratch disease, tularemia). Vision is not usually affected unless central corneal involvement is present. Scleral involvement is a nonspecific finding that is not limited to viral infections.

Table 10–3 summarizes clinical findings that may be helpful in distinguishing among viral, bacterial, and allergic conjunctivitis.

A variety of clinical findings can provide clues to a specific virus as the cause of conjunctivitis in a patient. Adenoviral conjunctivitis is usually bilateral, although onset in the second eye may not occur for 2 to 3 days after onset in the first eye. Herpes simplex virus (HSV) conjunctivitis is usually unilateral and may have less lid swelling and tearing than adenoviral disease. The simultaneous presence of cold sores also suggests HSV infection. Clusters of vesicles near the eye should create suspicion for HSV or varicella-zoster virus (VZV). VZV should be suspected if the vesicles are in a dermatomal distribution, although full dermatomal involvement might not always be present. A truly hemorrhagic conjunctivitis is suggestive of disease caused by enteroviruses such as enterovirus 70 or coxsackievirus A24. Appropriate systemic manifestations should alert the clinician to influenza-, measles-, or mumps-associated conjunctivitis. The presence of painless nodules that are waxy, round, and sometimes umbilicated should suggest molluscum contagiosum virus (MCV). Verrucous or papillomatous masses are suggestive of human papillomavirus (HPV) infection. Contact with birds should suggest infection with Newcastle disease virus (NDV).

Corneal Infections

The viruses most frequently associated with corneal infection are HSV, VZV, adenovirus, and measles virus. Nonsuppurative corneal ulceration characterized by epithelial defects, dendritic or geographic patterns of involvement, and decreased corneal sensitivity is highly suggestive of HSV or VZV. Chronic corneal infection with HSV may be associated with *neurotrophic ulcers*, which are painless, grayish, and oval. In contrast, *corneal ulcers* caused by bacteria or fungi are almost always painful and suppurative. In bacterial corneal ulcers a predisposing cause is often present (e.g., trauma, contact lens use, chronic topical corticosteroid therapy, prior surgery, concurrent infection of ocular adnexae). Single or multiple, round corneal opacities with no overlying epithelial defects (as demonstrated by the absence of fluorescein staining) can be seen in infections caused by adenoviruses, HSV, VZV, and EBV. Similar lesions can also be seen in chlamydial infection,

Table 10.1	Viruses that Infect Different Ocular Locations
Location	**Viruses**
Periocular tissue, lids	HSV, VZV, MCV, HPV
Conjunctiva	Adenovirus, enterovirus 70, coxsackievirus A24, HSV, VZV, NDV, influenza, measles, mumps, MCV, HPV, vaccinia
Cornea	HSV, VZV, EBV, adenovirus, mumps, rubella, vaccinia
Retina	CMV, VZV, HSV, HIV

HSV, Herpes simplex virus; *VZV,* varicella-zoster virus; *MCV,* molluscum contagiosum virus; *NDV,* Newcastle disease virus; *HPV,* human papillomavirus; *CMV,* cytomegalovirus; *HIV,* human immunodeficiency virus.

Table 10.2   Clinical Syndromes and Diagnostic Tests for Different Ocular Viral Infections

Virus	Clinical syndromes	Specimens	Diagnostic tests
Adenovirus	Epidemic keratoconjunctivitis Pharyngoconjunctival fever Acute follicular conjunctivitis	Conjunctival swabs	Viral isolation Immunofluorescence Enzyme immunoassay PCR

Herpes simplex	Vesicular blepharodermatitis
	Follicular conjunctivitis
	Dendritic, geographic ulcers
	Interstitial keratitis, stromal
	  necrosis
	Iridocyclitis, trabeculitis,
	  endotheliitis
	Acute retinal necrosis
	Progressive outer retinal
	  necrosis syndromes
		Conjunctival/corneal swabs
		Tear sample
		Impression debridement
		Vesicular fluid
		Aqueous humor
		Vitreous humor
		Corneal biopsy/button
		Retinal biopsy
			Viral isolation
			Immunofluorescence
			Enzyme immunoassay
			Cytology
			PCR

Varicella-zoster	Primary varicella infection
	Congenital varicella
	  syndrome
	Herpes zoster ophthalmicus
	Acute retinal necrosis
	  syndrome
	Progressive outer retinal
	  necrosis syndrome
		Vesicle scrapings and
		  aspirates
		Tear sample
		Corneal/conjunctival
		  scrapings
		Impression debridement
		Corneal biopsy/button
		Aqueous humor
		Vitreous humor
		Retinal biopsy
			Viral isolation
			Immunofluorescence
			Cytology
			PCR

Cytomegalovirus	Retinitis (edematous or
	  granular)
	Optic neuritis
	Acute retinal necrosis
	  syndrome
		Aqueous humor
		Vitreous humor
		Subretinal fluid
		Retinal biopsy
			Viral isolation
			Histology
			Immunofluorescence
			PCR

Epstein-Barr	Infectious mononucleosis Acute dacryocystitis Parinaud's syndrome Dendritic keratitis Subepithelial infiltrates Nummular stromal keratitis Uveitis, retinitis, choroiditis	Serum	Serology

Poxviruses	Molluscum contagiosum
	  lesions
	Chronic follicular conjunc-
	  tivitis
	Ocular orf virus infection
	  (contagious ecthyma)
	Ocular vaccinia
		Excisional biopsy
		Vesicular fluid
		Lesion scrapings
		Corneal/conjunctival
		  scrapings
			Histology
			Immunocytochemical
			  methods
			In situ hybridization
			Electron microscopy
			Culture
			Cytology
			Viral isolation

Enterovirus 70 Coxsackie-
  virus A24
	Acute hemorrhagic conjunc-
	  tivitis
		Conjunctival swabs	Viral isolation
			PCR

Human papillomavirus	Verrucae Conjunctival papillomas Conjunctival dysplasias and carcinomas	Excisional biopsy	Histology In situ hybridization PCR
Newcastle disease virus	Acute follicular conjunctivitis	Conjunctival swabs	Cytology Viral isolation Serology

PCR, Polymerase chain reaction.

Table 10.3 | Clinical Signs Differentiating Viral, Bacterial, and Allergic Conjunctivitis

Clinical signs	Viral	Bacterial	Allergic
Onset	Acute	Subacute to hyperacute	Chronic
Redness	Common	Common	Common
Discharge	Watery	Mucopurulent to purulent	Stringy
Itchiness	Mild	None	Marked
Bilateral involvement	Common	Uncommon	Common
Preauricular adenopathy	Present	Absent	Absent
Conjunctival follicles	Prominent	Mild	Mild
Course	<1-2 weeks	>1-2 weeks	Recurrent

tuberculosis (TB), syphilis, leprosy, and nummular (Dimmer's) or Padi keratitis.

Retinitis and Other Intraocular Infections

Many of the findings of intraocular viral infection are nonspecific and can occur in infections caused by a variety of viral or nonviral pathogens. Progressive decrease in visual acuity, particularly in an immunocompromised patient with no external manifestations of disease, should always alert the clinician to a possible intraocular infection. Ocular structures that may be involved include the iris, ciliary bodies, choroid, retina, vitreous, and optic nerve.

The most common viruses implicated are CMV, VZV, and HSV. Eye pain and redness are not prominent, but the patient may complain of significant photophobia and floaters. CMV retinitis, the most common form of intraocular infections in patients with acquired immunodeficiency syndrome (AIDS), may be accompanied by systemic signs and symptoms similar to those of infectious mononucleosis, but it may also occur without other symptoms. HSV and VZV can also cause iritis, iridocyclitis, choroiditis, retinitis, and neuritis. These infections may occur in immunocompetent as well as in immunocompromised patients. Findings of vitreous haze, retinal whitening or opacities, retinal hemorrhages, and retinal vascular sheathing visible on dilated funduscopic (ophthalmoscopic) examination are important signs of infectious retinitis. Posterior segment infections of nonviral origin (e.g., TB, syphilis, toxoplasmosis, pneumocystosis, cryptococcosis, other fungal infections) must also be considered in AIDS patients and those with other forms of immunosuppression.

SPECIMEN COLLECTION AND TRANSPORT

The method of collection and type of specimen depend on the anatomic localization of the disease. As a general rule, collection of specimens from the external surfaces of the eye can be done by the primary physician, except when sight-threatening disease is present (e.g., corneal ulcers, which might perforate with improper scraping). An ophthalmologist should perform tissue biopsies, aspiration of fluid, and procedures requiring magnification or special instruments and should obtain specimens from inside the eye.

The two methods most often used for collection of specimens from the ocular surface are *spatula debridement* (or *conjunctival scraping*), in which a sample is mechanically removed from the ocular surface with a blunt-tip spatula, and *minimal wiping debridement*, in which a Dacron or rayon swab is employed. Calcium alginate swabs should not be used because this material may inhibit the growth of some viruses.

When conjunctivitis is present, the specimen of choice for viral diagnostic studies is the *conjunctival swab*. The easiest and most accessible means of specimen collection is by swabbing the inferior cul-de-sac of the lower lid (Figure 10–1). After moistening the swab with transport medium or sterile water, the conjunctiva is exposed by pulling down the lower lid and gently swabbing from one end to the other, making at least two

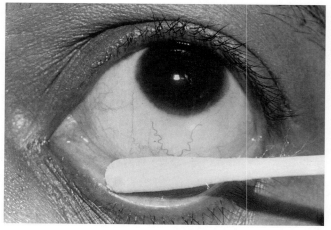

Figure 10.1 To obtain conjunctival specimen for laboratory diagnosis of viral infection, lower lid is pulled down to expose inferior cul-de-sac, which is swabbed with applicator stick.

passes. Topical anesthetic is not generally needed for conjunctival swabs, but patients should be warned that they may experience brief discomfort. Alternatively, a drop of proparacaine or tetracaine can be administered onto the conjunctiva before swabbing. If rose bengal stain is used, it should be applied after specimen collection, since the dye may inhibit viral growth and lead to a false-negative culture.

Immediately after conjunctival swabbing, the shaft of the applicator stick is cut or broken off after the tip is immersed in viral transport medium, with care taken to avoid contamination (Figure 10–2). If antigen detection is to be performed, some laboratories prefer that material be placed directly on glass microscope slides by rolling the swabs on the slides. If the same swab is to be used for culture, the glass slide should be decontaminated with alcohol and completely dry before the swab is applied. Specimens for viral isolation should be transported promptly and placed on ice if more than 60 minutes will elapse before arrival at the laboratory.

An alternative method used to collect samples from the ocular surface is *impression debridement*. This procedure involves the application of sterile cellulose acetate filter paper or a Schirmer strip directly to the conjunctival or corneal lesion.[1] Part of the filter paper strip can be sent for cell culture and part used for other diagnostic tests, such as polymerase chain reaction (PCR). Tear samples collected in capillary tubes or on Schirmer strips have also been used to detect viral antigens, quantify viral antibodies, and detect viral nucleic acid.

Conjunctival biopsies are usually done only for removal of papillomas or molluscum contagiosum lesions or when less invasive means have failed to yield a diagnosis and the disease process is progressive or recalcitrant.

If vesicular skin lesions are present around the eye, *vesicular fluid* should be collected using a sterile small-gauge needle. Scrapings from the base of the lesion should also be obtained. Both the fluid and the scrapings are excellent samples for viral culture; the scrapings are also appropriate for antigen detection procedures.

When keratitis or corneal ulcers are present, it may be necessary to collect specimens directly from the cornea (*corneal swab*). The eye should first be anesthetized with a drop of topical anesthetic. The lids should be held apart or a lid speculum placed. The moistened applicator tip is then applied to the corneal lesion, and the base and edges of the ulcer are gently swabbed. When corneal integrity is uncertain or visualization is poor, corneal scraping and swabbing should be avoided. Keratectomy and corneal biopsy specimens are not collected routinely but may be needed when the disease condition requires a lamellar or penetrating corneal transplant, as in corneal perforation.

The specimen of choice for PCR in determining the etiologic agent of infectious retinitis is *vitreous fluid*,

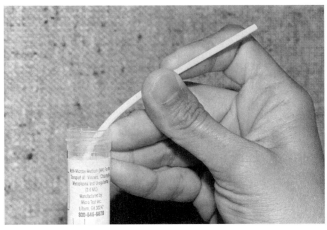

Figure 10.2 Conjunctival swab is immersed in viral transport medium, and shaft of applicator stick is broken off. Vial is recapped, with applicator tip and swab remaining immersed in medium and ready for transport.

which should be transported to the laboratory in a sterile container on ice. Very small volumes of fluid may be useful, and no amount should be considered too neglible to submit. Diluted vitreous washings may also be useful. In some patients, *aqueous humor* may substitute for vitreous; the relative sensitivity of these fluids in cases of viral retinitis is still under investigation. PCR has also been performed on corneal tissue and on tear fluid; these applications are still investigational in most clinics. When PCR testing is required, the clinician first must contact the laboratory to confirm the viruses being sought and the method of specimen collection and transport.

SPECIFIC VIRAL TESTING

Indications

The experienced clinician can accurately diagnose many viral infections of the eye using clues from the history, clinical presentation, or appearance of the lesions. Viral diagnostic tests are not routinely ordered unless factors are present that can obscure the diagnosis, such as prior treatment, presence of concurrent infections or eye diseases, and immunologic dysfunction that can cause atypical presentation. Other reasons for ordering specific diagnostic tests are unresponsiveness to therapy, suspicion of drug resistance, the need to rule in or rule out certain masquerade syndromes, and the need for laboratory confirmation of a presumed diagnosis to institute specific antiviral therapy.

Diagnostic Tests

The main tests used for making a specific viral diagnosis of ocular infection are viral culture; antigen detection usually by fluorescent antibody (FA) staining; and PCR.

Viral culture. Adenoviruses, HSV, VZV, and the enteroviruses grow well in cell culture and can be detected by most diagnostic virology laboratories without special notification. An innovative culture method for the detection of ocular viral pathogens is a shell vial culture with double-label immunofluorescent antibody staining used to detect HSV and adenovirus simultaneously after a 2-day incubation period.[2] This assay is not yet widely implemented in diagnostic laboratories.

Antigen assays. Antigen detection methods performed directly on the specimen can provide same-day results and do not require the presence of viable virus. This can be particularly advantageous when conditions for specimen transport are not optimal. FA staining of exfoliated cells from the conjunctiva or cornea may provide a rapid diagnosis and is widely available for adenoviruses, HSV, and VZV. This technique should be discussed with the laboratory in advance because laboratories (1) may require prior notification, (2) may vary in their capability to perform antigen detection tests for these viruses, (3) may require specification of the individual viruses to be detected, and (4) may have special requirements for collection and transport of specimens.

Polymerase chain reaction. PCR is rapidly becoming accepted as the method of choice for the diagnosis of intraocular infections such as iridocyclitis and retinitis. An important asset is the need for only a small amount of specimen. PCR can also detect the presence of fastidious and slow-growing viruses (e.g., CMV, VZV) more rapidly than culture techniques. Some aqueous and vitreous fluids have been found to contain substances that are inhibitory to PCR.[3] A variety of specimen-processing techniques, including dilution, chloroform extraction, or processing through a silica gel column, can remove the inhibitory material and allow PCR to be carried out.

Special considerations. MCV cannot be cultured, and infection with this agent is diagnosed clinically or by histopathology in unusual cases. HPV also cannot be cultured; when necessary, presence of this virus can be confirmed by histopathology or by PCR, which can also be used to type the virus. NDV and vaccinia virus are unusual viruses for diagnostic laboratories, and notification should be provided if these viruses are suspected.

SPECIFIC VIRAL AGENTS

Adenovirus

Adenoviruses are the most common cause of *viral conjunctivitis.* Clinical manifestations of adenoviral ocular infections include epidemic keratoconjunctivitis (EKC), pharyngoconjunctival fever (PCF), and non-

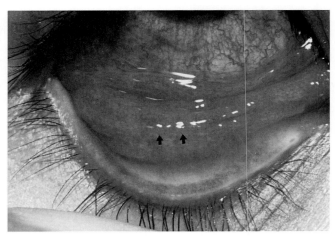

Figure 10.3 Acute follicular conjunctivitis seen in adenoviral ocular infection. Note enlarged follicles in inferior fornix (*arrows*) and conjunctival congestion and hyperemia.

specific acute follicular conjunctivitis (Figure 10–3). Commonly referred to as "pinkeye," adenoviral conjunctivitis frequently becomes bilateral, with tearing, redness, photophobia, and lid swelling. Many patients develop epithelial keratitis, followed 2 weeks later by subepithelial corneal infiltrates. Approximately one third of the 49 human adenovirus serotypes, especially 1 to 11, 14, 19, and 37, have been associated with one or more of the common forms of adenoviral ocular infections.[4]

Adenoviruses are nonenveloped double-stranded deoxyribonucleic acid (DNA) viruses that are very stable. They can be transmitted by water and fomites. Numerous cases of transmission by contaminated ophthalmologic equipment have been reported. Laboratory studies have demonstrated prolonged recoverability of desiccated adenovirus type 19 for up to 35 days from nonporous plastic.[5] Studies report that adenovirus type 8 can survive for up to 9 days on a tonometer and up to 7 days in a laboratory setting.[6]

The clinical diagnosis of adenoviral ocular infections is usually not difficult because of the characteristic presentation. The most consistent finding is acute follicular conjunctivitis. However, the proper diagnosis may be missed in atypical cases or when the initial examination is done by individuals unfamiliar with the characteristic signs and symptoms. Early, accurate diagnosis is important to prevent outbreaks by removing the infectious individual from the environment, thereby reducing the exposure of susceptible individuals. Laboratory diagnosis can also facilitate recognition of outbreaks related to contaminated medical equipment or other common sources.

The gold standard for detection of adenoviral infections is isolation of the virus in *cell culture.* Cell cultures may become positive as early as 1 day after inoculation and are positive by the seventh day in 95% of patients when the specimen is obtained within 1 week of the onset of symptoms.[6] The main disadvantages of cell culture are expense and the time required for detection of the virus.

The primary rapid diagnostic test used to detect adenoviruses is *antigen detection* by FA staining of virally infected conjunctival cells.[7] Other antigen detection techniques have also been used, including enzyme immunoassay (EIA),[6] radioimmunoassay (RIA) or dot blot technique,[8] immunofiltration,[9] and electron microscopy. Vastine et al[7] reported that direct immunofluorescence had a sensitivity and specificity of 100% in detecting adenoviral antigens in epithelial cells or conjunctival scrapings from 25 patients with a clinical diagnosis of EKC or PCF, including four whose cultures were negative. All these patients had adenovirus types 7, 8, or 19. As with all antigen detection procedures, high sensitivity depends on obtaining an adequate sample. Currently available reagents detect all adenoviral serotypes.

A commercial EIA, *Adenoclone* (Cambridge Bio-Science, Hopkinton, Mass), has been used to detect adenovirus in ocular specimens.[7] The Adenoclone assay is rapid (1 hour), is easy to perform, requires no expensive equipment, and can be performed in an office. This test is less sensitive than FA staining or culture. One study found that Adenoclone had a sensitivity of 77% and a specificity of 100% for samples collected within 1 week of the onset of clinical symptoms. Swabs taken more than one week after onset were usually negative.[6]

PCR has also been applied to the diagnosis of ocular adenoviral infections and appears to have a sensitivity equal to or greater than viral culture. In one study, PCR was positive on all specimens that were positive by both Adenoclone and culture and on 79% of specimens negative by Adenoclone and positive by culture. Only 1 of 38 nonadenoviral ocular swab samples was positive (specificity of 97%).[4] In another study, PCR was more sensitive than an RIA for adenoviral antigen. The sensitivity of PCR was largely independent of adenovirus serotype.[10] In a third study, PCR was more sensitive than culture and could be modified to provide identification of the adenovirus type in addition to detecting the virus.[11] Because of its complexity and expense, PCR should presently be viewed as a research tool for diagnosis of adenoviral infections.

Herpes Simplex Virus

HSV is the most common cause of *corneal blindness* in industrial nations and the most common cause of unilateral infectious corneal blindness in the world.

Ocular HSV infection has a variety of clinical manifestations. Primary infection may present as a periocular vesiculopustular or ulcerative blepharodermatitis, which is nondermatomal in distribution (Figure 10–4). A follicular or pseudomembranous conjunctivitis

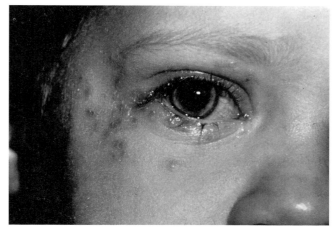

Figure 10.4   Primary herpes simplex in child with periocular vesiculopustular and ulcerative nondermatomal blepharodermatitis.

may be present alone or may be accompanied by an ulcerative keratitis, which may be punctate, dendritic, or geographic in appearance. Recurrent disease usually presents as superficial corneal ulcers. After multiple attacks, this process can lead to corneal scarring, vascularization, and thinning. Recurrent disease also has considerably more corneal stromal involvement, which can include disciform stromal keratitis, interstitial keratitis, and stromal necrosis.

Granulomatous iridocyclitis, trabeculitis, and endotheliitis have also been associated with HSV. HSV is also one of the causes of infectious retinitis seen in either immunologically competent or immunosuppressed individuals. Almost all ocular infections, except for some cases of retinitis and most neonatal infections are caused by HSV type 1. Neonatal disease can involve all structures of the eye as well as numerous other organs.

Corneal HSV infections are usually diagnosed by their typical dendritic appearance (Figure 10–5) or geographic pattern (Figure 10–6). In typical cases,

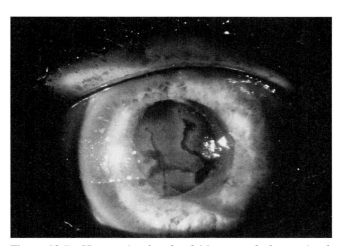

Figure 10.5   Herpes simplex dendritic corneal ulcer stained with rose bengal.

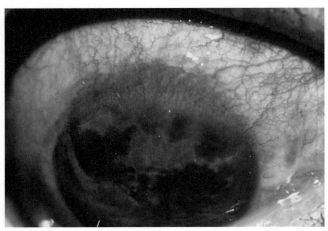

Figure 10.6 Geographic herpes simplex corneal ulcer stained with fluorescein.

clinical diagnosis by an experienced ophthalmologist is as accurate as viral culture. However, atypical cases may not be recognized by clinical examination. Laboratory tests are usually limited to patients with atypical presentations, such as concurrent infection, partial treatment, possible drug resistance, and corneal trauma or surgery, and to cases in which it is necessary to differentiate infectious dendrites from pseudodendrites. Viral culture, antigen detection methods, and cytology are positive only in the active phase of herpetic disease; between episodes when the virus is latent, these techniques are not positive. The question of whether HSV DNA can be detected in corneal tissue during latency is controversial.

Cytology is a traditional means for diagnosing herpetic ocular infections. Scrapings of corneal and conjunctival epithelial lesions obtained by a blunt-tip spatula or blade can be stained with Giemsa or Wright's stain to look for multinucleated giant cells and eosinophilic intranuclear inclusions (*Tzanck smear*). Conjunctival impression smears generally show an even distribution of polymorphonuclear cells and monocytes. The sensitivity of Tzanck smear is only about 40%, less than that of well-performed antigen detection methods. Another disadvantage is that the Tzanck smear cannot differentiate between infections caused by different herpesviruses.

Viral culture is the most definitive method for the diagnosis of ocular HSV infection, but even this method may underestimate the frequency of HSV ocular disease, particularly in patients with inactive herpetic keratitis, in whom only latent and nonviable virus may be present. Culture is useful for vesicular lesions involving the skin around the eye. These vesicles are punctured, and the vesicular fluid is absorbed on a swab. Scrapings from the base of the lesion are also a rich source of viable virus and can be used for FA staining as well. Corneal and conjunctival ulcers can be swabbed with a sterile cotton- or Dacron-tipped applicator after

topical anesthetic is applied but before topical rose bengal stain. Calcium alginate swabs should not be used because they have inhibitory activity against HSV.[12]

In patients with suspected *HSV retinitis*, a retinal biopsy specimen taken at the advancing border of the infected tissue can be placed in culture, or a sample of vitreous fluid can be tested for HSV DNA by PCR. Specimens for culture should be placed in appropriate media and promptly transported to the laboratory. Cell culture for HSV is very sensitive, and most isolates are detected within 72 hours (see Chapters 1 and 6).

A variety of methods have been used to detect HSV antigens in ocular specimens, including FA staining, EIA, immunofiltration, RIA, and latex agglutination (LA). FA staining of cells obtained by corneal swab or scraping has had high sensitivity compared with viral culture in some studies.[13-15] Cells were obtained in one study by applying a Biopore membrane to the cornea.[14] Interpretation of corneal FA stains requires skill, and the laboratory's experience with the technique can greatly affect the sensitivity and specificity of results.

A commercial EIA, *HerpChek* (DuPont Medical Products, Boston), has been evaluated for detection of ocular HSV infection. This assay is the first nonculture assay to have been approved by the U.S. Food and Drug Administration (FDA) for detection of HSV without culture backup. Two studies have shown HerpChek to have sensitivity comparable to culture in patients with ocular HSV infections.[16, 17]

PCR shows promise for the diagnosis of a variety of manifestations of ocular HSV infection, especially keratitis, iridocyclitis, and retinitis. Cassinotti et al[18] detected HSV-1 DNA in a corneal button from a patient with clinically suspected HSV disciform keratitis and from the corneal swab of another patient 1 week after onset of keratitis. Kowalski et al[17] compared EIA (improved HerpChek) and PCR with clinical examination for diagnosing ocular HSV disease. They found that laboratory diagnosis was more accurate than clinical examination in atypical cases. Interestingly, PCR was less sensitive than the HerpChek assay, but this may have been related to the larger sample volume used with HerpChek. PCR should still be viewed as investigational for the diagnosis of HSV corneal disease until the relationship between the detection of HSV DNA and the presence of active HSV keratitis has been clarified.

PCR has also been used to detect HSV DNA in vitreous fluid from patients with *acute retinal necrosis syndrome* (ARN).[19] Because of the absence of other good methods, PCR is rapidly becoming the method of choice for the diagnosis of ARN.

Varicella-zoster Virus

Varicella, the manifestation of primary infection with VZV, is a familiar exanthematous disease that afflicts most humans during childhood or adolescence and has the unique ability to cause a distinct clinical syndrome, *zoster* (shingles), on reactivation. Ocular manifestations of varicella include eyelid lesions, conjunctival vesicles, dendritic keratitis (Figure 10–7), iritis, internal ophthalmoplegia, extraocular muscle palsies, cataracts, chorioretinitis, and optic neuritis. Involvement by zoster of the ophthalmic branch of the trigeminal nerve is termed *herpes zoster ophthalmicus* (Figure 10–8) and results from reactivation of VZV in the distribution of the ophthalmic branch of the trigeminal ganglion. Involvement of this dermatome accounts for 10% to 25% of all episodes of zoster. Ocular involvement occurs in 50% to 72% of patients with herpes zoster ophthalmicus and can present as conjunctivitis, episcleritis, scleritis, keratitis, uveitis, secondary glaucoma, cataract, cranial nerve palsies, Horner's syndrome, postherpetic neuralgia, and orbital apex and inflammatory syndromes.

Infection by VZV may involve the posterior segment of the eye, causing ARN syndrome (Figure 10–9) and *progressive outer retinal necrosis* (PORN) syndrome (Figure 10–10). Congenital varicella syndrome may be associated with ocular abnormalities, including chorioretinitis, optic atrophy or hypoplasia, congenital cataracts, microphthalmos, and Horner's syndrome.

The diagnosis of zoster is almost always based on clinical findings without laboratory confirmation. Rarely, laboratory tests are needed to diagnose cases of VZV infection that lack cutaneous involvement (*zoster sine herpete*). Laboratory testing is also used to differentiate VZV disease from other entities that mimic it, including zosteriform HSV, hypersensitivity reactions, vesicular enteroviral infections, and contact dermatitis. AIDS patients may present with atypical ocular manifestations of VZV infection that may be misdiagnosed as

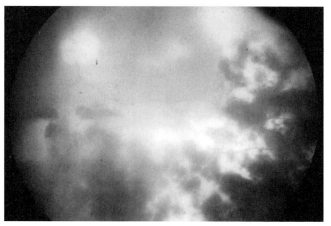

Figure 10.9 Acute retinal necrosis (ARN) syndrome caused by varicella-zoster virus in immunocompetent patient. Note severe vitreous haze, retinal necrosis, and opacification outside of major vascular arcades, with occlusive vasculopathy and retinal hemorrhages.

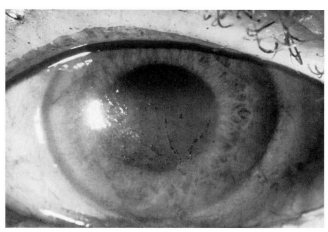

Figure 10.7 Dendriform (dendritic) keratitis stained with rose bengal in patient with acute varicella-zoster virus infection.

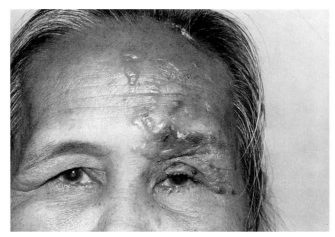

Figure 10.8 Acute herpes zoster ophthalmicus in elderly patient. Vesicular eruptions are seen along dermatomal distribution of ophthalmic branch of trigeminal nerve.

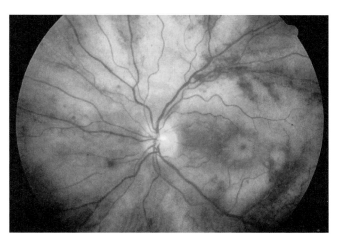

Figure 10.10 Severe progressive outer retinal necrosis (PORN) syndrome in AIDS patient caused by varicella-zoster virus. This is characterized by multifocal, deep retinal opacification. Retinitis rapidly progresses outward to periphery and becomes confluent. Vitreous haze or inflammation is minimal or absent, in contrast to ARN syndrome (Figure 10–9).

HSV, CMV, or ocular toxoplasmosis. Prompt diagnosis in these patients is essential to prevent chronic morbidity requiring prolonged drug treatment, which can increase the chance of emergence of antiviral resistance.

Cytology has been a traditional method for identification of ocular VZV infection. A *Tzanck smear* can be prepared as described for HSV. Scrapings from the base of vesicles are smeared on a glass slide and stained with Giemsa or Wright's stain. Examination by light microscopy reveals multinucleated giant cells, a mononuclear cellular reaction, eosinophilic intranuclear inclusion bodies, and margination of nuclear chromatin. This technique is positive in about 70% of vesicles and 55% of pustules and is almost always negative in crusted lesions. The Tzanck smear does not differentiate between VZV and HSV.[20]

Viral isolation in cell culture is the benchmark test for VZV but is less sensitive than antigen detection techniques. Infectious virus is present in highest titer in the clear vesicle stage. Vesicular lesions should be aspirated gently through a small-gauge needle into a small-volume syringe and sent immediately to the laboratory on ice. Alternatively, a small volume of viral transport medium can be drawn into the syringe after aspirating the vesicle. Scrapings may be taken from the base of two or three lesions and placed in viral transport media. If FA staining will be performed, a portion of the scrapings should be placed on glass microscope slides. Detection of growth in cell culture usually requires 4 to 7 days. Use of the shell vial technique may decrease this time to 1 to 2 days. In patients with suspected VZV retinitis, vitreous samples or retinal biopsy specimens may be directly inoculated into cell culture or used for PCR.

As for adenovirus and HSV, FA staining is the most widely used technique for detection of VZV antigen and is more sensitive than cell culture for VZV. Other techniques, as described for adenovirus and HSV, have also been used. Unlike HSV, no commercially available EIA kit suitable for office use has been developed. In addition to being used to analyze material from cutaneous lesions, antigen detection techniques have been used to detect virus-specific antigens in cells of vitreous humor aspirates collected at vitrectomy in patients with VZV-associated ARN syndrome. The vitreous specimen is pelleted by centrifugation onto glass slides and stained by the FA technique. Soushi et al[21] found antigen-positive cells in the vitreous humor aspirates of two of four patients with ARN from suspected VZV infection. Cultures of aspirates from all four patients were negative.

PCR is particularly useful in the diagnosis of early VZV retinitis, which can be difficult to distinguish from other causes of infectious retinitis (e.g., HSV, CMV, toxoplasmosis). In the most comprehensive study to date, Short et al[22] performed PCR on vitreous samples and were able to detect VZV DNA in 11 of 14 samples

from AIDS patients with PORN syndrome. All three negative samples came from eyes that had been treated aggressively with antiviral drugs and had clinically inactive disease at vitreous biopsy. VZV DNA was detected in only 2 of 75 control vitreous samples from immunosuppressed patients with vitreoretinal disease and 2 of 88 control vitreous samples from patients with AIDS and vitreoretinal inflammatory disease not related to PORN syndrome. PCR has also been used to detect VZV DNA in samples of aqueous or vitreous humor from patients with ARN.[23, 24] Experience is still too limited to provide estimates of sensitivity and specificity or to evaluate the utility of aqueous versus vitreous samples, but PCR appears much more sensitive than culture for the diagnosis of intraocular infections caused by VZV.

PCR has also been performed in cases of anterior uveitis and keratitis related to VZV. VZV DNA has been detected in the excised corneal button from a 6-year-old child with a perforated corneal ulcer. Yamamoto et al[25] detected VZV DNA in samples of aqueous humor from a patient with zoster sine herpete iridocyclitis. Pavan-Langston et al[26] detected VZV DNA by PCR in both tear samples and corneal impressions collected with Schirmer strips in four patients clinically diagnosed with delayed herpes zoster ophthalmicus-associated pseudodendrites. VZV DNA was not found in two cases of neurotrophic ulcers believed to be secondary to herpes zoster ophthalmicus. Mietz et al[27] were able to detect VZV DNA by PCR in 7 of 14 corneal buttons from patients with a confirmed history of herpes zoster ophthalmicus. In one specimen the interval between initial appearance and detection of VZV DNA was 51 years. These studies suggest that active viral replication may have a greater role than previously suspected in corneal disease associated with VZV. The significance of detecting VZV DNA in corneal specimens is still under investigation.[28]

Cytomegalovirus

Ocular involvement by CMV is mainly retinal, involving all layers of the retina and at times the retinal pigment epithelium. Occasionally, CMV can affect other ocular tissues, including conjunctiva, caruncle, tears, cornea, iris, and lens. CMV is the most common viral cause of *retinitis*. Apart from newborns with congenital CMV, of whom 5% to 30% have CMV retinitis, the disease is seen almost exclusively in severely immunocompromised patients. CMV retinitis occurs in up to 15% to 30% of patients with AIDS, usually appearing late in the course of HIV infection when the CD4 count is less than $50/\mu l$.[29, 30]

The diagnosis of CMV retinitis is based on the presence of characteristic lesions seen on ophthalmoscopic examination in an immunocompromised patient. Untreated disease can have various clinical

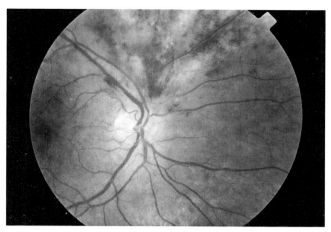

Figure 10.11   Cytomegalovirus retinitis involving superonasal quadrant of right eye with granular, white retinal opacification, retinal hemorrhages, and vascular sheathing.

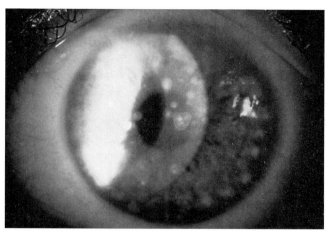

Figure 10.12   Multifocal nummular stromal lesions in cornea presumed to be caused by Epstein-Barr virus (EBV) in patient with diagnostic change in serial EBV serology.

presentations, with variable amounts of retinal whitening or opacification (edema or necrosis), retinal hemorrhage, and vascular sheathing (Figure 10–11). The two ends of the spectrum are known as the *fulminant/edematous* and *indolent/granular* types. CMV has also been found to produce a clinical picture similar to ARN syndrome.[31]

Laboratory diagnosis of CMV retinitis is usually limited to patients with unusual or puzzling clinical features. PCR is the only useful laboratory test to establish this diagnosis. Efforts have been made to demonstrate intraocular antibody production as a diagnostic technique, expressing the result as the Witmer-Goldmann coefficient, but studies have shown low sensitivity compared with PCR.[32-34]

PCR has been used to detect CMV DNA in aqueous humor, vitreous humor, subretinal fluid, and formalin-fixed ocular tissue sections.[35] McCann et al[34] reported an estimated sensitivity of 95% in detecting untreated CMV retinitis and a sensitivity of 48% in detecting CMV retinitis treated with systemic ganciclovir or foscarnet. Most importantly, their assay did not yield false-positive results when performed on vitreous humor from patients with other intraocular disorders or from AIDS patients with vitreous inflammation from other causes. Studies are still being done to determine the usefulness of aqueous humor compared with vitreous biopsy as a specimen for PCR.[36]

Detection of CMV DNA in an ocular sample does not rule out presence of another infectious agent. Dual infections of the retina with CMV and HSV or HIV have been described.[37, 38]

Epstein-Barr Virus

Ocular disease associated with EBV is uncommon but usually temporally associated with systemic EBV infection, as documented by EBV-specific serology (see Chapter 12). Ocular disease associated with EBV includes acute dacryocystitis, Parinaud's oculoglandular syndrome, conjunctival mass, Sjögren's syndrome, dendritic keratitis, subepithelial infiltrates, multifocal nummular nonsuppurative stromal keratitis (Figure 10–12), peripheral infiltrative keratitis, uveitis, retinitis, choroiditis, and a variety of neuroophthalmologic abnormalities. Because the serologic diagnosis provides only presumptive evidence that ocular manifestations are attributable to EBV, the clinician must rule out other potential causes before accepting EBV as the etiology.

No diagnostic tests other than serology are currently available for the diagnosis of EBV ocular disease. PCR is of interest for this purpose, but studies are required to determine whether it might sometimes detect EBV DNA in ocular specimens in the absence of disease. We are aware of one case in which PCR showed the presence of EBV DNA in vitreous fluid in a patient with EBV-associated lymphoma involving the eye.

Poxviruses

Poxviruses are large, morphologically complex viruses that contain linear, double-stranded DNA. The enveloped virion is brick shaped. Four poxviruses have been associated with ocular or eyelid infections: variola (smallpox virus), vaccinia virus, orf virus, and MCV. Of these, *molluscum contagiosum virus* is the most common cause of ocular disease. *Variola virus* was a major cause of ulcerative keratitis but is no longer a threat since its eradication in 1979. *Vaccinia conjunctivitis* is a well-recognized complication of smallpox vaccine. *Orf virus* primarily causes disease in sheep and other ungulates but can also cause disease in humans (contagious ecthyma) through contact with an infected animal.

The clinical manifestations of the different ocular poxvirus infections are distinct from one another. Molluscum contagiosum lesions are typically pale,

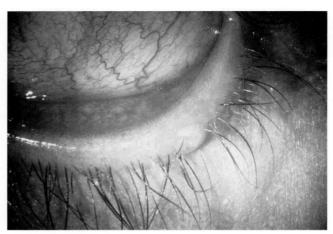

Figure 10.13 Molluscum contagiosum lesion on margin of lower lid. Note umbilicated center and presence of secondary follicular conjunctivitis.

flesh-colored, waxy, round, raised, painless skin nodules measuring 2 to 5 mm in diameter. The lesions usually have an umbilicated center (Figure 10–13). The distribution may be widespread, although the virus typically infects the face, including the eyelid margins, leading to toxic chronic follicular conjunctivitis, superficial keratitis, and pannus formation.[39, 40] The virus is spread by direct contact and by fomites. Infection is usually spread by sexual contact, with subsequent autoinoculation leading to ocular or adnexal involvement. Molluscum lesions are more common in immunocompromised patients, including those with AIDS. Treatment, when necessary, involves excision of the lesions.

Ocular involvement in orf is rare but usually seen in conjunction with characteristic epidermal skin lesions. Ocular vaccinia is a complication of smallpox vaccination in which the virus reaches the eye from the vaccination site by autoinoculation. Clinical manifestations vary depending on the host's specific immune status and include mucopurulent blepharoconjunctivitis, vesicle and pustule formation involving the eyelid and conjunctiva, superficial and stromal keratitis, ulcerative keratitis, and keratouveitis.[41]

The diagnosis of ocular poxvirus infections is usually based on the characteristic appearance of the lesions. MCV has never been cultured, and the laboratory diagnosis is based on characteristic histologic findings, including eosinophilic hyaline inclusions called *molluscum bodies*. The lesions have an eccentric location in the cytoplasm, displacing the nucleus. Thinly spread smears of material expressed from the core of the lesions can be stained with Papanicolaou, Wright's, Giemsa, or Gram stain to show numerous infected, inclusion-bearing cells. Use of supravital dyes allows visualization of the large poxvirus virions by light microscopy. MCV infection can also be demonstrated by immunocytochemical methods and by in situ or dot-blot hybridization.[40]

Vaccinia virus is present in vesicular fluid, scrapings of a vesicle's base, corneal and conjunctival scrapings,[41] and biopsy specimens. Stains of scrapings show eosinophilic cytoplasmic inclusion bodies known as *Guarnieri's bodies*. Vesicular fluid for culture should be collected using a fine needle and syringe or a capillary tube. Specimens can also be placed in viral transport media. Vaccinia virus grows readily in a variety of cell culture types widely used in diagnostic virology laboratories. Confirmation of vaccinia virus in infected cell cultures requires electron microscopy, which reveals virions with the characteristic poxvirus morphology. Identification of the specific poxvirus requires either inoculation of the chorioallantoic membrane of hen's eggs or restriction endonuclease analysis of DNA purified from infected cells. Laboratories should be notified whenever vaccinia virus is suspected, since most are no longer familiar with the virus and might not recognize its cytopathic effect in inoculated cell cultures.

Orf virus can be visualized by negative-staining electron microscopy. Most diagnostic virology laboratories are not prepared to carry out this procedure. Therefore, if orf is suspected, the laboratory should be contacted for instructions concerning specimen collection, since the specimen may have to be transported to a reference laboratory. Orf virus also grows in some cell cultures, including the primary monkey kidney cells used in many diagnostic virology laboratories. Laboratory notification of potential orf virus is essential to ensure that the sample is inoculated onto the appropriate cell culture types.

Enteroviruses

Among the 67 known enteroviral serotypes, *enterovirus 70* and *coxsackievirus A24* are the only two closely associated with ocular disease. Both these serotypes have been associated with the syndrome of *acute hemorrhagic conjunctivitis* (AHC). This entity was first recognized in 1969 and has occurred in epidemic and pandemic proportions since then in Asia, Europe, Africa, the South Sea Islands, Central and South America, and some parts of the United States.[42, 43] AHC can be differentiated clinically from adenoviral keratoconjunctivitis by its shorter incubation period, more rapid time course, and lack of subepithelial infiltrates.

The diagnostic test of choice for AHC is viral culture of the conjunctiva. Conjunctival swabs or scrapings must be obtained within 1 to 2 days after onset of symptoms.[42] A variety of cell culture types used in diagnostic virology laboratories can support the growth of the causative agents, but the laboratory should be notified to ensure that the specimen is inoculated onto the most appropriate cell culture types. Enterovirus PCR should also be applicable to the diagnosis of AHC. Enterovirus 70 can also be detected by FA staining using a monoclonal antibody to the virus.[44] A simple and rapid immunoassay for IgM antibodies to enterovirus 70 has been shown to have high sensitivity and specificity but is not widely available.[45]

Human Papillomavirus

The HPVs are members of the family Papovaviridae. Ocular manifestations include verrucae, which involve the skin of the lids and lid margins, and conjunctival papillomas, which are soft and usually pedunculated (Figure 10–14). A prominent vascular corkscrew pattern is also present. Inverted papillomas are usually seen in the lacrimal sac. HPV has also been associated with conjunctival dysplasias, epithelial neoplasias, and carcinomas.

HPV cannot be cultured, and no reliable serologic assay exists to diagnose acute or past infection. The diagnosis is usually made clinically and confirmed by histopathologic findings. Microscopically, pedunculated papillomas of the conjunctiva are composed of multiple fronds with fibrovascular cores covered by acanthotic epithelium.[46] Immunohistochemical techniques have been used to detect papillomavirus-specific capsid antigens. However, this approach is not as sensitive as the detection of HPV DNA by nucleic acid hybridization or PCR. These techniques are currently considered the gold standard for the diagnosis of HPV and can be used to type the virus as well as to confirm its presence[47] (see Chapter 7).

Newcastle Disease Virus

NDV is a paramyxovirus that mainly affects birds and poultry but can infect humans, presenting as an acute papillary or follicular conjunctivitis. Most infected patients have contact with birds; poultry workers, veterinarians, and laboratory workers are at risk. Human infections frequently occur in clusters paralleling avian epizootics. The virus is transmitted by aerosols or dust of respiratory or fecal origin, by hand-to-eye contact, or by live vaccine sprays. Clinical symptoms appear 12 to 48 hours after contact. The illness in humans is usually unilateral, and a tender, palpable preauricular lymph node is almost always present on the same side as the affected eye. Ocular secretions are scanty and nonpurulent. Fever, headache, and malaise occur at the onset but subside within 2 days. The illness is self-limited, with a usual course of 7 to 10 days.

The laboratory diagnosis of NDV is difficult. Conjunctival smears stained with Wright's or Giemsa stains show inflammatory cells consisting almost entirely of lymphocytes. The virus can be cultured from conjunctival swabs and washings. Specimens must be placed on ice and transported to the laboratory immediately. Embryonated hen's eggs are the preferred method of isolation. Cell culture isolation has been accomplished using chick embryo fibroblasts, but these cells are not

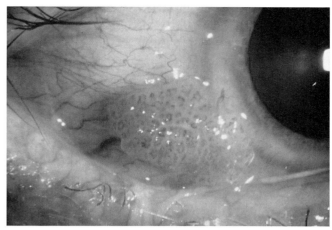

Figure 10.14 Bulbar conjunctival papilloma caused by human papillomavirus. Fleshy appearance with prominent vascular corkscrew pattern is typical.

routinely available in many diagnostic virology laboratories. The laboratory should be contacted in advance if the diagnosis is suspected so that arrangements can be made to send the specimen to a veterinary laboratory that has experience with this virus. The serologic response is inconsistent and is not useful for diagnosis.[48]

References

1. Pepose JS: Application of immunologic technology to the diagnosis of viral infections of the ocular surface, *Cornea* 7:36, 1988.
2. Walpita P, Darougar S: Double-label immunofluorescence method for simultaneous detection of adenovirus and herpes simplex virus from the eye, *J Clin Microbiol* 27:1623, 1989.
3. Wiedbrauk DL, Werner JC, Drevon AM: Inhibition of PCR by aqueous and vitreous fluids, *J Clin Microbiol* 33:2643, 1995.
4. Kinchington PR, Turse SE, Kowalski RP, Gordon YJ: Use of polymerase chain amplification reaction for the detection of adenoviruses in ocular swab specimens, *Invest Ophthalmol Vis Sci* 35:4126, 1994.
5. Nauheim RC, Romanowski EG, Araullo-Cruz T, et al: Prolonged recoverability of desiccated adenovirus type 19 from various surfaces, *Ophthalmology* 97:1450, 1990.
6. Gordon YJ, Aoki K, Kinchington PR: Adenovirus keratoconjunctivitis. In Pepose JS, Holland GN, Wilhelmus KR, editors: *Ocular infection and immunity*, St. Louis, 1996, Mosby.
7. Vastine DW, Schwartz HS, Yamashiroya HM, et al: Cytologic diagnosis of adenoviral epidemic keratoconjunctivitis by direct immunofluorescence, *Invest Ophthalmol Vis Sci* 16:195, 1977.
8. Killough R, Klapper PE, Bailey AS, et al: An immune dot-blot technique for the diagnosis of ocular adenovirus infection, *J Virol Methods* 30:197, 1990.

9. Cleveland PH, Richman DD: Enzyme immunofiltration staining assay for immediate diagnosis of herpes simplex virus and varicella-zoster virus directly from clinical specimens, *J Clin Microbiol* 25:416, 1987.

10. Morris DJ, Bailey AS, Cooper RJ, et al: Polymerase chain reaction for rapid detection of ocular adenovirus infection, *J Med Virol* 46:126, 1995.

11. Saitoh-Inagawa W, Oshima A, Aoki K, et al: Rapid diagnosis of adenoviral conjunctivitis by PCR and restriction fragment length polymorphism analysis, *J Clin Microbiol* 34:2113, 1996.

12. Thomson RB: Laboratory methods in basic virology. In Baron EJ, Peterson LR, Finegold SM, editors: *Diagnostic microbiology*, ed 9, St. Louis, 1994, Mosby.

13. Schwab IR, Raju VK, McClung J: Indirect immunofluorescent antibody diagnosis of herpes simplex with upper tarsal and corneal scrapings, *J Ophthalmol* 93:752, 1986.

14. Simon MW, Miller D, Pflugfelder SC, et al: Comparison of immunocytology to tissue culture for diagnosis of presumed herpesvirus dendritic epithelial keratitis, *Ophthalmology* 99:1408, 1992.

15. Gardner PS, McQuillin J: *Rapid virus diagnosis: application of immunofluorescence*, ed 2, London, 1980, Butterworths.

16. Dunkel EC, Pavan-Langston D, Fitzpatrick K, Cukor G: Rapid detection of herpes simplex virus antigen in human ocular infections, *Curr Eye Res* 7: 661, 1988.

17. Kowalski RP, Gordon YJ, Romanowski EG, et al: A comparison of enzyme immunoassay and polymerase chain reaction with the clinical examination for diagnosing ocular herpetic disease, *Ophthalmology* 100:530, 1993.

18. Cassinotti P, Mietz H, Siegl G: Suitability and clinical application of a multiplex nested PCR assay for the diagnosis of herpes simplex virus infections, *J Med Virol* 50:75, 1996.

19. Cunningham ET, Short GA, Irvine AR, et al: Acquired immunodeficiency syndrome–associated herpes simplex virus retinitis, *Arch Ophthalmol* 114:834, 1996.

20. Pavan-Langston D, Dunkel EC: Varicella-zoster virus diseases: anterior segment of the eye. In Pepose JS, Holland GN, Wilhelmus KR, editors: *Ocular infection and immunity*, St. Louis, 1996, Mosby.

21. Soushi S et al: Demonstration of varicella-zoster virus antigens in the vitreous aspirates of patients with acute retinal necrosis syndrome, *Ophthalmology* 95:1394, 1988.

22. Short GA, Margolis TP, Kuppermann BD, et al: A polymerase chain reaction–based assay for diagnosing varicella-zoster virus retinitis in patients with acquired immunodeficiency syndrome, *Am J Ophthalmol* 123:157, 1997.

23. Figueroa MS, Garabito I, Gutierrez C, Fortun J: Famciclovir for the treatment of acute retinal necrosis (ARN) syndrome, *Am J Ophthalmol* 123: 255, 1997.

24. Usui M et al: Polymerase chain reaction for diagnosis of herpetic intraocular inflammation, *Ocular Immunol Inflammation* 1:105, 1993.

25. Yamamoto S, Tada R, Shimomura Y, et al: Detecting varicella-zoster virus DNA in iridocyclitis using polymerase chain reaction: a case of zoster sine herpete, *Arch Ophthalmol* 113:1358, 1995.

26. Pavan-Langston D, Yamamoto S, Dunkel EC: Delayed herpes zoster pseudodendrites: polymerase chain reaction detection of viral DNA and the role of antiviral therapy, *Arch Ophthalmol* 113:1381, 1995.

27. Mietz H, Eis-Hubinger AM, Sundmacher R, et al: Detection of varicella-zoster virus DNA in keratectomy specimens by use of polymerase chain reaction, *Arch Ophthalmol* 115:590, 1997.

28. Liesegang TJ: The use of polymerase chain reaction techniques to detect varicella-zoster virus in corneal transplant tissue, *Arch Ophthalmol* 115:664, 1997.

29. Dunn JP, Jabs DA: Cytomegalovirus retinitis in AIDS: natural history, diagnosis, and treatment, *AIDS Clin Rev,* 1995-96, p 99.

30. Holland GN, Tufail A, Jordan MC: Cytomegalovirus diseases. In Pepose JS, Holland GN, Wilhelmus KR, editors: *Ocular infection and immunity*, St. Louis, 1996, Mosby.

31. Silverstein BE, Conrad D, Margolis TP, Wong IG: Cytomegalovirus-associated acute retinal necrosis syndrome, *Am J Ophthalmol* 123:257, 1997.

32. De Boer JH, Verhagen C, Bruinenberg M, et al: Serologic and polymerase chain reaction analysis of intraocular fluids in the diagnosis of infectious uveitis, *Am J Ophthalmol* 121:650, 1996.

33. Doornenbal P, Seerp Baarsma G, Quint WGV, et al: Diagnostic assays in cytomegalovirus retinitis: detection of herpesvirus by simultaneous application of the polymerase chain reaction and local antibody analysis on ocular fluid, *Br J Ophthalmol* 80:235, 1996.

34. McCann JD, Margolis TP, Wong MG, et al: A sensitive and specific polymerase chain reaction–based assay for the diagnosis of cytomegalovirus retinitis, *Am J Ophthalmol* 120:219, 1995.

35. Garcia-Ferrer FJ, Blatt AN, Laycock KA, Pepose JS: Molecular biologic techniques in ophthalmic pathology, *Ophthalmol Clin North Am* 8:25, 1995.

36. Mitchell SM, Fox JD: Aqueous and vitreous humor samples for the diagnosis of cytomegalovirus retinitis, *Am J Ophthalmol* 120:252, 1995.

37. Rummelt V, Rummelt C, John G, et al: Triple retinal infection with human immunodeficiency virus type 1, cytomegalovirus and herpes simplex virus type 1: light and electron microscopy, immunohistochemistry, and in situ hybridization, *Ophthalmology* 101:270, 1994.

38. Skolnik PR, Pomerantz RJ, de la Monte SM, et al: Dual infection of retina with human immunodeficiency virus type 1 and cytomegalovirus, *Am J Ophthalmol* 107:361, 1989.

39. Charteris DG, Bonshek RE, Tullo AB: Ophthalmic molluscum contagiosum: clinical and immunopathological features, *Br J Ophthalmol* 79:476, 1995.

40. Pepose JS, Esposito JJ: Molluscum contagiosum, orf, and vaccinia. In Pepose JS, Holland GN, Wilhelmus KR, editors: *Ocular infection and immunity*, St. Louis, 1996, Mosby.

41. Lee SF, Buller R, Chansue E, et al: Vaccinia keratouveitis manifesting as a masquerade syndrome, *Am J Ophthalmol* 117:480, 1994 .

42. Rosa RH, Alfonso EC: Enterovirus keratoconjunctivitis.

In Pepose JS, Holland GN, Wilhelmus KR, editors: *Ocular infection and immunity*, St. Louis, 1996, Mosby.

43. Rotbart HA: Enteroviruses. In Murray PR, editor: *Manual of clinical microbiology*, ed 7, Washington, DC, 1999, ASM Press.

44. Anderson SO, Bjorksten B, Burman LA: Detection of enterovirus 70 with monoclonal antibodies, *J Clin Microbiol* 20:405, 1984.

45. Wulff H et al: Diagnosis of enterovirus 70 infection by demonstration of IgM antibodies, *J Med Virol* 21:231, 1987.

46. McLean IW, Burnier MN, Zimmerman LE, Jakobiec FA: Tumors of the eye and ocular adnexa. In *Atlas of tumor pathology*, Washington, DC, 1994, Armed Forces Institute of Pathology.

47. Kiviat NB: Human papillomaviruses. In Murray PR, editor: *Manual of clinical microbiology*, ed 7, Washington, DC, 1999, ASM Press.

48. Wood TR: Newcastle disease. In Pepose JS, Holland GN, Wilhelmus KR, editors: *Ocular infection and immunity*, St. Louis, 1996, Mosby.

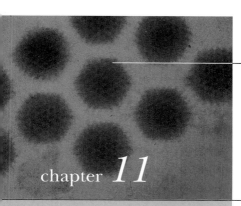

Gregory A. Storch

chapter *11*

Urinary Tract Infections

OVERVIEW

Viruses that can be detected in urine include adenovirus, polyomaviruses BK and JC, cytomegalovirus (CMV), herpes simplex virus, enteroviruses, mumps virus, and the human hantaviruses. Of these, only adenovirus, BK virus, and the hantaviruses cause significant urinary tract disease, whereas detection of the other viruses in urine is most often associated with infection at a site outside the urinary tract.

The most common urinary tract disease associated with both adenovirus and BK virus is *hemorrhagic cystitis.* Adenovirus hemorrhagic cystitis occurs in normal children and in immunocompromised individuals; BK virus hemorrhagic cystitis occurs almost exclusively in the latter. The hantaviruses cause *hemorrhagic fever with renal syndrome*, which is extremely rare in the United States but common in other parts of the world (see Chapter 16).

BK VIRUS

BK virus is a polyomavirus that was discovered in 1971 in the urine of a renal transplant recipient.[1] Its name derives from the initials of the patient from whom it was first isolated. The polyomaviruses are small deoxyribonucleic acid (DNA) viruses that are in the family Papovaviridae, which also includes the papillomaviruses. The only polyomavirus other than BK virus that is known to be a human pathogen is *JC virus*, the cause of progressive multifocal leukoencephalopathy (see Chapter 3). The only well-defined diseases attributable to BK virus involve the urinary tract. Most cases occur in immunocompromised patients, although a few cases of BK virus cystitis have been described in normal children.[2, 3]

Although they rarely cause disease, both BK and JC viruses are very common human viruses that usually produce infection with no recognizable disease manifestations. Serologic surveys reveal that nearly all children have antibodies to BK virus by age 10 or 11 years.[2, 4] BK virus has been demonstrated in the respiratory tract, suggesting a respiratory mode of transmission.[5] The virus is believed to produce latent infection with persistence in the kidneys and the central nervous system.[6] BK viruria is detected only rarely in the absence of immunosuppression, with reported frequencies of 0% in studies based on culture, 4% in a study based on DNA hybridization,[7] and 0% and 18% in studies based on PCR.[8, 9] The latter study used ultracentrifugation to concentrate large volumes of urine. In immunocompromised individuals, any of the methods can reveal BK virus in the absence of disease, and therefore the findings of laboratory tests must be interpreted in conjunction with the clinical findings.

Specific Patient Populations

Bone marrow transplant recipients. BK virus is an important cause of hemorrhagic cystitis in bone marrow transplant recipients. Hemorrhagic cystitis from any cause occurs in up to 25% of bone marrow transplant recipients and is most often caused by toxicity from drugs or by viral infection. After the early posttransplant period, BK virus infection is the most common cause, affecting both allogeneic and autologous marrow recipients.[10-12]

In a survey of bone marrow transplant recipients, 53% had BK virus detected by polymerase chain reaction (PCR) in one or more serial posttransplant urine specimens.[12] More than half the patients with BK viruria developed hemorrhagic cystitis, which did not occur in any patient without BK viruria. The onset of BK viruria occurred 2 to 15 weeks after transplantation (median of 21 days), typically in close temporal association with the onset of hemorrhagic cystitis. BK viruria was present in only 3% of pretransplant specimens. In the same study, adenovirus type 11 was detected in the urine of one patient.

Kidney transplant recipients. In renal transplant recipients, BK virus infection produces a uroepitheliitis that can cause ureteral obstruction.[1, 13] Basophilic intranuclear inclusions characteristic of papovavirus infection have been seen in epithelial cells of the ureter, renal pelvis, and tubules.[13, 14]

Molecular studies to define the prevalence of BK virus in renal transplant recipients have not been performed. One prospective study, however, using serology, viral culture, and urine cytology, showed evidence of BK virus infection in 44% of patients, of whom more than 50% had positive cytologic findings.[15]

Immunodeficient patients. Renal failure attributable to BK virus infection has been reported in patients with the hyper-IgM syndrome[16] and cartilage-hair hypoplasia.[17] Renal biopsies showed tubulointerstitial inflammation with intranuclear inclusions containing papovavirus particles on electron microscopy (EM). BK virus was present in the urine in both cases.

BK viruria has been detected by PCR in 23% to 24% of HIV-infected subjects.[8, 9] In both studies the prevalence of viruria increased with increasing immunodeficiency. Renal disease associated with BK virus has not been identified in patients with human immunodeficiency virus (HIV).

Laboratory Detection

A number of methods have been used to detect BK virus in patient samples, including urine cytology, EM, fluorescent antibody (FA) staining of urinary cells, enzyme immunoassay, viral culture, DNA hybridization, and PCR. All these methods can reveal evidence of BK virus infection in the absence of disease. The most important methods for clinical diagnosis are cytology and PCR.

Cytology. Urine cytology has been useful as a screening test. Papovavirus infection produces characteristic basophilic inclusions that almost or completely fill the nucleus of transitional epithelial cells[18] (see Figure 1–3). Identical inclusions can occur with either BK or JC virus infection. The inclusions are made up of masses of papovavirus particles, which can be identified by EM. In contrast to CMV inclusions, which can be cytoplasmic as well as nuclear, papovavirus inclusions occur only in the nucleus. Cytology is less sensitive for detecting BK viruria than PCR.

Viral culture. BK virus can be cultivated using a variety of cell culture types, including human embryonic or neonatal kidney cells, human embryonic fibroblast cells, and human fetal glial cells. Only the latter are useful for cultivating JC virus, which is more difficult to grow. BK virus grows slowly in culture, often requiring several weeks before cytopathic effect is apparent. Therefore culture is of use mainly in research laboratories or to recover an isolate for special studies. A shell vial assay has been developed[19] but is much less sensitive than PCR.[20]

Polymerase chain reaction. PCR can be used to detect BK virus DNA. Several assays that amplify different regions of the viral genome have been reported.[9, 21, 22] Some of these assays also amplify JC virus. The identity of the amplified product can be determined by differential hybridization probes or by digestion of the product with restriction endonucleases that can distinguish between the two viruses.[21]

Special considerations. Of the assays described, cytology and PCR are the most practical, although for both assays, detection of virus does not always correspond to clinically important disease. In the setting of bone marrow transplantation, however, detection of BK virus DNA by PCR in a urine sample from a patient with hemorrhagic cystitis should be considered presumptive evidence that BK virus is the cause.

ADENOVIRUS

Adenoviruses are a well-recognized cause of hemorrhagic cystitis. The disease is closely linked with adenovirus type 11, which is otherwise an unusual serotype. Other adenovirus serotypes, including 21, 34, and 35, have also been occasionally implicated.[23, 24] Adenovirus hemorrhagic cystitis occurs both in normal children[25, 26] and in immunocompromised adults. The

manifestations of the disease in children are abrupt onset of dysuria, urinary frequency, suprapubic pain, and gross hematuria. The urine contains leukocytes as well as erythrocytes. The disease is self-limited, usually lasting less than 2 weeks.

Specific Patient Populations

Most cases of adenovirus hemorrhagic cystitis in immunocompromised patients have been reported in bone marrow transplant recipients[27-29] and in renal transplant recipients.[24, 30, 31] Most of the cases in renal transplant recipients have occurred in the first week after transplantation. The clinical manifestations are similar to those in normal hosts, except serum creatinine may be transiently elevated, and the disease lasts approximately 1 week longer.[24] Detection of adenovirus 11 in the urine of renal transplant recipients in the absence of disease manifestations has been reported but appears to be unusual.[30, 31]

In bone marrow transplant recipients, adenovirus is a much less common cause of hemorrhagic cystitis than BK virus,[11, 12] although one study from Japan found adenovirus to account for the majority of cases.[29] The disease usually occurs within the first 100 days after transplantation, is often associated with graft-versus-host disease, may include involvement of the kidneys as well as the bladder, and may be a manifestation of disseminated adenovirus infection that can be lethal.[27, 28, 32, 33] Ribavirin has been used for treatment, but its efficacy is unproved.[34, 35]

Diagnosis of Hemorrhagic Cystitis

Adenovirus hemorrhagic cystitis should be suspected in normal hosts, especially children, or in immunocompromised individuals when they experience acute onset of hematuria plus symptoms of cystitis and when a bacterial culture is negative. The disease can be confirmed by a viral urine culture. Communication with the laboratory is essential when isolation of adenovirus from urine is desired. In some laboratories the routine setup of urine specimens may be directed toward detection of CMV and may not be optimal for adenovirus.

Rapid diagnosis of adenovirus hemorrhagic cystitis has been accomplished by FA staining of cells from the urinary sediment.[36] Use of PCR did not increase the detection of adenovirus in the urine in one study of bone marrow transplant recipients.[11] Further studies are required to evaluate PCR in this setting.

References

1. Gardner SD, Field AM: New human papovavirus (B.K.) isolated from urine after renal transplantation, *Lancet* 1:1253, 1971.

2. Shah KV, Daniel RW, Warszawski RM: High prevalence of antibodies to BK virus, an SV40-related papovavirus, in residents of Maryland, *J Infect Dis* 128:784, 1973.

3. Saitoh K, Sugae N, Koike N, et al: Diagnosis of childhood BK virus cystitis by electron microscopy and PCR, *J Clin Pathol* 46:773, 1993.

4. Vago L, Cinque P, Sala E, et al: JCV-DNA and BKV DNA in the CNS tissue and CSF of AIDS patients and normal subjects: study of 41 cases and review of the literature, *J AIDS* 12:139, 1996.

5. Goudsmit J, Wertheim-van Dillen P, van Strein A, van der Noordaa J: The role of BK virus in acute respiratory tract disease and the presence of BKV DNA in tonsils, *J Med Virol* 10:91, 1982.

6. Heritage J, Chesters PM, McCance DJ: The persistence of papovavirus BK DNA sequences in normal human renal tissue, *J Med Virol* 8:143, 1981.

7. Kitamura T, Aso Y, Kuniyoshi N, et al: High incidence of urinary JC virus excretion in nonimmunosuppressed older patients, *J Infect Dis* 161:1128, 1990.

8. Sundsfjord A, Flaegstad T, Flø R, et al: BK and JC viruses in human immunodeficiency virus type 1–infected persons: prevalence, excretion, viremia, and viral regulatory regions, *J Infect Dis* 169:485, 1994.

9. Markowitz R-B, Thompson HC, Mueller JF, et al: Incidence of BK virus and JC virus viruria in human immunodeficiency virus–infected and –uninfected subjects, *J Infect Dis* 167:13, 1993.

10. Arthur RR, Shah KV, Baust SJ, et al: Association of BK viruria with hemorrhagic cystitis in recipients of bone marrow transplants, *N Engl J Med* 315:230, 1986.

11. Azzi A, Fanci R, A, Ciappi S, et al: Monitoring of polyomavirus BK viruria in bone marrow transplantation patients by DNA hybridization assay and by polymerase chain reaction: an approach to assess the relationship between BK viruria and hemorrhagic cystitis, *Bone Marrow Transplant* 14:235, 1994.

12. Bedi A, Miller CB, Hanson JL, et al: Association of BK virus with failure of prophylaxis against hemorrhagic cystitis following bone marrow transplantation, *J Clin Oncol* 13:1103, 1995.

13. Coleman DV, Mackenzie EFD, Gardner SD, et al: Human polyomavirus (BK) infection and ureteric stenosis in renal allograft recipients, *J Clin Pathol* 31:338, 1978.

14. Purighalla R, Shapiro R, McCauley J, Randhawa P: BK virus infection in a kidney allograft diagnosed by needle biopsy, *Am J Kidney Dis* 26:671, 1995.

15. Gardner SD, MacKenzie EFD, Smith C, Porter AA: Prospective study of the human polyomaviruses BK and JC and cytomegalovirus in renal transplant recipients, *J Clin Pathol* 37:578, 1984.

16. de Silva LM, Bale P, de Courcy J, et al: Renal failure due to BK virus infection in an immunodeficient child, *J Med Virol* 45:192, 1995.

17. Rosen S, Harmon W, Krensky AM, et al: Tubulointerstitial nephritis associated with polyomavirus (BK type) infection, *N Engl J Med* 308:1192, 1983.

18. Coleman DV: The cytodiagnosis of human polyomavirus infection, *Acta Cytol* 19:93, 1975.

19. Marshall WF, Telenti A, Proper J, et al: Rapid detection of polyomavirus BK by a shell vial cell culture assay, *J Clin Microbiol* 28:1613, 1990.

20. Marshall WF, Telenti A, Proper J, et al: Survey of urine from transplant recipients for polyomaviruses JC and BK using the polymerase chain reaction, *Mol Cell Probes* 5:125, 1991.

21. Arthur RR, Dagostin S, Shah KV: Detection of BK virus and JC virus in urine and brain tissue by the polymerase chain reaction, *J Clin Microbiol* 27:1174, 1989.

22. Flaegstad T, Sundsfjord A, Arthur RR, et al: Amplification and sequencing of the control regions of BK and JC virus from human urine by polymerase chain reaction, *Virology* 180:553, 1991.

23. Mufson MA, Zollar LM, Mankad VN, Manalo D: Adenovirus infection in acute hemorrhagic cystitis, *Am J Dis Child* 121:281, 1971.

24. Koga S, Shindo K, Matsuya F, et al: Acute hemorrhagic cystitis caused by adenovirus following renal transplantation: review of the literature, *J Urol* 149:838, 1993.

25. Numazaki Y, Shigeta S, Kumasaka T, et al: Acute hemorrhagic cystitis in children: isolation of adenovirus type 11, *N Engl J Med* 278:700, 1968.

26. Mufson MA, Belshe RB: A review of adenoviruses in the etiology of acute hemorrhagic cystitis, *J Urol* 115:191, 1976.

27. Ambinder RF, Burns W, Forman M, et al: Hemorrhagic cystitis associated with adenovirus infection in bone marrow transplantation, *Arch Intern Med* 146:1400, 1986.

28. Shields AF, Hackman RC, Fife KH, et al: Adenovirus infections in patients undergoing bone-marrow transplantation, *N Engl J Med* 312:529, 1985.

29. Miyamura K, Takeyama K, Kojima S, et al: Hemorrhagic cystitis associated with urinary excretion of adenovirus type 11 following bone marrow transplantation, *Bone Marrow Transplant* 4:533, 1989.

30. Fiala M, Payne JE, Berne TV, et al: Role of adenovirus type 11 in hemorrhagic cystitis secondary to immunosuppression, *J Urol* 112:595, 1974.

31. Shindo K, Kitayama T, Ura T, et al: Acute hemorrhagic cystitis caused by adenovirus type 11 after renal transplantation, *Urol Int* 41:152, 1986.

32. Londergan TA, Walzak MP: Hemorrhagic cystitis due to adenovirus infection following bone marrow transplantation, *J Urol* 151:1013, 1994.

33. Flomenberg P, Babbitt J, Drobyski WR, et al: Increasing incidence of adenovirus disease in bone marrow transplant recipients, *J Infect Dis* 169:775, 1994.

34. Cassano WF: Intravenous ribavirin treatment for adenovirus cystitis after allogeneic bone marrow transplantation, *Bone Marrow Transplant* 7:247, 1991.

35. Murphy GF, Wood DPJ, McRoberts JW, Henslee-Downey PJ: Adenovirus-associated hemorrhagic cystitis treated with intravenous ribavirin, *J Urol* 149:565, 1993.

36. Belshe RB, Mufson MA: Identification by immunofluorescence of adenoviral antigen in exfoliated epithelial bladder epithelial cells from patients with acute hemorrhagic cystitis, *Proc Soc Exp Biol Med* 146:754, 1974.

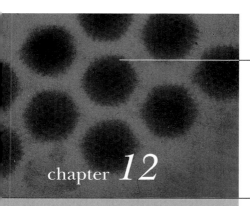

Gregory A. Storch

chapter *12*

Infectious Mononucleosis

OVERVIEW

Infectious mononucleosis is a common clinical syndrome that usually results from acute infection with *Epstein-Barr virus* (EBV). A small number of cases are caused by infection with other viruses, especially *cytomegalovirus* (CMV) and *human immunodeficiency virus* (HIV). The presence of *heterophile antibodies* is a marker of EBV infection, and tests for heterophile antibodies are generally sufficient for diagnostic purposes. In some patients, however, particularly those with a negative heterophile test or those with unusual clinical manifestations, specific viral testing is warranted.

This chapter is divided into three sections: (1) the diagnosis of infectious mononucleosis based on clinical findings and heterophile antibody assays, (2) EBV-specific tests, and (3) the main viral infections that account for cases of "heterophile-negative" infectious mononucleosis. EBV infection in immunocompromised hosts, including the posttransplant lymphoproliferative syndrome, is discussed in Chapter 15.

DIAGNOSIS OF INFECTIOUS MONONUCLEOSIS

Clinical Findings

The characteristic clinical findings in infectious mononucleosis are fever, malaise, exudative pharyngitis, lymphadenopathy, and atypical lymphocytosis in peripheral blood. The illness is most often encountered in adolescents but also occurs in younger children and in young adults. Cases in adults over age 30 are well recognized but unusual.

The presenting symptoms may be similar to those of streptococcal pharyngitis or pharyngitis caused by other viruses, especially adenovirus. Infectious mononucleosis should be suspected when fever is prolonged

(more than 3 days) and exudative pharyngitis accompanied by marked lymphadenopathy and/or splenomegaly is present. Other common but not universal findings include hepatomegaly with or without right upper quadrant tenderness, mild jaundice, and a transient erythematous maculopapular rash. Many unusual manifestations and complications can occur, including splenic rupture, autoimmune hemolytic anemia, severe thrombocytopenia, and neurologic complications such as encephalitis, meningitis, Bell's palsy, and Guillain-Barré syndrome.

Atypical Lymphocytes

A complete blood count (CBC) and a test for heterophile antibodies are usually adequate for establishing the diagnosis of infectious mononucleosis. The characteristic hematologic finding is lymphocytosis of 50% or greater and atypical lymphocytosis of 10% or greater of total leukocytes. The atypical lymphocytes are T cells that are reacting against EBV-infected B cells (Figure 12–1). In occasional cases, atypical lymphocytes and heterophile antibodies are absent early in the illness, but both are usually detectable within 1 to 2 weeks.

Heterophile Antibodies

Heterophile antibodies produced in acute EBV infection are also known as *Paul-Bunnell antibodies* and consist of immunoglobulin M (IgM) antibodies that agglutinate the erythrocytes of sheep, oxen, and horses. The presence of heterophile antibodies is diagnostic of acute EBV infection, and no further diagnostic testing is required. They are usually present in older children and adults with EBV infectious mononucleosis but are often absent in young children. For example, one study found that heterophile antibodies were present in 96% of college students with EBV-infectious mononucleosis.[1] In a study of children, heterophile antibodies were detected in more than 80% of cases in children and

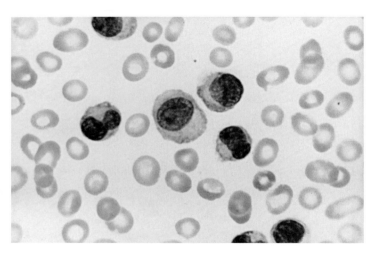

Figure 12.1 Atypical lymphocytes. Compared with normal small lymphocytes, which are slightly larger than erythrocytes, these cells are enlarged and have paler blue cytoplasm and finer nuclear chromatin. (Courtesy Teresa Vietti, MD, Department of Pediatrics, Washington University, St Louis.)

adolescents age 4 and older but in fewer than 50% of children under 4 years.[2]

The persistent absence of heterophile antibodies in an individual with the clinical syndrome of infectious mononucleosis, including atypical lymphocytosis, should prompt consideration of infection with CMV, HIV, or other agents (see later discussion).

Heterophile Antibody Assays

The classic heterophile antibody assay is the *Paul-Bunnell test*, which tests serum for agglutination of sheep erythrocytes. The heterophile antibody titer is defined as the highest dilution of serum that produces agglutination of sheep erythrocytes after absorption with guinea pig kidney. Absorption with beef erythrocytes and guinea pig kidney is used to distinguish EBV-associated heterophile antibodies from other antibodies that can also agglutinate erythrocytes. These include Forssman antibodies and antibodies that can occur with serum sickness, both of which are absorbed by guinea pig kidney.

Horse erythrocytes can be substituted for sheep erythrocytes and are more sensitive for the detection of heterophile antibodies. Heterophile antibodies usually persist for 2 to 3 months when measured using sheep erythrocytes but may be detectable for 1 year or more in 75% of patients when using horse erythrocytes (Figure 12–2).[3]

A related test is the *ox cell hemolysin test*. An ox cell hemolysin titer of 1:40 or greater is considered equivalent to a positive heterophile test.

Currently, most testing for heterophile antibodies is performed using *qualitative slide tests,* and few laboratories perform the Paul-Bunnell test or the ox cell hemolysin assay. Most of the slide tests use horse erythrocytes and do not require differential absorptions. The slide tests are generally highly specific for acute EBV infection, and most false-positives are related to errors in performing the tests. Slide tests are slightly less sensitive than classic tube tests, especially in children less than 4 years of age, who typically have lower levels of heterophile antibodies.[2]

SPECIFIC TESTING FOR EPSTEIN-BARR VIRUS

Virology and Associated Diseases

EBV is a member of the Herpesviridae family and is classified as a gamma herpesvirus based on its tropism for lymphoid cells. EBV also infects epithelial cells, notably those present in the oropharynx. Two viral variants, EBV-1 and EBV-2, have been recognized. These types are more closely related than herpes simplex virus types 1 and 2 but have consistent differences in some of the EBV nuclear antigens (EBNAs), especially EBNA-2.

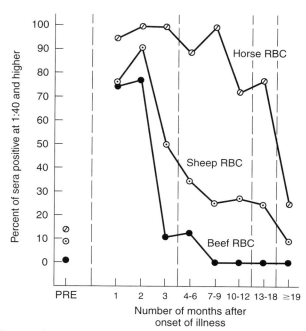

Figure 12.2 Persistence of heterophile antibodies during infectious mononucleosis. *RBC,* Red blood cells. (From Evans AS, Niederman JC, Cenabre LC, et al: *J Infect Dis* 132:546, 1975.)

EBV-1 is much more common than EBV-2 in the United States. As with other herpesviruses, EBV establishes a latent state after primary infection.

EBV is common in all human populations. Primary infection is often asymptomatic or unrecognized when it occurs in early childhood but often results in infectious mononucleosis when it occurs in older children or adolescents. Therefore infectious mononucleosis tends to be more common in developed societies, where primary EBV infection is often delayed, than in underdeveloped countries, where a large percentage of the population become infected with EBV during early childhood.

EBV is also associated with several malignancies, notably Burkitt's lymphoma, nasopharyngeal carcinoma, and Hodgkin's disease. In immunocompromised individuals, especially those with acquired immunodeficiency syndrome (AIDS), EBV is associated with primary central nervous system lymphoma (see Chapter 3), non-Hodgkin's lymphoma, leiomyosarcoma, and oral hairy leukoplakia. After solid organ or bone marrow transplantation, EBV is associated with lymphoproliferative syndromes that are collectively referred to as *posttransplant lymphoproliferative disorder* (PTLD) (see Chapter 15).

Viral Life Cycle and Relationship to Infectious Mononucleosis

As with the other herpesviruses, EBV is capable of both active and latent infection. During *active* (also termed *lytic* or *productive*) *infection*, most of the viral genes are expressed, complete viral particles are released from infected cells, and the infected cell eventually dies as a result of infection. During *latent infection*, a restricted number of genes are expressed (see Chapter 15). Lymphoid cells that are latently infected by EBV are stimulated to proliferate and are also "immortalized." This process is also referred to as *transformation*. EBV-1 is more efficient than EBV-2 at inducing transformation.

The initial event in infectious mononucleosis is lytic infection of epithelial cells in the oropharynx. Release of infectious virus particles from these cells is believed to lead to infection of B lymphocytes. Early in infectious mononucleosis, five per 10^4 peripheral blood mononuclear cells are EBV infected.[4] Within a short time, a cytotoxic T-lymphocyte response develops and limits the proliferation of infected B cells, so that by the third month after infection, the number of infected leukocytes declines to 1 to 5 per 10^7 peripheral blood cells. A small number of infected B cells persist for the individual's lifetime. Shedding of infectious EBV particles in the saliva occurs during infectious mononucleosis and may recur periodically. Approximately 10% to 20% of healthy EBV-seropositive individuals are found to have positive cultures for EBV in prevalence surveys.

Laboratory Detection

EBV does not grow in routine cell cultures used in diagnostic virology laboratories. It can be cultivated by incubating cells from the patient in cell culture media along with uninfected lymphocytes (usually derived from umbilical cord blood) from another individual. Infection of the donor cells is detected by observing proliferation of these cells, with expression of EBV antigens.[5] This technique is not practical for clinical diagnosis, and therefore serologic tests have been the main diagnostic tests available for the specific virologic diagnosis of EBV infection. EBV deoxyribonucleic acid (DNA) can be detected by polymerase chain reaction (PCR) in peripheral blood leukocytes in patients with EBV infectious mononucleosis.[6] This testing is not necessary in routine cases of infectious mononucleosis.

Epstein-Barr Virus–Specific Serology

Acute EBV infection can be diagnosed using serologic tests specific for EBV. EBV-specific serologic tests are more complicated and expensive than heterophile tests. They should be used only (1) when clinical suspicion of EBV infection persists despite a negative heterophile test, (2) in cases with unusual clinical manifestations, and (3) in young children who may have heterophile-negative EBV infection.

Currently used EBV serologic tests detect antibodies to three different groups of EBV antigens: *viral capsid antigen* (VCA), *early antigen* (EA), and *nuclear antigen* (EBNA). Antibodies to these antigens have different times of appearance and duration (Figure 12–3). Therefore analysis of all three can provide information about whether infection is recent or remote.

Table 12–1 outlines EBV antibody profiles in different disease states, including those in the EBV-associated malignancies Burkitt's lymphoma and nasopharyngeal carcinoma.

Antibodies to viral capsid antigen. The antigen used in this test is derived from lymphoid cell lines that are chronically infected with EBV. These cells produce fully formed infectious viral particles, and the "antigen" is thus a complex mixture of structural proteins of the virus. Both indirect immunofluorescence and enzyme immunoassay (EIA) formats are available for detection of antibodies to VCA, and either can be used to differentiate between IgG and IgM antibodies.

Immunoglobulin G and M antibodies to VCA (VCA-IgG, VCA-IgM) are usually present at high levels at the onset of symptomatic illness and are uniformly present by the third week of illness.[2, 3] Therefore the best serologic evidence of acute infection is the presence of VCA-IgM, since it may not be possible to demonstrate seroconversion or a fourfold increase in titer of VCA-IgG.[7] The height of the VCA-IgG titer is also not useful for diagnosing recent infection. After infection, VCA-IgG persists for the individual's lifetime. VCA-IgM is present at high levels for 1 to 2 months, then declines rapidly, but may remain detectable by sensitive tests for 12 months or more in a few patients.[3]

Antibodies to early antigen. EAs are antigens expressed early in the life cycle of EBV. The antigen preparation used in the test is prepared from *Raji cells*, which are EBV-infected lymphoid cells originally derived from a patient with Burkitt's lymphoma. The production of EBV EAs in the cells is induced by superinfection of the cells with EBV or by exposure to certain inhibitors of DNA synthesis.

Testing for antibodies to EA uses indirect immunofluorescence. Antibodies to two different EA components, termed *diffuse* (EA-D) and *restricted* (EA-R), can be distinguished. EA-D is present in both the nucleus and the cytoplasm of infected cells, whereas EA-R is present only in cytoplasmic aggregates.

Antibodies to the two components, anti-EA-D and anti-EA-R can be further distinguished because EA-R, but not EA-D, is destroyed by methanol fixation of the cells used as antigenic substrate. Anti-EA-D is present during approximately 70% of cases of infectious mononucleosis and tends to appear a few weeks later than anti-VCA.[8] Anti-EA-D declines rapidly and is only rarely detectable after 12 months.[9] Anti-EA-R is not usually detectable during infectious mononucleosis but ap-

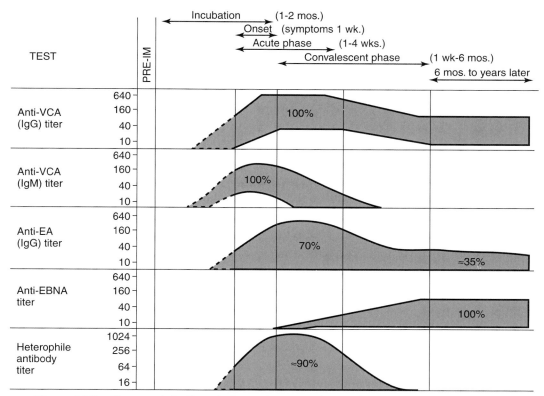

Figure 12.3 Characteristic Epstein-Barr virus–specific antibody responses observed in young adults with acute infectious mononucleosis. *VCA*, Viral capsid antigen; *EA*, early antigen; *EBNA*, Epstein-Barr nuclear antigen. (From Henle W, Henle G, Horowitz C: Epstein-Barr virus specific diagnostic tests in infectious mononucleosis, *Hum Pathol* 5:551, 1974.)

pears during convalescence. It is most likely to be detectable in individuals with high levels of antibodies to VCA. Anti-EA-R may persist for years after uncomplicated infectious mononucleosis[9] and is also detected in some normal individuals without a recent history of mononucleosis. The presence of anti-EA-R has been described as indicating reactivation of latent EBV infection,[10] but this concept has not been rigorously validated and is not useful clinically.

Many clinical laboratories do not distinguish between EA-D and EA-R.

Antibodies to nuclear antigen. EBNA actually consists of six different viral antigens (EBNA 1, 2, 3A, 3B, 3C, and leader protein [LP]) found in the nucleus of infected cells. Antibodies to EBNA are detectable at low levels, using the *anti-complement immunofluorescence* method.[7] These antibodies to EBNA (anti-EBNA) rise

Table 12.1   Epstein-Barr Virus (EBV) Antibody Profiles

Clinical setting	VCA-IgG	VCA-IgM	Anti-EA-D	Anti-EA-R	Anti-EBNA
Acute infectious mononucleosis	+	+*	+	−	−
Convalscent mononucleosis	+	+/−	−	+	+
Past EBV infection (immune)	+	−	−	−	+
No EBV infection (susceptible)	−	−	−	−	−
Burkitt's lymphoma	+	−	−	+†	+
Nasopharyngeal carcinoma	+‡	−	+†	+/−	−

VCA, Viral capsid antigen; *EA-D, EA-R*, early antigen—diffuse, restricted; *EBNA*, Epstein-Barr nuclear antigen
*Detected in 75% of patients.
†Present at very high levels.
‡IgA antibodies to VCA may also be present.

later after infection than anti-VCA and anti-EA. In a few patients, anti-EBNA may be detectable in the first 2 weeks after infection. In more than half of all patients with infectious mononucleosis, however, anti-EBNA is not detectable for more than 1 month, and in occasional patients it is not detectable until 6 months after onset.[11] Anti-EBNA persists for life.

Antibody profiles. In acute EBV infection, VCA-IgG, VCA-IgM, and anti-EA-D are present (VCA-IgM and anti-EA-D are not detected in every case), and anti-EBNA is absent (see Table 12–1). Patients with past infection are positive for VCA-IgG and anti-EBNA.

In my experience the tests for VCA antibodies are often useful for defining past or recent EBV infection, whereas the tests for antibodies to EA and EBNA provide useful information only in very selected clinical circumstances.

Chronic Infection

A syndrome of *chronic fatigue*, variably accompanied by low-grade fever, pharyngitis, and malaise, has been attributed to chronic EBV infection.[12, 13] Chronic EBV infection was suggested as the cause, because some patients with the syndrome were found to have high levels of VCA-IgG and anti-EA with absent VCA-IgM. A subgroup of patients also lacked anti-EBNA, and this unusual finding was thought to indicate an abnormal immune response to EBV. In fact, persisting high levels of IgG anti-VCA plus anti-EA are found in some patients years after an uncomplicated episode of infectious mononucleosis.[9] In addition, subsequent studies did not find significantly higher EBV antibody levels in patients with chronic fatigue syndrome compared with controls,[14, 15] raising doubts about whether a causative relationship exists between EBV infection and chronic fatigue syndrome.

Although unusual EBV infections undoubtedly exist, no validated serologic criteria are currently available to make a reliable diagnosis of chronic EBV infection.

Box 12.1   Etiology of Heterophile-negative Infectious Mononucleosis

Early Epstein-Barr virus (EBV) infection
EBV infection in young children
Cytomegalovirus (CMV)
Human immunodeficiency virus (HIV)
Toxoplasma gondii (rare)
Rubella (rare)

HETEROPHILE-NEGATIVE MONONUCLEOSIS

Some patients with a prolonged febrile illness and atypical lymphocytosis have a negative heterophile test. Box 12–1 lists the causes of heterophile-negative infectious mononucleosis. EBV infection can be excluded by repeating the heterophile test after 3 to 5 days and by performing EBV-specific serologic tests.

The most well-recognized cause of truly heterophile-negative infectious mononucleosis is acute CMV infection. Acute HIV infection can have similar manifestations and should be considered as an alternative diagnosis.

Cytomegalovirus

The cardinal features of CMV mononucleosis are fever (lasting 2 to 3 weeks in many patients), malaise, atypical lymphocytosis, and mildly abnormal liver function tests. Adenopathy and splenomegaly occur less often than in EBV infectious mononucleosis, and exudative pharyngitis is rare.[16-18] The atypical lymphocytes are indistinguishable from those present in EBV infection.

The simplest way to implicate CMV as the cause is to test for CMV IgM antibodies, which are usually detectable at the onset of illness or within a short time.[17, 19] These antibodies persist at high levels for approximately 3 months, then decline, but may be detectable by sensitive tests for several more months. A negative test for CMV-IgM does not absolutely rule out CMV as the cause. For example, in one study of pregnant women with primary CMV infection who were tested using a commercially available EIA for CMV-IgM, the sensitivity of detection was only 77% on specimens obtained within 8 weeks of seroconversion.[20]

An important caveat related to the serodiagnosis of acute CMV infection is that a false-positive test for CMV IgM antibodies can occur in acute EBV infection. This is a one-way cross-reaction because patients who truly have acute CMV infection do not have false-positive tests for EBV.[21, 22] Therefore, when CMV IgM antibody testing is performed, it is important to test also for EBV VCA-IgM to rule out acute EBV infection as the cause of a positive test for CMV IgM. The cross-reaction does not affect IgG antibodies,[21] so seroconversion or a rising titer of IgG CMV antibodies can also be used to prove that CMV is the cause.

The diagnosis of acute CMV infection can also be made by culture, antigen detection, or DNA detection. Extensive comparative data regarding sensitivity of urine and blood cultures are not available, but urine cultures apparently are positive in most patients, with culture positivity persisting for months.[23] The frequency of positive blood cultures has varied in different reports from 26% to 100%[24, 25] and may depend on the laboratory's skill in isolating CMV. In a recent report the pp65 antigenemia assay was positive in 57% and PCR performed on leukocytes was positive in 100% of immunocompetent patients with CMV mononucleosis.[24] The pp65 assay was negative by 3 months after onset in all patients; PCR was still positive in 47% after 3 months but was always negative in samples taken 6 months or more after onset.

Human Immunodeficiency Virus

Acute HIV infection can present as an infectious mononucleosis–like syndrome with a negative heterophile test.[26] The importance of recognizing this syndrome has been emphasized because of the possible efficacy of early treatment.

Standard HIV antibody tests may be negative because the symptoms associated with acute infection often occur before anti-HIV antibodies have developed. The p24 antigen test typically becomes positive approximately 6 days earlier than HIV antibody tests (see Chapter 17) and thus can be used for the diagnosis of acute HIV infection. HIV RNA is typically detectable in plasma even before p24 antigen,[27] and therefore HIV plasma RNA assays are the most sensitive tests for detecting acute HIV infection. However, an important caveat is that HIV RNA assays are not licensed for use in diagnosis of HIV infection and false positive tests have occurred in this setting.[28] The levels of HIV RNA in the false positive cases reported were all less than 2000 copies per milliliter, whereas levels are typically much higher in true acute HIV infection. The diagnosis of HIV infection should never be based solely on the plasma HIV RNA assay, but should be supported by the finding of a positive HIV antibody test in a later serum specimen.

References

1. Evans AS, Niederman JC, McCollum RW: Seroepidemiologic studies of infectious mononucleosis with EB virus, *N Engl J Med* 279:1121, 1968.
2. Sumaya CV, Ench Y: Epstein-Barr virus infectious mononucleosis in children. II. Heterophile antibody and viral-specific responses, *Pediatrics* 75:1011, 1985.
3. Evans AS, Neiderman JC, Cenabre LC, et al: A prospective evaluation of heterophile and Epstein-Barr virus–specific IgM antibody tests in clinical and subclinical infectious mononucleosis: specificity and sensitivity of these tests and persistence of antibody, *J Infect Dis* 132:546, 1975.
4. Rocchi G, De Felici A, Ragona G, Heinz A: Quantitative evaluation of Epstein-Barr virus–infected mononuclear peripheral blood leukocytes in infectious mononucleosis, *N Engl J Med* 296:132, 1977.
5. Lennette ET: Epstein-Barr virus (EBV). In Lennette EH, Lennette DA, Lennette ET, editors: *Diagnostic procedures for viral, rickettsial, and chlamydial infections,* ed 7, Washington, DC, 1995, American Public Health Association.
6. Kenagy DN, Schlesinger Y, Weck K, et al: Epstein-Barr virus DNA in peripheral blood leukocytes of patients with posttransplant lymphoproliferative disease, *Transplantation* 60:547, 1995.
7. Henle W, Henle G, Horowitz C: Epstein-Barr virus specific diagnostic tests in infectious mononucleosis, *Hum Pathol* 5:551, 1974.
8. Henle W, Henle G, Niederman JC, et al: Antibodies to early antigens induced by Epstein-Barr virus in infectious mononucleosis, *J Infect Dis* 124:58, 1971.
9. Horwitz CA, Henle W, Henle G, et al: Long-term serological follow-up of patients for Epstein-Barr virus after recovery from infectious mononucleosis, *J Infect Dis* 151:1150, 1985.
10. Sumaya C: Endogenous reactivation of Epstein-Barr virus infections, *J Infect Dis* 135:374, 1977.
11. Henle G, Henle W, Horwitz CA: Antibodies to Epstein-Barr virus–associated nuclear antigen in infectious mononucleosis, *J Infect Dis* 130:231, 1974.
12. Jones JF, Ray CG, Minnich LL, et al: Evidence for active Epstein-Barr virus infection in patients with persistent unexplained illnesses: elevated anti-early antigen antibodies, *Ann Intern Med* 102:1, 1985.
13. Straus SE, Tosato G, Armstrong G, et al: Persisting illness and fatigue in adults with evidence of Epstein-Barr virus infection, *Ann Intern Med* 102:7, 1985.
14. Holmes GP, Kaplan JE, Stewart JA, et al: A cluster of patients with a chronic mononucleosis-like syndrome: is Epstein-Barr virus the cause? *JAMA* 257:2297, 1987.
15. Buchwald D, Sullivan JL, Komaroff AL: Frequency of 'chronic active Epstein-Barr virus infection' in a general medical practice, *JAMA* 257:2303, 1987.
16. Cohen JI, Corey GR: Cytomegalovirus infection in the normal host, *Medicine* 64:100, 1985.
17. Horwitz CA, Henle W, Henle G, et al: Clinical and laboratory evaluation of cytomegalovirus-induced mononucleosis in previously healthy individuals, *Medicine* 65:124, 1986.
18. Klemola E, von Essen R, Wager O, et al: Cytomegalovirus mononucleosis in previously healthy individuals, *Ann Intern Med* 71:11, 1969.
19. Rasmussen L, Kelsall D, Nelson R, et al: Virus-specific IgG and IgM antibodies in normal and immunocompromised subjects infected with cytomegalovirus, *J Infect Dis* 145:191, 1982.
20. Stagno S, Tinker MK, Elrod C, et al: Immunoglobulin M antibodies detected by enzyme-linked immunosorbent assay and radioimmunoassay in the diagnosis of cytomegalovirus infections in pregnant women and newborn infants, *J Clin Microbiol* 21:930, 1985.
21. Hanshaw JB, Niederman JC, Chessin LN: Cytomegalovirus macroglobulin in cell-associated herpesvirus infections, *J Infect Dis* 125:304, 1972.
22. Horwitz CA, Henle W, Henle G, et al: Heterophile-negative infectious mononucleosis and

mononucleosis-like illnesses: laboratory confirmation of 43 cases, *Am J Med* 63:947, 1977.

23. Jordan MC, Rousseau W, Stewart JA, et al: Spontaneous cytomegalovirus mononucleosis: clinical and laboratory observations in nine cases, *Ann Intern Med* 79:153, 1973.

24. Revello MG, Zavattoni M, Sarasini A, et al: Human cytomegalovirus in blood of immunocompetent persons during primary infection: prognostic implications for pregnancy, *J Infect Dis* 177:1170, 1998.

25. Rinaldo CR Jr, Black PH, Hirsch MS: Interaction of cytomegalovirus with leukocytes from patients with

mononucleosis due to cytomegalovirus, *J Infect Dis* 136: 667, 1977.

26. Schacker T, Collier AC, Hughes J, et al: Clinical and epidemiologic features of primary HIV infection, *Ann Intern Med* 125:257, 1996.

27. Daar ES, Moudgil T, Meyer RD, Ho DD: Transient high levels of viremia in patients with primary human immunodeficiency virus infections, *N Eng J Med* 324:961, 1991.

28. Rich JD, Merriman NA, Mylonakis E, et al: Misdiagnosis of HIV infection by HIV-1 plasma viral load testing: a case series, *Ann Intern Med* 130:37, 1999.

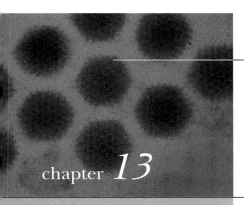

Richard L. Hodinka, Karyn L. Moshal

chapter *13*

Childhood Infections

Outline continued

OVERVIEW

Almost any viral infection that occurs in adults can occur in the pediatric population as well. The most common infections in children are those that involve the respiratory and gastrointestinal tracts. The traditional viral infections of childhood, however, are those that occur predominantly in the pediatric population, as discussed in this chapter. These include diseases caused by *measles, mumps,* and *rubella* viruses, *human parvovirus B19; human herpesvirus type 6* (HHV-6) and *type 7* (HHV-7), and the *nonpolio enteroviruses.* The diagnosis of varicella is discussed in Chapter 6.

Diagnosis of illness related to these agents involves a well-documented history of exposure and vaccination, clinical signs and symptoms, and laboratory testing. A variety of methods are now available for laboratory diagnosis of each virus, including viral isolation in cell culture, demonstration of viral antigens or nucleic acids in body fluids or tissues, and serology for detection of virus-specific antibodies. This has allowed for more rapid and sensitive identification of these viruses but has made testing choices and interpretation of results more complex.

The following sections discuss unique features of the individual viruses; the incidence, epidemiology, and clinical presentation of disease; and the current laboratory tests available for diagnosis, their use and interpretation, the most appropriate specimens needed for each test, and assays under development. Table 13–1 summarizes the approach to the rapid diagnosis of the childhood viral infections. Diagnosis of localized manifestations or infections in immunocompromised hosts is discussed in other chapters (e.g., Chapter 15 for HHV-6/7 infections). The discussion of enteroviral infections in this chapter is limited to generalized infections with nonpolio enteroviruses, since central nervous system, cutaneous, and cardiac manifestations

Table 13.1	Rapid Diagnosis of Childhood Viral Infections

Virus	Preferred rapid diagnostic test(s)
Measles	FA stain of nasopharyneal/throat specimen* Measles IgM antibody titer†
Rubella	Rubella IgM antibody titer
Mumps	Mumps IgM antibody titer
Parvovirus B19	Parvovirus B19 IgM antibody titer
Human herpesvirus type 6 (HHV-6)	PCR plus HHV-6 antibody titer‡
Nonpolio enteroviruses	PCR§

*FA, Fluorescent antibody. Positive from shortly before to several days after onset of rash.
†IgM, Immunoglobulin M. Positive starting about 6 days after onset of rash.
‡PCR, Polymerase chain reaction. Combination of positive PCR of blood plus negative HHV-6 antibody titer indicates current infection. May not be applicable in infants under 3 months of age, in whom maternal antibody may be detectable.
§RT-PCR, Reverse transcription polymerase chain reaction. Sensitivity and specificity of RT-PCR performed on serum or urine for diagnosis of generalized enteroviral infection are unknown.

of enteroviral infections are discussed in Chapters 3, 6, and 9, respectively. Diagnosis of congenital infections caused by rubella, parvovirus, and enteroviruses is discussed in Chapter 14.

MEASLES (RUBEOLA)

Virology

Measles virus is a member of the Paramyxoviridae family and belongs to the genus *Morbillivirus*, which includes the closely related canine distemper and rinderpest viruses. Table 13–2 summarizes the common features of measles virus.

Measles particles are 150 to 300 nm in diameter and consist of an internal helical nucleocapsid containing a single-stranded ribonucleic acid (RNA) genome and an outer lipoprotein envelope. The virus contains projections of hemagglutinin and fusion glycoproteins within the envelope, but it differs from other paramyxoviruses in that it possesses no neuraminidase activity. One antigenic serotype of measles virus exists, and humans are the only natural host. A live attenuated virus vaccine has been successful in controlling measles in the United States and many other countries.

Epidemiology

Despite more than 80% of children worldwide immunized against measles, 1 million infants and children

Table 13.2   Common Characteristics of Measles, Mumps, and Rubella Viruses

Common features	Measles	Mumps	Rubella
Classification			
Family	Paramyxoviridae	Paramyxoviridae	Togaviridae
Genus	*Morbillivirus*	*Paramyxovirus*	*Rubivirus*
Properties	ss RNA genome	ss RNA genome	ss RNA genome
	Lipid envelope, 150-300 nm, 1 antigenic type	Lipid envelope, 200 nm, 1 antigenic type	Lipid envelope, 60 nm, 1 antigenic type
Natural host	Humans	Humans	Humans
Transmission	Respiratory droplets	Respiratory droplets	Respiratory droplets
Epidemiology			
Distribution	Worldwide	Worldwide	Worldwide
Prevaccine era	Epidemics in children ages 5-9 every 2-5 yr in winter and spring	Epidemics in children ages 5-9 every 2-4 yr in winter and spring	Minor epidemics every 6-9 yr Pandemics every 30 yr in children ages 5-9 in winter and spring
Vaccine era	Shift in age incidence to children up to age 4, adolescents, and young adults	Shift in age incidence to adolescents and young adults	Highest attack rates in young, unvaccinated adults
Clinical illness	Cough, coryza, conjunctivitis, rash, fever	Parotitis	Postnatal: rash, low-grade fever, lymphadenopathy CRS
Incubation period	8-12 days	16-18 days	16-18 days
Communicability	3-5 days before to 4 days after rash	1-2 days before to 5 days after parotitis	5 days before to 6 days after rash Children with CRS can be contagious for up to a year or more

CRS, Congenital rubella syndrome.

still die from this disease and its complications every year. Mortality rates of 15% to 25% have been reported in developing countries, and localized epidemics of measles continue to be observed in developed nations.

In the era before widespread vaccine use, urban-centered measles epidemics occurred in children ages 5 to 9 every 2 to 5 years in winter and spring and lasted 3 to 4 months. In the late 1980s and early 1990s measles outbreaks have occurred in many large U.S. metropolitan areas. The age incidence has changed from the prevaccine era, with most cases in the outbreaks occurring in unvaccinated preschool children, inadequately immunized persons of high school and college age, and groups with religious or philosophic exemption to vaccination. Since the implementation of a two-dose schedule of measles immunization, measles incidence in the United States has been extremely low, with a large proportion of cases related to international importation.

Measles is one of the most contagious of communicable diseases and is transmitted by direct contact with aerosolized droplets from respiratory secretions of infected persons. The virus remains infective in droplet form in air for several hours, and airborne spread of measles has occurred in physician offices. The incubation period is approximately 8 to 12 days from exposure to onset of symptoms.

Clinical Manifestations

Figure 13–1 shows the timing of clinical findings in a typical case of measles. The disease is characterized by a prodrome that lasts for 3 to 5 days and consists of cough, coryza, conjunctivitis, malaise, anorexia, and an ascending fever to 39.5°C. *Koplik spots* can be detected on the buccal or labial mucosa during the prodromal period and are pathognomonic of measles. The spots appear gray to white on a bright-red mucosal surface and persist for several days.

The typical rash of measles generally occurs on about day 14 after exposure (4 to 5 days after onset of symptoms) and is erythematous and maculopapular. It usually begins behind the ears and on the face and spreads progressively over the chest, trunk, and limbs. The rash resolves slowly, with temporary pigmentation and desquamation of the skin. Patients are most contagious during the prodrome and up to 4 days after appearance of the rash. The disease can be particularly severe and sometimes fatal in infants less than 2 years of

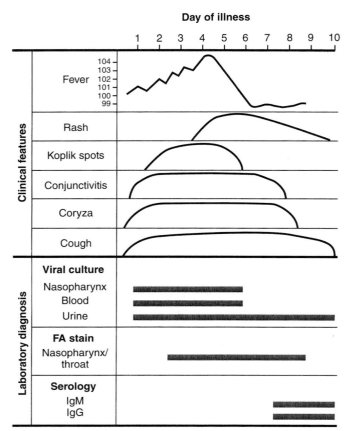

Figure 13.1   Timing of clinical findings and diagnostic test results in measles. *FA*, Fluorescent antibody.

age, in immunocompromised and chronically ill patients, and in malnourished persons.

Complications

Complications of measles include otitis media, croup, bronchitis, primary viral and secondary bacterial pneumonias, and encephalitis. Transient postmeasles immunosuppression can leave a patient vulnerable to other infections circulating in the community in the months after acute infection.

Subacute sclerosing panencephalitis (SSPE), a rare but fatal degenerative neurologic disease secondary to persistent replication of defective measles virus, can appear years after primary measles infection or immunization. SSPE is characterized by progressive intellectual, physical, and behavioral deterioration. No treatment exists for SSPE, and the disease is uniformly fatal (see Chapter 3).

Atypical and modified measles are other unusual manifestations of measles virus infection. *Atypical measles* is seen in people who received the formalin-killed measles vaccine that was in use between 1963 and 1968 and are then exposed to live measles virus. The disease is characterized by pneumonia with nodular pulmonary infiltrates and rash that begins on the extremities and progressively involves the trunk and face. *Modified measles* is a mild form of typical measles that occurs in individuals with preexisting measles antibody levels below that required for protection but sufficient to modify the illness on exposure to measles virus.

Diagnosis

Diagnosis of a typical case of measles seldom requires the assistance of the diagnostic virology laboratory and is usually based on clinical presentation. Fewer physicians now recognize the clinical features of measles, however, and the disease can be modified by prior immunization. Also, measles infection in patients with impaired cellular immune responses can be atypical, with the development of life-threatening giant cell pneumonia or encephalitis without evidence of fever or rash. In such patients, it may be difficult or impossible to establish a clinical diagnosis. The transmission of measles in the community and to health care workers in medical settings is also a concern.

Therefore the laboratory must provide a prompt and accurate diagnosis of measles to assist in the management of these patients and to institute appropriate infection control measures. Laboratory confirmation of measles is also necessary to control community outbreaks and for epidemiologic surveillance. Figure 13–1 shows the time periods when various diagnostic tests are positive in relation to clinical findings. Early in the course of illness, the best means for making a rapid diagnosis is by fluorescent antibody (FA) staining of cellular material obtained from combined nasopharyngeal (NP) and throat specimens. If testing is delayed until 5 or more days after onset of rash, a rapid diagnosis is best made by detection of measles-specific immunoglobulin M (IgM) antibodies.

Viral culture.   Measles virus can be isolated in conventional cell culture from NP and conjunctival secretions, blood, urine, cerebrospinal fluid (CSF), and tissue specimens. Primary cultures of human neonatal or monkey kidney cells are considered the best cell lines for growth of measles virus from clinical specimens. Cytopathic effect (CPE) includes formation of multinucleated giant cells (*syncytia*) and spindle-shaped single cells. Further identification of measles virus in culture is accomplished by hemadsorption of Old World monkey red blood cells and FA staining using specific monoclonal antibodies. Isolation of the virus is technically difficult, however, and the rate of virus recovery is particularly low. The virus grows slowly in culture and may produce little to no discernible CPE.

A centrifugation-assisted shell vial culture assay using human lung carcinoma cells (A549) and antigen detection by immunofluorescence allows for identification of measles virus within 1 to 2 days of inoculation of clinical specimens.[1] More recently, B95-8 cells, an

Epstein-Barr virus–transformed marmoset B-lymphoblastoid cell line, have been shown to be highly sensitive for the isolation of measles virus using conventional culture methods.[2, 3]

The optimal time for recovery of measles virus from NP secretions and blood is during the prodromal period and up to 1 to 2 days after the onset of rash. Virus can be isolated from urine for a week or more after the appearance of rash, making this a useful clinical specimen.[4] Measles virus is not easily isolated from the CSF or brain tissue of patients with central nervous system (CNS) disease.

Serology. The most practical method for confirming a diagnosis of measles is the demonstration of a fourfold rise in measles-specific immunoglobulin G (IgG) antibody in paired acute and convalescent sera or the detection of IgM antibody in a single serum. Detection of IgM antibody provides a more rapid diagnosis of acute measles virus infection than IgG determinations. A concern with viral IgM assays is the occurrence of false-positive and false-negative reactions caused by, respectively, high levels of rheumatoid factor and competing specific IgG antibodies. Separation of IgG and IgM fractions or the use of reverse-capture solid-phase IgM assays has been used to avoid these problems. In addition, cross-reactions with antibodies to parvovirus B19 have been observed in at least one commercial measles IgM assay.[5]

The sensitivity of measles-specific IgM testing depends on the time at which specimens are collected relative to the onset of the rash. The optimal time during the illness for antibody detection is 3 to 11 days after onset of rash. Before this, measles antibodies are detected in only 77% or less of patients. IgM positivity decreases rapidly from 4 to 5 weeks after onset of rash and can decline earlier in previously immunized patients.

The presence of measles IgG antibodies is evidence of past infection with measles virus and signifies immunity to measles. Historically, complement fixation, hemagglutination inhibition, and neutralization tests have been used for detection of measles antibodies. These have largely been replaced by faster, more sensitive and specific enzyme immunoassays (EIAs) and indirect fluorescent antibody (IFA) tests that can be adapted to detection of measles IgG and IgM antibodies.[6, 7] Both measles IgM and IgG kits are commercially available. Serologic diagnosis is retrospective, however, and antibody responses may be delayed or absent in immunocompromised patients despite clinical symptoms suggesting measles infection.

Oral fluid specimens have been used as a noninvasive alternative to the collection of blood for the detection of measles-specific IgM antibodies in large groups of patients during acute outbreaks and for postvaccination antibody testing,[8] but this testing is not widely available

at present. Also, EIAs using recombinant proteins produced in baculovirus and mammalian expression systems have been recently developed as less expensive and more sensitive alternatives to conventional assays based on whole virus as the antigen source.[9, 10] In patients with SSPE and other neurologic diseases caused by measles virus, CSF may be tested for intrathecal synthesis of viral antibody if paired with a serum specimen from the same date (see Chapter 3).[11]

Cytology and FA staining. Rapid detection of measles can be accomplished by direct cytologic examination of cellular material from respiratory secretions, urine, conjunctivae, buccal mucosa, and tissue for characteristic multinucleated giant cells containing eosinophilic intranuclear and cytoplasmic inclusions. This method is not specific, however, and has not been widely employed.

A more direct approach is to use FA staining for the detection of measles antigen.[1, 12, 13] Measles-specific monoclonal antibodies are now commercially available and have been used for the rapid identification of measles antigen from urine and NP secretions of infected patients. Combined throat and NP swab specimens were used in one study.[1] In laboratories that are skilled in FA staining, this method can be very useful for providing a rapid viral diagnosis.

RT-PCR. RT-PCR has been used successfully for the direct detection of measles viral RNA in a variety of clinical specimens. These include NP aspirates, peripheral blood mononuclear cells, and plasma of patients with natural measles infection;[14, 15] CSF and brain tissue of patients with acute measles encephalitis and SSPE;[14, 16] urine of individuals after vaccination;[17] and frozen tissues from apparently healthy individuals.[18] Conserved sequences of the matrix, nucleocapsid, phosphoprotein, fusion, and hemagglutinin genes have been used for amplification. RT-PCR is a rapid, sensitive, and specific test for the detection of measles virus, although the availability of the assay is limited.

MUMPS

Virology

Mumps virus belongs to the genus *Paramyxovirus* in the family Paramyxoviridae (see Table 13–2). The genus includes parainfluenza and Newcastle disease viruses. Mumps virus is pleomorphic with a diameter of 150 to 200 nm and possesses a single-stranded RNA genome surrounded by a helical nucleocapsid and lipid envelope. The envelope contains surface projections of two glycoproteins; the *hemagglutinin-neuraminidase protein* facilitates attachment of the virus to a host cell and viral release, and the *fusion protein* mediates fusion of lipid membranes and penetration of the neucleocapsid into the cell. Humans are the only known reservoir, and only one antigenic type of mumps virus exists. The virus is spread by the respiratory route. A live attenuated virus vaccine is highly effective and is given in combination with measles and rubella vaccines.

Epidemiology

The epidemiology of mumps is similar to that observed for measles infections. Before use of the mumps vaccine, the disease usually occurred in the winter and spring in intervals of 2 to 4 years. The incidence rates of mumps were highest in children 5 to 9 years of age in the prevaccine era, but most cases in the United States are now seen in adolescents and young infants. Because of the success of mumps immunization, the incidence of mumps in the United States is currently very low. The disease has an incubation period of 16 to 18 days, and infected individuals are contagious from 2 days before to 5 days after the development of clinical symptoms.

Clinical Manifestations

The most common clinical presentation of mumps is swelling of the salivary glands, particularly the parotid glands.[19] Patients typically have low-grade fever, fatigue, and a tender parotid gland that enlarges over 2 to 3 days to obscure the angle of the mandible. The swelling is usually bilateral and remains for 7 to 10 days. Unilateral swelling can occur in 25% of infected individuals. Most cases of mumps are mild and self-limited, and approximately 30% of mumps infections are subclinical. Severe illness is more likely to occur in infected adults.

Complications

Complications of mumps typically involve the CNS. Mumps is the second leading cause of *aseptic meningitis* worldwide, and approximately 10% to 30% of patients will have a meningitic component to their illness (see Chapter 3). Meningitis can occur in the absence of parotitis. Epididymo-orchitis, oophoritis, and mastitis occur in postpubertal patients; sterility and impaired fertility are uncommon. Pancreatitis, polyarthritis, and encephalitis are rare but important complications of mumps.

Diagnosis

A typical case of mumps usually does not require laboratory confirmation, although other infectious and noninfectious causes of parotitis can be confused with mumps. A laboratory diagnosis is required in the absence of parotitis or with features other than salivary gland manifestations. In general, requests for diagnostic testing to detect mumps virus are infrequent in most countries where immunization for mumps is routine.

However, mumps remains a common infection in developing countries worldwide. A definitive diagnosis of mumps is normally achieved by isolation of the virus in cell culture or serologic testing.

Viral culture. Mumps virus can be isolated from saliva, urine, CSF, and swabbings of the area around Stensen's duct. A variety of primary and continuous cell lines will support the growth of mumps virus, although primary rhesus monkey kidney and human neonatal kidney cells are used most often. Isolation of mumps virus from respiratory secretions is possible from 9 days before to 8 days after the onset of clinical illness. Virus can be recovered from the CSF within 8 to 9 days of the beginning of CNS disease and from urine for as long as 2 weeks after symptoms have begun. Mumps virus induces the formation of syncytia in cell culture, although not all primary isolates will produce a recognizable CPE. Hemadsorption with guinea pig red blood cells (see Chapter 1) is used for presumptive identification, and FA staining using specific monoclonal antibodies is used to confirm the growth of mumps virus in culture. Mumps virus grows slowly and can be difficult to detect; isolation rates from CSF and urine specimens vary considerably, and false-negative results are common due to the lability of the virus.

Whenever mumps virus is suspected, it is important to notify the virology laboratory to ensure that the appropriate cell cultures are inoculated and that hemadsorption is performed to detect positive cultures.

Serology. Serologic diagnosis of mumps virus infection is the method of choice in most clinical settings. Complement fixation, hemagglutination inhibition, hemolysis-in-gel, and neutralization assays have been used traditionally for the detection of antibodies to mumps. These methods are technically demanding, require rigid standardization and preparation of reagents, and have a long turnaround time. More sensitive, rapid, and cost-effective EIAs and IFAs are now routinely used, and commercial kits are available.

A fourfold or greater rise in mumps-specific IgG antibody between acute and convalescent sera or the presence of virus-specific IgM in a single serum is diagnostic of primary infection. The patient's immune status can be determined by screening a single serum specimen. As with the serodiagnosis of other viral illnesses, care must be taken when interpreting mumps-specific IgM antibody assays, since false results may occur in the presence of rheumatoid factor or high levels of mumps-specific IgG antibody. Solid-phase IgM capture assays are now being used more often, however, and are generally a rapid and accurate means of detecting mumps-specific IgM antibody.[20]

A definitive diagnosis of mumps infection based on measurements of IgG antibodies to mumps virus may be hampered by the production of cross-reactive antibodies between mumps virus and parainfluenza viruses.[21] This is not usually a practical problem if the clinical findings are compatible with mumps. The detection of elevated mumps-specific IgG antibody in CSF compared with serum or the finding of mumps-specific IgM antibodies in a single CSF specimen can be diagnostic in patients with aseptic meningitis.[11, 20] Mumps-specific IgM has been detected in saliva specimens 1 to 5 weeks after the onset of infection, making this specimen a useful alternative to the collection of serum.[8] However, salivary antibody testing is not widely available at present.

FA staining. FA staining and a time-resolved fluoroimmunoassay have been developed for rapid and direct detection of mumps virus antigens from exfoliated cells of NP secretions.[22, 23] Availability of commercial reagents is limited, however, and these methods have not been widely applied to the diagnosis of mumps.

RT-PCR. RT-PCR has been successfully used for the direct detection of mumps virus RNA in urine, respiratory, and CSF specimens of patients with clinical disease.[24-27] Conserved nucleotide sequences encoding the F protein, hemagglutinin-neuraminidase protein, and the small hydrophilic protein of mumps virus have been selected as targets for amplification. This method is also suitable for epidemiologic studies to distinguish circulating strains of mumps virus from one another and to differentiate wild-type virus from vaccine strains, particularly when aseptic meningitis develops after immunization with mumps vaccine.[25-27]

Although RT-PCR has proved to be a rapid, sensitive, and specific assay for detection of mumps virus, it is not routinely available in most diagnostic laboratories.

RUBELLA (GERMAN MEASLES)

Virology

Rubella virus is a single-stranded RNA virus that belongs to the genus *Rubivirus* in the family Togaviridae (see Table 13–2). The virus is spheric with a diameter of 60 to 70 nm and is surrounded by a lipid envelope containing projections of hemagglutinin. Only one antigenic type of rubella virus exists, and humans are the only known natural host. A live attenuated virus vaccine effectively controls infections with rubella virus and is given in combination with measles and mumps vaccines.

Epidemiology

Before the widespread use of rubella vaccine, epidemics most often occurred in the winter and spring in children 5 to 9 years of age. Postnatal rubella now occurs more often in young, unvaccinated adults.

Approximately 10% to 20% of persons in this age group in the United States are susceptible to infection. Currently, the incidence of rubella virus in the United States is very low because of the success of rubella immunization. Postnatally acquired rubella is spread through respiratory droplets, and the incubation period is 14 to 21 days.

Clinical Manifestations

Figure 13–2 shows the timing of clinical manifestations of rubella. Rubella virus characteristically causes a mild, self-limited, febrile disease of children and young adults with the development of a discrete maculopapular, erythematous rash and generalized lymphadenopathy. The illness resembles a mild case of measles. Approximately 25% to 50% of infections are asymptomatic. Transient arthritis or arthralgia occurs most frequently in adolescent and adult females and may involve the joints of the fingers, wrists, elbows, knees, and ankles.

Complications

Severe complications of postnatal rubella are uncommon but may include encephalitis and thrombocytopenia. The importance of rubella virus as an agent of human disease, however, lies in its ability to cause transplacental infection of the fetus when the infection occurs during pregnancy. This can lead to stillbirth, spontaneous abortion, resorption of the embryo, or

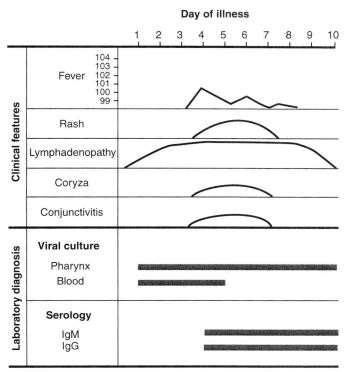

Figure 13.2 Timing of clinical findings and diagnostic test results in rubella.

infants born with *congenital rubella syndrome* (CRS). The risk of intrauterine transmission with fetal damage is greatest during the first trimester of pregnancy. The most common abnormalities in CRS include ophthalmologic defects, cardiac malformations, mental disability, and hearing loss. Initial presentation at birth can mimic sepsis, with jaundice, hepatosplenomegaly, thrombocytopenia, and purpuric skin lesions. Growth retardation and radiolucent bone disease also occur, and delayed manifestations of CRS may be seen up to 5 years of age (see Chapter 14).

Diagnosis

The clinical diagnosis of rubella is unreliable because symptoms and signs in infancy and childhood can be mild, nonspecific, and similar to those of other viral infections. Outbreaks of rubella also continue to occur, particularly in countries with less effective immunization programs. Therefore a definitive laboratory diagnosis is necessary and usually depends on the isolation of the virus in cell culture or the detection of rubella-specific IgG or IgM antibodies (see Figure 13–2).

Viral culture. Rubella virus can be grown in cell culture and has been isolated from respiratory secretions, blood, urine, stool, tears, CSF, lens and cataract material, and tissue from autopsy, as well as from amniotic fluid and placental and fetal tissue. Primary African green monkey kidney cells are most widely used for this purpose. Virus may be found in NP secretions from 7 days before to 14 days after onset of the rash in postnatal rubella. However, it can be difficult to isolate rubella virus in cell culture. Also, the method is slow and requires special techniques to recognize viral growth because most primary isolates of the virus do not produce CPE in infected cells (see Chapter 1). For these reasons, culture is rarely used in the routine diagnosis of rubella infection.

Isolation of rubella virus may be helpful to confirm infection in a newborn infant with suspected CRS or in patients with serious complications of rubella, but the method cannot be used to exclude infection. Infants with CRS may excrete virus in respiratory secretions and urine for months to years after birth and can transmit the virus to susceptible contacts. Persistent infection can lead to continued damage and severe sequelae. Viral isolation is useful to determine the duration of viral shedding and contagiousness in these infants.

Serology. Serologic testing is the method of choice for the diagnosis of rubella infections. The detection of rubella-specific antibodies is also useful for determining the immune status of patients and contacts and for verifying the immune response to vaccination. Rubella antibody testing is often performed in women of childbearing age before or during pregnancy to determine rubella immune status.

Commercially available latex agglutination (LA) tests, passive hemagglutination assays, and EIAs provide rapid results in the detection of rubella antibodies. EIAs based on recombinant and synthetic rubella antigens have been recently introduced to enhance the accuracy of rubella serodiagnosis.[28-30] Demonstration of seroconversion from a negative to a positive IgG antibody response or detection of rubella-specific IgM is diagnostic of primary infection. Sensitive and specific IgM capture EIAs have been used successfully for the diagnosis of primary rubella infection in serum and saliva.[8] Rubella-specific IgM antibodies can be detected in serum within a few days of the onset of rash. Fourfold or greater rises in rubella-specific IgG antibodies between acute and convalescent sera also may support a recent rubella infection. The presence of IgG to rubella virus in a single serum specimen indicates past rubella infection or previous immunization. IgM antibodies to rubella can sometimes persist at low levels for 6 months to 1 year after acute infection.

False-positive IgM results are possible, depending on the methods used for testing. When uncertain, the finding of rubella-specific IgM antibodies should be confirmed by obtaining acute and convalescent specimens to test for rubella-specific IgG antibodies or by performing cultures for rubella virus.

Detection of rubella RNA. Conventional *nucleic acid hybridization* techniques have been developed for the direct detection of rubella virus RNA in clinical specimens.[31, 32] This method is superior to virus isolation and has successfully confirmed congenital rubella infections when applied to products of conception and to the examination of chorionic villus biopsies. The assay is cumbersome and labor intensive, however, and is not routinely available for diagnostic use.

More recently, *RT-PCR* has replaced conventional nucleic acid hybridization as a rapid, sensitive, and specific method for rubella virus RNA detection. Gene sequences encoding the E1 membrane glycoprotein of rubella virus have been selected for amplification.[33] The method has been used to detect virus in chorionic villi, placenta, amniotic fluid, fetal blood, lens tissue, and products of conception for prenatal and postnatal diagnosis of congenital rubella. RT-PCR is also used to identify rubella virus in pharyngeal secretions from infected patients or vaccine recipients (see Chapter 14).[34-38] Additional work is needed to determine the value of RT-PCR for prenatal diagnosis of rubella infection, since rubella virus has been detected in the placenta when the fetus was uninfected and was not found in the placenta when the fetus was infected.[36]

The clinician must remember that in utero detection of rubella RNA indicates infection of the mother and fetus but does not necessarily predict disease or an adverse outcome for the fetus.

HUMAN PARVOVIRUS B19

Virology

Human parvovirus B19 is classified in the genus *Erythrovirus* in the family Parvoviridae. It is a single-stranded deoxyribonucleic acid (DNA) virus that possesses an icosahedral capsid but lacks a lipid envelope. The virus is one of the smallest DNA viruses, with a diameter of 18 to 26 nm; the genome codes for only three structural proteins. Humans are the only known host, and parvoviruses known to cause disease in other mammals and insects are not known to infect humans.

Virus-Host Interaction

Human parvovirus B19 is unusual in its extreme tissue tropism; the natural target of infection is the nucleus of immature dividing erythroid progenitor cells. Infected cells cease to proliferate, resulting in an impairment of normal erythrocyte development. In healthy children this loss of red cell production is of little consequence, and infection with parvovirus B19 leads to a mild, self-limited febrile illness referred to as *erythema infectiosum*, or *fifth disease*. Many cases are never recognized.

Immunocompromised individuals may be unable to limit the infection and may develop chronic infection that presents as pure red cell aplasia. Likewise, infection during pregnancy can lead to persistent infection in the fetus associated with fetal anemia and hydrops fetalis.

Epidemiology

Human parvovirus B19 has a worldwide distribution and is spread by the respiratory route, transfusion of blood or blood products, and vertically from mother to fetus. Approximately 50% of the population is infected during childhood. The highest incidence of infection occurs in children 4 to 7 years of age, and outbreaks of fifth disease are typically seen in schools and households during late winter and spring. Nosocomial spread of parvovirus B19 to hospital staff has been documented.[39] Parvovirus B19 is quite contagious, and spread from an index case to susceptible household and school contacts is common. The period of contagiousness precedes the appearance of rash, and individuals with fifth disease are considered noncontagious.

Clinical Manifestations

Table 13–3 lists the most common clinical manifestations of infection with human parvovirus B19. Acute parvovirus B19 infection (erythema infectiosum, fifth

Table 13.3	Common Clinical Manifestations of Human Parvovirus B19 Infection
Host state	**Clinical syndrome(s)**
Immunocompetence	Erythema infectiosum (fifth disease)
	Nonspecific febrile illness
	Arthritis and arthralgia
Chronic hemolytic anemia	Transient aplastic crisis
Acquired or congenital immunodeficiency	Pure red cell aplasia from chronic bone marrow suppression
Pregnancy	Fetal or congenital anemia
	Spontaneous abortion, stillbirth
	Nonimmune hydrops fetalis

disease) is characterized by a confluent, erythematous, maculopapular rash that appears on the face in a "slapped-cheek" pattern and then spreads in 1 to 2 days to the trunk and limbs. The rash on the arms and legs is usually lacy or reticular in appearance. Other symptoms include cough, headache, sore throat, vomiting, diarrhea, and anorexia. The incubation period is 6 to 18 days, and the illness lasts for 1 to 2 weeks. The rash may recur for an additional 2 to 4 weeks on exposure to sunlight, heat, or cold and may be exacerbated by physical activity and stress.

Asymptomatic infections, as well as a nonspecific, influenza-like illness without rash, are common in children. Arthritis and arthralgias occur frequently in infected adults, particularly women, sometimes without rash. Rare dermatologic manifestations include vesiculopustular eruptions, purpura with or without thrombocytopenia, and an erythematous rash on the hands and feet referred to as "socks-and-gloves" syndrome.

Complications

Infection in patients with chronic hematologic diseases (e.g., sickle cell anemia, hereditary spherocytosis, β-thalassemia) can result in an acute, severe, and occasionally fatal aplastic crisis. The aplastic anemia is transient and the result of a rapid fall in hemoglobin with a loss of reticulocytes from the peripheral blood and the absence of erythrocyte precursors from the bone marrow.

Patients with acquired or congenital immunodeficiency, including those infected with human immunodeficiency virus (HIV), can develop a pure red cell aplasia as the result of chronic bone marrow suppression with persistent anemia or a remitting and relapsing anemia with reticulocytopenia. Infection during pregnancy can cause fetal or congenital anemia, spontaneous abortion, stillbirth, and nonimmune hydrops fetalis. Although fetal hydrops is a well-recognized complication of maternal parvovirus B19 infection, the overall risk is low (see Chapter 14).

Diagnosis

Figure 13–3 shows the relationships among virologic and clinical events in acute human parvovirus B19 infection. Table 13–4 summarizes the most useful tests for diagnosing specific syndromes associated with parvovirus B19 infection. A useful culture system for parvovirus B19 does not currently exist, and most diagnosis depends on molecular methods for the direct detection of the viral DNA in clinical specimens or the detection of specific antiviral antibodies produced in response to infection.

In immunocompetent individuals, including pregnant women and patients with erythema infectiosum or transient aplastic crisis, the most practical method for detecting parvovirus B19 infection involves testing a single serum specimen for B19-specific IgM antibodies. Because aplastic crisis occurs earlier after infection than does fifth disease, parvovirus IgM antibodies may not be detectable until some days after onset of the crisis, whereas they are usually detectable in patients with fifth disease. B19 DNA is detectable by molecular methods in the blood of these patients during the aplastic crisis. Detection of fetal infection or chronic infection in immunocompromised patients is best accomplished by molecular methods for detection of parvovirus B19 DNA because a serologic response to B19 infection may not occur in these settings.

Serology. Both IgG and IgM antibodies to human parvovirus B19 are present soon after onset of disease. IgM to parvovirus B19 can be detected by the third day

Table 13.4	Diagnosis of Human Parvovirus B19 Infection
Syndrome	**Preferred diagnostic test**
Fifth disease (erythema infectiosum)	Parvovirus B19 IgM
Acute arthritis	Parvovirus B19 IgM
Aplastic crisis	Serum PCR, Parvovirus B19 IgM*
Red cell aplasia (immunocompromised individuals)	Serum PCR
Hydrops fetalis	Amniotic fluid PCR
Determination of immune status	Parvovirus B19 IgG

PCR, Polymerase chain reaction.
*A test for parvovirus B19 IgM antibodies serology may be negative at presentation but will become positive within a few days.

of symptoms, peaks at 30 days, and becomes undetectable by 60 to 90 days; specific IgG is usually present by the seventh day of illness and persists for years.[40] Therefore a positive IgM result for parvovirus B19 antibody suggests current or very recent infection, and the detection of IgG antibody indicates previous exposure and probable immunity to reinfection. A diagnosis also can be made by detecting a seroconversion or a significant increase in B19-specific IgG antibody between acute and convalescent sera, if collection of specimens is done early in the disease process.

IFAs, EIAs, radioimmunoassays (RIAs), and hemadherence assays have been developed that detect parvovirus B19–specific IgG and IgM antibodies.[41-44] Antibody capture EIAs are generally the preferred method for measuring B19-specific IgM antibody responses. Initially, high titers of virus in the serum of patients with aplastic crisis were used as the source of antigen for parvovirus B19 serologic assays. However, this source

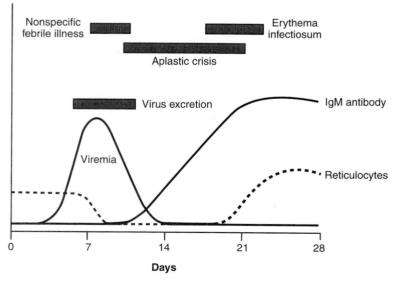

Figure 13.3 Virologic, immunologic, hematologic, and clinical events in human parvovirus B19 infection. (From Cherry JD: In Feigin RD, Cherry JD, editors: *Textbook of pediatric infectious diseases*, ed 4, Philadelphia, 1998, WB Saunders.)

could not be sustained in large quantities for diagnostic purposes. Parvovirus B19 structural proteins were subsequently expressed in various mammalian and baculovirus expression systems, and peptides can now be synthesized for use as antigens in the development of immunoassays. Several kits are now commercially available.

Recently, *saliva* has been shown to be a convenient alternative to serum for serodiagnosis of parvovirus B19 infections.[45] Approximately 60% of patients with acute infection can be diagnosed within the first 5 days of illness using saliva as a specimen. The most appropriate time in the course of illness for the collection of saliva for optimal sensitivity of antibody determinations is not yet known.

Detection of parvovirus B19 DNA. Antibodies to human parvovirus B19 are not detectable in some immunodeficient patients with chronic, persistent infection. Also, serologic assays for prenatal diagnosis of infection in the fetus may have limited usefulness. B19-specific IgG can represent passively acquired maternal antibody, and production of viral IgM in the fetus can be delayed or absent (see Chapter 14).

Conventional nucleic acid hybridization assays or polymerase chain reaction (PCR) for parvovirus B19 DNA are best suited for these clinical situations. A variety of *dot blot hybridization* assays have been developed using either isotopic probes or nonisotopic probes labeled with biotin or digoxigenin for the detection of B19 DNA in serum, blood and blood products, tissue, and amniotic fluid.[46-48] In most cases of persistent parvovirus B19 infection, levels of viremia are high, and dot blot hybridization is sufficient to make a diagnosis. *In situ hybridization* (ISH) assays have been used successfully to localize parvovirus B19 DNA within bone marrow cells and tissue specimens of patients, particularly the infected fetus and patients in aplastic crisis or with chronic bone marrow supression.[49, 50] In one study the detection of parvovirus B19 DNA in cord blood by ISH proved to be more sensitive than a nested PCR for the diagnosis of fetal infection.[51]

In general, PCR assays are more sensitive and practical than traditional DNA hybridization techniques. Oligonucleotide sequences that code for either the viral capsid or the nonstructural proteins of the virus have been used as primers for viral amplification.[52-55] Parvovirus B19 DNA has been detected by PCR in serum, urine, CSF, pleural fluid, respiratory secretions, peripheral blood mononuclear cells, bone marrow cells, tissue, synovial fluid, and amniotic fluid. PCR performed on serum is very useful for the recognition of chronic parvovirus B19 infection in immunocompromised individuals and, when performed on amniotic fluid, for the diagnosis of intrauterine infection (see Chapter 14). Parvovirus B19 DNA can also be detected by PCR in peripheral blood of almost all patients with fifth disease,

whereas the level of virus in blood is not readily detected by dot blot hybridization.[52, 56]

Recently, PCR has been advocated for screening donated blood to prevent transmission of parvovirus B19 during transfusion. In situ PCR has been used to detect small quantities of viral DNA in individual cells and tissue sections and may play an important role in studies of the natural history of parvovirus B19 infections.[57, 58] Currently, molecular methods for the detection of parvovirus B19 DNA are investigational and have limited availability.

Other diagnostic methods. Attempts to grow human parvovirus B19 in conventional cell culture have been unsuccessful. The virus has been propagated in human erythroid leukemic cell lines and primary cell cultures of erythroid precursor cells obtained from human peripheral blood, fetal liver and bone marrow, but such culture systems are impractical for diagnostic use.

Electron microscopic examination of negatively stained clinical specimens has been used for the direct detection of viral particles. *Immune electron microscopy* and the technique of *pseudoreplication* also have been employed to enhance visualization of the virus. These methods are labor intensive, however, and lack sensitivity compared with other assays used in the diagnostic laboratory. They also require specialized equipment and a high level of technical expertise.

EIAs and RIAs also have been developed for the detection of parvovirus B19 antigens in the serum of infected patients. These assays are generally less sensitive than direct DNA hybridization or PCR. Recently, a *dot immunoperoxidase* assay, which uses monoclonal antibodies directed against parvovirus B19 capsid proteins, has shown promise as a rapid, sensitive, and specific test for large-scale screening of serum samples for the detection of viral antigens.[59]

HUMAN HERPESVIRUS TYPE 6

Virology

Human herpesvirus type 6 (HHV-6) is an ubiquitous, T-lymphotrophic virus that was first isolated in 1986 from the peripheral blood mononuclear cells of patients with acquired immunodeficiency syndrome (AIDS) and lymphoproliferative disorders.[60] The virus is a member of the family Herpesviridae and is similar in morphology to other herpesviruses but is genetically and serologically distinct. Primary infection with HHV-6 results in the establishment of latent or persistent infection, and reactivation may occur in response to different stimuli. The virus has a diameter of 160 to 200 nm and consists of an internal core containing double-stranded DNA and an icosahedral nucleocapsid surrounded by an amorphous tegument and an envelope.

Two distinct but closely related variants of HHV-6 have been described. *Variant B* is found most often in patients with symptomatic primary infections. *Variant A* has not been definitively associated with human disease or independently isolated during primary infection. Humans are the only known natural host for HHV-6, and the virus is presumed to be spread by person-to-person contact through respiratory secretions. Intrauterine or perinatal transmission has been suggested.

Clinical Manifestations

Infections with HHV-6 are common and often mild or inapparent; nearly 100% of children have been infected with the virus and display antibodies to it by school age. The most commonly recognized manifestation of HHV-6 in children ages 6 months to 3 years is *roseola* (*roseola infantum, exanthem subitum, sixth disease*). The illness begins abruptly with a high fever (39° to 40°C) that continues for 3 to 5 days, followed by an erythematous, blanching, maculopapular, nonpruritic rash beginning on the face or trunk and spreading to other areas. The rash usually lasts for 1 to 3 days with no subsequent desquamation or pigment changes. Interestingly, most cases of acute HHV-6 infection in young children do not result in an illness recognizable as roseola. Studies have revealed that acute viremic HHV-6 infection accounted for 14% of febrile children under 2 years of age seen in an emergency room, most of whom had a nonspecific febrile illness without a rash[61, 62] (see Complications).

Primary HHV-6 infection in adults is rare but may result in prolonged lymphadenopathy, hepatitis, or an illness resembling mononucleosis. Reactivated infection in healthy persons is asymptomatic. It remains to be established whether HHV-6 causes or contributes to disease in the immunocompromised host, although reactivation in organ transplant recipients has been associated with fever, hepatitis, bone marrow suppression, and pneumonia (see Chapter 15). Evidence also suggests that HHV-6 infection may contribute to disease progression with HIV and may interact with other viruses, such as Epstein-Barr virus (EBV), cytomegalovirus (CMV), human papillomaviruses, to affect their behavior.

Complications

Febrile convulsions are a common complication of roseola; approximately one third of all febrile convulsions in childhood have been attributed to HHV-6 infection. Other complications of primary infection include rash without fever, intussusception, infectious mononucleosis-like syndrome, bulging of the anterior fontanelle, hepatitis, lymphadenopathy, aseptic meningitis, meningoencephalitis, and encephalitis.

Diagnosis

A typical case of exanthem subitum in a child can be made clinically without involving the laboratory. However, a laboratory diagnosis may be necessary (1) to diagnose HHV-6 infection that presents without rash, (2) to exclude other agents that may cause similar clinical presentations, and (3) to detect atypical and more severe manifestations of HHV-6 infection. Laboratory methods may also function in defining the role of HHV-6 in disease of adults and immunocompromised hosts and to link this virus to other clinical conditions.

Diagnostic methods for the detection of HHV-6 are still under development, however, and only recently have commercial reagents been made available for use by diagnostic laboratories.[63, 64] The sensitivity, specificity, and clinical relevance of each assay remain to be firmly established.

Viral culture. HHV-6 can be isolated from patients' peripheral blood mononuclear cells grown in primary culture or by co-cultivation of these cells with stimulated umbilical cord mononuclear cells or donor peripheral blood mononuclear cells.[64, 65] Saliva and other body fluids and tissues can be co-cultured with activated donor cells for isolation of the virus as well. One study found that the virus could not be cultured from saliva during acute infection.[66]

The optimal time for collection of specimens in children with roseola is during the febrile phase, before the development of rash. Infected peripheral blood mononuclear cells show a specific CPE, with intracytoplasmic and intranuclear inclusion bodies appearing within 7 to 10 days. The CPE can be subtle and difficult to recognize, but growth can be confirmed by immunofluorescence or EIA for the detection of HHV-6 antigens. FA staining reveals a characteristic granular nuclear and cytoplasmic fluorescence in infected cells. This culture method is slow, labor intensive, requires a high level of technical expertise, and is not performed routinely in most clinical laboratories.

Positive culture results are most useful to diagnose primary infection but can be difficult to interpret in immunocompromised hosts and during reactivation of the virus, when finding virus may be unrelated to the clinical presentation.

Human diploid lung fibroblasts (MRC-5) can support the growth of HHV-6 and have been used in a centrifugation-assisted *shell vial amplification assay* for the detection of the immediate-early antigen of the virus in peripheral blood mononuclear cells obtained from patients.[67] Polyclonal and monoclonal antibodies specific for both or either variant of HHV-6 are commercially available and stain the nucleus of infected MRC-5 cells as early as 12 hours after infection; maximum staining is observed within 48 to 72 hours.

The shell vial assay is more rapid and less labor intensive than conventional culture. The sensitivity and specificity of this test for HHV-6 have yet to be clearly defined, however, and this test is currently not offered as a routine service in most virology laboratories.

Serology. Various methods have been developed for serodiagnosis of HHV-6 infection, including IFA tests, EIAs, and neutralization assays.[60, 63, 64] IFA tests are used most often, although EIAs are slightly more sensitive. Commercial IFA and EIA kits for the detection of HHV-6-specific IgG and IgM are now available. These assays have been used mainly for the diagnosis of primary infection with HHV-6 in children with acute illnesses and to study the epidemiology, pathology, and natural history of infection. Western immunoblots and radioimmunoprecipitation assays have been used mostly for research purposes to define the immune response to specific viral proteins.

Demonstration of seroconversion from a negative to a positive IgG antibody response or detection of HHV-6-specific IgM antibody during a primary infection establishes HHV-6 as the causative agent. A fourfold or greater rise in HHV-6-specific IgG between acute and convalescent sera indicates recent infection due to reactivation or reinfection. If HHV-6-specific IgG is present in both acute and convalescent sera but the titer is unchanged, the result is interpreted as HHV-6 infection in the past. Detection of IgG antibody to HHV-6 in a single serum specimen can provide evidence of previous exposure to the virus and identify those individuals at risk for infection.

Results of serologic tests for antibody to HHV-6 should be interpreted with extreme caution. Variations in the detection of HHV-6-specific antibodies have been observed and may be related to the assay used and the need for further standardization of methods and reagents. The detection of IgG or IgM antibodies to HHV-6 may not always indicate primary infection, and serologic studies have limited value in establishing an association of reactivation or latent infection with disease. An increase in HHV-6-specific IgG antibody can occur during infections with other herpesviruses (e.g., EBV, CMV, HHV-7), and determining the relative importance of each virus in causing disease can be difficult. Serologic tests for HHV-6-specific IgM also should be carefully interpreted, since IgM can appear during both primary and reactivated HHV-6 infections and can persist for extended periods after a primary infection. Also, some children may not develop detectable IgM responses during primary infection.

Antigen assays and PCR. Numerous oligonucleotide primers have been described and used in PCR assays for the direct detection of HHV-6 DNA from respiratory specimens, peripheral blood mononuclear cells, tissues, and genital secretions.[68-70] CSF specimens also have been examined by PCR to diagnose HHV-6-related febrile seizures and other neurologic diseases (see Chapter 3).[71, 72]

More recently, HHV-6 antigens also have been directly detected from clinical specimens using monoclonal antibodies in an immunofluorescence assay or using a newly developed antigen capture EIA.[73] With these procedures, HHV-6 has been found in most populations studied, including patients with roseola, transplant recipients, individuals with AIDS or lymphoproliferative disorders, and latently infected healthy children and adults.

Therefore the ubiquitous distribution of HHV-6 may necessitate the use of methods that measure active viral replication, since qualitative detection of viral antigens or DNA may simply indicate the presence of HHV-6 but may not be predictive of symptomatic disease. A more accurate assessment of the involvement of HHV-6 in a given disease may be provided by the detection of cell-free virus in serum or plasma by PCR,[74, 75] by qualitative amplification of specific HHV-6 messenger RNA (mRNA) transcripts, by detection of viral antigen expression in tissues by immunohistochemistry (IHC),[76] or by quantitative measures of viral load by DNA PCR.[77] The usefulness of these methods in the accurate diagnosis of HHV-6 disease requires further study.

Special considerations in young children. Unfortunately, no practical diagnostic test currently allows rapid diagnosis of acute HHV-6 infection in children. Demonstration of antibody seroconversion or a fourfold increase in titer is a good indication of acute infection but requires a convalescent specimen. HHV-6-specific IgG and IgM antibodies are first detectable 5 to 7 days after onset.[78] Serodiagnosis is complicated by (1) increases in antibody titer with viral reactivation and (2) inability to demonstrate a serologic response in infants less that 3 months of age because of maternal antibodies in the acute specimen.[61]

The presence of HHV-6-specific IgM antibodies also has less than optimal sensitivity and specificity for acute infection. A positive culture of HHV-6 from peripheral blood mononuclear cells correlated with serologic evidence of acute infection and occurred only in children during the acute phase of illness.[61, 62] However, HHV-6 cultures are not widely available in diagnostic laboratories. PCR performed on peripheral blood mononuclear cells was uniformly positive but was also frequently positive in follow-up convalescent specimens, as well as in 25% of children who did not have acute HHV-6 infection.

Chiu et al[78] recently found that the combination of a positive PCR on peripheral blood and a negative HHV-6 antibody test was diagnostic of acute infection. This interesting concept requires further validation. Because of the confounding effect of maternal antibody, this approach is not applicable to infants less than 3 months of age. Antibody testing was carried out on a 1:50 dilution of plasma to avoid oversensitive detection of maternal antibody in children over 3 months of age. In the same study, PCR detection of high levels of HHV-6 DNA in peripheral blood mononuclear cells and detection of HHV-6 DNA in plasma had sensitivities of 100% and 90% for the diagnosis of acute infection. Occasionally, however, these results were also found in patients with other infections who may have been experiencing HHV-6 reactivation. The finding of HHV-6 DNA in peripheral blood mononuclear cells but not in saliva may indicate acute infection because of the late appearance of HHV-6 in saliva.[78, 79]

HUMAN HERPESVIRUS TYPE 7

Virology and Clinical Manifestations

Human herpesvirus type 7 (HHV-7) is a recently described member of the herpesvirus family that was first isolated in 1989 from peripheral blood mononuclear cells of a healthy adult.[80] As with HHV-6, this virus is an ubiquitous beta herpesvirus with a tropism for CD4+ lymphocytes and the capability for latency and reactivation after primary infection. Although closely related to HHV-6, it is genetically and immunologically distinct.[81-83] The prevalence of antibody to HHV-7 is more than 85% in U.S. and European populations.

Infection with HHV-7 occurs early in life, usually after 24 months of age, but later than infection with HHV-6.[82, 84] HHV-7 has been associated with up to 10% of roseola cases and, as with HHV-6, is thought to be responsible for seizures and other neurologic events in children. Its role in other human diseases has not been defined.

Diagnosis

Diagnosis of HHV-7 infection is essentially the same as for HHV-6.[63, 80] HHV-7 can be grown in peripheral blood mononuclear cells or cord blood cells and produces a CPE that is indistinguishable from that of HHV-6.[81, 85] A continuous T-cell line (Sup-T1) supports the growth of HHV-7 with variable success. The virus can be frequently and consistently isolated from the saliva and peripheral blood cells of infected individuals.[85, 86]

IFA tests, EIAs, and Western blot assays have been developed for the serodiagnosis of HHV-7 infection, using HHV-7-infected cells as the antigen source.[82, 84, 87] Seroconversion to HHV-7 is independent of that for HHV-6 and is diagnostic for primary infection. A simultaneous rise in antibody to HHV-6 can occur, however, during seroconversion to HHV-7 resulting from antigenic cross-reactivity.[78] Conversely, primary infection with HHV-6 does not cause a rise in antibody titers to HHV-7. PCR primers that amplify HHV-7 DNA have been developed for the detection and quantitation of this virus from clinical specimens.[77, 83, 88, 89]

As with HHV-6, the laboratory diagnosis of HHV-7 is confounded by its ubiquitous distribution. A combination of laboratory methods and patient assessment may be necessary to provide a reliable diagnosis of HHV-7 infection and to establish a relationship between infection and human disease. As in HHV-6 infection, when an effort is made to link the virus to unusual disease manifestations, the demonstration of viral antigen and nucleic acid by IHC and ISH is highly desired.

NONPOLIO ENTEROVIRUSES

Virology and Epidemiology

Enteroviruses belong to the family Picornaviridae and are a diverse group that includes *poliovirus* types 1 to 3, *coxsackievirus A* (Coxsackie A virus) types 1 to 24 (A23 does not exist), *coxsackievirus B* (Coxsackie B virus) types 1 to 6, *echovirus* types 1 to 31 (types 10 and 28 do not exist), and the numbered enterovirus types 68 to 71. They are small (20 to 29 nm in diameter), nonenveloped viruses that possess a single-stranded RNA genome surrounded by an icosahedral capsid. Transmission is by the fecal-oral and respiratory routes, and humans are the only known reservoir. Replication occurs in the gastrointestinal (GI) tract, although enteroviruses rarely cause significant enteric disease.

The distribution of enteroviruses is worldwide, with a year-round prevalence in tropical and semitropical areas and epidemics observed mainly during the summer months in temperate climates. Several serotypes circulate at one time, and different serotypes are prevalent in different years. The incidence of infection is highest in lower socioeconomic groups; overcrowding and inadequate sanitation are important factors. Asymptomatic infection is common, and spread to nonimmune family members is high.

Clinical Manifestations

Nonpolio enteroviruses are responsible for an estimated 5 to 10 million symptomatic infections each year in the United States. The incidence and severity of these infections is highest in neonates and young children, and a variety of clinical manifestations involving all organ systems has been described (Table 13–5). These include aseptic meningitis, encephalitis, pericarditis, myocarditis, hepatitis, various respiratory and GI illnesses, acute hemorrhagic conjunctivitis, and exanthemas and enanthemas. Chronic and often fatal me-

Table 13.5	Clinical Manifestations Associated with Nonpolio Enteroviruses

Organ system	Clinical syndromes
Respiratory	Common cold
	Pharyngitis
	Tonsillitis
	Croup
	Bronchitis
	Bronchiolitis
	Parotitis
	Herpangina
	Stomatitis
	Hand-foot-and-mouth disease
	Pneumonia
	Pleurodynia
Cardiac	Pericarditis
	Myocarditis
Neurologic	Aseptic meningitis
	Encephalitis
	Paralysis
	Guillain-Barré syndrome
	Transverse myelitis
	Cerebellar ataxia
	Peripheral neuritis
Ocular	Acute hemorrhagic conjunctivitis
Skin	Exanthems
	Enanthems
Gastrointestinal	Gastroenteritis
	Hepatitis
	Peritonitis
	Mesenteric adenitis
	Intussusception
	Appendicitis
	Pancreatitis
	Reye's syndrome
	Diabetes mellitus
Genitourinary	Orchitis
	Epididymitis
Other	Nonspecific febrile illness
	Neonatal sepsis

ningoencephalitis can occur in immunocompromised patients, especially those with agammaglobulinemia.

The most common manifestation of nonpolio enterovirus infection in infants and children is *nonspecific febrile illness*. This illness is responsible for hospitalization of many infants each summer. The disease begins with an abrupt onset of fever (38.3° to 40°C) with malaise, anorexia, and occasionally generalized myalgia. The fever may last for 3 days but may be biphasic, with 1 day of fever followed by 2 to 3 days of apparent recovery, then recurrence of fever for an additional 2 to 4 days. Complaints of a sore throat are common and conjunctivitis is possible; older children may experience headache. Although considered to be mild and self-limiting, the severity of the illness varies depending on the host and viral serotype.

A variety of respiratory manifestations also have been observed in infants and children infected with nonpolio enteroviruses. These include common cold symptoms, pharyngitis, herpangina, stomatitis, croup, bronchiolitis, pneumonia, and pleurodynia. Nausea, diarrhea, vomiting, and abdominal pain are often part of the systemic illness with enteroviral infections.

In newborns, disseminated infections with the nonpolio enteroviruses can result in fulminant hepatitc failure, fatal myocarditis and meningoencephalitis, and a clinical presentation mimicking bacterial sepsis. The sepsislike illness can be severe and is characterized by fever, irritability, rash, lethargy, hypotonia, abdominal distension, and poor feeding. Vomiting, diarrhea, seizures, and apnea also may occur.

Diagnosis

Infections with the nonpolio enteroviruses are difficult to distinguish from other infectious and noninfectious diseases that have overlapping clinical features. Therefore the clinical diagnosis of enteroviral illness is imprecise and is often one of exclusion or presumption based on negative bacterial cultures and a suggestive clinical presentation. Patients are often hospitalized and treated with antibacterial agents. Laboratory testing can provide an accurate diagnosis of enteroviral infection and is useful in assessing the need for continued hospital admission and antimicrobial use.

Viral culture. Isolation in cell culture remains the standard for the laboratory diagnosis of enteroviruses, although false-negative results are common. Primary monkey kidney and human embryonic lung fibroblast cells are used routinely for culture and support the growth of most clinically important enteroviruses. Recovery rates for coxsackievirus types A and B may be enhanced by the addition of human rhabdomyosarcoma and Buffalo green monkey kidney cells, respectively. Most Coxsackie A viruses will not grow using conventional cell culture techniques and must be detected by inoculation into suckling mice. This practice is cumbersome, however, and has been discontinued by most diagnostic laboratories.

Growth in cell culture usually occurs in 1 to 4 days and is characterized by a CPE of rounded, refractile cells that degenerate to lysis. Virus may be recovered from the stool, CSF, throat, serum, white blood cells, urine, and biopsy or postmortem specimens. Stool specimens are preferred over rectal swabs because they produce a higher yield of virus.[90] Blood is a useful specimen to culture in infants less than 3 months of age.[91] Other specimens, including pericardial fluid, vesicle fluid, pleural fluid, and ocular discharge, may also be useful depending on the patient's clinical presentation.

Culturing multiple sites enhances the chances of isolating an enterovirus because of the generalized nature of most enteroviral infections. After growth in cell culture the specific enterovirus serotype can be determined by antibody neutralization or by FA staining using appropriate monoclonal antibodies. Typing is rarely necessary for clinical purposes because diseases caused by these viruses are usually not serotype specific.

The isolation of enteroviruses from stool specimens and respiratory secretions must be interpreted with care. First, the laboratory must determine whether the isolate is a vaccine strain of poliovirus, especially if the child has a history of recent immunization. Vaccine strains of poliovirus can be isolated from both stool and respiratory secretions for several months after receipt of the live attenuated oral poliovirus vaccine. The CPE of these viruses cannot be reliably distinguished from that of the nonpolio enteroviruses, although the viruses can be distinguished in the laboratory by FA staining or neutralization with specific antisera. In addition, nonpolio enteroviruses can be found in asymptomatic individuals and can be excreted in the stool for long periods after infection. For these reasons, isolation of these viruses from the feces may not be related to a patient's current illness. This consideration is somewhat less important during the first few months of life; isolation of an enterovirus is usually associated with current illness in these infants.[91]

Serology. Serologic tests have limited use in the diagnosis of enteroviruses. Enteroviral serologies rely on the demonstration of a fourfold or greater rise in virus type-specific antibody titers between acute and convalescent sera. Because many antigenically different enteroviruses exist with no common group antigen, serologic testing without isolation of the virus or knowledge of the serotypes circulating in the community is impractical. Recently, enterovirus-specific antibody capture EIAs have been developed and have shown promise for the early detection of IgM antibodies during infection with certain coxsackievirus B serotypes.[92-94] The assays appear to lack the appropriate specificity for diagnostic use, however, and their availability remains limited.

Antigen assays. The absence of a shared antigen among the enteroviruses has hampered the development and use of FA staining and EIA for the direct detection of enteroviral antigens in clinical specimens.[95] Currently, no commercial antigen assays are available for diagnostic use. Recently, "cocktails" of monoclonal antibodies specific for each of the major enteroviral groups and individual antibodies to certain serotypes have been produced commercially. These reagents have been used in FA staining methods for identification and typing of enteroviruses grown in conventional tube cultures and centrifugation-assisted shell vial culture systems.[96-98] The use of these antibodies for the direct detection of enteroviruses in clinical specimens has not been evaluated.

Nucleic acid assays and RT-PCR. Conventional nucleic acid hybridization assays using complementary DNA (cDNA) or RNA probes have been developed for direct detection of enteroviruses from clinical specimens.[99] Such assays lack the necessary sensitivity to be clinically useful, however, because of the limited quantity of virus in many body fluids and tissues.

The development of RT-PCR is more promising for the rapid and sensitive amplification of enteroviral DNA[100, 101] (see Chapters 3 and 9). The 5' noncoding region of the enterovirus genome is highly conserved across all the enterovirus groups, and oligonucleotide primers and probes have been selected from this site for RT-PCR. Assays have been developed for universal detection of all known serotypes and for the detection of particular enterovirus groups, serotypes, and strains. RT-PCR has been used to diagnose the presence of enteroviruses in a number of different specimens, including respiratory secretions, serum, blood, urine, CSF, and tissue.[102] The most extensively evaluated application of RT-PCR is in the diagnosis of enteroviral infections of the CNS, where the viral load in CSF is low and the yield from cell culture particularly poor.[103, 104] RT-PCR is potentially useful for the diagnosis of other enteroviral diseases, such as myocarditis,[105] chronic meningoencephalitis,[106] and acute febrile illness in children. In neonatal enteroviral infections, RT-PCR has been shown to be more sensitive than culture when performed on specimens of serum and urine.[107]

A commercial RT-PCR has been developed and evaluated[108] but is currently not available for diagnostic use.

References

1. Minnich LL, Goodenough F, Ray CG: Use of immunofluorescence to identify measles virus infections, *J Clin Microbiol* 29:1148, 1991.
2. Kobune F, Sakata H, Sugiura A: Marmoset lymphoblastoid cells as a sensitive host for isolation of measles virus, *J Virol* 64:700, 1990.
3. Forthal DN, Blanding J, Aarnaes S, et al: Comparison of different methods and cell lines for isolating measles virus, *J Clin Microbiol* 31:695, 1993.
4. Laboratory diagnosis of measles infection and monitoring of measles immunization: memorandum from a WHO meeting, *Bull World Health Organ* 72:207, 1994.
5. Jeckerson SA, Beller M, Middaugh JP, Erdman DD: False positive rubeola IgM tests, *N Engl J Med* 332:1103, 1995.

6. Erdman DD, Anderson LJ, Adams DR, et al: Evaluation of monoclonal antibody–based capture enzyme immunoassays for detection of specific antibodies to measles virus, *J Clin Microbiol* 29:1466, 1991.

7. Rossier E, Miller H, McCulloch B, et al: Comparison of immunofluorescence and enzyme immunoassay for detection of measles-specific immunoglobulin M antibody, *J Clin Microbiol* 29:1069, 1991.

8. Perry KR, Brown DWG, Parry JV, et al: Detection of measles, mumps and rubella antibodies in saliva using antibody capture radioimmunoassay, *J Med Virol* 40: 235, 1993.

9. Hummel KB, Erdman DD, Heath J, et al: Baculovirus expression of the nucleoprotein gene of measles virus and utility of the recombinant protein in diagnostic enzyme immunoassays, *J Clin Microbiol* 30:2874, 1992.

10. Bouche F, Ammerlaan W, Berthet F, et al: Immunosorbent assay based on recombinant hemagglutinin protein produced in a high-efficiency mammalian expression system for surveillance of measles immunity, *J Clin Microbiol* 36:721, 1998.

11. Andiman WA: Organism-specific antibody indices, the cerebrospinal fluid–immunoglobulin index and other tools: a clinician's guide to the etiologic diagnosis of central nervous system infection, *Pediatr Infect Dis J* 10: 490, 1991.

12. Smaron MF, Saxon E, Wood L, et al: Diagnosis of measles by fluorescent antibody and culture of nasopharyngeal secretions, *J Virol Methods* 33:223, 1991.

13. Hodinka RL, Stetser RL, Wainwright J: Rapid detection of measles virus using immunofluorescence, Abstracts of the 92nd annual meeting of the American Society for Microbiology, p. 449, 1992.

14. Nakayama T, Mori T, Yamaguchi S, et al: Detection of measles virus genome directly from clinical samples by reverse transcriptase–polymerase chain reaction and genetic variability, *Virus Res* 35:1, 1995.

15. Shimizu H, McCarthy CA, Smaron MF, Burns JC: Polymerase chain reaction for detection of measles virus in clinical samples, *J Clin Microbiol* 31:1034, 1993.

16. Godec MS, Asher DM, Swoveland PT, et al: Detection of measles virus genomic sequences in SSPE brain tissue by the polymerase chain reaction, *J Med Virol* 30: 237, 1990.

17. Rota PA, Khan AS, Durigon E, et al: Detection of measles virus RNA in urine specimens from vaccine recipients, *J Clin Microbiol* 33:2485, 1995.

18. Katayama Y, Kohso K, Nishimura A, et al: Detection of measles virus mRNA from autopsied human tissues, *J Clin Microbiol* 36:299, 1998.

19. Philip RN, Reinhard KR, Lackman DB: Observations on a mumps epidemic in a "virgin" population, *Am J Epidemiol* 142:233, 1995.

20. Glikmann G, Pedersen M, Mordhorst CH: Detection of specific immunoglobulin M to mumps virus in serum and cerebrospinal fluid samples from patients with acute mumps infection, using an antibody-capture enzyme immunoassay, *Acta Pathol Microbiol Immunol Scand* 94:145, 1986.

21. Nicolai-Scholten, ME, Ziegelmaier R, Behrens F, et al: The enzyme-linked immunosorbent assay (ELISA) for determination of IgG and IgM antibodies after infection with mumps virus, *Med Microbiol Immunol* 168: 81, 1980.

22. Minnich L, Ray CG: Comparison of direct immunofluorescent staining of clinical specimens for respiratory virus antigens with conventional isolation techniques, *J Clin Microbiol* 12:391, 1980.

23. Hierholzer JC, Bingham PG, Castells E, et al: Time-resolved fluoroimmunoassays with monoclonal antibodies for rapid identification of parainfluenza type 4 and mumps virus, *Arch Virol* 130,335, 1993.

24. Boriskin YS, Booth JC, Yamada A: Rapid detection of mumps virus by the polymerase chain reaction, *J Virol Methods* 42:23, 1993.

25. Afzal MA, Buchanan J, Dias JA, et al: RT-PCR based diagnosis and molecular characterization of mumps viruses derived from clinical specimens collected during the 1996 mumps outbreak in Portugal, *J Med Virol* 52: 349, 1997.

26. Cusi MG, Bianchi S, Valassina M, et al: Rapid detection and typing of circulating mumps virus by reverse transcription/polymerase chain reaction, *Res Virol* 147: 227, 1996.

27. Kashiwagi Y, Kawashima H, Takekuma K, et al: Detection of mumps virus genome directly from clinical samples and a simple method for genetic differentiation of the Hoshino vaccine strain from wild strains of mumps virus, *J Med Virol* 52:195, 1997.

28. Grangeot-Keros L, Enders G: Evaluation of a new enzyme immunoassay based on recombinant rubella virus–like particles for the detection of immunoglobulin M antibodies to rubella virus, *J Clin Microbiol* 35: 398, 1997.

29. Grangeot-Keros L, Pustowoit B, Hobman T: Evaluation of Cobas core rubella IgG EIA recomb, a new enzyme immunoassay based on recombinant rubella-like particles, *J Clin Microbiol* 33:2392, 1995.

30. Mitchell LA, Zhang T, Ho M, et al: Characterization of rubella virus–specific antibody responses by using a new synthetic peptide–based enzyme-linked immunosorbent assay, *J Clin Microbiol* 30:1841, 1992.

31. Ho-Terry L, Terry GM, Londesborough P, et al: Diagnosis of fetal rubella infection by nucleic acid hybridization, *J Med Virol* 24:175, 1988.

32. Cradock-Watson JE, Miller E, Ridehalgh MK, et al: Detection of rubella virus in fetal and placental tissues and in the throats of neonates after serologically confirmed rubella in pregnancy, *Prenat Diagn* 9:91, 1989.

33. Eggerding FA, Peters J, Lee RK, et al: Detection of rubella virus gene sequences by enzymatic amplification and direct sequencing of amplified DNA, *J Clin Microbiol* 29:945, 1991.

34. Ho-Terry L, Terry GM, Londesborough P: Diagnosis of foetal rubella virus infection by polymerase chain reaction, *J Gen Virol* 71:1607, 1990.

35. Bosma TJ, Corbett KM, O'Shea S, et al: PCR for detection of rubella virus RNA in clinical samples, *J Clin Microbiol* 33:1075, 1995.

36. Bosma TJ, Corbett KM, Eckstein MB, et al: Use of PCR for prenatal and postnatal diagnosis of congenital rubella, *J Clin Microbiol* 33:2881, 1995.

37. Tanemura M, Suzumori K, Yagami Y, et al: Diagnosis of fetal rubella infection with reverse transcription and nested polymerase chain reaction: a study of 34 cases diagnosed in fetuses, *Am J Obstet Gynecol* 174:578, 1996.

38. Revello MG, Bandanti F, Sarasini A, et al: Prenatal diagnosis of rubella virus infection by direct detection and semiquantitation of viral RNA in clinical samples by reverse transcription–PCR, *J Clin Microbiol* 35:708, 1997.

39. Bell LM, Naides SJ, Stoffman P, et al: Human parvovirus B19 infection among hospital staff after contact with infected patients, *N Engl J Med* 321:485, 1989.

40. Anderson LJ: Role of parvovirus B19 in human disease, *Pediatr Infect Dis J* 6:711, 1987.

41. Anderson LJ, Tsou C, Parker RA, et al: Detection of antibodies and antigens of human parvovirus B19 by enzyme-linked immunosorbent assay, *J Clin Microbiol* 24:522, 1986.

42. Brown CS, van Bussel MJ, Wassenaar AL, et al: An immunofluorescence assay for the detection of parvovirus B19 IgG and IgM antibodies based on recombinant viral antigen, *J Virol Methods* 29:53, 1990.

43. Salimans MM, van Bussel MJ, Brown CS, et al: Recombinant parvovirus B19 capsid as a new substrate for detection of B19-specific IgG and IgM antibodies by an enzyme-linked immunosorbent assay, *J Virol Methods* 39:247, 1992.

44. Wang Q-Y, Erdman DD: Development and evaluation of capture immunoglobulin G and M hemadherence assays by using human type O erythrocytes and recombinant parvovirus B19 antigen, *J Clin Microbiol* 33:2466, 1995.

45. Cubel RC, Oliveira SA, Brown DWG, et al: Diagnosis of parvovirus B19 infection by detection of specific immunoglobulin M antibody in saliva, *J Clin Microbiol* 34:205, 1996.

46. Clewley JP: Detection of human parvovirus using a molecularly cloned probe, *J Med Virol* 15:173, 1985.

47. Mori J, Field AM, Clewley JP, et al: Dot blot hybridization assay of B19 virus DNA in clinical specimens, *J Clin Microbiol* 27:459, 1989.

48. Zerbini M, Musiani M, Venturoli S, et al: Rapid screening for B19 parvovirus DNA in clinical specimens with a digoxigenin-labeled DNA hybridization probe, *J Clin Microbiol* 28:2496, 1990.

49. Nascimento JP, Hallam NF, Mori J, et al: Detection of B19 parvovirus in human fetal tissues by in situ hybridization, *J Med Virol* 33:77, 1991.

50. Musiani M, Roda A, Zerbini M, et al: Detection of parvovirus B19 DNA in bone marrow cells by chemiluminescence in situ hybridization, *J Clin Microbiol* 34:1313, 1996.

51. Zerbini M, Musiani M, Gentilomi G, et al: Comparative evaluation of virological and serological methods in prenatal diagnosis of parvovirus B19 fetal hydrops, *J Clin Microbiol* 34:603, 1996.

52. Clewley JP: Polymerase chain reaction assay of parvovirus B19 DNA in clinical specimens, *J Clin Microbiol* 27:2647, 1989.

53. Koch WC, Adler SP: Detection of human parvovirus B19 DNA by using the polymerase chain reaction, *J Clin Microbiol* 28:65, 1990.

54. Sevall JS: Detection of parvovirus B19 by dot-blot and polymerase chain reaction, *Mol Cell Probes* 4:237, 1990.

55. Torok TJ, Wang QY, Gary GW Jr, et al: Prenatal diagnosis of intrauterine infection with parvovirus B19 by the polymerase chain reaction technique, *Clin Infect Dis* 14:149, 1992.

56. Erdman DD, Usher MJ, Tsou C, et al: Human parvovirus B19 specific IgG, IgA, and IgM antibodies and DNA in serum specimens from persons with erythema infectiosum, *J Med Virol* 35:110, 1991.

57. McOmish F, Yap PL, Jordan A, et al: Detection of parvovirus B19 in donated blood: a model system for screening by polymerase chain reaction, *J Clin Microbiol* 31:323, 1993.

58. Gallinella G, Young NS, Brown KE: In situ hybridisation and in situ polymerase chain reaction detection of parvovirus B19 DNA within cells, *J Virol Methods* 50:67, 1994.

59. Gentilomi G, Musiani M, Zerbini M, et al: Dot immunoperoxidase assay for the detection of parvovirus B19 antigens in serum samples, *J Clin Microbiol* 35:1575, 1997.

60. Braun DK, Dominguez G, Pellett PE: Human herpesvirus 6, *Clin Microbiol Rev* 10:521, 1997.

61. Pruksananonda P, Hall CB, Insel RA, et al: Primary human herpesvirus 6 infection in young children, *N Engl J Med* 326:1445, 1992.

62. Hall CB, Long CE, Schnabel KC, et al: Human herpesvirus-6 infection in children: a prospective study of complications and reactivation, *N Engl J Med* 331:432, 1994.

63. Hodinka RL: Human herpesvirus 6 and 7. In Rose NR, Conway de Marcario E, Folds JD, et al, editors: *Manual of clinical laboratory immunology,* ed 5, Washington, DC, 1997, ASM Press.

64. Krueger GRF, Ablashi DV, Josephs SF, et al: Clinical indications and diagnostic techniques of human herpesvirus-6 (HHV-6) infection, *In Vivo* 5:287, 1991.

65. Salahuddin SZ, Ablashi DV, Markham PD, et al: Isolation of a new virus, HBLV, in patients with lymphoproliferative disorders, *Science* 234:596, 1986.

66. Suga S, Yazaki T, Kajita Y, et al: Detection of human herpesvirus 6 DNA in samples from several body sites of patients with exanthem subitum and their mothers by polymerase chain reaction assay, *J Med Virol* 46:52, 1995.

67. Luka J, Okano M, Thiele G: Isolation of human herpesvirus-6 from clinical specimens using human fibroblast cultures, *J Clin Lab Anal* 4:483, 1990.

68. Kondo K, Hayakawa Y, Mori H, et al: Detection by polymerase chain reaction amplification of human herpesvirus 6 DNA in peripheral blood of patients with exanthem subitum, *J Clin Microbiol* 28:970, 1990.

69. Jarrett RF, Clark DA, Josephs SF, et al: Detection of human herpesvirus-6 DNA in peripheral blood and saliva, *J Med Virol* 32:73, 1990.

70. Leach CT, Newton ER, McParlin S, et al: Human herpesvirus 6 infection of the female genital tract, *J Infect Dis* 169:1281, 1994.

71. Kondo K, Nagafuji H, Hata A, et al: Association of human herpesvirus 6 infection of the central nervous system with recurrence of febrile convulsions, *J Infect Dis* 167:1197, 1993.

72. Yoshikawa T, Nakashima T, Suga S, et al: Human herpesvirus-6 DNA in cerebrospinal fluid of a child with exanthem subitum and meningoencephalitis, *Pediatrics* 89:888, 1992.

73. Marsh S, Kaplan M, Asano Y, et al: Development and application of HHV-6 antigen capture assay for the detection of HHV-6 infections, *J Virol Methods* 61:103, 1996.

74. Huang LM, Kuo PF, Lee CY, et al: Detection of human herpesvirus-6 DNA by polymerase chain reaction in serum or plasma, *J Med Virol* 38:7, 1992.

75. Secchiero P, Carrigan DR, Asano Y, et al: Detection of human herpesvirus 6 in plasma of children with primary infection and immunosuppressed patients by polymerase chain reaction, *J Infect Dis* 171:273, 1995.

76. Krueger GRF, Klueppelberg U, Hoffman A, et al: Clinical correlates of infection with human herpesvirus-6, *In Vivo* 8:457, 1994.

77. Secchiero P, Zella D, Crowley RW, et al: Quantitative PCR for human herpesviruses 6 and 7, *J Clin Microbiol* 33:2124, 1995.

78. Chiu SS, Cheung CY, Tse CYC, Peiris M: Early diagnosis of primary human herpesvirus 6 infection in childhood: serology, polymerase chain reaction, and virus load, *J Infect Dis* 178:1250, 1998.

79. Clark DA, Kidd IM, Collingham KE, et al: Diagnosis of primary human herpesvirus 6 and 7 infections in febrile infants by polymerase chain reaction, *Arch Dis Child* 77:42, 1977.

80. Ablashi DV, Berneman ZN, Kramarsky B, et al: Human herpesvirus-7 (HHV-7): current status, *Clin Diagn Virol* 4:1, 1995.

81. Frenkel N, Schirmer EC, Wyatt LS, et al: Isolation of a new herpesvirus from human CD4$^+$ T cells, *Proc Natl Acad Sci USA* 87:748, 1990.

82. Wyatt LS, Rodriguez WJ, Balachandran N, et al: Human herpesvirus 7: antigenic properties and prevalence in children and adults, *J Virol* 65:6260, 1991.

83. Berneman ZN, Ablashi DV, Li G, et al: Human herpesvirus 7 is a T-lymphotropic virus and is related to, but significantly different from, human herpesvirus 6 and human cytomegalovirus, *Proc Natl Acad Sci USA* 89:10552, 1992.

84. Clark DA, Freeland JML, Mackie PLK, et al: Prevalence of antibody to human herpesvirus 7 by age, *J Infect Dis* 168:252, 1993.

85. Wyatt LS, Frenkel N: Human herpesvirus 7 is a constitutive inhabitant of adult human saliva, *J Virol* 66:3206, 1992.

86. Hidaka Y, Liu Y, Yamamoto M, et al: Frequent isolation of human herpesvirus 7 from saliva samples, *J Med Virol* 40:343, 1993.

87. Foa-Tomasi L, Avitabile E, Ke L, et al: Polyvalent and monoclonal antibodies identify major immunogenic proteins specific for human herpesvirus 7–infected cells and have weak cross-reactivity with human herpesvirus 6, *J Gen Virol* 75:2719, 1994.

88. Sada E, Yasukawa M, Ito C, et al: Detection of human herpesvirus 6 and human herpesvirus 7 in the submandibular gland, parotid gland, and lip salivary gland by PCR, *J Clin Microbiol* 34:2320, 1996.

89. Gautheret-Dejean A, Aubin J-T, Poirel L, et al: Detection of human *Betaherpesvirinae* in saliva and urine from immunocompromised and immunocompetent subjects, *J Clin Microbiol* 35:1600, 1997.

90. Mintz L, Drew WL: Relation of culture site to the recovery of nonpolio enteroviruses, *Am J Clin Pathol* 74:324, 1980.

91. Dagan R, Jenista JA, Prather SL, et al: Viremia in hospitalized children with enterovirus infections, *J Pediatr* 106:397, 1985.

92. Bell EJ, McCartney RA, Basquill D, et al: μ-antibody capture ELISA for the rapid diagnosis of enterovirus infections in patients with aseptic meningitis, *J Med Virol* 19:213, 1986.

93. Swanink CM, Veenstra L, Poort YAG, et al: Coxsackievirus B1–based antibody-capture enzyme-linked immunosorbent assay for detection of immunoglobulin G (IgG), IgM, and IgA with broad specificity for enteroviruses, *J Clin Microbiol* 31:3240, 1993.

94. Goldwater PN: Immunoglobulin M capture immunoassay in investigation of coxsackievirus B5 and B6 outbreaks in south Australia, *J Clin Microbiol* 33:1628, 1995.

95. Herrmann JE, Hendry RM, Collins MF: Factors involved in enzyme-linked immunoassay of viruses and evaluation of the method for identification of enteroviruses, *J Clin Microbiol* 10:210, 1979.

96. Yagi S, Schnurr D, Lin J: Spectrum of monoclonal antibodies to coxsackievirus B-3 includes type- and group-specific antibodies, *J Clin Microbiol* 30:2498, 1992.

97. Trabelsi A, Grattard F, Nejmeddine M, et al: Evaluation of an enterovirus group–specific anti-VP1 monoclonal antibody, 5-D8/1, in comparison with neutralization and PCR for rapid identification of enteroviruses in cell culture, *J Clin Microbiol* 33:2454, 1995.

98. Klespies SL, Cebula DE, Kelley CL, et al: Detection of enteroviruses from clinical specimens by spin amplification shell vial culture and monoclonal antibody assay, *J Clin Microbiol* 34:1465, 1996.

99. Rotbart HA: Nucleic acid detection systems for enteroviruses, *Clin Microbiol Rev* 4:156, 1991.

100. Rotbart HA: Enzymatic RNA amplification of the enteroviruses, *J Clin Microbiol* 28:438, 1990.

101. Chapman NM, Tracy S, Gauntt CJ, et al: Molecular detection and identification of enteroviruses using enzymatic amplification and nucleic acid hybridization, *J Clin Microbiol* 28:843, 1990.

102. Rotbart HA, Ahmed A, Hickey S, et al: Diagnosis of enteroviral infection by polymerase chain reaction of multiple specimen types, *Pediatr Infect Dis J* 16:409, 1997.

103. Sawyer MH, Holland D, Aintablian N, et al: Diagnosis of enteroviral central nervous system infection by polymerase chain reaction during a large community outbreak, *Pediatr Infect Dis J* 13:177, 1994.

104. Rotbart HA: Enteroviral infections of the central nervous system, *Clin Infect Dis* 20:971, 1995.

105. Martin AB, Webber S, Fricker J, et al: Acute myocarditis rapid diagnosis by PCR in children, *Circulation* 90: 330, 1994.
106. Rotbart HA, Kinsella JP, Wasserman RL: Persistent enterovirus infection in culture-negative meningoencephalitis: demonstration by enzymatic RNA amplification, *J Infect Dis* 161:787, 1990.
107. Abzug MJ, Loeffelholz M, Rotbart HA: Diagnosis of neonatal enterovirus infection by polymerase chain reaction, *J Pediatr* 126:447, 1995.
108. Rotbart HA, Sawyer MH, Fast S, et al: Diagnosis of enteroviral meningitis by using PCR with a colorimetric microwell detection assay, *J Clin Microbiol* 32:2590, 1994.

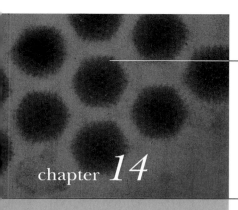

Jerome Yankowitz, Charles Grose

chapter *14*

Congenital Infections

OVERVIEW

Diagnostic virology is of critical importance in congenital infection. Several ribonucleic and deoxyribonucleic acid (RNA, DNA) viruses are now known to cause clinically significant fetal infection that results in miscarriage, intrauterine death, or fetopathy secondary to structural and neurodevelopmental abnormalities. The viruses discussed in this chapter include *cytomegalovirus* (CMV), *herpes simplex* (HSV), *varicella-zoster* (VZV), *human parvovirus B19, human immunodeficiency* (HIV), *rubella, lymphocytic choriomeningitis* (LCM), the *enteroviruses,* and *adenovirus* (Box 14–1). The diagnosis of the hepatitis viruses is discussed in Chapter 8. A brief background is provided for each virus, but the focus of the chapter is the approach to diagnosis, both in utero (where appropriate) and postnatal.

TECHNIQUES FOR PRENATAL DIAGNOSIS

Prenatal diagnosis of fetal infection continues to make enormous strides since a previous review in 1989.[1] One reason is the increased use of imaging technology such as *ultrasonography* (US). A viral etiology should be considered for most fetal US abnormalities.[2] These include but are not limited to fetal growth restriction, amniotic fluid volume disorders, intracranial or intrahepatic calcifications, hydrocephaly or microcephaly, isolated ascites, pericardial or pleural effusions, and nonimmune hydrops. Another reason for improved diagnosis is the incorporation of the *polymerase chain reaction* (PCR) as part of diagnostic protocols to detect viral DNA or RNA without the need to isolate the virus. The availability of *prenatal diagnosis* at many medical centers has also improved detection of fetal infection. Invasive techniques in widespread use include amnio-

centesis, chorionic villus sampling (CSV), and fetal blood sampling (cordocentesis).

Amniocentesis

Amniocentesis was first performed in 1952 by Bevis[3] to detect the presence of bilirubin derivatives in the amniotic fluid of fetuses at risk for immune hemolytic anemia. Since then, amniocentesis has been used to obtain amniotic fluid cells for the prenatal diagnosis of hereditary disorders such as hemoglobinopathies and enzyme deficiencies. It was originally performed blindly, but now amniocentesis is generally done with constant US visualization. The amniotic fluid is aspirated after percutaneous insertion of a small-gauge (narrow-bore) abdominal needle (Figure 14–1). As much as 36 ml of amniotic fluid (5% to 10% of the total volume) can be removed safely between 15 and 20 weeks of gestation.[4] The risk of fetal loss is less than 1%.[5, 6] Although complications are rare, they include leakage of amniotic fluid and vaginal bleeding. When amniocentesis is performed before 15 weeks of gestation (*early amniocentesis*), approximately 1 ml of fluid is removed per week of gestation.

Chorionic Villus Sampling

Transcervical CVS was first attempted in the late 1960s,[7] but the technique was not used often because of a high incidence of fetal loss (3% to 5%). The procedure has been coupled with high-resolution US with resulting improvement in the fetal loss rate.[8, 9] For the two main techniques, transcervical and transabdominal, the placenta and fetus are localized by real-time sector-scanner US.

In *transcervical CVS* a narrow-bore catheter is inserted transcervically under sterile conditions into the decidua-chorion space with the use of continuous US surveillance. Suction is applied and the biopsy sample aspirated. CVS is safest when performed between 7 and 12 weeks of gestation for the prenatal diagnosis of hereditary metabolic disorders. Brambati et al[10] reported that 72% of 283 women who underwent CVS had fetomaternal hemorrhage, demonstrated by marked elevation of the alpha-fetoprotein (AFP) level in maternal sera.

In some patients, transcervical CVS is not feasible for technical or obstetric reasons. Contraindications include vaginitis, vaginismus, inaccessible cervical canal, twin pregnancy, and a previous technical failure.[11] Under such circumstances, *transabdominal CVS* may be performed, which carries a lower risk of fetal loss and bleeding complications.[12, 13]

In a multicenter study conducted by the National Institute of Child Health and Human Development, Rhoads et al[14] compared the efficacy and safety of transcervical CVS with amniocentesis in two groups of women who had prenatal diagnosis because of ad-

---

Box 14.1   Viruses that Cause Congenital Infection

Human immunodeficiency (HIV)
Cytomegalovirus (CMV)
Parvovirus B19
Hepatitis B (HBV)
Hepatitis C (HCV)
Herpes simplex (HSV)
Varicella-zoster (VZV)
Rubella
Lymphocytic choriomeningitis (LCM)
Lassa fever
Enteroviruses (rare)
Adenoviruses (rare)

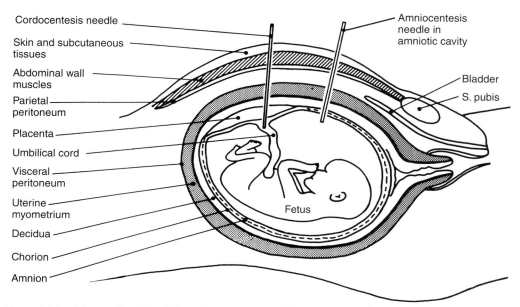

Figure 14.1   Maternal and fetal tissue layers traversed during amniocentesis and prenatal umbilical cord sampling (cordocentesis). *S.,* symphysis. (From Grose C, Oussama I, Weiner CP: *Pediatr Infect Dis J* 8:459, 1989.)

vanced maternal age. Cytogenetic diagnoses were made in 97.8% of 2235 women using CVS and 99.4% of 651 women using amniocentesis. Multiparous women reported more frequent obstetric complications after CVS (19.0%) than after amniocentesis (14.8%). Although CVS offers the advantage of first-trimester prenatal diagnosis, the study results show that amniocentesis is associated with lower incidences of procedural failure and ambiguous diagnosis. For example, CVS was unsuccessful in 40 patients, 17 (0.8%) of whom underwent amniocentesis because of uncertain cytogenetic diagnoses. The overall incidence of fetal loss from spontaneous abortion after CVS was about 2%, whereas that for amniocentesis was about 1%.

A syndrome of malformed extremities and cavernous hemangioma is associated with CVS performed early in gestation.[15, 16]

Cordocentesis

In 1985, Daffos et al[16] published their method of fetal blood sampling via the umbilical cord, now known as cordocentesis. Cordocentesis is usually performed after a gestational age of 17 weeks as an outpatient procedure, which can be completed in minutes.[17] Sedation and local anesthesia are not needed. The patient lies in a comfortable supine position to facilitate relaxation of the abdominal wall musculature. Using high-resolution real-time ultrasound, the clinician locates the insertion of the placental origin of the umbilical cord. The abdominal wall is cleaned aseptically, the US transducer (in a sterile bed) is placed on the abdomen, and the umbilical cord placental origin is relocated. A spinal needle (20 to 25 gauge, 3½ to 7 inches long) is inserted

along the sonographic plane down to the umbilical cord (see Figure 14–1). The umbilical cord is punctured and fetal blood (1 to 8 ml) obtained for diagnostic studies.[18, 19]

Pure fetal blood is almost always obtained at cordocentesis. However, contamination of the sample by maternal blood should be ruled out by several tests based on the characteristics of fetal red blood cells (RBCs) and hemoglobin. These tests include (1) a determination of RBC mean corpuscular volume because fetal RBCs are larger than adult RBCs, (2) a Kleihauer-Betke acid elution technique because fetal RBCs resist alkaline pH more than adult RBCs; and (3) an antiagglutination test that differentiates between fetal and adult RBCs by demonstrating specific marker antigens on RBC membranes.

The complications of cordocentesis have been extensively evaluated. Incidence of fetal loss was 1.7% and 1.9% in two studies,[16, 17] but fetal loss often cannot be attributed solely to the procedure itself. The severity of fetal disease (e.g., marked fetal hydrops, multiple chromosomal anomalies) has a major effect on the likelihood of intrauterine fetal demise or spontaneous abortion.

ANTIBODY SYNTHESIS IN THE FETUS AND NEWBORN

A knowledge of the timing and kinetics in the transfer of maternal antibodies and the fetal synthesis of antibodies is crucial for understanding serologic testing in the fetus and newborn (Figure 14–2). Specific antibodies are synthesized by the fetus starting at about

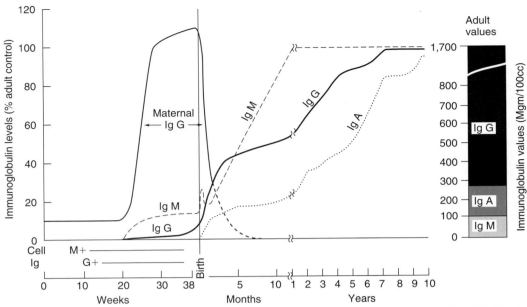

Figure 14.2 Kinetics of fetal and neonatal immunoglobulins. (From Alford CA: *Pediatr Clin North Am* 18:99, 1971.)

20 weeks of gestation but may not reach detectable levels for 1 or 2 more weeks. These antibodies are of the immunoglobulin M (IgM) isotype. Maternal antibodies are actively transferred to the fetus by the placenta beginning in the middle of gestation, reaching peak levels about week 26 or 27 of gestation.[20] These antibodies are exclusively of the immunoglobulin G (IgG) isotype. Therefore detection of virus-specific IgM antibodies in the fetus or newborn is diagnostic of congenital infection. At birth the infant's serum IgG level is slightly higher than the maternal level. Maternally derived immunoglobulins in the infant's serum decline, with a half-life of 30 days. Specific maternal antibodies can be detected for 1 year or more in some cases. The neonate continues synthesis of IgM antibodies after birth and begins to synthesize IgG and immunoglobulin A (IgA) as well.

Because congenital infection usually results in an elevation of total IgM level in the serum of the fetus or newborn, total IgM level in cord blood has been used to screen for congenital infection. The upper limit of normal is approximately 20 mg/dl; this value may vary in different laboratories. In one study, IgM levels were measured in cord blood of 5951 infants.[20] Elevated levels were found in 192, of whom 69 (36%) were found to have congenital infections. The infections diagnosed included 13 cases of CMV infection, eight cases of toxoplasmosis, five cases of rubella, and four cases of syphilis, 13 with aseptic meningitis, five with bacteremia, and a group with localized infections. IgM levels were highest in infants with rubella or syphilis and somewhat lower in those with toxoplasmosis, CMV, or enteroviral infection. Screening for total IgM level has been largely

replaced by more specific tests for congenital infection (see following sections).

An important caveat related to serodiagnosis of congenital infection is that infants with a variety of congenital infections can produce *rheumatoid factor* (RF; IgM antibodies directed against IgG).[21, 22] RF can bind to pathogen-specific IgG antibodies (derived from the mother) to form complexes that may be falsely detected in some assays as pathogen-specific IgM antibodies. The amount of RF required to produce a false-positive pathogen-specific IgM assay is below the level of detection of standard commercial assays for RF. Another caveat regarding pathogen-specific IgM tests is that high levels of virus-specific IgG antibodies can lead to false-negative assays for virus-specific IgM antibodies because of competition. Specific measures can be taken in the laboratory to avoid problems related to RF and IgG competition (see Chapter 1).

CYTOMEGALOVIRUS

Virology and Epidemiology

CMV is a double-stranded DNA virus of the herpesvirus family. The virus may be excreted for weeks, months, or years after a primary infection. A latency period eventually occurs, but reactivation and reinfection both occur. The prevalence of *seropositivity*, reflecting past exposure, varies by age and demographic factors. One study of more than 21,000 women attending a prenatal clinic in London revealed marked variation in the rate by race (white 46%, Asian 88%, black 77%), parity (increasing seropositivity with increasing parity), and socioeconomic status.[23] Among mostly middle-income women in Alabama, 54% were seropositive, with white women having a lower rate than black women.[24] The incidence of *seroconversion,* signifying primary infection, in women of childbearing age approximates 2% per year in higher socioeconomic groups and up to 6% per year in lower socioeconomic groups.[25]

Serologic or culture evidence of in utero CMV infection is present in 0.2% to 2.2% of all live-born infants, making CMV the most common cause of congenital infection in the United States.[26] The risk of transmission to the fetus is much higher with primary maternal infection (40% to 50%) than with recurrent infection (less than 1%).[27] Also, the risk of symptomatic infection is much higher with primary maternal infection. For example, in the studies from Birmingham, Ala, symptomatic congenital infection was seen only in infants infected as a result of primary maternal infection.[28] In this group, 18% were symptomatic at birth. The rates of any symptomatic manifestation observed either at birth or in the first few years of life were 25% in infants infected as a result of primary infection versus 8% in the infants infected as a result of recurrent infection.

Clinical Manifestations

Maternal CMV infection is generally asymptomatic. Occasionally it manifests as a mononucleosis-like syndrome with lymphocytosis, abnormal liver function tests, spiking fever and malaise, myalgias, and chills. Congenital infection is asymptomatic at birth in 90% of cases. The remaining 10% of newborns with symptomatic disease have signs such as hepatosplenomegaly, jaundice, microcephaly, deafness, chorioretinitis, cerebral calcifications followed by mental disability, thrombocytopenia, and abnormal liver function tests. CMV is the most common cause of congenital sensorineural hearing loss, which may not be detected initially in neonates with no other stigmata of congenital CMV infection.

Diagnosis

If a woman of reproductive age has no CMV antibody, she is susceptible to a primary CMV infection. If she has a low titer of CMV-specific IgG antibody, she could have either a long-past infection or a very recent primary infection. Paired serum specimens may be needed to resolve this question. A fourfold or greater rise in titer is consistent with a primary infection but also can occur in those with past infection.[28a] IgM-specific antibody is usually present for 4 to 8 months after a primary infection but can increase periodically or persist at low titer for years. In one study the sensitivity of a widely used commercial enzyme immunoassay (EIA) for CMV

IgM used for the detection of primary infection in pregnant women was 73%. The assay was also positive in 4% of women with recurrent infection.[29]

Prenatal diagnosis. Isolation of CMV in culture and detection of CMV DNA from amniotic fluid are currently considered the standard methods for the prenatal diagnosis of congenital CMV infection. Studies at the University of Iowa Prenatal Diagnostic Unit clearly showed that CMV can be isolated from amniotic fluid.[30, 31] This observation was confirmed by a prospective evaluation of 1771 pregnant Belgian women with an initial CMV seroprevalence of 49%. They were followed by serial serology and culture of urine, saliva, and cervical secretions at each prenatal visit. Seroconversion occurred in 20 susceptible women (2.3%). Seven of the 20 agreed to a fetal evaluation by cordocentesis and amniocentesis. Five of the seven had positive amniotic fluid cultures for CMV, three of whom had fetal CMV IgM antibodies. Pathologic confirmation of CMV in fetal tissue after termination supported amniotic fluid culture being superior to measurements of fetal CMV IgM antibodies in diagnosing fetal infection.[32] Others have subsequently made similar observations.[33-40] Attempts to culture CMV from fetal blood have usually been unsuccessful.[33, 37, 40]

PCR can also be performed to detect CMV DNA in amniotic fluid and appears to be slightly more sensitive than culture.[33, 34] In three series that performed both culture and PCR, PCR was positive in 75% to 92% of infected patients and culture in 56% to 100%.[33, 34, 38] Explanations for the failure of either technique to detect in utero infection include sampling too early in gestation and too soon after infection.[39, 41, 42] Sampling before 21 weeks of gestation has been associated with lower sensitivity.[33, 41, 42] The minimum time between maternal infection and sampling has not been determined. Repeat sampling over several-week intervals is advised when a high likelihood exists of primary maternal infection. PCR may be particularly advantageous compared with culture when amniotic fluid specimens must be transported, because a delay in processing the specimen is more detrimental to culture than to PCR.

A positive result of either culture or PCR is a reliable indicator of fetal infection but does not predict which infants with in utero infection will have symptomatic infection. Some infants with congenital infection documented by culture or PCR have been delivered and have been normal.[34, 38, 39, 42] The ability of US to determine which infants have symptomatic infection has not been extensively evaluated. Lipitz et al[38] performed prenatal US in six pregnancies in which in utero infection was documented. One fetus was found to have growth restriction and ventriculomegaly on US and after birth had deafness and cerebral palsy. One other fetus had a hyperechogenic bowel on prenatal US but had no apparent abnormality at birth. The other four fetuses had normal US results and were normal at birth, with no apparent abnormalities after a median follow-up of 24 months.

Postnatal diagnosis. Postnatal diagnosis of congenital CMV is best made by viral culture obtained within the first week of life. Obtaining the culture early in life is important to support that the infection was acquired in utero, since positive cultures after the second week can occur in infants infected during the peripartum period as well as in those with in utero acquisition.[43] Cultures are uniformly positive and are often positive very rapidly because infants with congenital infection shed large amounts of virus in the urine that is readily detected by either shell vial or conventional culture[44] (see Chapters 1 and 15). The level of virus is higher in infants with symptomatic infection than in asymptomatic infants. The level of viruria remains high for approximately 9 months; after that time it reaches a plateau at a lower level and may continue at that level for years after infection.

PCR has also been used successfully to detect CMV in the urine of infants with congenital infection.[45] Culture of saliva has been shown to provide comparable sensitivity to urine culture.[46] Viremia is present in some infants with congenital infection, especially those who are symptomatic, and can be detected by culture,[47] the pp65 antigenemia assay,[48] or PCR.[49]

The detection of CMV-specific IgM antibodies in a newborn is also diagnostic of congenital infection, but this method is less reliable than culture. The performance of assays for CMV-specific IgM depends on the test method. The immunofluorescent antibody (IFA) assay should not be used because of poor sensitivity and specificity.[22] A radioimmunoassay (RIA) showed excellent performance, with a sensitivity of 89% and a specificity of 100%,[50] but is not commercially available. A commercially available EIA had a sensitivity of only 69% in a large series, with a 6% false-positive rate.[29] In general, serologic diagnoses of congenital CMV should be supported by a positive culture.

VARICELLA-ZOSTER VIRUS

Virology and Epidemiology

VZV is a human herpesvirus. Primary VZV infection, *varicella* (or *chickenpox*), is a contagious disease characterized by an exanthem consisting of vesicles that evolve into pustules, crusts, and scabs and occurring 10 to 21 days after exposure. Patients are contagious 1 or 2 days before the onset of the rash and for 4 or 5 days after it first appears.[51] This generally mild childhood disease is much more severe in adults. Only 1.8% of cases are reported in adults, but 25% of deaths occur after the

second decade of life.[52] *Herpes zoster*, or *shingles*, is caused by reactivation of virus that has lain dormant in dorsal root ganglia since childhood chickenpox. It usually affects segmental dermatomes on reactivation.

From 70% to 80% of young adults report a history of varicella.[53] Among adults with no history of varicella, only about 25% are actually susceptible; in other words, 75% have had extremely mild chickenpox, that went unrecognized during childhood. Among pregnant women with a negative or indeterminate history of varicella, 80% have positive serology indicative of previous infection.[54] An estimated 7000 to 9000 cases of varicella occur during pregnancy in the United States annually. One study of more than 250,000 members of the Harvard Community Health Program showed a higher incidence of varicella in persons over 14 years of age, with more complications than previously reported.[55]

Clinical Manifestations

Congenital VZV infection occurs when a woman contracts chickenpox during the first half of gestation. Laforet and Lynch[56] first reported the fetopathy in a mother who developed chickenpox during the eighth week of pregnancy. The neonate was born at term with well-defined cicatricial lesions on a leg, as well as bony hypoplasia. Hydrocephalus was present along with optic atrophy. Subsequent reports have convincingly documented that congenital varicella is associated with a syndrome of skin scarring, limb hypoplasia, and eye and brain damage (Table 14–1). Atrophy of an extremity, most often a leg ("peg leg"), is the most distinguishing feature. Specific central nervous system (CNS) findings,

Table 14.1 Stigmata of Fetal Varicella Infection

Structures affected	Stigmata
Sensory nerves	Cutaneous manifestations
	Zigzag (cicatricial) skin lesions
	Hypopigmentation
Optic stalk, optic cup, and lens vesicle	Microphthalmia
	Cataracts
	Chorioretinitis
	Optic atrophy
Brain (encephalitis)	Microcephaly
	Hydrocephalus
	Intracranial calcifications
	Hydranencephaly
Cervical and lumbosacral cord	Hypoplasia of lower extremities
	Motor and sensory deficits
	Absent muscle stretch reflexes
	Horner's syndrome and anisocoria
	Anal and vesical sphincter dysfunction

including cerebral atrophy, hydranencephaly, and cerebellar aplasia, can be visualized prenatally. A large retrospective study found that the risk of the syndrome was approximately 2% when maternal infection occurred during the first 20 weeks of pregnancy.[57] This risk of congenital VZV infection does not appear to be reduced by administration of varicella-zoster immune globulin (VZIG) to the mother.[58]

Maternal chickenpox between 20 and 40 weeks of gestation causes fewer fetal problems. VZV reactivation (herpes zoster) poses little or no risk of causing embryopathy.[51]

Diagnosis

Chickenpox in a pregnant woman can often be diagnosed by visual inspection without the need for virus-specific tests (see Chapter 6). A fluorescent antibody (FA) stain using a monoclonal antibody against VZV can be performed on a scraping if necessary. Serologic tests are available to measure both IgM and IgG antivaricella antibodies. Culture of the virus from vesicle fluid is slow but remains the classic means of diagnosis. DNA diagnostic methods are emerging as powerful tools.[59] The same techniques can be used to diagnose chickenpox if it occurs in the newborn.

Prenatal diagnosis. Total IgM can be elevated in a fetus with VZV infection, and the VZV-specific fraction can be measured. This procedure is only available in selected laboratories with a special interest in VZV. Experience with PCR for the prenatal diagnosis of VZV infection is limited. In one study, PCR was positive for VZV DNA in specimens obtained by CVS from two women with varicella during pregnancy. One fetus was aborted and the other was born at term. Neither had evidence of fetal varicella syndrome.[60]

In the most extensive study reported to date, 107 pregnancies complicated by varicella were analyzed.[61] Amniocentesis was performed in all and analyzed by PCR and culture. VZV-specific IgM antibodies were measured in fetal blood specimens from 82 women. PCR was positive for VZV DNA in nine amniotic fluids, of which only two were positive by culture. VZV-specific IgM antibodies were not detected in any of the fetal blood specimens. Of the nine amniotic fluids positive for VZV DNA, two fetuses had evidence of fetal varicella syndrome. One was aborted at 24 weeks' gestation, and examination was compatible with fetal varicella syndrome. The other was born at term with bilateral microphthalmia that had not been detected by prenatal US. This infant developed zoster at age 4 months. One fetus died in utero and was found to have an unrelated chromosomal abnormality. One pregnancy was terminated by therapeutic abortion; the fetus was anatomically normal but positive for VZV DNA. The remaining five pregnancies went to term and the babies were normal, but two developed zoster within 1 year after birth.

The conclusion from this study is that a positive PCR result strongly suggests fetal infection but does not necessarily predict fetal varicella syndrome, whereas a negative result on amniotic fluid indicates a favorable outcome. Pregnancies in which VZV DNA is detected in amniotic fluid should have close morphologic monitoring by US and possibly magnetic resonance imaging (MRI), focusing on the limbs and cerebral and ocular structures.

We recommend that in all cases of maternal varicella during pregnancy, if an early US is normal, a second US should be performed 8 to 10 weeks after maternal infection to detect later fetal sequelae.

Postnatal diagnosis. Documentation of congenital varicella is difficult at term because virus is no longer excreted postpartum and cultures are negative. VZV-specific IgM is diagnostic if present, but may not persist postpartum.[62]

HERPES SIMPLEX VIRUS

Virology and Epidemiology

HSV types 1 and 2 are closely related human herpesviruses, one with a tropism for the oropharynx (type 1) and the other for the genital mucosa (type 2) (see Chapter 6). Both form latent infections that may reactivate periodically throughout life. *HSV-1 infections* are very common, and a majority of children become infected. *HSV-2 infections* are sexually transmitted and therefore usually occur during adolescence and early adulthood. Approximately 20% of the U.S. adult population is infected with HSV-2.

When a primary HSV-2 infection is contracted during pregnancy, the fetus is at high risk of acquiring HSV-2 infection at delivery. The perinatal form of transmission has received considerable attention in the last decade. Intrauterine transmission also can occur but is much less common and often misdiagnosed as perinatal transmission.[63]

Congenital infection

Fetopathy secondary to HSV-2 infection closely resembles the VZV fetopathy described earlier. South et al[64] first described the HSV syndrome. In 1987 the participants in the National Institutes of Health–sponsored collaborative trial of antiviral therapy published a definitive analysis of 13 infants with intrauterine HSV-2 infection.[65] They reaffirmed that most neonatal HSV infections are acquired at parturition by fetal

Table 14.2	Findings in Congenital Herpes Simplex Virus (HSV) Infection

Finding	Number (%)
Low birth weight	22/26 (85)
Small for gestational age	9/25 (36)
Microcephaly, seizures, diffuse brain damage, intrancranial calcification	20/30 (67)
Chorioretinitis, microphthalmia	17/30 (57)
Culture-positive vesicles or bullae	28/30 (93)
HSV type 2 infection	24/27 (89)
Other findings: retinal dysplasia, scars on skin or digits, cataracts, pneumonitis, hepatomegaly	

Data from Hutto C, Arvin A, Jacobs R, et al: *J Pediatr* 110:97, 1987.

contact with infected maternal genital secretions. A few infants still have abnormalities noted in utero, an indication that infection can occur before delivery. In the study population of almost 200 infants, an estimated 5% of neonatal HSV infections were intrauterine.

The principal sites of fetal involvement were the skin, eyes, and CNS (Table 14–2). Of the 13 infants, 12 had skin lesions. In eight, vesicles or bullae were observed at birth; the other four had scarring over the scalp, face, trunk, or extremities. Occasionally, vesicular lesions appeared postpartum around the areas of scarring. Even the one infant without vesicles in the perinatal period developed skin lesions by 2 weeks of age. CNS abnormalities were also seen in two infants. Microcephaly was the most common sign, present in seven infants. Computed tomography (CT) often showed hydranencephaly or atrophy of the brain. Many of the neurologic sequelae are identical to those found in congenital VZV infection (see Table 14–1). Chorioretinitis was seen in eight infants, two of whom had microphthalmia. In addition to the previous stigmata, three infants had hepatitis with elevated liver enzymes, and one infant had calcifications in the lungs and adrenal glands. Four of the infants died in early infancy.

With regard to maternal gestational data, four of the 13 women had a documented primary HSV-2 infection, and one woman had a recurrent episode of genital herpes. Virologic results from the other eight women were inconclusive as to serologic status.[65]

Natal Infection

Infants infected with HSV during birth or shortly thereafter become symptomatic within the first month of life, most often toward the end of the first week or early in the second week. Approximately 75% have cutaneous vesicles. Neonatal disease has been divided into three categories: disease limited to the skin, eyes, and mucous membranes (40%); disease limited to the CNS (35%); and disseminated disease (25%).[66] The

prognosis is worst for those with disseminated disease, followed by those with CNS disease. Those with disease limited to the skin, eyes, and mucous membranes have a much better outcome.[67]

Common sites of lesions are at sites of trauma, such as scalp electrode and circumcision sites, the eyes, the mouth, and the presenting part of the infant's body. Isolated CNS disease often becomes evident during the third week of life; these infants may present with or without cutaneous lesions. The cerebrospinal fluid (CSF) usually contains a lymphocytic pleocytosis. Electroencephalograms (EEGs) and CNS imaging techniques are abnormal, with evidence of a process that can involve the temporal lobe but is often diffuse or multifocal. Patients with disseminated infection can have a clinical picture resembling bacterial sepsis. Pneumonitis, hepatitis, and evidence of disseminated intravascular coagulation may be present.

Diagnosis

Prenatal diagnosis of congenital HSV-2 infection has not been well studied but should not be difficult. Presumably, some stigmata of the fetopathy can be visualized by US and the virus detected by either culture or PCR analysis of the amniotic fluid or cord blood cells. In one reported case, US at 19 weeks' gestation revealed possible ventriculomegaly, echogenic bowel, and persistent flexion of the legs. A culture of amniotic fluid was positive for HSV-2, and HSV IgM antibodies were detected in cord blood obtained by cordocentesis.[68]

Intrauterine HSV infection usually can be differentiated from intrapartum infection by physical examination and the date of onset of lesions after birth. HSV fetopathy should be readily apparent at parturition, and in most cases, HSV-2 can be cultured from vesicular lesions that are present at birth or appear within the first 2 days of life. In those patients who do not have fresh vesicles, detection of HSV IgM antibodies in the blood of the neonate during the first week of life is also diagnostic of in utero HSV infection.

Viral culture and serology. Diagnosis of HSV infection in infants who acquire HSV in the peripartum period can usually be accomplished by isolation of HSV from cutaneous lesions. Other useful sites to culture include conjunctiva, nasopharynx, CSF, and blood. The diagnosis of infants without cutaneous lesions bears special mention.[69] The blood is a particularly important site to culture in infants suspected of having the disseminated form of the disease, especially when cutaneous lesions are not present. The frequency of viremia in disseminated disease is not known, but positive blood cultures have been diagnostic in some patients.[69, 70]

Polymerase chain reaction. The potential for PCR performed on blood to improve the recognition of HSV cases has not yet been extensively evaluated. In one report, however, HSV DNA was detected in the serum of all three patients with disseminated HSV infection, one of two with CNS disease, and one of two with skin, eye, and mucous membrane disease.[71] Corresponding cultures were positive only in one patient.

The largest experience with PCR in neonatal HSV infection has been for testing CSF.[71-73] In a recent series, PCR performed on CSF was positive in 76% of infants with CNS disease, 93% of those with disseminated infection, and 24% of those with disease apparently limited to the skin, eyes, and mucous membranes.[73] Some of the negative specimens were obtained more than 4 days after initiation of acyclovir therapy, which may explain the relatively low sensitivity in patients with CNS disease. CSF results from three infants were negative before starting acyclovir, however, suggesting that a negative PCR alone should not be taken as ruling out CNS disease. The concept that a positive PCR on CSF can identify subclinical CNS infection in infants without clinical evidence of CNS disease requires further study. Likewise, the role of PCR for evaluating the duration of antiviral therapy is also under investigation. A negative PCR performed on CSF does not rule out the presence of HSV at other body sites.

HUMAN PARVOVIRUS B19

Virology and Clinical Manifestations

A member of the family Parvoviridae, human parvovirus B19 is a single-stranded DNA virus discovered in 1975.[74] It infects only humans and is transmitted via aerosolized droplets. B19 preferentially replicates in actively dividing cells such as erythroid progenitors. From 30% to 50% of reproductive-age women have serologic evidence of past infection. The incubation period of primary infection is 4 to 20 days. The childhood exanthem is called *erythema infectiosum* (*fifth disease*, slapped-cheek disease) (see Chapter 13). Most adult infection is asymptomatic. Viremia occurs 6 to 8 days after exposure and persists for 4 to 7 days. The rash develops 16 days after exposure, or 8 days after viremia. The exanthem begins on the face but can spread to the trunk or extremities. A drop in hematocrit can be detected 2 to 3 weeks after exposure in the adult or about a week after the viremia. The associated reticulocytopenia lasts for 7 to 10 days. Arthritis is also a common manifestation, affecting as many as 80% of adults but only 10% of children.

Parvovirus B19 infection during pregnancy can be associated with fetal infection, which has been linked to *hydrops fetalis* and fetal death.[1] In a recent study, parvovirus B19 accounted for 18% of cases of idiopathic nonimmune hydrops.[75] Hydrops results from fetal anemia presumably caused by parvovirus B19 infection of fetal erythroid precursors. *Fetal myocarditis* has also been documented and may contribute in some cases.[76]

Stillbirth resulting from maternal parvovirus B19 infection has occurred 1 to 12 weeks after infection. Hydrops is unlikely to occur later, however, if fetal anemia and hydrops have not become evident by 8 weeks after infection. For this reason, weekly US evaluations for 4 to 8 weeks after maternal exposure or infection are often performed. A careful history must be obtained because adults can have two symptomatic periods after exposure: (1) fever, malaise, and other flulike symptoms occur during the viremia and (2) rash, which occurs 16 to 18 days after exposure.[77] Intrauterine transfusion can be done when necessary, but some cases of fetal infection resolve spontaneously.[78]

No consistent pattern of congenital abnormalities have been reported in infants born after in utero parvovirus B19 infection, although examples of isolated malformations have been reported.[79]

Epidemiology

The magnitude of the risk to the fetus posed by maternal parvovirus B19 has been studied extensively. During community outbreaks, infection rates in pregnant women as high as 3.7% have been documented.[80] In another study, 16.7% of pregnant women with known exposure became infected,[81] and infection rates as high as 50% after household exposure have been reported.[82] The rate of transmission to the fetus was 27% in one study.[83] Estimates of the rates of fetal loss vary from less than 1% up to 9%.[80, 83-85] The risk of fetal death is confined to the first 20 weeks of gestation.

Diagnosis

Human parvovirus B19 cannot be cultured in the laboratory, and therefore the available diagnostic tests are limited to serology, dot blot hybridization, and PCR (see Chapter 13). B19-specific IgM is a marker of recent primary infection that appears 14 days after infection or 3 days after onset of symptoms and remains for 3 to 4 months.[86] B19-specific IgG appears in the third week after infection and remains throughout life. Table 14–3 shows the interpretation of parvovirus B19 serologic profiles.

Prenatal diagnosis of fetal infection should be

Table 14.3		Parvovirus B19 Serologic Profiles
IgG	**IgM**	**Interpretation**
–	–	Susceptible
+	–	Past infection (at least 4 mo), immune status
–	+	Very recent infection (past 7 days)*
+	+	Recent infection (7 days–4 mo)

*This pattern is also occasionally seen in immunocompromised patients with chronic B19 infection.

performed in cases of unexplained nonimmune hydrops or when acute parvovirus B19 infection has been documented in the mother and fetal hydrops is detected by US. PCR amplification of B19 DNA or DNA dot blot hybridization techniques can detect B19 DNA in maternal serum, fetal blood, or amniotic fluid.[78, 87-89] PCR is more sensitive than dot blot hybridization and is also more sensitive than detection of parvovirus-specific IgM antibodies in fetal blood.[89] One study found higher sensitivity for PCR performed on amniotic fluid than on fetal blood.[89] The detection of parvovirus B19 DNA in either specimen is presumptive evidence of fetal infection. By itself, however, detection of B19 DNA in amniotic fluid or fetal blood does not provide information about the consequences of that infection, which must be judged by frequent US evaluation.

LYMPHOCYTIC CHORIOMENINGITIS VIRUS

Virology and Epidemiology

Lymphocytic choriomeningitis (LCM) virus is an arenavirus that is closely related to Lassa fever virus of West Africa. Mice become chronically infected with LCM virus and are the source of infection for humans. Transmission occurs by human contact with excreta of rodents; in temperate climates, human exposure often occurs during the winter months, when mice live in older houses to escape the cold weather. Seroprevalence studies in Baltimore found LCM antibodies in almost 5% of adults; further trapping studies documented the presence of infected rodents in houses of humans with LCM antibodies.[90] Primary infection in humans often resembles a "flu syndrome" with fever and malaise.

Because LCM infection usually occurs in the winter months when influenza virus is prevalent, specific diagnostic studies are rarely performed. When a pregnant woman contracts primary LCM infection, fetal infection can occur. Interestingly, a predilection for infection of the fetus with high rates of fetal wastage has also been noted in infection with other arenaviruses, including Lassa fever and Junin.[91]

Although recognized in the past, LCM disease has often been overlooked in investigations of virus-induced fetopathy.[92] Recently at the University of Iowa Hospital, we have documented LCM congenital infection in two neonates and confirmed the disease in a third neonate from Chicago.[93]

Clinical Manifestations

Certain clinical features of congenital LCM infection closely mimic those of congenital toxoplasmosis. In each disorder, chorioretinitis affects 50% of infected infants, and hydrocephalus rather than microcephaly is the more common CNS abnormality. A few infants with congenital LCM infection exhibit microcephaly and intracranial calcifications, which are reminiscent of congenital CMV infection. Because of the relatively high incidence of CMV infection in the United States, however, congenital microcephaly and intracranial calcifications are more often the result of CMV infection. The findings of hepatosplenomegaly, jaundice, or petechial rash support the diagnosis of CMV infection and not congenital LCM infection. Data on the outcome of congenital LCM infection indicate that more than 40% of the reported infants died, and the majority of survivors had severe neurodevelopmental sequelae. Case selection, however, could impart bias toward a more severe syndrome and outcome.

LCM virus infection should be recognized as an important potential cause of congenital viral infection among infants born in the United States, especially among infants who have congenital hydrocephalus and chorioretinitis without jaundice or hepatosplenomegaly.

Diagnosis

At present, LCM virus infection is usually diagnosed by serologic methods, including LCM-specific IgM and IgG antibody titers.[92, 93] A reverse-transcription polymerase chain reaction (RT-PCR) assay for LCM virus has been described.[94] In the future, RNA amplification techniques likely will be applied to detect genomic sequences in the tissues of the fetus.

HUMAN IMMUNODEFICIENCY VIRUS

HIV type 1 is the most common human retrovirus; HIV-2 is a less virulent agent. HIV-1 infection causes severe disease by affecting the immune system; more specifically, the virus replicates in the CD4+ helper T lymphocytes.

Clinical manifestations are complex and varied depending on the stage of the disease. The patient may be completely asymptomatic for several years after primary HIV infection. Women with HIV infection may transmit the infection to their fetus in 25% or more of pregnancies if they are not receiving antiviral therapy.[95, 96] Treatment of the pregnant woman with antiviral medication reduces the transmission rate to 8% or lower.[97] Most cases of vertical transmission of HIV are thought to occur during parturition.

With this marked decrease in transmission, prenatal diagnosis has become less important. Prenatal diagnosis of HIV infection has been approached with extreme caution because of the concern about inadvertent transmission of maternal virus to the fetus during the diagnostic procedure.[1] Cordocentesis has been preformed successfully to culture virus from the fetal cells,[98] but this procedure is considered contraindicated under routine circumstances. The postnatal diagnosis of HIV infection in the exposed infant is made by culture or PCR performed on peripheral blood mononuclear cells[98] (see Chapter 17).

RUBELLA VIRUS

Rubella is a togavirus whose teratogenic effects on the human fetus are well known. The stigmata include a constellation of cardiovascular anomalies (patent ductus arteriosus, pulmonary artery stenosis), auditory defects (bilateral hearing loss), ocular defects (cataracts, glaucoma, retinitis), neurologic impairment (transient meningoencephalitis, hypotonia, mental disability), purpura, growth delay, and hepatosplenomegaly.[1]

The virus is transplacentally transmitted to the fetus from a newly infected susceptible mother. The risk of fetal infection varies with the gestational age at exposure: 81% (first 12 weeks); 54% (13 to 16 weeks); 36% (17 to 22 weeks); 30% (23 to 30 weeks); 60% (31 to 36 weeks); and 100% (last week of pregnancy). The risk of fetal malformation is highest in the first 12 weeks of gestation (85%), lower in weeks 13 to 16 (35%), and minimal after 16 weeks.[99]

Diagnosis

Laboratory tests for the detection of rubella virus include culture, serology (IgG and IgM), and molecular detection. Rubella virus is difficult to culture in the laboratory because it may not produce cytopathic effect (CPE) in some cell culture types (see Chapter 1). Accordingly, serology has been widely used.

Prenatal diagnosis. The prenatal diagnosis of congenital rubella has been made by isolation of rubella virus from amniotic fluid samples obtained by amniocentesis between 17 and 21 weeks of gestation in women with clinical rubella[100, 101] (see Chapter 13). Because of the difficulties in isolating rubella virus in cell culture, however, most effort has been directed at diagnosis by detection of rubella-specific IgM in fetal blood.

Because rubella continues to be a problem in European populations, European workers have performed a number of studies. Daffos et al[102] were successful in using rubella-specific IgM assays on fetal blood to diagnose congenital rubella. They concluded that the fetal immune system first elaborated rubella-specific IgM by 21 weeks of gestation.[103] In a similar study in Germany, Enders and Jonatha[104] obtained fetal blood by cordocentesis between 21 and 23 weeks of gestation and diagnosed fetal infection in 28 of 31 fetal blood samples after testing for rubella-specific IgM by

three different IgM EIAs. In the two cases of rubella embryopathy at birth with rubella-specific IgM presumably a false-negative result, the fetal blood samples had been drawn at 22 and 23 weeks of gestation.

Morgan-Capner et al[105] obtained fetal blood by fetoscopy from four fetuses of mothers with confirmed rubella infection between 19 and 25 weeks of gestation and tested for rubella-specific IgM by capture RIA. Three specimens had rubella-specific IgM; in each case the fetus had congenital rubella. One specimen was negative, and the newborn was unaffected by rubella. This study showed that rubella-specific IgM can be elaborated by the fetal immune system in detectable amounts as early as 19 weeks' gestation. Some of the apparently false-negative assays for rubella-specific IgM in other studies may have occurred because of competition from large amounts of rubella-specific IgG.

Molecular techniques have also been investigated for prenatal diagnosis of congenital rubella. Terry et al[106] reported a 36-year-old woman who developed preconceptual rubella infection (2 days after her last menstrual period); rubella-specific IgM was demonstrated in maternal serum by specific IgM capture assay. CVS was done at 12 weeks of gestation in an attempt to diagnose fetal infection. The fetal tissue suspensions induced characteristic CPE in permissive cell line cultures (Vero cells). The virus was also isolated from fetal tissues and placenta after abortion. The same authors also reported on the use of DNA-RNA hybridization. When RNA extracted from fetal tissues obtained by CVS was dotted onto nitrocellulose filter, hybridization with a cloned radiolabeled rubella complementary DNA (cDNA) probe gave a strong signal.

RT-PCR assays to detect rubella RNA have been developed and used on chorionic villus tissue, fetal tissue samples, and amniotic fluid.[107, 108] In one study, rubella RNA was detected in amniotic fluid from all eight fetuses with congenital rubella and from none of eight uninfected fetuses.[108] One sample from an infected fetus obtained at 15 weeks of gestation was negative, but a second sample obtained at 22 weeks was positive.

Postnatal diagnosis. The diagnosis of congenital rubella can be confirmed postnatally by culture or serology. Infants with congenital rubella are culture positive for many months after birth. At 1 year of age, 2% to 20% of infected infants still shed virus.[99] The best sites to culture are the pharynx, urine, conjunctiva, feces, CSF, and blood.

Congenitally infected infants are born with rubella antibody titers in the blood comparable to those of the mother. These levels persist or even increase during the first few years of life. The diagnosis can also be made from a single specimen by testing for rubella-specific IgM antibodies. Rubella-specific IgM persists for at least 6 months in almost all congenitally infected infants and has been detected in 29% of blood samples obtained between 6½ months and 2 years.[109] False-positive rubella-specific IgM tests can occur with acute Epstein-Barr virus, with human parvovirus B19 infection, or for no apparent reason.[110] Therefore rubella-specific IgM assays should be considered only preliminary evidence of congenital rubella. They should be confirmed by serial determinations of rubella-specific IgG or total antibodies, to show a stable or rising titer, or by culture or PCR.

ENTEROVIRUSES

The role of enteroviruses in causing fetal infection and congenital disease has been extensively evaluated. Based on serologic assessment for *coxsackieviruses* and *echoviruses* in stored blood samples from more than 800 pregnancies complicated by congenital abnormalities, as well as from 23,000 control samples, virologists discovered a relationship between congenital heart disease, urogenital abnormalities, and digestive system anomalies in the neonate and increased titers in the mother.[111, 112] This relationship, however, has not been confirmed.

Other investigators showed that a high percentage of infants with histologic evidence of interstitial myocarditis had infection with *Coxsackie B virus*.[113] *Echovirus 11* has been implicated in a fetal death at 29 weeks.[114] The 18-month-old sibling had a confirmed echovirus 11 infection 3 weeks before the fetal death; the same virus was isolated from multiple fetal tissues at autopsy. Congenital echovirus infection has been demonstrated by growing the virus from amniotic fluid obtained at 34 weeks of gestation; the twin fetuses were found to have enteroviral infection at birth.[115]

PCR would presumably have increased sensitivity for prenatal diagnosis of enteroviral infections but has not yet been evaluated for this purpose.

Enteroviral infections are common in the first month of life. Some of these infections, especially those with onset in the first week of life, may be transmitted from the mother in the peripartum period. They can be diagnosed by culture of the infant's stool and oropharyngeal secretions (see Chapter 13).

ADENOVIRUS

Adenovirus infection has not been associated with fetopathy in the past.[1] Adenovirus was implicated, however, in a case of fetal anasarca with massive ascites, scalp and skin edema, and pericardial and pleural effusions. US evaluation suggested a cardiomyopathic process. Delivery occurred at 34 weeks due to preterm labor. Cardiomyopathy was documented after delivery.

Adenoviral genomic material was found in maternal, fetal, and neonatal blood by PCR amplification.[116]

CONCLUSION

A strong association may exist between viral genomic material in pregnancies and abnormal ultrasound results. Virologic prenatal diagnosis is clearly in early stages despite extensive investigations of congenital viral infections over the past 30 years. We anticipate rapid strides in diagnosis of intrauterine viral infection as a result of development of powerful techniques (e.g., PCR) and easier access to the fetus. Clinicians must be vigilant, however, not to cause harm to the fetus by the invasive technique itself.[15] These developments should also result in efficacious treatments to reduce the sequelae of intrauterine viral infection.

References

1. Grose C, Oussama I, Weiner CP: Prenatal diagnosis of fetal infection: advances from amniocentesis to cordocentesis—congenital toxoplasmosis, rubella, cytomegalovirus, varicella virus, parvovirus and human immunodeficiency virus, *Pediatr Infect Dis J* 8:459, 1989.
2. Weiner CP, Grose C, Naides SJ: Diagnosis of fetal infection in the patient with an ultrasonographically detected abnormality but a negative clinical history, *Am J Obstet Gynecol* 168:6, 1993.
3. Bevis DCA: The antenatal prediction of hemolytic disease of the newborn, *Lancet* 1:395, 1952.
4. Hanson FW, Tennant FR, Zorn EM, Samuels S: Analysis of 2136 genetic amniocenteses: experience of a single physician, *Am J Obstet Gynecol* 152:436, 1985.
5. Johnson A, Godmilow L: Genetic amniocentesis at 14 weeks or less, *Clin Obstet Gynecol* 31:345, 1988.
6. Cao A, Furbetta M, Angius A, et al: Haematological and obstetric aspects of antenatal diagnosis of beta-thalassaemia: experience with 200 cases, *J Med Genet* 19:81, 1982.
7. Rodeck CH, Nicolaides KH: Fetoscopy, *Br Med Bull* 42:296, 1986.
8. Hahneman N, Mohr J: Genetic diagnosis in the embryo by means of biopsy from extra embryo membranes, *Bull Eur Soc Hum Genet* 2:23, 1968.
9. Lilford RJ, Linton G, Irving HC, Mason MK: Transabdominal chorion villus biopsy: 100 consecutive cases, *Lancet* 1:1415, 1987.
10. Brambati B, Oldrini A, Lanzani A: Transabdominal chorionic villus sampling: a freehand ultrasound-guided technique, *Am J Obstet Gynecol* 157:134, 1987.
11. Brambati B, Guercilena S, Bonacchi I, et al: Feto-maternal transfusion after chorionic villus sampling: clinical implications, *Hum Reprod* 1:37, 1986.
12. Brambati B, Oldrini A, Ferrazzi E, Lanzani A: Chorionic villus sampling: an analysis of the obstetric experience of 1,000 cases, *Prenat Diagn* 7:157, 1987.

13. Evans MI, Koppich FC 3d, Nemitz B, et al: Early genetic amniocentesis and chorionic villus sampling: expanding the opportunities for early prenatal diagnosis, *J Reprod Med* 33:450, 1988.

14. Rhoads GG, Jackson LG, Schlesselman SE, et al: The safety and efficacy of chorionic villus sampling for early prenatal diagnosis of cytogenetic abnormalities, *N Engl J Med* 320:609, 1989.

15. Burton BK, Schulz CJ, Burd LI: Spectrum of limb disruption defects associated with chorionic villus sampling, *Pediatrics* 91-989, 92:722 (erratum), 1993.

16. Daffos F, Capella-Pavlovsky M, Forestier F: Fetal blood sampling during pregnancy with use of a needle guided by ultrasound: a study of 606 consecutive cases, *Am J Obstet Gynecol* 153:655, 1985.

17. Weiner CP: Cordocentesis, *Obstet Gynecol Clin North Am* 15:283, 1988.

18. Habibi B, Bretagne M, Bretagne Y, et al: Blood group antigens on fetal red cells obtained by umbilical vein puncture under ultrasound guidance: a rapid hemagglutination test to check for contamination with maternal blood, *Pediatr Res* 20:1082, 1986.

19. Forestier F, Cox WL, Daffos F, Rainaut M: The assessment of fetal blood samples, *Am J Obstet Gynecol* 158:1184, 1988.

20. Alford CA: Immunoglobulin determinations in the diagnosis of fetal infection, *Pediatr Clin North Am* 18:99, 1971.

21. Reimer CB, Black CM, Phillips DJ, et al: The specificity of fetal IgM: antibody or anti-antibody? *Ann NY Acad Sci* 254:77, 1975.

22. Stagno S, Pass RF, Reynolds DW, et al: Comparative study of diagnostic procedures for congenital cytomegalovirus infection, *Pediatrics* 65:251, 1980.

23. Tookey PA, Ades AE, Peckham CS: Cytomegalovirus prevalence in pregnant women: the influence of parity, *Arch Dis Child* 67:779, 1992.

24. Stagno S, Pass RF, Cloud G, et al: Primary cytomegalovirus infection in pregnancy: incidence, transmission to fetus, and clinical outcome, *JAMA* 256:1904, 1986.

25. Yow MD, Williamson DW, Leeds LJ, et al: Epidemiologic characteristics of cytomegalovirus infection in mothers and their infants, *Am J Obstet Gynecol* 158:1189, 1988.

26. Demmler GJ: Congenital cytomegalovirus infection and disease; *Rep Pediatr Infect Dis* 7:17, 1997.

27. Stagno S, Pass RF, Dworsky ME, et al: Congenital cytomegalovirus infection: the relative importance of primary and recurrent maternal infection, *N Engl J Med* 306:945, 1982.

28. Fowler KB, Stagno S, Pass RF, et al: The outcome of congenital cytomegalovirus infection in relation to maternal antibody status, *N Engl J Med* 326:663, 1992.

28a. Waner JL, Weller TH, Kevy SV: Patterns of cytomegaloviral complement-fixing antibody activity: a longitudinal study of blood donors, *J Infect Dis* 127:538, 1973.

29. Stagno S, Tinker MK, Elrod C, et al: Immunoglobulin M antibodies detected by enzyme-linked immunosorbent assay and radioimmunoassay in the diagnosis of cytomegalovirus infections in pregnant women and newborn infants, *J Clin Microbiol* 21:930, 1985.

30. Weiner CP, Grose C: Prenatal diagnosis of congenital cytomegalovirus infection by virus isolation from amniotic fluid, *Am J Obstet Gynecol* 163:1253, 1990.

31. Grose C, Meehan T, Weiner CP: Prenatal diagnosis of congenital cytomegalovirus infection by virus isolation after amniocentesis, *Pediatr Infect Dis J* 11:605, 1992.

32. Lamy ME, Mulongo KN, Gadisseux JF, et al: Prenatal diagnosis of fetal cytomegalovirus infection, *Am J Obstet Gynecol* 166:91, 1992.

33. Donner C, Liesnard C, Content J, et al: Prenatal diagnosis of 52 pregnancies at risk for congenital cytomegalovirus infection, *Obstet Gynecol* 82:481, 1993.

34. Revello MG, Baldanti F, Furione M, et al: Polymerase chain reaction for prenatal diagnosis of congenital human cytomegalovirus infection, *J Med Virol* 47:462, 1995.

35. Hogge WA, Buffone GJ, Hogge JS: Prenatal diagnosis of cytomegalovirus (CMV) infection: a preliminary report, *Prenat Diagn* 13:131, 1993.

36. Xu W, Sundqvist VA, Brytting M, Linde A: Diagnosis of cytomegalovirus infections using polymerase chain reaction, virus isolation and serology, *Scand J Infect Dis* 25:311, 1993.

37. Hohlfeld P, Vial Y, Maillard-Brignon C, et al: Cytomegalovirus fetal infection: prenatal diagnosis, *Obstet Gynecol* 78:615, 1991.

38. Lipitz S, Yagel S, Shalev E, et al: Prenatal diagnosis of fetal primary cytomegalovirus infection, *Obstet Gynecol* 89:763, 1997.

39. Nicolini U, Kustermann A, Tassis B, et al: Prenatal diagnosis of congenital human cytomegalovirus infection, *Prenat Diagn* 14:903, 1994.

40. Lynch L, Daffos F, Emanuel D, et al: Prenatal diagnosis of fetal cytomegalovirus infection, *Am J Obstet Gynecol* 165:714, 1991.

41. Catanzarite V, Dankner WM: Prenatal diagnosis of congenital cytomegalovirus infection: false-negative amniocentesis at 20 weeks' gestation, *Prenat Diagn* 13:1021, 1993.

42. Donner C, Liesnard C, Brancart F, Rodesch F: Accuracy of amniotic fluid testing before 21 weeks' gestation in prenatal diagnosis of congenital cytomegalovirus infection, *Prenat Diagn* 14:1055, 1994.

43. Reynolds DW, Stagno S, Hosty TS, et al: Maternal cytomegalovirus excretion and perinatal infection, *N Engl J Med* 289:1, 1973.

44. Stagno S, Reynolds DW, Tsiantos A, et al: Comparative serial virologic and serologic studies of symptomatic and subclinical congenitally and natally acquired cytomegalovirus infections, *J Infect Dis* 132:568, 1975.

45. Demmler GJ, Buffone GJ, Schimbor CM, May RA: Detection of cytomegalovirus in urine from newborns by using polymerase chain reaction DNA amplification, *J Infect Dis* 158:1177, 1988.

46. Balcarek KB, Warren W, Smith RJ, et al: Neonatal screening for congenital cytomegalovirus infection by detection of virus in saliva, *J Infect Dis* 167:1433, 1993.

47. Lang DJ, Noren B: Cytomegaloviremia following congenital infection, *J Pediatr* 73:812, 1968.

48. Barbi M, Binda S, Primache V, Novelli C: Cytomegalovirus in peripheral blood leukocytes of infants with

congenital or postnatal infection, *Pediatr Infect Dis J* 15: 898, 1996.

49. Nelson CT, Istas AS, Wilkerson MK, Demmler GJ: PCR detection of cytomegalovirus DNA in serum as a diagnostic test for congenital cytomegalovirus infection, *J Clin Microbiol* 33:3317, 1995.

50. Griffiths PD, Stagno S, Pass RF, et al: Congenital cytomegalovirus infection: diagnostic and prognostic significance of the detection of specific immunoglobulin M antibodies in cord serum, *Pediatrics* 69:544, 1982.

51. Grose C: Varicella-zoster virus infections: chickenpox, shingles, and varicella vaccine. In Glaser R, Jones JF, editors: *Herpesvirus infections*, New York, 1994, Marcel Dekker.

52. Chapman S, Duff P: Varicella in pregnancy, *Semin Perinat* 17:403, 1993.

53. Struewing JP, Hyans KC, Tueller JE, Gray GC: The risk of measles, mumps, and varicella among young adults: a serosurvey of US Navy and Marine Corps recruits, *Am J Public Health* 83:1717, 1993.

54. McGregor JA, Mark S, Crawford GP, Levin MJ: Varicella zoster antibody testing in the care of pregnant women exposed to varicella, *Am J Obstet Gynecol* 157:281, 1987.

55. Choo PW, Donahue JG, Manson JE, Platt R: The epidemiology of varicella and its complications, *J Infect Dis* 172:706, 1995.

56. Laforet EG, Lynch CL: Multiple congenital defects following maternal varicella, *N Engl J Med* 236:534, 1947.

57. Pastuszak AL, Levy M, Schick B, et al: Outcome after maternal varicella infection in the first 20 weeks of pregnancy, *N Engl J Med* 330:901, 1994.

58. Grose C: Varicella-zoster immune globulin, *Rep Pediatr Infect Dis* 7:13, 1997.

59. Puchhammer-Stöckl E, Kunz C, Wagner G, Enders G: Detection of varicella zoster virus DNA in fetal tissue by polymerase chain reaction, *J Perinat Med* 22:65, 1994.

60. Isada NB, Paar DP, Johnson MP, et al: In utero diagnosis of congenital varicella zoster virus infection by chorionic villus sampling and polymerase chain reaction, *Am J Obstet Gynecol* 165:1727, 1991.

61. Mouly F, Mirlesse V, Meritet JF, et al: Prenatal diagnosis of fetal varicella-zoster virus infection with polymerase chain reaction of amniotic fluid in 107 cases, *Am J Obstet Gynecol* 177:894, 1997.

62. Cuthbertson G, Weiner CP, Giller RH, Grose C: Prenatal diagnosis of second-trimester congenital varicella syndrome by virus-specific immunoglobulin M, *J Pediatr* 111:592, 1987.

63. Grose C: Congenital infections caused by varicella zoster virus and herpes simplex virus, *Semin Pediatr Neurol* 1:43, 1994.

64. South MA, Tompkins WA, Morris CR, Rawls WE: Congenital malformation of the central nervous system associated with genital type (type 2) herpesvirus, *J Pediatr* 75:13, 1969.

65. Hutto C, Arvin A, Jacobs R, et al: Intrauterine herpes simplex virus infections, *J Pediatr* 110:97, 1987.

66. Whitley RJ, Corey L, Arvin A, et al: Changing presentation of herpes simplex virus infection in neonates, *J Infect Dis* 158:109, 1988.

67. Whitley R, Arvin A, Prober C, et al: Predictors of morbidity and mortality in neonates with herpes simplex virus infections: the National Institute of Allergy and Infectious Diseases Collaborative Antiviral Study Group, *N Engl J Med* 324:450, 1991.

68. Lanouette JM, Duquette DA, Jacques SM, et al: Prenatal diagnosis of fetal herpes simplex infection, *Fetal Diagn Ther* 11:414, 1996.

69. Arvin AM, Yeager AS, Bruhn FW, Grossman M: Neonatal herpes simplex infection in the absence of mucocutaneous lesions, *J Pediatr* 100:715, 1982.

70. Golden S: Neonatal herpes simplex viremia, *Pediatr Infect Dis J* 7:425, 1988.

71. Kimura H, Futamura M, Kito H, et al: Detection of viral DNA in neonatal herpes simplex virus infections: frequent and prolonged presence in serum and cerebrospinal fluid, *J Infect Dis* 164:289, 1991.

72. Troendle-Atkins J, Demmler GJ, Buffone GJ: Rapid diagnosis of herpes simplex virus encephalitis by using the polymerase chain reaction, *J Pediatr* 123:376, 1993.

73. Kimberlin DW, Lakeman FD, Arvin AM, et al: Application of the polymerase chain reaction to the diagnosis and management of neonatal herpes simplex virus disease: National Institute of Allergy and Infectious Diseases Collaborative Antiviral Study Group, *J Infect Dis* 174:1162, 1996.

74. Anderson LJ: Role of parvovirus B19 in human disease, *Pediatr Infect Dis J* 6:711, 1987.

75. Jordan JA: Identification of human parvovirus B19 infection in idiopathic nonimmune hydrops fetalis, *Am J Obstet Gynecol* 174:37, 1996.

76. Naides SJ, Weiner CP: Antenatal diagnosis and palliative treatment of non-immune hydrops fetalis secondary to fetal parvovirus B19 infection, *Prenat Diagn* 9:105, 1989.

77. Anderson MJ: Parvoviruses as agents of human disease, *Prog Med Virol* 34:55, 1987.

78. Torok TJ, Wang QY, Gary GW Jr, et al: Prenatal diagnosis of intrauterine infection with parvovirus B19 by the polymerase chain reaction technique, *Clin Infect Dis* 14:149, 1992.

79. Katz VL, McCoy MC, Kuller JA, Hansen WF: An association between fetal parvovirus B19 infection and fetal anomalies: a report of two cases, *Am J Perinatol* 13:43, 1996.

80. Gratacos E, Torres PJ, Vidal J, et al: The incidence of human parvovirus B19 infection during pregnancy and its impact on perinatal outcome, *J Infect Dis* 171: 1360, 1995.

81. Harger JH, Adler SP, Koch WC, Harger GF: Prospective evaluation of 618 pregnant women exposed to parvovirus B19: risks and symptoms, *Obstet Gynecol* 91:413, 1998.

82. Anderson LJ, Hurwitz ES: Human parvovirus B19 and pregnancy, *Clin Perinatol* 15:273, 1988.

83. Public Health Laboratory Service Working Party on Fifth Disease: Prospective study of human parvovirus (B19) infection in pregnancy, *Br Med J* 300:1166, 1990.

84. Miller E, Fairley CK, Cohen BJ, Seng C: Immediate and long term outcome of human parvovirus B19 infection in pregnancy, *Br J Obstet Gynaecol* 105:174, 1998.

85. Rodis JF, Quinn DL, Gary GW Jr, et al: Management and outcomes of pregnancies complicated by hu-

man B19 parvovirus infection: a prospective study, *Am J Obstet Gynecol* 163:1168, 1990.

86. Torok TJ: Parvovirus B19 and human disease, *Adv Intern Med* 37:431, 1992.

87. Kovacs BW, Carlson DE, Shahbahrami B, Platt LD: Prenatal diagnosis of human parvovirus B19 in nonimmune hydrops fetalis by polymerase chain reaction, *Am J Obstet Gynecol* 167:461, 1992.

88. Nikkari S, Ekblad U: A rapid and safe method to detect fetal parvovirus B19 infection in amniotic fluid by polymerase chain reaction: report of a case, *Am J Perinatol* 12:447, 1995.

89. Zerbini M, Musiani M, Gentilomi G, et al: Comparative evaluation of virological and serological methods in prenatal diagnosis of parvovirus B19 fetal hydrops, *J Clin Microbiol* 34:603, 1996.

90. Childs JE, Glass GE, Ksiazek TG, et al: Human-rodent contact and infection with lymphocytic choriomeningitis and Seoul viruses in an inner-city population, *Am J Trop Med Hyg* 44:117, 1991.

91. Peters CJ: Arenaviruses. In Richman DD, Whitley RJ, Hayden FG, editors: *Clinical virology*, New York, 1997, Churchill Livingstone.

92. Barton LL, Budd SC, Morfitt WS, et al: Congenital lymphocytic choriomeningitis virus infection in twins, *Pediatr Infect Dis J* 12:942, 1993.

93. Wright R, Johnson D, Neumann M, et al: Congenital lymphocytic choriomeningitis virus syndrome: a disease that mimics congenital toxoplasmosis or cytomegalovirus infection, *Pediatrics* 100:E9, 1997.

94. Park JY, Peters CJ, Rollin PE, et al: Development of a reverse transcription–polymerase chain reaction assay for diagnosis of lymphocytic choriomeningitis virus infection and its use in a prospective surveillance study, *J Med Virol* 51:107, 1997.

95. Peckham C, Gibb D: Mother-to-child transmission of the human immunodeficiency virus, *N Engl J Med* 333:298, 1995.

96. Boyer PJ, Dillon M, Navaie M, et al: Factors predictive of maternal-fetal transmission of HIV-1: preliminary analysis of zidovudine given during pregnancy and/or delivery, *JAMA* 271:1925, 1994.

97. Connor EM, Sperling RS, Gelber R, et al: Reduction of maternal-infant transmission of human immunodeficiency virus type 1 with zidovudine treatment: Pediatric AIDS Clinical Trials Group Protocol 076 Study Group, *N Engl J Med* 331:1173, 1994.

98. Pizzo PA, Wilfert CM: *Pediatric AIDS*, ed 3, Baltimore, 1998, Williams and Wilkins.

99. Cooper LZ, Preblud SR, Alford CAJ: Rubella. In Remington JS, Klein JO, editors: *Infectious diseases of the fetus & newborn infant*, ed 4, Philadelphia, 1995, WB Saunders.

100. Levin MJ, Oxman MN, Moore MG, et al: Diagnosis of congenital rubella in utero, *N Engl J Med* 290:1187, 1974.

101. Alestig K, Bartsch FK, Nilsson LA, Strannegard O: Studies of amniotic fluid in women infected with rubella, *J Infect Dis* 129:79, 1974.

102. Daffos F, Forestier F, Grangeot-Keros L, et al: Prenatal diagnosis of congenital rubella, *Lancet* 2:1, 1984.

103. Grangeot-Keros L, Pillot J, Daffos F, Forestier F: Prenatal and postnatal production of IgM and IgA antibodies to rubella virus studied by antibody capture immunoassay, *J Infect Dis* 158:138, 1988.

104. Enders G, Jonatha W: Prenatal diagnosis of intrauterine rubella, *Infection* 15:162, 1987.

105. Morgan-Capner P, Rodeck CH, Nicolaides KH, Cradock-Watson JE: Prenatal detection of rubella-specific IgM in fetal sera, *Prenat Diagn* 5:21, 1985.

106. Terry GM, Ho-Terry L, Warren RC, et al: First trimester prenatal diagnosis of congenital rubella: a laboratory investigation, *Br Med J (Clin Res Ed)* 292:930, 1986.

107. Bosma TJ, Corbett KM, Eckstein MB, et al: Use of PCR for prenatal and postnatal diagnosis of congenital rubella, *J Clin Microbiol* 33:2881, 1995.

108. Revello MG, Baldanti F, Sarasini A, et al: Prenatal diagnosis of rubella virus infection by direct detection and semiquantitation of viral RNA in clinical samples by reverse transcription–PCR, *J Clin Microbiol* 35:708, 1997.

109. Cradock-Watson JE, Ridehalgh MK: Specific immunoglobulins in infants with the congenital rubella syndrome, *J Hyg (Lond)* 76:109, 1976.

110. Morgan-Capner P: False positive tests for rubella-specific IgM, *Pediatr Infect Dis J* 10:415, 1991 (letter).

111. Brown GC, Evans TN: Serologic evidence of coxsackievirus etiology of congenital heart disease, *JAMA* 199:183, 1967.

112. Brown GC, Karunas RS: Relationship of congenital anomalies and maternal infection with selected enteroviruses, *Am J Epidemiol* 95:207, 1972.

113. Burch GE, Sun SC, Chu KC et al: Interstitial and coxsackievirus B myocarditis in infants and children: a comparative histologic and immunofluorescent study of 50 autopsied hearts, *JAMA* 203:1, 1968.

114. Johansson ME, Holmstrom S, Abebe A, et al: Intrauterine fetal death due to echovirus 11, *Scand J Infect Dis* 24:381, 1992.

115. Strong BS, Young SA: Intrauterine coxsackie, group B type 1, infection: virus cultivation from amniotic fluid in the third trimester, *Am J Perinatol* 12:78, 1995.

116. Towbin JA, Griffin LD, Martin AB, et al: Intrauterine adenoviral myocarditis presenting as nonimmune hydrops fetalis: diagnosis by polymerase chain reaction, *Pediatr Infect Dis J* 13:144, 1994.

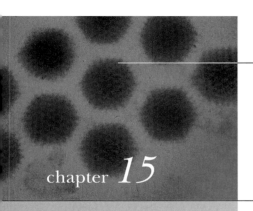

Gregory A. Storch

Viral Infections in Immunocompromised Patients

Outline continued

OVERVIEW

Certain viruses are important as opportunistic pathogens that cause serious infections in patients with congenital or acquired immunodeficiencies (Table 15–1). The causative agents can be divided into two categories. The first are true opportunistic pathogens, viruses that are usually or always nonpathogenic in individuals with a normal immune system but that cause severe illness in immunocompromised patients. Prominent members of this group are human *cytomegalovirus* (CMV) and the polyomaviruses JC and BK. The second category includes those viruses that characteristically cause self-limited illness in normal individuals but cause unusually severe or persistent infection in immunocompromised patients. Examples include herpes simplex virus or common respiratory viruses such as respiratory syncytial virus and the parainfluenza viruses. The causative viruses vary depending on the nature of the immune compromise (Table 15–2).

This chapter discusses disseminated infection caused by CMV, *Epstein-Barr virus* (EBV), *human herpesviruses 6 to 8* (HHV-6, HHV-7, HHV-8), and *adenovirus*. Localized viral infections in immunocompromised patients (e.g., from common respiratory viruses) are discussed in the chapters dealing with infections of the affected organ system. Chapters 3 and 11 discuss diagnosis of JC virus infection, the cause of progressive multifocal leukoencephalopathy (PML), and BK virus infection, a cause of hemorrhagic cystitis. Chapter 13 discusses diagnosis of human parvovirus B19 chronic infection as a cause of persistent red blood cell aplasia.

CYTOMEGALOVIRUS

Virology

Human cytomegalovirus (CMV) is a member of the family Herpesviridae. Based on its slow growth in culture and its specificity for humans, it is classified in the beta herpesvirus subfamily, along with human herpesviruses 6 and 7 (HHV-6, HHV-7). Although different strains can be identified by genomic analysis, no well-defined subtypes exist, and the human immune

Table 15.1	Viral Infections in Immunocompromised Hosts
Virus	**Syndrome(s)**
Cytomegalovirus	Disseminated infection
	Pneumonia
	Colitis, esophagitis, gastritis, other gastrointestinal tract manifestations
	Hepatitis
	Retinitis
	Encephalitis, radiculomyelitis, peripheral neuritis, other nervous system manifestations
	Adrenalitis
Epstein-Barr	Posttransplant lymphoproliferative disorder
	Primary central nervous system lymphoma
Herpes simplex	Severe mucocutaneous infection
	Esophagitis
	Pneumonia
	Retinitis
	Meningoencephalitis
Varicella-zoster	Zoster (localized or disseminated)
	Retinitis
	Myelitis, encephalitis
Human herpesvirus 6	Encephalitis
	Bone marrow suppression
	Hepatitis
Human herpesvirus 8	Kaposi's sarcoma
	AIDS-related body-cavity-based lymphoma
Adenovirus	Disseminated infection
	Hepatitis
	Hemorrhagic cystitis
JC	Progressive multifocal leukoencephalopathy (PML)
BK	Hemorrhagic cystitis
Parvovirus B19	Chronic red blood cell aplasia
Vaccinia	Progressive vaccinia (vaccinia necrosum)
Respiratory syncytial	Pneumonia
Parainfluenza	Pneumonia
	Persistent respiratory infection
Measles	Pneumonia
	Encephalitis
	Disseminated infection
Enteroviruses	Chronic meningoencephalitis

response is cross-reacting with all strains. The CMV virion has icosahedral symmetry with 162 capsomeres and is surrounded by a lipid-containing envelope. The genome includes more than 200,000 base pairs and has been completely sequenced.

CMV genes are classified as alpha (α), beta (β), and gamma (γ), based on the timing and dependence of expression on preceding synthesis of viral proteins and deoxyribonucleic acid (DNA). The α (*immediate-early*) genes are the first genes expressed after CMV infects a cell. The expression of these genes can occur in the presence of inhibitors of viral protein synthesis. The β (*early*) genes are next and can be expressed in the presence of inhibitors of viral DNA synthesis, although they depend on synthesis of immediate-early viral proteins. The α and β gene products are involved with viral DNA synthesis. The γ (*late*) genes are expressed last and encode structural CMV proteins.

Epidemiology and Host-Virus Interaction

CMV infection is extremely widespread. In the United States, 30% to 50% of middle-class adults and 50% to 90% of adults from lower socioeconomic groups are seropositive, indicating past infection. Approximately 1% of infants are born with congenital infection, of which approximately 10% are symptomatic.[1] Infection occurs in the early postpartum period in an additional 5% to 10% of infants. Seroprevalence increases during early childhood, then levels off, but increases again with the onset of sexual activity. During active infection the virus is shed in saliva, urine, and genital fluids and can be transmitted by close personal contact, including but not limited to sexual contact. It can also be transmitted by blood transfusion. Active infection during pregnancy can result in congenital infection (see Chapter 14). Congenital infection is much more likely with primary rather than reactivation infection during pregnancy.

As with the other human herpesviruses, CMV is associated with primary, latent, and reactivation infection. *Primary infection* is usually not recognized clinically but can be associated with an infectious mononucleosis syndrome, especially when it occurs in adults (see Chapter 12). *Latency* is established after primary infection and persists for the individual's lifetime. The site of latent infection is thought to include cells of myeloid lineage.[2, 3] Only a small proportion of circulating leukocytes are latently infected. *Reactivation* can occur in immunologically normal individuals but is more likely to occur in those with immune compromise. When it occurs in normal individuals, reactivation is virtually always asymptomatic. In contrast, when reactivation occurs in the immunocompromised individual, illness frequently occurs, ranging in severity from minimal to life threatening. Reinfection with new strains of CMV has also been recognized in immunocompromised individuals.[4]

Clinical Illnesses

Primary CMV infection in normal individuals beyond infancy is associated with an infectious mononucleosis-like syndrome (see Chapter 12). Congenital CMV infection ranges from severely symptomatic in approximately 0.5% of patients to asymptomatic in 90%[1] (see Chapter 14). The clinical manifestations of CMV infection in immunocompromised patients vary with the nature of the immune compromise (Table 15–3).

In organ transplant recipients the most common manifestation is a systemic syndrome that occurs in the second through fourth month after transplantation and

Table 15.2	Types of Immune Compromise and Associated Viral Infections
Type of immune compromise	**Virus(es)**
Acquired immunodeficiency syndrome (AIDS)	CMV, HSV, VZV, EBV (central nervous system lymphoma, lymphocytic interstitial pneumonitis [LIP]), Kaposi's sarcoma (HHV-8), adenovirus, JC virus, parvovirus B19, HBV, HCV
Organ transplantation	CMV, HSV, VZV, EBV (posttransplant lymphoproliferative disorder [PTLD]), HHV-6, adenovirus, BK virus, parvovirus B19, HBV, HCV
Other immunosuppressive therapy	HSV, VZV, CMV
Congenital infection	
Hypogammaglobulinemia	Enteroviruses (chronic meningoencephalitis, dermatomyositis-like syndrome), poliovirus (vaccine strain), rotavirus
Severe combined immunodeficiency	CMV, HSV, VZV Measles (wild type and vaccine strain) Poliovirus (vaccine strain) RSV, parainfluenza viruses, adenovirus, rotavirus, vaccinia
Common variable immunodeficiency	CMV, EBV
X-linked lymphoproliferative syndrome	EBV (overwhelming infection, aplastic anemia, hypogammaglobulinemia, agranulocytosis, hemophagocytic syndrome, lymphoma)
Cartilage-hair hypoplasia	VZV, vaccinia

CMV, Cytomegalovirus; *HSV,* herpes simplex; *VZV,* varicella-zoster; *EBV,* Epstein-Barr; *HHV-6* and *HHV-8,* human herpesvirus 6 and 8; *HBV* and *HCV,* hepatitis B and C; *RSV,* respiratory syncytial.

Table 15.3	Manifestations of Symptomatic Cytomegalovirus Infection in Immunocompromised Patients	
Manifestation/area infected	Transplant recipients	AIDS patients
Systemic syndrome	3+	1+
Pneumonia	1+	Rare
Retina	Rare	3+
Gastrointestinal tract		
Colon	2+	2+
Esophagitis	1+	1+
Other	1+	1+
Liver	2+	1+
Nervous system		
Brain	Rare	1+
Spinal cord and nerve roots	Rare	1+
Peripheral nerves	Rare	1+
Kidneys	1+	Rare
Adrenal glands	Rare	1+

resembles CMV mononucleosis in immunologically normal individuals. The major clinical manifestations are fever, malaise, leukopenia, thrombocytopenia, and abnormal liver function tests. Localized infection may complicate the systemic syndrome or may occur without preceding systemic illness. Sites of localized infection include lungs, colon, esophagus, other locations within the gastrointestinal (GI) tract, liver, and kidneys. Clinically important involvement of the retina, the central nervous system (CNS), or the adrenal glands is unusual in transplant recipients. In patients immunocompromised because of acquired immunodeficiency syndrome (AIDS), the most common manifestations are retinitis, colitis, esophagitis, pneumonia, radiculomyelitis, and encephalitis.

Antiviral agents used for CMV infection include ganciclovir, foscarnet, and cidofovir.

Diagnostic Tests

A wide variety of laboratory methods are available for the diagnosis of CMV infection (Box 15–1). Viral culture is used to detect the presence of infectious virus, which defines active (as opposed to latent) CMV infection. Tests for CMV antigens and nucleic acids are other approaches to the direct detection of CMV in clinical specimens. Culture and tests to detect CMV antigens or nucleic acids can be performed on many different specimens, including tissue. Visualization of the virus by electron microscopy is an alternative approach to direct detection of the virus but is rarely used in patient diagnosis at present. Histologic examination looking microscopically at tissue sections for characteristic CMV inclusions can be uniquely useful by providing information concerning the relationship between the presence of CMV and evidence of disease in the tissue under examination (see Chapter 1). Tests for CMV antibodies can be used to define current or recent infection, either by demonstrating a rising titer or the presence of immunoglobulin M (IgM)–specific CMV antibodies. Serologic testing can also be used to identify patients with past CMV infection.

All efforts to make a laboratory-based diagnosis of CMV disease are complicated by the potential presence of active infection without disease manifestations; therefore detection of CMV is not equivalent to the identification of CMV disease. The choice of specimen for testing is critical, since the presence of CMV in blood, cerebrospinal fluid (CSF), or ocular fluid usually indicates disease, whereas presence in urine or saliva often occurs without disease. Table 15–4 summarizes the advantages and disadvantages of methods to detect CMV in blood specimens.

Viral culture. Viral isolation in cell culture is the traditional standard for the diagnosis of CMV infection. A significant drawback of conventional culture is the slow growth of the virus, which often requires 14 days or more before it can be detected. Human fibroblasts are the cell type required for the growth of CMV in the laboratory. Numerous well-established fibroblast cell lines can be used (e.g., MRC-5, WI-38). Many laboratories establish their own fibroblast cultures, starting from a variety of human sources, including foreskin, other skin, and tonsil tissue. Appropriate specimens for culture include blood (from which leukocyte or buffy coat fraction is used), urine, saliva or throat swab, bronchial wash or bronchoalveolar lavage (BAL) fluid, and amniotic fluid.

After specimens are inoculated, the cultures are observed for the development of cytopathic effect (CPE). The CPE caused by CMV is usually sufficiently distinct to allow confident identification of the virus, but when uncertain a fluorescent antibody (FA) stain

Box 15.1	Diagnostic Tests for Cytomegalovirus Infection

Viral culture
pp65 antigenemia assay
Polymerase chain reaction (PCR)
Electron microscopy (EM)
Histology
    Immunohistochemistry (IHC)
    In situ hybridization (ISH)
Serology
    Immunoglobulin G (IgG)
    Immunoglobulin M (IgM)

Table 15.4   Advantages and Disadvantages of Methods for Detection of CMV in Blood

Method	Advantages	Disadvantages
Conventional culture	Relatively specific for symptomatic infection Versatile (can be performed on multiple specimen types Provides isolate for susceptibility testing and further characterization	Slow (typically 7-21 days) Requires virus viability in specimen
Shell vial culture	Rapid Can be performed on multiple specimen types	Requires virus viability in specimen Cytotoxicity can interfere with result Low sensitivity in some laboratories
pp65 antigenemia assay	Rapid Sensitive Quantitative Does not require viable virus	Labor intensive Antigen not stable with ex vivo storage
Polymerase chain reaction (PCR)	Sensitive Does not require viable virus Target is stable Lends itself to instrumentation Can be made quantitative	Qualitative PCR is too sensitive for many applications
Hybrid capture assay	Convenient Quantative Relatively specific for symptomatic disease	Less sensitive than PCR

or a shell vial culture can be performed on cells from the culture to confirm the presence of CMV. A positive culture signifies active CMV infection but is not diagnostic of CMV disease. Growth of the virus from blood is closely associated with disease, although asymptomatic CMV viremia can occur in immunocompromised individuals. Positive cultures of saliva or urine have little predictive value for the presence of current CMV disease in most clinical settings.

A unique aspect of the conventional viral culture is that it provides a viral isolate that can be maintained or stored in the laboratory and used for phenotypic antiviral susceptibility testing as well as further characterization that may be useful for epidemiologic purposes.

Shell vial culture. The shell vial culture revolutionized the diagnostic approach to CMV by allowing detection of the virus within 1 to 2 days from receipt of the specimen[5-7] (see Chapter 1). The essential components of this procedure include inoculation of the specimen onto cultured fibroblast cells, centrifugation to enhance uptake of virus by the fibroblasts, and detection of virus infection of the cells using FA staining, usually performed 16 to 40 hours after inoculation. The FA stain typically employs a monoclonal antibody specific for the CMV major immediate-early antigen. The significance of a shell vial culture is the same as that of a conventional culture. Although the traditional shell vial assay is a qualitative test, it can be made quantitative by

counting the number of leukocytes inoculated into the culture and the number of fluorescent foci detected.[8]

The sensitivity of the shell vial culture compared with conventional culture varies according to the specimen type. Substantial variation also occurs from laboratory to laboratory. In our laboratory the shell vial culture detects CMV in 40% more urine specimens than conventional culture, in 10% more respiratory specimens, but in 20% fewer blood specimens (Table 15–5). Numerous variables affect the sensitivity of shell vial cultures, including procedures used for specimen processing, number of shell vial cultures inoculated, conditions of centrifugation, age of fibroblast cells, duration of incubation before antibody staining, monoclonal antibody employed, quality of fluorescent microscope, and experience of personnel.[9-11] Toxic effects of the specimen on the fibroblast cells in the shell vial culture can decrease sensitivity by making the cell monolayer unreadable.

For culturing CMV from the blood, the number of leukocytes inoculated into culture also has an important effect on the ability to detect CMV.[8] Use of too few leukocytes can compromise sensitivity, whereas use of too many may produce toxicity. Use of a blood volume of 5 ml versus 2.5 ml has been shown to increase the yield, as has culturing two or three blood samples obtained at different times.[12, 13] For maximum detection from blood, use of both shell vial cultures and conventional cultures is advised.[11, 12] For urine, saliva, and BAL specimens, laboratories with a sensitive shell

Table 15.5 Relative Detection of CMV from Different Specimen Types by Shell Vial and Conventional Culture Techniques

Specimen	Total detected*	Detected by shell vial (%)†	Detected by conventional culture (%)†	Shell vial/conventional‡
Urine	367	341 (93)	248 (68)	1.4
Blood (leukocytes)	147	99 (67)	124 (84)	0.8
Respiratory	126	105 (83)	98 (78)	1.1

Modified from Arens M, Owen J, Hagerty CM, et al: *Diagn Microbiol Infect Dis* 14:125, 1991.
*Total number of cultures positive by either technique.
†Percent of total number detected.
‡Number of positive shell vial cultures divided by number of positive conventional cultures.

vial culture technique may use the shell vial culture in place of conventional culture without compromising sensitivity.

Regardless of whether convention culture or shell vial culture is being used, conditions of specimen transport are important for detecting CMV. Our laboratory has found that detection of CMV in blood by the shell vial culture is not affected by a 6-hour delay in inoculation of the specimen but is much less effective after 24 hours.[14]

pp65 antigenemia assay. This assay is an alternative method to viral culture for detecting the presence of CMV in blood, first described by investigators in the Netherlands[15] and Italy[16] in 1988 and 1989. The pp65 antigenemia assay is based on the direct detection of CMV antigen in circulating leukocytes through the use of either FA or *immunoperoxidase* (IP) staining. Current preference in most laboratories is for FA staining, which has been found to be more sensitive.[17, 18] The best sensitivity has been achieved using monoclonal antibodies to the CMV lower matrix protein, a 65-kilodalton phosphoprotein designated pp65.[19]

The pp65 antigenemia assay has several practical attributes. First, it requires only about 5 hours to perform, so results can be available the same day the specimen is obtained. Second, it is more sensitive than viral culture for detecting the presence of CMV in the blood.[20-23] Third, it can be quantitative, providing a measure of the intensity of infection. Commercial kits are now available for performing the pp65 antigenemia assay, although many laboratories have also performed the assay using components that they assembled themselves. The commercial kits currently licensed in the United States are CMV Brite (Biotest Diagnostics, Denville, NJ) for immunofluorescence and CMV-vue (Incstar, Stillwater, Minn) for immunoperoxidase. The current licensure is only for qualitative testing. Both these kits use the monoclonal antibodies C10 and C11.[24]

Performance of the assay begins with isolation of leukocytes from whole blood, usually by dextran sedimentation. The leukocytes are then counted using a hemocytometer or a Coulter counter, and a standardized number (usually 50,000 to 200,000) are spotted onto a microscope slide by cytocentrifugation or by spotting a drop of cell suspension onto the slide and allowing the cells to settle. The cells are fixed with formaldehyde or paraformaldehyde, which have been shown to be more effective than acetone or acetone-methanol,[17, 22, 25] and permeabilized by treatment with the nonionic detergent Nonidet P-40. FA or IP staining is performed using the appropriate monoclonal antibody and detection system, and the stained slides are viewed by microscopy to detect antigenic foci. To obtain a quantitative result, the antigenic foci are counted and expressed in relation to the number of cells spotted on the slide as antigenic foci per 200,000 cells. Several studies suggest that the number of foci is affected by the anti-pp65 monoclonal antibody used, with several other monoclonals yielding higher totals than the C10 and C11 antibodies.[17, 23, 26, 27] Because many variables may affect the number of antigenic foci detected, comparisons of quantitative data obtained in different laboratories can be difficult.

The predominant cell in which pp65 antigen is detected is the *polymorphonuclear neutrophil leukocyte* (PMN, Figure 15–1). The detection of CMV pp65 in circulating leukocytes indicates active infection and is closely associated with significant disease, although

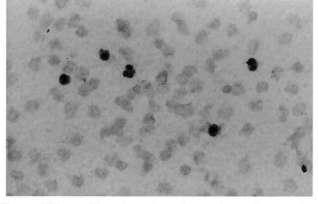

Figure 15.1 pp65 antigen in polymorphonuclear neutrophils (PMNs) demonstrated by immunoperoxidase staining.

asymptomatic antigenemia may occur after organ transplantation or in AIDS. Levels of antigenemia in patients with asymptomatic infection are usually low.[28-31] The question of whether the antigen detected represents replicating virus within the cell or ingested viral particles is controversial, but CMV immediate-early and late transcripts have been detected in PMNS,[32, 33] indicating that CMV can replicate within these cells. pp65 has also been detected in circulating endothelial cells. Some investigators have suggested that this finding indicates organ involvement,[34, 35] but the association has not been corroborated by others.[36]

Transport and processing of specimens for the pp65 antigenemia assay are important steps. Ethylenediaminetetraacetic acid (EDTA), heparin, or acid-citrate-dextrose (ACD) blood collection tubes have been shown to be suitable.[37, 38] The CMV-Brite kit specifies use of heparin or EDTA tubes, and the CMV-vue kit specifies use of EDTA tubes. Prompt transport is required because of degradation of the pp65 antigen. The degree of degradation is modest; for example, the number of antigenic foci has been shown to decrease by 13% to 62% in 24 hours.[25, 39, 40] This does not usually result in failure to detect pp65 antigenemia unless the level of antigenemia is very low, but it can affect the accuracy of quantitation, especially when the level of antigenemia is being monitored in serial specimens. For delays of greater than 24 hours, storage at 4°C is preferred. Reasonable processing guidelines for qualitative testing are that blood specimens should be processed within 24 hours whenever possible and always within 48 hours. For quantitative testing, processing should take place within 6 to 8 hours of collection.

Polymerase chain reaction. One of the early applications of PCR in diagnostic virology was for the detection of CMV. PCR has been used to detect CMV DNA in a wide variety of body fluids, including blood, urine, BAL fluid, ocular fluid, and CSF. Testing of blood is most relevant for the diagnosis of systemic CMV infection. A number of different CMV genes have been used as the target for amplification. For diagnostic purposes the most important criteria for selecting an amplification target within the CMV genome are that (1) the primer binding sites allow amplification only of CMV DNA, and (2) those sites are conserved across different strains so that all strains are detected. PCR and other nucleic acid amplification techniques are the most sensitive means for detecting the presence of CMV in patient specimens, and therefore their use may exacerbate the problem of differentiating between presence of CMV and CMV disease.

A fundamental issue concerning the application of PCR to the detection of CMV in blood is whether PCR detects CMV DNA in the blood of individuals with latent CMV. CMV can be transmitted by blood transfusion from donors with latent CMV infection, indicating that CMV genomes must be present in peripheral blood of at least some normal individuals. Although some studies have reported positive PCR results in normal CMV-seropositive and CMV-seronegative individuals, more recent studies have detected CMV DNA only in the blood of patients with active infection.[41, 42] This has also been the experience in our laboratory. CMV DNA cannot be detected in the blood of normal individuals with latent infection probably because the frequency of latently infected cells is too low to be detected by typical PCR protocol, which usually involves testing of 100,000 to 1 million leukocytes.

The extreme sensitivity of PCR is both its main advantage and a potential disadvantage. Although a positive PCR of leukocytes is unusual in individuals who do not have active CMV infection, detection of CMV DNA in blood does not correlate well with symptomatic infection. Quantitative PCR methods probably will be necessary to improve the relationship between PCR and symptomatic disease. At present, qualitative PCR performed on blood is largely limited to two applications. First, it can provide the earliest detection of CMV after solid organ or bone marrow transplantation (see following sections). Second, when systemic CMV is a concern, a negative PCR performed on blood has high negative predictive value for ruling out systemic CMV disease.

Another issue relates to which component of blood should be used to perform PCR. Peripheral blood leukocytes, plasma, serum, and whole blood have all been used. The largest experience to date is with peripheral blood leukocytes. The question of whether presence of CMV in plasma or serum is a unique indicator of active infection has not been resolved.

Studies have also reported on detection of CMV DNA in serum[43, 44] or plasma.[45-50] The levels of CMV DNA in leukocytes and plasma are correlated, with higher levels in leukocytes.[47, 51, 52] As expected, several studies have shown lower sensitivity for plasma assays than for leukocyte-based assays.[48, 50, 52, 53] Plasma or serum may be preferable when lower sensitivity is desired and in leukopenic patients, who may have inadequate leukocytes for sensitive detection of PCR.[50]

Reverse-transcription polymerase chain reaction. RT-PCR distinguishes between active and latent infection by using PCR or other amplification techniques to detect CMV ribonucleic acid (RNA) rather than DNA. This approach is based on the concept that many CMV genes, especially those encoding structural proteins, are transcribed during active infection but not during latency. Thus detection of these specific CMV RNA sequences indicates active infection. The use of PCR to detect RNA requires the use of *reverse transcriptase* to convert the target RNA into its complementary DNA (cDNA), which can serve as a substrate for PCR.

Other amplification reactions, such as *nucleic acid sequence–based amplification* (NASBA), can be used as alternatives to RT-PCR for detection of CMV RNA. The

NASBA technique is used for measurement of human immunodeficiency virus (HIV) RNA (see Chapter 17). RNA detection reactions have more stringent requirements for specimen handling and processing because of the much greater lability of RNA compared with DNA.

A potential concern with any specific RNA detection assay is whether the amplified product truly indicates the presence of the specific RNA in the specimen or whether it could result from amplification of DNA that was also present in the initial reaction mixture. With RT-PCR the standard approach to this problem is to treat nucleic acid from the specimen with deoxyribonuclease (DNase) before the amplification reaction is carried out, to inactivate any contaminating DNA. In addition, a control reaction in which the RT step is omitted can be performed. Another innovative approach is to select as the target for amplification a CMV RNA molecule that is produced after splicing of the template DNA.[54] Using this approach, the size of the final amplified product distinguishes between product amplified from spliced RNA (shorter length) and that from contaminating DNA (longer length).

Several reports describing detection of CMV RNA in peripheral blood leukocytes have appeared,[54-60] but these assays are not yet in use in clinical laboratories. A commercial NASBA assay to detect CMV RNA is under development but is not yet available. No clinical studies have yet been performed to assess the relative detection capability of CMV RNA versus DNA.

bDNA and hybrid capture assays. Two assays for direct detection of specific nucleic acid segments that rely on amplification of *signal* rather than amplification of target nucleic acid have been applied to the detection of CMV DNA. The branched-chain DNA (bDNA) assay (Bayer Diagnostics, Emeryville, Calif) has been extensively used to measure HIV RNA (see Chapter 17). It has not yet been evaluated for CMV.

The hybrid capture assay (Hybrid Capture System, Digene Corporation, Silver Spring, Md) is a novel technique for the detection of specific DNA that has been applied to several viruses, including CMV, human papillomavirus (HPV), and hepatitis B virus (HBV). The assay provides direct detection of specific DNA and can also provide quantitative information on DNA in the specimen. Results can be available in 1 day. The hybrid capture assay for CMV was recently licensed by the U.S. Food and Drug Administration (FDA) for the qualitative detection of CMV. The same assay is marketed in Europe (Murex Diagnostics, Dartford, UK).

The hybrid capture assay is performed on whole blood collected in EDTA or ACD tubes (see Figure 1-10). A 3.5-ml aliquot of blood is treated with a lysing agent to release and denature CMV DNA from leukocytes. A mixture of RNA probes complementary to 17% of the CMV genome is added to the lysed specimen, then incubated under conditions that allow hybridiza-

tion with any CMV DNA present in the specimen, resulting in the formation of RNA-DNA hybrid molecules. Hybrids are captured by an antibody, which is bound to the walls of the reaction tubes and recognizes DNA-RNA hybrids. Captured hybrids are then detected using an alkaline phosphatase–labeled antibody to RNA-DNA hybrids plus a chemiluminescent substrate. The resulting light emission is read in a luminometer. Several alkaline phosphatase molecules are bound to each antibody molecule, and multiple enzyme-conjugated antibody molecules are bound to each RNA-DNA hybrid. This results in amplification of the signal generated from detection of hybrids.

Because the total amount of light emitted is proportional to the amount of CMV DNA present in the specimen, the hybrid capture assay can be used to estimate the amount of CMV DNA present in the specimen. In the quantitative assay the result is expressed as picograms (pg) of CMV DNA per milliliter or CMV genomes per milliliter. To convert from pg/ml to genomes/ml, the result in pg/ml is multiplied by 689. The limit of detection of the first-generation hybrid capture assay was 5000 copies/ml of whole blood, which has been reduced to 700 copies for a second-generation assay.[61] A concern regarding the quantitative assay is that the assay is performed on a constant volume of blood without regard to the leukocyte count, potentially causing variability in the measurement of CMV DNA in blood, most of which is in leukocytes.

Only limited information is available on the clinical performance of the CMV hybrid capture assay, especially the licensed second-generation assay. The first-generation assay was more sensitive than culture but less sensitive than the pp65 antigenemia assay or PCR.[62-64] Levels of DNA detected by the first-generation hybrid capture assay correlated closely with levels of pp65 antigenemia.[62, 65] The second-generation assay appears to have sensitivity comparable to the pp65 antigenemia assay.[66] The assay has been used to monitor DNA levels in renal,[67] liver,[68] and bone marrow transplant[64] recipients (see later discussion).

Quantitation of Blood Level

Quantitation of the level of CMV in blood has been proposed as a means to distinguish between significant and nonsignificant infection and to assess the response to treatment. Numerous studies in organ transplant recipients and AIDS patients using quantitative culture techniques, the pp65 antigenemia assay, the hybrid capture assay, and quantitative PCR show a statistical relationship between higher CMV blood levels and significant disease.* This is a strong but not absolute relationship, and levels of CMV in patients with symptomatic and asymptomatic infection overlap. CMV

---

*References 28, 52, 61, 64, 65, 67–76.

levels decline with effective therapy, and persistent high levels have been associated with antiviral drug resistance.[77] Similarly, a slowly declining CMV level after initiation of therapy has been proposed as an early warning of antiviral resistance.[71]

Each of the assays used for direct detection of CMV can provide quantitative data. Quantitation of antigenemia using the pp65 assay or of infectious viremia using the shell vial assay is achieved by determining the number of cells analyzed and the number of positive foci detected. Unfortunately, the pp65 antigenemia assay has the following relative disadvantages as a quantitative measure:

1. Lability of the pp65 antigen imposes strict handling requirements for accurate quantitation.
2. Failure of a proportion of leukocytes to adhere to the microscope slide can affect the accuracy of quantitation, and current methods do not evaluate the actual number of cells examined.
3. Range of values detected is relatively narrow.
4. Quantitation by the antigenemia assay is laborious and potentially subjective because it requires counting of antigenic foci by microscopy.

The quantitative shell vial assay[8] has some of the same disadvantages as the antigenemia assay. Nucleic acid–based detection methods, including PCR and the hybrid capture assay, are the most promising. The advantages of these assays include stability of DNA[14, 78] and a large range of measurable values.[69] These advantages are being realized in the successful widespread use of quantitative RT-PCR assays for measurement of HIV and hepatitis C virus (HCV) RNA (see Chapters 8 and 17). Although quantitative PCR assays for CMV are not yet standardized and cutoffs for defining significant infection not yet well defined, these assays likely will have an important role in future management strategies for CMV infection.

Diagnosis after Bone Marrow Transplantation

CMV is the most important opportunistic infection in patients who undergo bone marrow transplantation. Without prophylactic antiviral therapy, approximately 50% of all allogeneic transplant recipients develop active infection, and approximately 20% to 25% develop symptomatic CMV disease.[79] CMV seropositivity of either the recipient or the donor is a risk factor. The risks of both CMV infection and disease are much lower after autologous transplantation. The highest risk period occurs shortly after engraftment, during the second and third months after the transplant. CMV infections during the preengraftment period and long after the high-risk period are also increasingly recognized.

Frequent manifestations of CMV infection after bone marrow transplantation include fever and malaise, often accompanied by leukopenia and thrombocytope-

nia. CMV pneumonia is a common complication and is associated with a high fatality rate. Other common sites of localized involvement infection are the GI tract and liver.

Antiviral agents with activity against CMV, especially ganciclovir, have greatly improved the outcome of CMV infection in the bone marrow transplant (BMT) recipient. Current efforts are directed at prophylactic and preemptive regimens to minimize CMV-related morbidity and mortality.

Relationship between virologic findings and CMV disease. The purpose of testing for CMV in the BMT recipient may be to diagnose current CMV disease or to identify patients at risk of future CMV disease so that they can receive preemptive therapy. For either purpose, an understanding of the temporal relationship between viral detection and occurrence of CMV disease manifestations is important (Figure 15–2).

An important principle is that virologic events precede clinical manifestations. Engraftment occurs approximately 3 weeks after transplantation, and CMV is usually first detected in the ensuing weeks. PCR performed on leukocytes is the first test to become positive, followed by the pp65 antigenemia assay, then by culture. Quantitative aspects of CMV viremia have not been as well studied in BMT recipients as in solid organ transplant recipients (see later discussion) because any detection of viremia in BMT recipients has usually led to initiation of antiviral therapy. The CMV viral load may be lower in BMT recipients than in solid organ transplant recipients or in AIDS patients.[80]

Diagnostic tests for CMV in BMT recipients are described next, and Table 15–6 lists preferred tests for various purposes.

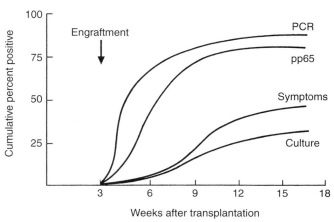

Figure 15.2 Temporal relationship between onset of symptoms and diagnostic tests for CMV in bone marrow transplant recipients, showing cumulative percentage of patients positive for each diagnostic test by week after transplantation. *PCR*, Polymerase chain reaction; *pp65*, antigenemia assay.

Table 15.6	Preferred Tests for CMV Diagnosis and Surveillance in Bone Marrow Transplant Recipients

Purpose of diagnostic test	Preferred test(s)
Diagnosis of current disease	
CMV syndrome	pp65 antigenemia assay or leukocyte (buffy coat) culture
Pneumonia	Histology of lung tissue or culture of broncho-alveolar lavage (BAL) fluid
Gastrointestinal tract	Histology and culture of mucosal tissue
Surveillance	Leukocyte polymerase chain reaction (PCR)

Viral culture. The evolution of viral cultures after bone marrow transplantation has been thoroughly described by Myers et al[79] at the Fred Hutchinson Cancer Research Center in Seattle. In their experience, cultures of blood, urine, and oropharyngeal secretions typically became positive 7 to 8 weeks after transplantation, approximately 14 days before the onset of localized disease manifestations (e.g., pneumonia). Blood cultures were more useful than cultures of other specimens for distinguishing between patients with and without symptomatic CMV disease, but they were still not completely satisfactory. The sensitivity, specificity, positive predictive value, and negative predictive value of serial blood cultures for invasive disease were 45%, 92%, 60%, and 86%, respectively. Thus, although a positive blood culture identified a patient as being at increased risk of invasive CMV disease (relative risk 5.5), the predictive value was low, and more than half the patients who developed invasive disease were not identified by detection of viremia. The discriminatory power of a positive blood culture for identifying patients at risk for invasive disease could be greatly increased by simultaneous consideration of clinical risk factors, such as graft-versus-host (GVH) disease, CMV seropositivity, and older age. The relative risk of CMV pneumonia in patients with viremia plus these risk factors compared with patients without viremia, and none of the risk factors was greater than 50.

pp65 antigenemia assay and PCR. The use of the pp65 antigenemia assay and PCR have both been investigated extensively in BMT recipients.[18, 81, 82] The pp65 antigenemia assay is clearly more sensitive than viral blood culture[18] but is not always positive before the onset of symptomatic CMV disease.[82] In contrast, PCR performed on leukocytes has had 100% sensitivity for

detection of symptomatic disease in several studies.[48, 80-85] The predictive value of a positive PCR result for CMV disease in these studies was 45% to 67%. PCR is almost always positive 10 days or more before the onset of symptoms, providing an opportunity to begin pre-emptive antiviral therapy. Experience with plasma PCR is limited but suggests that the sensitivity is similar to that of the pp65 antigenemia assay.[46, 48, 50] Plasma PCR is of special interest in patients with very low leukocyte counts in whom leukocyte PCR or the pp65 antigenemia assay may be insensitive.[50]

Diagnosis of current disease. CMV disease after bone marrow transplantation can produce systemic and localized disease manifestations. Unfortunately, no one test is ideal for the current diagnosis of symptomatic systemic disease. When localized disease is present, analysis of specimens from the site of disease is the best approach.

Systemic infection. Culture of the blood is neither sensitive nor specific and can be slow if conventional tube culture is being used. The pp65 antigenemia assay and PCR performed on blood are more sensitive but have positive predictive values of 50% or lower. Quantitative PCR or plasma PCR may improve the specificity for diagnosis of current disease, but further studies are required to document this. Serologic testing is not useful for the diagnosis of current disease because (1) some patients, especially those with the most severe illness, may not have a serologic response; (2) it may be difficult to distinguish current from past infection; and (3) the serologic response may lag behind the occurrence of disease.

Pneumonia. Biopsy of lung tissue and BAL fluid have both been evaluated extensively for the diagnosis of CMV pneumonia in BMT recipients. Histologic examination of lung tissue is the gold standard but may not be the most sensitive method. Open lung biopsy has greater sensitivity than transbronchial biopsy for histologic examination because of the larger tissue sample available for examination.[85] A number of other techniques can increase the sensitivity of detection of CMV in tissue samples, including detection of CMV antigens and DNA in lung tissue by immunohistochemistry (IHC) or in situ hybridization (ISH),[86-88] viral culture,[86, 89] and PCR.[90] The lack of histologic evidence of CMV pneumonia in some BMT patients may represent sampling error but in others may indicate low-level viral replication in the absence of CMV pneumonia.

BAL fluid is sometimes used in place of or in addition to biopsy to evaluate possible CMV pneumonia in BMT recipients. In one study of BMT recipients with pulmonary infiltrates, shell vial and conventional cultures of BAL fluid correlated closely with cultures of lung tissue obtained at open lung biopsy or autopsy.[91]

Culture results also correlated closely with histologic evidence of CMV pneumonia, although one patient who had positive cultures of both BAL fluid and lung tissue had histologic evidence of *Pneumocystis carinii* pneumonia without evidence of CMV pneumonia. FA staining and cytology of the same BAL fluid had sensitivities of only 29% and 59%, respectively, compared with conventional culture of lung tissue.[91]

PCR has also been used to detect CMV in BAL fluid from BMT recipients with pneumonia. In one study, PCR had a sensitivity of 100% but a low positive predictive value for CMV pneumonia.[92] The results of this study suggested that a negative PCR on BAL fluid may be useful for ruling out the diagnosis of CMV pneumonia.

If BAL is performed on BMT recipients without pneumonia, CMV is sometimes detected but does not necessarily signify the presence of current CMV pneumonia.[93] These patients are at risk for subsequent CMV pneumonia.[93, 94]

Gastrointestinal tract disease. Diagnosis of CMV disease of the GI tract in the BMT recipient is best accomplished using specimens obtained through endoscopic visualization. Because of the small samples obtained, both histology and culture should be performed. Adequate sensitivity requires the presence of subepithelial tissue in the biopsy, since CMV infection occurs in the underlying stroma rather than the epithelial lining of the esophagus. In a recent study, culture was the most sensitive method of detection, followed by IHC, then histology.[95]

Prediction of future disease. Recently, prophylactic and preemptive therapeutic programs have been evaluated to prevent symptomatic CMV infection in BMT recipients. Preemptive approaches require a diagnostic test that can identify patients at risk of CMV disease so that they can receive antiviral therapy before illness occurs. In the first major studies of preemptive therapy, viral cultures of blood or BAL fluid were used as triggers for starting therapy. Although the regimens studied decreased the frequency of CMV disease, they were not completely successful because some patients developed CMV disease without a preceding positive culture.[79, 94, 96]

The poor performance of culture for initiating preemptive therapy stimulated efforts to use instead the pp65 antigenemia assay and PCR. In one extensive evaluation the performance of the antigenemia assay was disappointing.[82] Patients were monitored weekly using the antigenemia assay and treated with ganciclovir for a positive culture or for antigenemia exceeding three positive cells per two slides (corresponding to one positive cell per 100,000 cells examined). Four of 10 patients with CMV disease before day 100 after transplantation developed their disease before the antigen-

emia assay was positive. Four additional patients progressed from low-level antigenemia to symptomatic CMV disease before treatment was started. Progression was significantly associated with the presence of GVH disease. In the same study, leukocyte PCR was always positive before the onset of either high-grade antigenemia or clinical disease.

In contrast, the use of PCR-based preemptive therapy has been demonstrated to reduce the incidence of CMV disease in BMT recipients.[75, 97, 98] The implication is that PCR is the best assay on which to base preemptive CMV treatment regimens in BMT recipients. The relative value of plasma, leukocytes, and whole blood as the specimen on which PCR is performed requires further study.

Future strategies may employ both quantitation of CMV load and assessment of CMV risk, with different virologic thresholds for initiating treatment based on the presence of other risk factors such as GVH disease.[98] For example, in a patient with significant GVH disease, any detection of CMV would lead to the initiation of therapy, whereas in a patient without GVH disease, therapy might be initiated only after a specific quantitative threshold (not yet defined) were exceeded.

Diagnosis after Solid Organ Transplantation

CMV is the most common opportunistic infection in recipients of solid organ transplants. Active CMV infection occurs in 60% to 100% of solid organ transplant recipients when either the donor or recipient is CMV seropositive before transplantation. Symptomatic disease occurs in 20% to 60% in the absence of prophylactic treatment.[99] As in BMT recipients, most cases occur in the second and third months after transplantation.

The clinical manifestations typically include a mononucleosis-like syndrome characterized by fever, leukopenia, thrombocytopenia, and abnormal liver function tests, often referred to as *CMV syndrome.* Pneumonia, GI tract involvement, and hepatitis may also occur, whereas retinitis and CNS involvement are rare. The transplanted organ is frequently involved, especially in lung, liver, and intestinal transplants. This may in part reflect frequent biopsy of the transplanted organ to monitor for rejection. CMV-seronegative recipients who receive organs from CMV-seropositive donors are at the highest risk for symptomatic CMV disease, followed by CMV-seropositive recipients of organs from CMV-seropositive donors. Increased immunosuppression is also a risk factor for symptomatic disease.

Ganciclovir is used to treat symptomatic infection and is also increasingly used in prophylactic or preemptive regimens designed to prevent symptomatic CMV infection.[100, 101] These regimens include prophylactic treatment before any evidence of infection is present, preemptive treatment triggered by a positive test before the onset of symptoms, and preemptive treatment given during periods of increased immunosuppressive medications used to treat allograft rejection.

Relationship between virologic findings and CMV disease. The principles governing the diagnosis of CMV infection in solid organ transplant recipients are largely similar to those described for BMT recipients. One difference is that primary CMV infection, which occurs when a CMV-seropositive donor organ is transplanted into a CMV-seronegative recipient, is an important risk factor for severe disease in solid organ transplant recipients. Although GVH disease is not a consideration in these patients, augmented immunosuppression used to treat allograft rejection is a risk factor for CMV disease.

Viremia occurs several weeks after transplantation, usually preceding the onset of CMV-related symptoms (Figure 15–3). The presence of CMV in blood can be detected earliest by PCR performed on leukocytes, followed by the pp65 antigenemia assay, then by culture.[20, 28, 102, 103] CMV-specific IgM antibodies are not detected until after the onset of symptoms in most patients.[104] The level of viremia is initially low but rises over several weeks, reaching peak levels that vary widely from patient to patient.[69, 71] Some patients have peak levels exceeding 100,000 genomes/10^5 leukocytes, as measured by quantitative PCR, or 1000 antigenic foci/10^5 leukocytes, as measured by the pp65 antigenemia assay. CMV-related symptoms tend to occur at or shortly before the peak level. Although patients with CMV disease tend to have higher levels than patients with asymptomatic infection, exceptions exist. Some patients develop CMV-related symptoms at relatively low levels, and some patients with high levels remain asymptomatic.[28, 71]

Diagnostic tests for CMV in solid organ transplant recipients are discussed next, and Table 15–7 lists preferred tests for various purposes.

Viral culture. In three studies that performed serial cultures on blood specimens from kidney and liver transplant recipients, the sensitivity, specificity, positive predictive value, and negative predictive value for symptomatic CMV disease were 56% to 61%, 47% to 88%, 42% to 46%, and 53% to 93%, respectively.[104-106] Blood cultures were more valuable than cultures of urine or oropharyngeal secretions because blood cultures became positive earlier and could better distinguish between symptomatic and asymptomatic patients. In one study, for example, patients with positive blood cultures had a relative risk of developing symptomatic disease of 7.1, compared with 2.1 for positive urine culture and 1.8 for positive throat swab culture.[105]

pp65 antigenemia assay and PCR. PCR performed on leukocytes and the pp65 antigenemia assay provide earlier and faster detection of viremia than blood cultures. Both assays are positive in almost all patients with symptomatic CMV infection, usually before the onset of symptoms. PCR is the most sensitive and becomes positive earlier than the antigenemia assay in most patients. Both assays are frequently positive in patients with asymptomatic infection as well as in those with CMV disease and thus have low positive predictive power.* The use of a specific antigenemia threshold such as 10 or 20 foci/100,000 cells increases the specificity and discriminatory power of the antigenemia assay but decreases the sensitivity.[31] Likewise, quantitative PCR may be capable of better discrimination

---

*References 20, 28, 65, 73, 102, 103

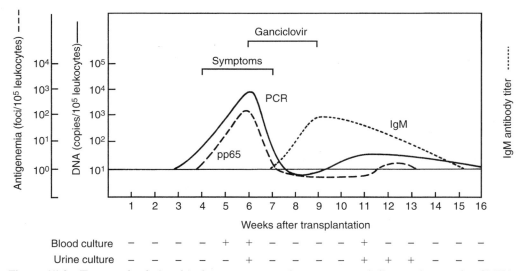

Figure 15.3 Temporal relationship between onset of symptoms and diagnostic tests for CMV in solid organ transplant recipients. *PCR*, Polymerase chain reaction; *pp65*, antigenemia assay; *IgM*, immunoglobulin M.

Table 15.7	Preferred Tests for CMV Diagnosis and Surveillance in Solid Organ Transplant Recipients

Purpose of diagnostic test	Preferred test(s)
Diagnosis of current disease	
CMV syndrome	pp65 antigenemia assay or leukocyte (buffy coat) culture
Pneumonia	Histology of lung tissue
Hepatitis	Histology of liver tissue
Enteritis	Histology and culture of intestinal mucosa
Surveillance	Leukocyte plasma polymerase chain reaction (PCR), hybrid capture assay, or pp65 antigenemia assay

between those with symptomatic and asymptomatic infection.[69, 71]

Diagnosis of current disease. As in BMT recipients, CMV disease after solid organ transplantation can be systemic and/or localized. The diagnosis of systemic disease is based on clinical suspicion and supported by the detection of CMV in the blood (see following discussion). The diagnosis of localized CMV infection is based on detecting histologic evidence of CMV in involved tissue. Many patients with localized CMV infection also have CMV in the blood, but analysis of tissue from the organ itself provides more specific evidence of CMV involvement of that organ. Frequently, the transplanted organ is the site of possible CMV infection. In these patients the manifestations of infection and those of graft rejection can be similar. Accurate diagnosis is crucial because the therapeutic approaches for infection and rejection are diametrically opposed. Infection requires antiviral therapy, with decreased immunosuppression if possible. In contrast, rejection requires augmentation of immunosuppression, which could worsen viral infection.

Systemic infection. No diagnostic test is ideal for the diagnosis of systemic CMV infection without organ localization (CMV syndrome). Cultures of blood are neither sensitive nor specific, since (1) single blood cultures are often negative in patients with symptomatic disease, and (2) if repeated blood cultures are performed, viremia is often detected in asymptomatic patients. Positive blood cultures, however, have a relatively high predictive value for current or impending disease in the first 3 months after transplantation when symptomatic infection is common.[104]

The pp65 antigenemia assay and PCR performed on leukocytes are almost always positive in patients with symptomatic disease but are also frequently positive in those without symptoms, resulting in a low positive predictive value but a high negative predictive value in the early posttransplant period. PCR may remain positive for a long period after first becoming positive, and thus its value for the diagnosis of current disease is even lower after the first few months after transplant.

In practice the diagnosis of CMV syndrome is often made on the basis of clinical suspicion when fever occurs in the second or third month after transplantation in the absence of other causes. As described earlier, the role of specific viral studies is to support the diagnosis, with failure to demonstrate CMV suggesting that other causes should be sought.

Pneumonia. CMV pneumonia is common in lung or heart-lung transplant recipients but unusual in recipients of other solid organ transplants. In lung transplant recipients, BAL and transbronchial biopsies are performed at regular intervals after transplantation to monitor for rejection and infection. Histologic evidence of CMV pneumonia is the most important criterion for the diagnosis of CMV pneumonia. Since the individual biopsy specimens obtained by transbronchial biopsy are small, the sensitivity of histologic diagnosis of either rejection or infection depends on performing multiple biopsies. A total of 10 biopsies is considered acceptable for the diagnosis of rejection and also provides ample material for diagnosis of infection.[107]

IP staining to detect CMV antigens may be helpful in selected cases that are suspicious but nondiagnostic, but routine screening by IP staining does not greatly increase the overall yield.[108, 109] Culture of biopsy tissue does not provide additional useful information. Culture of BAL fluid is often positive in the absence of histologic evidence of CMV pneumonia. In one study the predictive value of a positive BAL culture for histologic CMV pneumonia was 81% in the first 3 months after lung transplantation but only 5% thereafter.[110] Positive blood cultures were present in 26 of 28 lung transplant recipients with CMV pneumonia in one study. Patients with CMV pneumonia had higher levels of virus in blood than patients without pneumonia, but with considerable overlap.[72]

Hepatitis. In liver transplant patients, biopsy of the transplanted liver is performed at regular intervals to diagnose rejection or infection. Histology is the gold standard for the diagnosis of CMV hepatitis. CMV culture of biopsy tissue is less sensitive and is not routinely required.[111] Detection of CMV antigens in liver tissue by IP staining is more sensitive than conventional histology.[112-114] In contrast, detection of CMV DNA by ISH has not been shown to be more sensitive than histology.[112, 113, 115] PCR performed on liver tissue is both sensitive and specific for CMV hepatitis and can sometimes allow earlier diagnosis than histology.[116, 117] In one study, 9 of 13 patients with CMV hepatitis had positive blood cultures, and all 13 had positive urine cultures.[111]

Enteritis. Histology is also more sensitive than viral culture for diagnosis of CMV enteritis occurring after small intestinal transplantation. In one study, PCR performed on small intestinal biopsy specimens was more sensitive than histology, allowing earlier diagnosis after transplantation. Most episodes of CMV enteritis were not associated with detection of CMV in blood by shell vial culture.[118]

Prediction of future disease. The pp65 antigenemia assay, PCR, and possibly the hybrid capture assay are better suited than viral culture for prediction of future disease to initiate preemptive therapy. Any of these assays probably can be used, with PCR providing a longer interval between detection and onset of symptoms but at the price of lower specificity. As in BMT recipients, diagnostic tests may be used in conjunction with risk-adapted approaches for solid organ recipients. For example, high-risk patients might be screened with a qualitative PCR or antigenemia assay and receive antiviral therapy if any CMV is detected, whereas low-risk patients might be monitored with a quantitative test and receive treatment only when the level of viremia exceeds a specific threshold (not currently defined).

Diagnosis in AIDS Patients

CMV is one of the most important causes of opportunistic infection in patients with AIDS. In the era before highly active antiretroviral therapy, approximately 40% of AIDS patients experienced serious CMV infection during their illness.[119] With protease inhibitor therapy, however, the frequency of invasive CMV infections has decreased sharply. Most symptomatic disease occurs in individuals with far-advanced HIV infection and CD4+ counts less than 100 cells/mm^3.[120] The most common manifestations are retinitis, GI tract manifestations (e.g., colitis, esophagitis), hepatitis, pneumonia, radiculomyelitis, and encephalitis.

Diagnostic tests for CMV in patients with AIDS are discussed next, and Table 15–8 lists preferred tests for various purposes.

Tests in HIV-infected patients. The diagnosis of symptomatic CMV disease is complicated by the high prevalence of positive CMV tests in patients with advanced HIV. More than 90% of HIV-infected adults are CMV seropositive.[119] In a longitudinal study of CMV in homosexual males, CMV IgM antibodies were detected intermittently in 95% of men who were positive for CMV immunoglobulin G (IgG).[121] In a recent study from Denmark, 5.5% of HIV-seropositive individuals

Table 15.8	Preferred Tests for CMV Diagnosis and Surveillance in AIDS Patients
Purpose of diagnostic test	**Preferred test(s)**
Diagnosis of current disease	
CMV syndrome	pp65 antigenemia assay or leukocyte (buffy coat) culture
Pneumonia	Histology of lung tissue or culture of broncho-alveolar lavage (BAL) fluid*
Gastrointestinal tract	Histology of mucosal biopsy
Nervous system	PCR of cerebrospinal fluid
Retinitis	Clinical diagnosis (PCR of vitreous or aqueous fluid when clinical features are atypical)
Surveillance	Quantitative plasma or leukocyte PCR (investigational)

PCR, Polymerase chain reaction.
*Culture of BAL fluid in a patient who is not receiving anti CMV drugs has a low positive predictive value but a high negative predictive value for CMV pneumonitis.

with CD4+ counts less than 100 cells/mm^3 had CMV IgM antibodies.[122] Since individuals with HIV have been shown to be infected with multiple strains of CMV, the presence of CMV-specific IgM antibodies may signify recent infection with a new strain. The prevalence of positive cultures depends greatly on the degree of HIV-associated immunosuppression. In asymptomatic individuals with CD4+ lymphocyte counts greater than 100 cells/mm^3, positive urine cultures are found in approximately 10%[123] and positive blood cultures in 1% to 2%.[123, 124] In individuals with CD4+ counts less than 100 cells/mm^3, positive urine cultures have been reported in 42% to 70% and positive blood cultures in 2% to 41%.[123-126] The large range in these estimates results from whether or not studies included patients with symptomatic CMV infection. Approximately 10% to 30% of asymptomatic individuals with CD4+ counts less than 100 are positive by the pp65 antigenemia assay,[127, 128] and 20% to 60% are positive by PCR performed on leukocytes, serum, or plasma.[70, 129-131]

Diagnosis of current disease. CMV infection in AIDS patients most often presents as localized infection. Laboratory diagnosis of each of the forms of localized CMV disease depends on demonstrating the presence of CMV at the site of disease. Urine cultures, blood cultures, the pp65 antigenemia assay, PCR (on leukocytes, plasma, or serum), and serology are all of little use because of the high prevalence in asymptomatic individuals described earlier.

Retinitis and neurologic disease. CMV retinitis is usually diagnosed by clinical examination (see Chapter 10). PCR analysis of aqueous or vitreous fluid can be used to provide a laboratory diagnosis in occasional patients with unusual clinical features for whom the ophthalmologic examination is not diagnostic. CMV disease of the nervous system includes encephalitis, radiculomyelitis, and peripheral neuritis. CMV encephalitis and radiculomyelitis are effectively diagnosed by performing PCR on CSF (see Chapter 3).

Gastrointestinal tract disease. CMV can produce symptomatic infection at any level of the GI tract from the mouth to the rectum. Involvement of the esophagus, stomach, and colon are most common. Neither the symptoms nor the endoscopic appearance are specific for CMV. In attempting to diagnose CMV colitis, endoscopic examination of the entire colon is important, since up to 39% of cases may be limited to the cecum.[132, 133]

The standard for laboratory diagnosis is histologic examination of involved tissue obtained by endoscopic biopsy under direct visualization. CMV inclusions can be detected in a variety of cell types within lesions, including endothelial cells, fibroblasts, smooth muscle cells, macrophages, and epithelial cells.[134, 135] In CMV esophagitis, infection is limited to stromal cells rather than squamous epithelial cells, and thus it is important to biopsy the bed of ulcerative lesions.[136] Cells with characteristic inclusions can be difficult to locate and atypical in appearance.[137, 138] Therefore the sensitivity of histology depends greatly on the number of biopsy specimens examined and the pathologist's experience and diligence. Because endoscopic biopsy specimens are small, sampling error can be a problem. In one study, for example, only 13% of separate biopsy specimens from CMV-positive lesions were positive.[139] Examination of 10 separate biopsy specimens has been recommended to minimize sampling error.[140] CMV inclusions are only rarely detected in normal mucosa, even when sampled from patients with CMV lesions elsewhere in the GI tract.[139]

IP staining to detect CMV antigens may facilitate the detection of CMV infection, particularly when the appearance of CMV-infected cells is atypical.[136, 139-141] Use of IP staining has increased the overall detection of CMV in some studies.[136] It may be particularly helpful for pathologists who are less familiar with the histologic appearance of CMV infection. As with histology, IP staining is also subject to sampling error.

ISH and PCR have also been used to detect CMV DNA in biopsy samples from patients with CMV GI disease. ISH can be performed on formalin-fixed tissue.

It can be useful in a manner similar to IP staining for CMV antigens to document CMV infection of cells with atypical inclusions.[138, 142] The drawback of ISH is that it may be positive in biopsies with no histologic evidence of CMV,[143-146] and the clinical significance of this finding is unclear. Use of PCR on GI biopsy specimens increases the sensitivity of detection of CMV GI disease, but it can also be positive in specimens from normal mucosa in patients with CMV GI disease elsewhere.[139, 147] As with ISH, the significance of this finding is unclear, and PCR should still be considered investigational for the diagnosis of CMV GI disease.

The role of viral cultures in the diagnosis of CMV disease of the GI tract is problematic because results do not always correlate with histologic findings. Cultures of lesions are sometimes positive in the absence of histologic evidence of disease.[148] The significance of this finding is unclear, but since many patients with CMV GI disease also have CMV viremia, positive cultures could result from blood contamination of the specimen. Some of these cases, however, may represent significant GI infection in which histology is negative because of sampling error. Cultures can also be negative when histologic findings are diagnostic of CMV infection.[139, 142, 149] Finally, information obtained by culture is often delayed. For these reasons, culture of lesions is not generally recommended. Culture of stool, rectal swabs, or oropharyngeal secretions are likewise not recommended for the diagnosis of CMV GI disease because of poor sensitivity and specificity.[135, 142]

Pneumonia. CMV pneumonia is typically recognized only at autopsy in AIDS patients. Only a small proportion of findings are thought to represent symptomatic CMV pneumonia, however since other pathogens are present in most patients.[150] Another finding that casts doubt on the clinical significance of most CMV respiratory tract infections in patients with AIDS is that patients with *P. carinii* pneumonia who also have CMV detected in BAL fluid do no worse than patients with *P. carinii* alone even when no treatment for CMV is given.[151] Nevertheless, in a minority of those with positive cultures of respiratory specimens, clinically symptomatic CMV pneumonia has been identified, based on the absence of other pathogens and improvement with ganciclovir therapy.[152-154]

The most definitive laboratory evidence of CMV pneumonia is based on histologic examination of lung tissue, supplemented by IHC. A limitation is that tissue samples obtained by transbronchial biopsy are small, and sampling error can lead to failure to identify CMV pneumonia.[155] A positive culture of BAL fluid provides supportive evidence but must be interpreted with caution because positive cultures of BAL fluid occur in patients with AIDS who do not have CMV pneumonia.[150, 156] A negative BAL culture makes the diagnosis of CMV pneumonitis very unlikely.[156] As in patients with other forms of immune compromise, cytology is much less sensitive than culture for detection of CMV pneumonia in AIDS patients.[157, 158] PCR performed on BAL fluid is more sensitive than culture. This finding would not be expected to correlate with histologic evidence of CMV pneumonia. Nevertheless, detection of CMV DNA in BAL fluid by PCR has been shown to predict future extrapulmonary disease.[159]

Prediction of future disease. Diagnostic tests for CMV have been evaluated for their ability to predict future occurrence of symptomatic CMV disease in AIDS patients who are currently asymptomatic. This information could be used to guide the use of oral ganciclovir or other antivirals for prophylaxis of CMV. Oral ganciclovir has been shown to be effective in reducing the incidence of symptomatic CMV infection in HIV-infected patients[126] but is not recommended for routine use because of prohibitive cost.[160]

Tests that have been evaluated for their predictive ability include urine culture, blood culture, pp65 antigenemia assay, and PCR performed on leukocytes, whole blood, or plasma. In one study, qualitative PCR performed on plasma had sensitivity and specificity for future disease of 89% and 75%[161] (Table 15–9). Urine culture had comparable sensitivity but was much less specific. Leukocyte culture was much less sensitive. Increasing the threshold level of plasma DNA increased the specificity of prediction but decreased the sensitivity. Other studies have also shown clear relationships between the level of CMV DNA in plasma[131] or whole blood[70] and the likelihood of future disease (Figure 15–4). A positive antigenemia assay also predicts future disease, but the interval between test positivity and the onset of symptoms is shorter than for PCR.[122] As for PCR-based assays, higher levels of antigenemia are associated with a higher likelihood of future disease.[162]

Although several different assays provide predictive information about future likelihood of CMV disease, the need for such assays will be determined by therapeutic strategies that consider the efficacy, toxicity, and cost-effectiveness of CMV prophylactic therapy.

EPSTEIN-BARR VIRUS

Clinical Manifestations

As a member of the family Herpesviridae, Epstein-Barr virus (EBV) has a life cycle that includes a latent state after acute infection. Latency is maintained by cell-mediated immunity in the host. Disorders of cell-mediated immunity can change the balance between host and virus and may be associated with a variety of EBV-related diseases (Table 15–10). The most recognized disease in immunocompromised patients is *post-transplant lymphoproliferative disorder* (PTLD; see later discussion). *X-linked lymphoproliferative syndrome* is a congenital immunodeficiency selective for EBV in which affected males may experience fatal infectious mononucleosis, hemophagocytic syndrome, lymphoproliferative syndromes (including malignant lymphoma), hypogammaglobulinemia, aplastic anemia, and agranulocytosis. EBV is also associated with nasopharyngeal carcinoma, the African form of Burkitt's lymphoma, and some cases of Hodgkin's disease, but the relationship between these entities and prior immunosuppression is not clear.

Diagnostic Tests

The diagnosis of EBV infection in immunocompromised individuals poses special problems. Serologic testing, the mainstay of diagnosis in normal individuals (see Chapter 12), is usually not useful. Most adults are seropositive as a result of prior EBV infection. In immunocompromised patients the levels of antibodies to the EBV *viral capsid antigen* (VCA) and *early antigen* (EA) may be elevated and levels of antibodies to *Epstein-Barr nuclear antigen* (EBNA) decreased compared with normal individuals,[165] but these findings are

Table 15.9	Test Parameters for Diagnostic Tests Used to Predict Symptomatic CMV Infection in AIDS Patients			
Test	**Sensitivity (%)**	**Specificity (%)**	**Positive predictive value (%)**	**Negative predictive value (%)**
Urine culture	85	29	37	83
Leukocyte culture	42	93	69	81
Plasma PCR	89	75	58	94
Plasma PCR (threshold ≤100 copies/ml)	73	90	73	90
Plasma PCR (threshold ≤1000 copies/ml)	35	100	100	80

Data from Shinkai H, Bossette SA, Powderly W, et al: *J Infect Dis* 175:302, 1997.
PCR, Polymerase chain reaction.

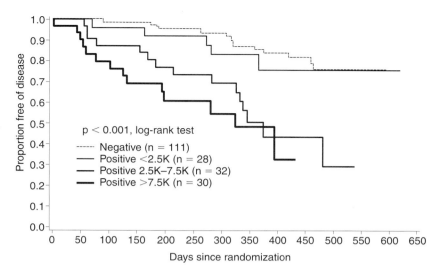

Figure 15.4 Kaplan-Meier curve showing relationship between level of CMV DNA detected in plasma by PCR and development of CMV disease in AIDS patients. *K*, ×1000 CMV DNA copies/ml. (From Spector SA, Wong R, Hsia K, et al: *J Clin Invest* 101:500, 1998.)

rarely diagnostic of current EBV disease in individual patients. Levels of infectious virus detectable by culture may be elevated in EBV-related disease in immunocompromised patients, but the culture method required for EBV is cumbersome and not done in routine diagnostic virology laboratories. Therefore the approach to diagnosis in immunocompromised patients often employs direct detection of EBV antigens or nucleic acids in blood or involved tissues (see PTLD discussion).

Life Cycle

Appropriate application of techniques for direct detection of EBV is based on an understanding of the behavior of EBV in cells. When EBV infects cells, it may enter either a lytic or a latent cycle. *Lytic infection,* also referred to as *active infection* or *productive infection,* is associated with production and release of infectious viral particles from infected cells. Lytic infection occurs in epithelial cells and some lymphoid cells and mani-

Table 15.10	Manifestations of EBV Infection in Immunocompromised Patients
Manifestation	**Immunodeficiency state**
Posttransplant lymphoproliferative disorder (PTLD)	Organ transplantation
Leiomyomas, leiomyosarcomas	AIDS in children[163] Organ transplantation[164]
Lymphomas	AIDS
Oral hairy leukoplakia	AIDS
Lymphocytic interstitial pneumonitis (LIP)	AIDS in children
X-linked lymphoproliferative syndrome	Selective congenital deficiency

AIDS, Acquired immunodeficiency syndrome.

fests in infectious mononucleosis and oral hairy leukoplakia. During lytic infection the EBV genome exists in a linear configuration within infected cells.

Latent infection, which occurs in B lymphocytes, results in transformation or "immortalization" of the infected cell. This means that latently infected EBV-infected cells will proliferate unless held in check by host immunity. During latent infection the EBV genome exists in infected cells in a circular configuration called an *episome.* In addition, integration of the EBV genome at random locations within host chromosomes also occurs. Expression of some EBV genes does occur during latency but is limited to the genes encoding six EBNAs (1, 2, 3A, 3B, 3C, and leader protein [LP]), three *latent membrane proteins* (LMP-1, LMP-2A, and LMP-2B), and two small, nonpolyadenylated, nontranslated transcripts called *Epstein-Barr–encoded RNAs* (EBER-1, EBER-2). EBER-1 and EBER-2 are the most abundant EBV ribonucleic acid (RNA) species produced during latent infection, with 10^7 copies per infected cell, followed by LMP-1, with 60 copies per infected cell.

The set of genes expressed as RNA transcripts and corresponding protein products during latent infection varies in different disease states. Latently infected lymphocytes in patients with infectious mononucleosis and patients with PTLD express the six EBNAs, three LMPs, and two EBERs. In Burkitt's lymphoma a more restricted form of latency is present, and only EBNA-1 is expressed. This down-regulation of viral gene expression is thought to be a mechanism by which virally infected cells elude host immune surveillance. Nasopharyngeal carcinoma cells express EBNA-1, LMP-1, and LMP-2.[166]

Posttransplant Lymphoproliferative Disorder

PTLD is defined as an abnormal proliferation of lymphoid tissue occurring after solid organ or bone marrow transplantation. Approximately 90% of cases are associated with EBV and involve proliferation of EBV-infected B lymphocytes. Most cases are thought to result from the failure of the host's cell-mediated immune system to control the proliferation of EBV-infected lymphocytes.

The most important risk factor for PTLD is primary EBV infection in the transplant recipient.[167] The period of highest risk is the first 6 months after transplantation, although PTLD can occur at any time after transplantation. The clinical presentation may be an infectious mononucleosis-like syndrome with swelling of lymph nodes or tonsillar tissue. Other patients may present with extranodal disease, most often involving the GI tract, lungs, and brain. The allograft itself can be involved, and the clinical manifestations can be confused with allograft rejection.

The lymphoid infiltrates of PTLD are usually composed of polymorphic collections of lymphoid cells, often with prominent areas of necrosis. The lymphoid cells involved can be polyclonal, oligoclonal, or monoclonal. The *clonality* of the lymphoid cells is usually defined by surface immunoglobulin expression, as detected by IHC stains, or by immunoglobulin gene rearrangements as detected by molecular studies. An alternative marker of clonality is based on molecular studies of the infecting strain of EBV. Different strains vary in the number of repeat copies of a 500–base-pair (bp) segment located at the terminus of the linear form of the genome.[168]

Because viral replication using the viral DNA polymerase is not occurring during lymphoproliferation, antiviral agents (e.g., acyclovir, ganciclovir) that act by inhibiting viral DNA polymerase probably have only a minor role in PTLD treatment. Some patients, especially those with infection early after transplantation, may respond to reduction of immunosuppression, whereas others require treatment with cytotoxic antitumor agents.

The diagnosis of PTLD is strongly supported by demonstrating latency-associated EBV antigens or RNA in proliferative lymphoid lesions.[169] Because not all PTLD is associated with EBV, failure to demonstrate EBV does not rule out PTLD. The EBV antigen frequently used as the target of detection is LMP-1,[170] which is most often detected by IP staining using a specific monoclonal antibody. Failure to detect LMP-1 does not rule out the presence of EBV because PTLD lesions can vary in LMP-1 expression.[171-174]

Detection of EBV nucleic acid is usually based on detection of EBERs by ISH.[174a] IHC for LMP and ISH for EBER RNA can be done on formalin-fixed tissue. Some caution must be used in interpreting the presence of EBV in tissue, since LMP and EBV DNA can also be detected in tonsils and cervical lymph nodes of patients with infectious mononucleosis.[175, 176] Also, small quantities of EBV RNA can occasionally be detected in normal lymphoid tissue or in lymphoid tissue occurring in variety of lymphoproliferative states.[177, 178] Detection of other EBV proteins and RNAs can be used to define the pattern of EBV gene expression and is available in some pathology departments with a special interest in EBV infection.

PCR has been used to detect EBV DNA in organs affected by PTLD. One study found high levels of EBV DNA in hepatic tissue from patients with PTLD but not in other liver transplant recipients.[179] Quantitation or semiquantitation is probably important because low levels of EBV DNA might be detected in tissues from patients without PTLD.

The need to obtain diagnostic information without an invasive procedure has stimulated efforts to use PCR on *peripheral blood leukocytes* (PBLs) for the diagnosis of PTLD. Although all patients who have experienced past infection with EBV are believed to have circulating B cells infected with EBV, the frequency of infected cells is low, ranging between one per 10^5 and one per 10^6 B cells.[166] Therefore PCR assays performed on PBLs are positive in only 10% to 20% of normal EBV-seropositive patients, and the quantity of EBV DNA present is low.[180] When the immune system is suppressed, the quantity of EBV DNA present in PBLs increases. Most patients with PTLD have very high levels of EBV DNA that can be distinguished by quantitative PCR assays from the levels measured in transplant recipients without PTLD.[180-183] Although this generalization applies to most patients with PTLD, a few patients with PTLD do not have elevated levels of EBV DNA, and conversely, some transplant recipients with elevated levels of EBV DNA in the range seen with PTLD do not develop clinically evident PTLD.[179, 180, 182]

Interestingly, high levels of EBV may be present before PTLD is recognized by its clinical manifestations.[180, 183] This observation has stimulated interest in serial monitoring of transplant recipients for leukocyte EBV levels after transplantation. Also, in patients with PTLD and elevated EBV DNA levels, these levels may decline with effective treatment,[180, 183] suggesting that this measurement may be used as a "tumor marker." These observations are provocative, but further work is required to define the clinical utility of EBV monitoring in transplant recipients before such monitoring is accepted as standard practice.

HUMAN HERPESVIRUSES 6 AND 7

Virology and Life Cycle

Human herpesviruses 6 and 7 (HHV-6, HHV-7) are members of the Herpesviridae family, first recognized in 1986 and 1990. Both are classified as beta herpesviruses related to human CMV. Two variants of HHV-6 have been recognized, designated A and B. *Variant B* appears to be much more common. The two variants share approximately 95% nucleotide homology. As with other herpesviruses, both HHV-6 and HHV-7 undergo latency after primary infection and can reactivate later in life. HHV-6 is susceptible in vitro to ganciclovir and foscarnet.

Clinical Manifestations

Both HHV-6 and HHV-7 have been implicated as causes of the common infant illness roseola (*exanthem subitum*), which represents primary infection with HHV-6 or HHV-7 (see Chapter 13). Virtually all cases of roseola associated with HHV-6 are caused by variant B. Not all primary HHV infections result in a roseola-like illness; some children experience a nonspecific febrile illness, whereas others have asymptomatic infection. Overall, infection with both HHV-6 and HHV-7 occurs in almost everyone in the first 2 years of life, and more than 95% of adults have circulating antibodies to both viruses, indicating past infection. Salivary shedding of both viruses is common in adults, signifying reactivated infection. Clinical illnesses attributed to HHV-6 infection in normal adults include a mononucleosis-like syndrome, hepatitis, and encephalomyelitis.

The role of HHV-6 and HHV-7 as causes of serious opportunistic infections is still incompletely defined, partly because of the high frequency of viral shedding in normal individuals. Because most adults are seropositive, disease in transplant recipients usually results from reactivation of latent infection. Virologic evidence of active infection after transplantation is common, but evidence of clinically significant disease is unusual. Among BMT recipients, 26% to 44% have serologic evidence of active HHV-6 infection.[184, 185] Viremia can be documented by culture in 40% to 46%[184-186] and by PCR in 61% to 70%.[187, 188] Moderate to severe GVH disease increases the risk of active infection.[187, 189, 190] The frequency of active HHV-6 infection is lower in solid organ transplant recipients. In this group, 24% to 54% have serologic evidence of active infection,[191-193] with viremia documented by culture in 14% to 19%[192, 194] and by PCR in 28% to 36%.[195, 196]

In immunocompromised patients, HHV-6 is most evident as a cause of disease in BMT recipients. Clinical

syndromes in this patient population include delayed engraftment,[188] late bone marrow suppression,[197] interstitial pneumonitis,[189] skin rashes resembling GVH disease,[184] and encephalitis.[198] In prospective studies the frequency of these syndromes has been low.[184, 185] Descriptions of clinical disease in solid organ transplant recipients are limited to case reports describing cytopenias, interstitial pneumonitis, a febrile dermatosis with encephalopathy in liver transplant recipients,[199, 200] and duodenitis and pancreatitis in a heart transplant recipient.[201] A role for HHV-6 as a cause of allograft rejection has been suggested but has not been well documented. HHV-6 infection has been more common in patients with evidence of active CMV infection,[193, 195, 202] but it is not yet known whether this reflects an interaction between the viruses or indicates that immunosuppression is a risk factor for both viruses.

Little information is currently available about disease caused by HHV-7 in immunocompromised patients, although evidence supports an association with CMV infection.[195] Disease caused by HHV-6 or HHV-7 in HIV-infected patients is not well defined, although possible involvement of HHV-6 in lymphoproliferative disease is a concern.

Diagnostic Tests

Tests available for detection of HHV-6 and HHV-7 include culture, PCR, and serology. Table 15–11 summarizes the results of the HHV-6 diagnostic tests in primary infection, normal children and adults, and reactivation in immunocompromised patients. Unlike CMV, HHV-6 does not characteristically produce inclusions in infected tissue, and no unique histologic footprint has been recognized. IHC has been used, however, to detect HHV-6 antigens in diseased tissue. Experience with ISH for HHV-6 DNA is more limited but has also been used to document unusual clinical manifestations.

Viral culture. Both HHV-6 and HHV-7 can be recovered in culture by placing cells from the patient specimen in

Table 15.11 Results of Diagnostic Tests for HHV-6

Patient group	Culture		Polymerase chain reaction		Serology	
	Saliva	PBMCs*	Saliva	PBMCs*	IgG	IgM
Primary infection	−	+	−	+	+†	+
Normal adult	Often +	−	Often +	−‡	+	−
Immunocompromised	+	+	+	+	+	+/−§

*Peripheral blood mononuclear cells.
†Seroconversion or rising titer.
‡5%-10% or more may be positive, depending on assay conditions and sensitivity.
§Variable.

culture without other cells, but best success has been achieved by cocultivation with human umbilical cord lymphocytes stimulated with phytohemagglutinin. Growth of virus is detected by a CPE consisting of balloonlike syncytia and is confirmed by FA staining with an appropriate monoclonal antibody or by PCR detection of specific viral DNA. After primary isolation, variant A of HHV-6 can be propagated in a line of immature T cells called *HSB-2. Peripheral blood mononuclear cells* (PBMCs) and saliva have been the specimens from which virus has been most readily isolated. A shell vial culture technique has been described for HHV-6.[199] Interestingly, this technique uses human fibroblast cells rather than PBMCs as the target cell for infection. Although studies cite good correlation with conventional culture techniques, more experience is required to evaluate this technique.

HHV-6 and HHV-7 can be isolated from blood during primary infection but are rarely recovered from the blood of nonimmunocompromised patients after recovery from primary infection.[203] In contrast, both viruses can frequently be cultured from the saliva of healthy individuals years after a primary infection. HHV-6 has been cultured from the blood of 40% to 50% of BMT recipients and from saliva of approximately 60%.[184, 185] Recovery of virus from the blood tends to occur in the first month after transplantation and is sporadic in most patients.[184] Because umbilical cord mononuclear cells are not in routine use in most diagnostic virology laboratories, cultures for HHV-6 or HHV-7 usually require special arrangements or involvement of a research laboratory with a specific interest in these viruses.

Polymerase chain reaction. PCR has been used for the detection of both HHV-6 and HHV-7. Specimens in which viral DNA has been detected include PBMCs, plasma, saliva, urine, and biopsy or autopsy tissue. HHV-6 DNA can be detected in PBMCs of 5% to 64% of normal individuals,[204, 205] depending on the sensitivity of the PCR assay. HHV-7 DNA has been detected by PCR in saliva from 96% of normal individuals and in peripheral blood from 83%.[206] Levels of HHV-7 DNA in peripheral blood are low, and thus the proportion of persons found to be positive is greatly affected by the amount of patient DNA included in the assay and the analytic sensitivity of the assay. HHV-6 and HHV-7 DNA have been detected in PBMCs or peripheral blood of individuals with HIV infection. The frequency of detection is less than with CMV, and surprisingly, detection is more common in individuals with high CD4+ counts.[207, 208]

Because the frequency of clinically significant HHV-6 or HHV-7 infection after bone marrow or solid organ transplantation is low, PCR performed on PBMCs is too sensitive for routine diagnosis and may be useful only for excluding current infection with these viruses.

Approaches to increasing the specificity of PCR for diagnosis of clinically significant infection include quantitative PCR and use of plasma as a specimen. One study showed that although HHV-6 could be almost always detected in lung tissue from BMT recipients and from normal individuals, high levels were much more likely in patients with interstitial pneumonitis of unknown etiology, suggesting that HHV-6 might be the cause of the pneumonitis in these patients.[189]

Serology. Serologic methods can also be used for the diagnosis of HHV-6 and HHV-7 infections. Assays that have been used include indirect immunofluorescence, enzyme-linked immunosorbent assay (ELISA), and neutralization. Commercial availability of these assays is still limited. Seroconversion can be documented in patients with primary infection, and a rising titer has been suggested as evidence of reactivation. Serologic assays do not distinguish between HHV-6 variants A and B, and some serologic cross-reaction seems to occur between HHV-6 and HHV-7.[209] Primary CMV infection has been shown to induce antibodies that cross-react with HHV-6, resulting in false-positive tests for HHV-6 antibodies.[210] Other studies, however, have not observed cross-reactivity.[211, 212]

In general, serologic diagnosis is not advised in immunocompromised patients because of the question of cross-reactivity with other viruses and because of poor sensitivity for detection of HHV-6 infection in this patient population.[183, 184]

Diagnostic Approach

Although the presence of HHV-6 or HHV-7 can be documented using culture, PCR, or serology, validated criteria do not currently exist for establishing the clinical significance of infection with these ubiquitous viruses. When a suggestive clinical syndrome is present, evidence of active infection can be sought using culture (if available) or PCR. Serology is not recommended because of questionable sensitivity and specificity. Because infection frequently occurs without symptoms, a positive culture or PCR does not prove that the clinical syndrome is caused by HHV-6 or HHV-7. Detection of viral antigens or nucleic acid in diseased tissue can provide stronger supportive evidence. In some patients, empiric therapy with an antiviral agent (e.g., foscarnet, ganciclovir) that has activity against HHV-6 or HHV-7 may be attempted. Resolution of the clinical manifestation and reversal of the positive culture or PCR to negative provide further evidence supporting a causative role for the suspected virus.

Until additional data are available, most diagnoses of clinical disease attributable to HHV-6 or HHV-7 must be considered tentative.

HUMAN HERPESVIRUS 8 (KAPOSI'S SARCOMA VIRUS)

Virology and Epidemiology

Human herpesvirus 8 (HHV-8) is a newly described herpesvirus that has been linked *to Kaposi's sarcoma* (KS). HHV-8 is classified as a gamma herpesvirus (lymphotropic herpesviruses) along with EBV and the simian virus *Herpesvirus saimiri*. The association of HHV-8 with KS was recognized originally in patients infected with HIV[213] and was subsequently extended to patients with classical KS[214] and to renal transplant patients with KS.[215] HHV-8 has also been implicated as the cause of multicentric *Castleman's disease*[216] and an unusual form of AIDS-related lymphoma called *body cavity lymphoma*.[217] Linkages between HHV-8 and multiple myeloma,[218] pemphigus,[219] and sarcoidosis[220] have been proposed but are not yet confirmed.

The epidemiology of HHV-8 is still incompletely understood. Serologic testing (see following discussion) has revealed evidence of past infection in 1% to 2% of blood donors, 25% to 35% of HIV-infected homosexual males, 2% to 3% of HIV-infected hemophiliac patients, and 3% to 4% of HIV-infected women.[221] Some evidence suggests a sexual mode of transmission.[222] Transmission through organ transplantation has recently been documented.[223]

Diagnostic Tests

Diagnostic tests for HHV-8 are research tools that are not currently available in routine diagnostic virology laboratories. Although these tests are clearly important for research on HHV-8, the clinical need for specific viral diagnosis of HHV-8 infection is undefined.

Viral culture. The behavior of HHV-8 in culture has some similarities to EBV. Certain cell lines such as *BCBL-1*, derived from body cavity lymphomas, contain latent HHV-8. Treatment with phorbol esters results in induction of lytic infection with release of viral particles into the medium.[224] Recently, an embryonal kidney epithelial cell line called *293 cells* has been used to culture HHV-8 from KS tissue.[225] Virus culture is not currently used in clinical diagnosis. It is useful for research, however, and may ultimately be useful for production of antigens in serologic tests.

Polymerase chain reaction. PCR can be used to detect HHV-8 DNA in the lesions of virtually all patients with KS.[213, 214] Most assays have used primers that amplify a 233-bp segment called *KS-330*. This segment is the portion of the HHV-8 genome detected in the original discovery of the virus[213] and is part of a gene analogous to the BLF-1 gene of EBV. Increased sensitivity has been achieved using a nested PCR assay (see Chapter 1).[226]

HHV-8 DNA can be detected by PCR in PBMCs of 30% to 50% of patients with KS, 7% to 8% of AIDS patients without KS, and no HIV-negative blood donors or volunteers.[226-229] The presence of HHV-8 DNA in PBMCs in AIDS patients has been shown to precede the development of KS.[226] One study showed that the blood cells harboring HHV-8 DNA were CD19+ B lymphocytes.[230] HHV-8 DNA has also been detected in semen,[231, 232] the prostate gland,[231] saliva and nasal secretions,[233] and CSF.[234]

Serology. Similar to EBV serology, HHV-8 serologic assays measure antibodies to antigens expressed during latency or expressed only during lytic infection. Assays for antibodies to latent antigens have used the indirect immunofluorescence format to measure antibodies to a *latency-associated nuclear antigen* (LANA) encoded by open reading frame (ORF) 73[235, 236] and to latent antigens expressed in the cell line BCP-1.[237] These assays have detected HHV-8 antibodies in 71% to 88% of patients with AIDS-related KS, 94% to 100% of patients with classic KS, 20% to 30% of homosexual males with AIDS, 3.5% of HIV-seropositive women, up to 3% of blood donors in the United States and the United Kingdom, and 51% of HIV-negative Ugandans without KS.[235, 237-239]

Assays for antibodies to VCAs include an IFA assay that uses BCBL-1 cells induced into a lytic cycle using phorbol esters and an ELISA to an antigen encoded by ORF 65. The prevalence of antibodies in blood donors detected by the phorbol-stimulated cell assay is higher than that found in other assays.[239] Whether this assay is truly more sensitive or is detecting antibodies that may be cross-reactive with other herpesviruses has not yet been determined.

Although the general patterns of antibody prevalence detected by different assays are similar, correlation of test results on individual specimens is poor.[240] Until assays are better standardized, they cannot be used to determine reliably an individual patient's HHV-8 antibody status.

ADENOVIRUS

Virology

Adenoviruses are double-stranded DNA viruses divided into 49 serotypes that have been grouped in six different subgenuses. The adenoviruses are common causes of respiratory and GI infection in normal individuals, especially children. Life-threatening infection in the normal host is unusual.[241]

Although sometimes mild or even asymptomatic, adenovirus infection in immunocompromised patients can be disseminated, with a high fatality rate.[241] Some differences related to the cause of immunosuppression can be delineated.

Epidemiology and Clinical Manifestations

Two comprehensive studies have documented adenovirus infections in 5% and 21% of BMT recipients, with rates of disease of 1% and 6.5%.[242, 243] Clinical manifestations included pneumonia, hepatitis, nephritis, colitis, and encephalitis. Infection was most common in the first 4 months after transplantation. Risk factors for infection were allograft transplantation, moderate to severe GVH disease, and pediatric age group. The most common serotypes were 11, 34, and 35. These three serotypes are members of *subgenus B* and are uncommon in normal individuals. Approximately 50% of invasive infections were fatal. Adenovirus infection has been detected in 10% of pediatric liver transplant patients, with hepatitis occurring in 2% to 3%, usually in the early posttransplant period.[244, 245] The hepatitis is severe, with a high fatality rate, and in one study was closely associated with *adenovirus type 5.* In renal transplant recipients the most notable manifestation of adenovirus infection has been *hemorrhagic cystitis,* although rare patients with pneumonia or hepatitis have been reported.

The source of adenovirus infections in transplant patients is thought to be reactivation of latent virus, although firm supportive evidence is lacking. Adenovirus infection has not been prominent in patients with HIV. Reported manifestations include hepatitis, pneumonitis, nephritis, colitis, encephalitis, and parotitis. In a prospective study, adenovirus infection was common in patients with HIV, with a 28% 1-year risk, but most infections were asymptomatic.[246] Most isolates were from stool specimens, and unusual serotypes in *subgenus D* were common. Disseminated adenovirus infection has occurred in patients with congenital immunodeficiency. The most common manifestations have been pneumonia and hepatitis, with a high fatality rate.[241]

Diagnostic Approach

The approach to diagnosis of adenovirus infection in immunocompromised patients is similar to that in normal individuals, relying primarily on culture and FA staining to detect adenoviral antigens directly in patient specimens. The most appropriate specimens are determined by the site of disease and include respiratory and stool specimens. The detection of adenovirus in urine or blood can be a clue to the presence of disseminated disease but asymptomatic viremia has been reported in pediatric HIV patients.[247]

Another important clue to the presence of disseminated disease is detection of adenovirus in specimens from multiple body sites. Detection in tissue by culture or histology provides documentation of invasive disease. Adenovirus infection is associated with characteristic "smudge cells" containing large intranuclear inclusions with an irregular outline. Basophilic intranuclear inclusions surrounded by a clear halo can also be seen. These inclusions have occasionally been confused with those caused by CMV infection. Electron microscopy of adenovirus-associated inclusions reveals regular arrays of characteristic icosahedral adenovirus virions.

References

1. Stagno S: Cytomegalovirus. In Remington JS, Klein JO, editors: *Infectious diseases of the fetus & newborn infant,* Philadelphia, 1995, WB Saunders.
2. Taylor-Weideman J, Sissons JG, Borysiewicz LK, Sinclair JH: Monocytes are a major site of persistence of human cytomegalovirus in peripheral blood mononuclear cells, *J Gen Virol* 72:2059, 1991.
3. Soderberg-Naucler C, Fish KN, Nelson JA: Reactivation of latent human cytomegalovirus by allogeneic stimulation of blood cells from healthy donors, *Cell* 91:119, 1997.
4. Grundy JE, Lui SF, Super M, et al: Symptomatic cytomegalovirus infection in seropositive kidney recipients; reinfection with donor virus rather than reactivation of recipient virus, *Lancet* 2:132, 1988.
5. Gleaves CA, Smith TF, Shuster EA, Pearson GR: Rapid detection of cytomegalovirus in MRC-5 cells inoculated with urine specimens by using low-speed centrifugation and monoclonal antibody to an early antigen, *J Clin Microbiol* 19:917, 1984.
6. Gleaves CA, Smith TF, Shuster EA, Pearson GR: Comparison of standard tube and shell vial cell culture techniques for the detection of cytomegalovirus in clinical specimens, *J Clin Microbiol* 21:217, 1985.
7. Griffiths PD, Panjwani DD, Stirk PR, et al: Rapid diagnosis of cytomegalovirus infection in immunocompromised patients by detection of early antigen fluorescent foci, *Lancet* 2:1242, 1984.
8. Buller RS, Bailey TC, Ettinger NA, et al: Use of a modified shell vial technique to quantitate cytomegalovirus viremia in a population of solid-organ transplant recipients, *J Clin Microbiol* 30:2620, 1992,
9. Shuster EA, Beneke JS, Tegtmeier GE, et al: Monoclonal antibody for rapid laboratory detection of cytomegalovirus infections: characterization and diagnostic application, *Mayo Clin Proc* 60:577, 1985.
10. Paya CV, Wold AD, Ilstrup DM, Smith TF: Evaluation of number of shell vial cell cultures per clinical specimen for rapid diagnosis of cytomegalovirus infection, *J Clin Microbiol* 26:198, 1988.
11. Arens M, Owen J, Hagerty CM, et al: Optimizing recovery of cytomegalovirus in the shell vial culture procedure, *Diagn Microbiol Infect Dis* 14:125, 1991.
12. Paya CV, Wold AD, Smith TF: Detection of cytomegalovirus infections in specimens other than urine by the shell vial assay and conventional tube cultures, *J Clin Microbiol* 25:755, 1987.
13. Reina J, Blanco I, Munar M: Determination of the number of blood samples needed for optimal detection of cytomegalovirus viremia in immunocompromised patients using a shell-vial assay, *Eur J Clin Microbiol Infect Dis* 16:318, 1997.

14. Roberts TC, Buller RS, Gaudreault-Keener M, et al: Effects of storage temperature and time on qualitative and quantitative detection of cytomegalovirus in blood specimens by shell vial culture and PCR, *J Clin Microbiol* 35:2224, 1997.

15. van der Bij W, Torensma R, van Son WJ, et al: Rapid immunodiagnosis of active cytomegalovirus infection by monoclonal antibody staining of blood leukocytes, *J Med Virol* 25:179, 1988.

16. Revello MG, Percivalle E, Zavattoni M, et al: Detection of human cytomegalovirus immediate early antigen in leukocytes as a marker of viremia in immunocompromised patients, *J Med Virol* 29:88, 1989.

17. Gerna G, Revello MG, Percivalle E, Morini F: Comparison of different immunostaining techniques and monoclonal antibodies to the lower matrix phosphoprotein (pp65) for optimal quantitation of human cytomegalovirus antigenemia, *J Clin Microbiol* 30:1232, 1992.

18. Boeckh M, Bowden R, Goodrich JM, et al: Cytomegalovirus antigen detection in peripheral blood leukocytes after allogeneic marrow transplantation, *Blood* 80: 1358, 1992.

19. Gerna G, Percivalle E, Revello MG, Morini F: Correlation of quantitative human cytomegalovirus pp65-, p72- and p150-antigenemia, viremia and circulating endothelial giant cells with clinical symptoms and antiviral treatment in immunocompromised patients, *Clin Diagn Virol* 1:47, 1993.

20. Gerna G, Zipeto D, Parea M, et al: Monitoring of human cytomegalovirus infections and ganciclovir treatment in heart transplant recipients by determination of viremia, antigenemia, and DNAemia, *J Infect Dis* 164, 1991.

21. Erice A, Holm MA, Gill PC, et al: Cytomegalovirus (CMV) antigenemia assay is more sensitive than shell vial cultures for rapid detection of CMV in polymorphonuclear blood leukocytes, *J Clin Microbiol* 30:2822, 1992.

22. Landry ML, Ferguson D: Comparison of quantitative cytomegalovirus antigenemia assay with culture methods and correlation with clinical disease, *J Clin Microbiol* 31:2851, 1993.

23. Brumback BG, Bolejack SN, Morris MV, et al: Comparison of culture and the antigenemia assay for detection of cytomegalovirus in blood specimens submitted to a reference laboratory, *J Clin Microbiol* 35:1819, 1997.

24. van der Bij W, Shirm J, Torensma R, et al: Comparison between viremia and antigenemia for detection of cytomegalovirus in blood, *J Clin Microbiol* 26:2531, 1988.

25. Boeckh M, Woodgerd PM, Stevens-Ayrs T, et al: Factors influencing detection of quantitative cytomegalovirus antigenemia, *J Clin Microbiol* 32:832, 1994.

26. Pérez JL, Niubò J, Ardunuy C, et al: Comparison of three commercially available monoclonal antibodies directed against pp65 antigen for cytomegalovirus antigenemia assay, *Diagn Microbiol Infect Dis* 21:21, 1995.

27. St George K, Rinaldo CR Jr.: Comparison of commercially available antibody reagents for the cytomegalovirus pp65 antigenemia assay, *Clin Diagn Virol* 7:147, 1997.

28. The TE, van der Ploeg M, van den Berg AP, et al: Direct detection of cytomegalovirus in peripheral blood leukocytes—a review of the antigenemia assay and polymerase chain reaction, *Transplantation* 54:193, 1992.

29. Gerna G, Revello MG, Percivalle E, et al: Quantification of human cytomegalovirus viremia by using monoclonal antibodies to different viral proteins, *J Clin Microbiol* 28:2681, 1990.

30. Landry ML, Ferguson D: Comparison of quantitative cytomegalovirus antigenemia assay with culture methods and correlation with clinical disease, *J Clin Microbiol* 31:2851, 1993.

31. Niubò J, Pérez JL, Martínez-Lacasa JT, et al: Association of quantitative cytomegalovirus antigenemia with symptomatic infection in solid organ transplant patients, *Diagn Microbiol Infect Dis* 24:19, 1996.

32. von Laer D, Serr A, Meyer-Konig U, et al: Human cytomegalovirus immediate early and late transcripts are expressed in all major leukocyte populations in vivo, *J Infect Dis* 172:365, 1995.

33. Gerna G, Zipeto D, Percivalle E, et al: Human cytomegalovirus infection of the major leukocyte subpopulations and evidence for initial viral replication in polymorphonuclear leukocytes from viremic patients, *J Infect Dis* 166:1236, 1992.

34. Percivalle E, Revello MG, Vago L, et al: Circulating endothelial giant cells permissive for human cytomegalovirus (HCMV) are detected in disseminated HCMV infections with organ involvement, *J Clin Invest* 92:663, 1993.

35. Grefte A, van der Giessen M, van Son W, The TH: Circulating cytomegalovirus (CMV)-infected endothelial cells in patients with an active CMV infection, *J Infect Dis* 167:270, 1993.

36. Salzberger B, Myerson D, Boeckh M: Circulating cytomegalovirus (CMV)-infected endothelial cells in marrow transplant patients with CMV disease and CMV infection, *J Infect Dis* 176:778, 1997.

37. Storch GA, Gaudreault-Keener M, Welby PC : Comparison of heparin and EDTA transport tubes for detection of cytomegalovirus in leukocytes by shell vial assay, pp65 antigenemia assay, and PCR, *J Clin Microbiol* 32: 2581, 1994.

38. Landry ML, Cohen S, Huber K: Comparison of EDTA and acid-citrate-dextrose collection tubes for detection of cytomegalovirus antigenemia and infectivity in leukocytes before and after storage, *J Clin Microbiol* 35:305, 1997.

39. Niubò J, Perez JL, Carvajal A, et al: Effect of delayed processing of blood samples on performance of cytomegalovirus antigenemia assay, *J Clin Microbiol* 32: 1119, 1994.

40. Landry ML, Ferguson D, Cohen S, et al: Effect of delayed specimen processing on cytomegalovirus antigenemia test results, *J Clin Microbiol* 33:257, 1995.

41. Bitsch A, Kirschner H, Dupke R, Bein G: Failure to detect human cytomegalovirus DNA in peripheral blood leukocytes of healthy blood donors by the polymerase chain reaction, *Transfusion* 32:612, 1992.

42. Wolff C, Skourtopoulos M, Hornschemeyer D, et al: Significance of human cytomegalovirus DNA detection

in immunocompromised heart transplant recipients, *Transplantation* 61:750, 1996.

43. Ishigaki S, Takeda M, Kura T, et al: Cytomegalovirus DNA in the sera of patients with cytomegalovirus pneumonia, *Br J Haematol* 79:198, 1991.

44. Brytting M, Xu W, Wahren B, Sundqvist V-A: Cytomegalovirus DNA detection in sera from patients with active cytomegalovirus infections, *J Clin Microbiol* 30:1937, 1992.

45. Spector SA, Merrill R, Wolf D, Dankner WM: Detection of human cytomegalovirus in plasma of AIDS patients during acute visceral disease by DNA amplification, *J Clin Microbiol* 30:2359, 1992.

46. Wolf DG, Spector SA: Early diagnosis of human cytomegalovirus disease in transplant recipients by DNA amplification in plasma, *Transplantation* 56:330, 1993.

47. Gerna G, Furione M, Baldanti F, Sarasini A: Comparative quantitation of human cytomegalovirus DNA in blood leukocytes and plasma of transplant and AIDS patients, *J Clin Microbiol* 32:2709, 1994.

48. Brytting M, Mousavi-Jazi M, Bostrom L, et al: Cytomegalovirus DNA in peripheral blood leukocytes and plasma from bone marrow transplant recipients, *Transplantation* 60:961, 1995.

49. Hebart H, Muller C, Loffler J, et al: Monitoring of CMV infection: a comparison of PCR from whole blood, plasma-PCR, pp65-antigenemia and virus culture in patients after bone marrow transplantation, *Bone Marrow Transplant* 17:861, 1996.

50. Boeckh M, Gallez-Hawkins GM, Myerson D, et al: Plasma polymerase chain reaction for cytomegalovirus DNA after allogeneic marrow transplantation: comparison with polymerase chain reaction using peripheral blood leukocytes, pp65 antigenemia, and viral culture, *Transplantation* 64:108, 1997.

51. Zipeto D, Morris S, Hong C, et al: Human cytomegalovirus (CMV) DNA in plasma reflects quantity of CMV DNA present in leukocytes, *J Clin Microbiol* 33:2607, 1995.

52. Boivin G, Handfield J, Toma E, et al: Comparative evaluation of the cytomegalovirus DNA load in polymorphonuclear leukocytes and plasma of human immunodeficiency virus–infected subjects, *J Infect Dis* 177:355, 1998.

53. Rasmussen L, Zipeto D, Wolitz RA, et al: Risk for retinitis in patients with AIDS can be assessed by quantitation of threshold levels of cytomegalovirus DNA burden in blood, *J Infect Dis* 176:1146, 1997.

54. Nelson PN, Rawal BK, Boriskin YS, et al: A polymerase chain reaction to detect a spliced late transcript of human cytomegalovirus in the blood of bone marrow transplant recipients, *J Virol Methods* 56:139, 1996.

55. Bitsch A, Kirchner H, Dupke R, Bein G: Cytomegalovirus transcripts in peripheral blood leukocytes of actively infected transplant patients detected by reverse transcription–polymerase chain reaction, *J Infect Dis* 167:740, 1993.

56. Gozlan J, Salord J-M, Chouaïd C, et al: Human cytomegalovirus (HCMV) late-mRNA detection in peripheral blood leukocytes of AIDS patients: diagnostic value for HCMV disease compared with those of viral culture and HCMV DNA detection, *J Clin Microbiol* 31:1943, 1993.

57. Meyer-Köning U, Serr A, von Laer D, et al: Human cytomegalovirus immediate early and late transcripts in peripheral blood leukocytes: diagnostic value in renal transplant recipients, *J Infect Dis* 171:705, 1995.

58. Randhawa PS, Manez R, Frye B, Ehrlich GD: Circulating immediate-early mRNA in patients with cytomegalovirus infections after solid organ transplantation, *J Infect Dis* 170:1264, 1994.

59. Patel R, Smith TF, Espy M, et al: A prospective comparison of molecular diagnostic techniques for the early detection of cytomegalovirus in liver transplant recipients, *J Infect Dis* 171:1010, 1995.

60. Gozlan J, Laporte JP, Lesage S, et al: Monitoring of cytomegalovirus infection and disease in bone marrow recipients by reverse transcription–PCR and comparison with PCR and blood and urine cultures, *J Clin Microbiol* 34:2085, 1996.

61. Boeckh M, Boivin G: Quantitation of cytomegalovirus: methodologic aspects and clinical applications, *Clin Microbiol Rev* 11:533, 1998.

62. Mazzulli T, Wood S, Chua R, Walmsley S: Evaluation of the Digene Hybrid Capture System for detection and quantitation of human cytomegalovirus viremia in human immunodeficiency virus–infected patients, *J Clin Microbiol* 34:2959, 1996.

63. Baldanti F, Zavattoni M, Sarasini A, et al: Comparative quantification of human cytomegalovirus DNA in blood of immunocompromised patients by PCR and Murex Hybrid Capture System, *Clin Diagn Virol* 8:159, 1997.

64. Hebart H, Gamer D, Loeffler J, et al: Evaluation of Murex CMV DNA hybrid capture assay for detection and quantitation of cytomegalovirus infection in patients following allogeneic stem cell transplantation, *J Clin Microbiol* 36:1333, 1998.

65. Rollag H, Sagedal S, Holter E, et al: Diagnosis of cytomegalovirus infection in kidney transplant recipients by a quantitative RNA-DNA hybrid capture assay for cytomegalovirus DNA in leukocytes, *Eur J Clin Microbiol Infect Dis* 17:124, 1998.

66. Schirm J, Kooistra A, van Son WJ, et al: Comparison of the Murex Hybrid Capture TM CMV DNA assay (V 2.0) and the CMV-antigenemia assay for the detection and quantitation of CMV in blood samples from immunocompromised patients. Presented at the Fourteenth Annual Meeting of the Pan American Society for Clinical Virology, Clearwater Beach, Fla, April 1998.

67. Imbert-Marcille BM, Cantarovich D, Ferre-Aubineau V, et al: Usefulness of DNA viral load quantification for cytomegalovirus disease monitoring in renal and pancreas/renal transplant recipients, *Transplantation* 63:1476, 1997.

68. Macartney M, Gane EJ, Portmann B, Williams R: Comparison of a new quantitative cytomegalovirus DNA assay with other detection methods, *Transplantation* 63:1803, 1997.

69. Cope AV, Sabin C, Burroughs A, et al: Interrelationships among quantity of human cytomegalovirus (HCMV) DNA in blood, donor-recipient serostatus, and administration of methylprednisolone as risk factors for HCMV disease following liver transplantation, *J Infect Dis* 176:1484, 1997.

70. Bowen EF, Sabin CA, Griffiths PD, et al: Cytomegalovirus (CMV) viraemia detected by polymerase chain reaction identifies a group of HIV-positive patients at high risk of CMV disease, *AIDS* 11:889, 1997.

71. Roberts TC, Brennan DC, Buller RS, et al: Quantitative polymerase chain reaction to predict occurrence of symptomatic cytomegalovirus infection and assess response to ganciclovir therapy in renal transplant recipients, *J Infect Dis* 178:626, 1998.

72. Bailey TC, Buller RS, Ettinger NA, et al: Quantitative analysis of cytomegalovirus viremia in lung transplant recipients, *J Infect Dis* 171:1006, 1995.

73. van den Berg AP, van der Bij W, van Son WJ, et al: Cytomegalovirus antigenemia as a useful marker of symptomatic cytomegalovirus infection after renal transplantation—a report of 130 consecutive patients, *Transplantation* 48:991, 1989.

74. van den Berg AP, Klompmaker IJ, Haagsma EB, et al: Antigenemia in the diagnosis and monitoring of active cytomegalovirus infection after liver transplantation, *J Infect Dis* 164:265, 1991.

75. Ljungman P, Loré K, Aschan J, et al: Use of a semiquantitative PCR for cytomegalovirus DNA as a basis for pre-emptive antiviral therapy in allogeneic bone marrow transplant patients, *Bone Marrow Transplant* 17:583, 1996.

76. Toyoda M, Carlos JB, Galera OA, et al: Correlation of cytomegalovirus DNA levels with response to antiviral therapy in cardiac and renal allograft recipients, *Transplantation* 63:957, 1997.

77. Boivin G, Chou S, Quirk MR, et al: Detection of ganciclovir resistance mutations and quantitation of cytomegalovirus (CMV) DNA in leukocytes of patients with fatal disseminated CMV disease, *J Infect Dis* 173:523, 1996.

78. Schafer P, Tenschert W, Gutensohn K, Laufs R: Minimal effect of delayed sample processing on results of quantitative PCR for cytomegalovirus DNA in leukocytes compared to results of an antigenemia assay, *J Clin Microbiol* 35:741, 1997.

79. Meyers JD, Ljungman P, Fisher LD: Cytomegalovirus excretion as a predictor of cytomegalovirus disease after marrow transplantation: importance of cytomegalovirus viremia, *J Infect Dis* 162:373, 1990.

80. Boivin G, Quirk MR, Kringstad BA, et al: Early effects of ganciclovir therapy on the quantity of cytomegalovirus DNA in leukocytes of immunocompromised patients, *Antimicrob Agents Chemother* 41:860, 1997.

81. Einsele H, Steidle M, Vallbracht A, et al: Early occurrence of human cytomegalovirus infection after bone marrow transplantation as demonstrated by the polymerase chain reaction technique, *Blood* 77:1104, 1991.

82. Boeckh M, Gooley TA, Myerson D, et al: Cytomegalovirus pp65 antigenemia-guided early treatment with ganciclovir versus ganciclovir at engraftment after allogeneic marrow transplantation: a randomized double-blind study, *Blood* 88:4063, 1996.

83. Schmidt CA, Oettle H, Wilborn F, et al: Demonstration of cytomegalovirus after bone marrow transplantation by polymerase chain reaction, virus culture and antigen detection in buffy coat leukocytes, *Bone Marrow Transplant* 13:71, 1994.

84. Yuen K-Y, Lo SK-F, Chiu EK-W, et al: Monitoring of leukocyte cytomegalovirus DNA in bone marrow transplant recipients by nested PCR, *J Clin Microbiol* 33:2530, 1995.

85. Springmeyer SC, Silvestri RC, Sale GE, et al: The role of transbronchial biopsy for the diagnosis of diffuse pneumonias in immunocompromised marrow transplant recipients, *Am Rev Respir Dis* 126:763, 1982.

86. Hackman RC, Myerson D, Meyers JD, et al: Rapid diagnosis of cytomegaloviral pneumonia by tissue immunofluorescence with a murine monoclonal antibody, *J Infect Dis* 151:325, 1985.

87. Myerson D, Hackman RC, Meyers JD: Diagnosis of cytomegaloviral pneumonia by in situ hybridization, *J Infect Dis* 150:272, 1984.

88. Jiwa M, Steenbergen RD, Zwaan FE, et al: Three sensitive methods for the detection of cytomegalovirus in lung tissue of patients with interstitial pneumonitis, *Am J Clin Pathol* 93:491, 1990.

89. Churchill MA, Zaia JA, Forman SJ, et al: Quantitation of human cytomegalovirus DNA in lungs from bone marrow transplant recipients with interstitial pneumonia, *J Infect Dis* 155:501, 1987.

90. Burgart LJ, Heller MJ, Reznicek MJ, et al: Cytomegalovirus detection in bone marrow transplant patients with idiopathic pneumonitis: a clinicopathologic study of the clinical utility of the polymerase chain reaction on open lung biopsy specimen tissue, *Am J Clin Pathol* 96:572, 1991.

91. Crawford SW, Bowden RA, Hackman RC, et al: Rapid detection of cytomegalovirus pulmonary infection by bronchoalveolar lavage and centrifugation culture, *Ann Intern Med* 108:180, 1988.

92. Cathomas G, Morris P, Pekle K, et al: Rapid diagnosis of cytomegalovirus pneumonia in marrow transplant recipients by bronchoalveolar lavage using the polymerase chain reaction, virus culture, and the direct immunostaining of alveolar cells, *Blood* 81:1909, 1993.

93. Ruutu P, Ruutu T, Volin L, et al: Cytomegalovirus is frequently isolated in bronchoalveolar lavage fluid of bone marrow transplant recipients without pneumonia, *Ann Intern Med* 112:913, 1990.

94. Schmidt GM, Horak DA, Niland JC, et al: A randomized, controlled trial of prophylactic ganciclovir for cytomegalovirus pulmonary infection in recipients of allogeneic bone marrow transplants, *N Engl J Med* 324:1005, 1991.

95. Hackman RC, Wolford JL, Gleaves CA, et al: Recognition and rapid diagnosis of upper gastrointestinal cytomegalovirus infection in marrow transplant recipients: a comparison of seven virologic methods, *Transplantation* 57:231, 1994.

96. Goodrich JM, Mori M, Gleaves CA, et al: Early treatment with ganciclovir to prevent cytomegalovirus disease after allogeneic bone marrow transplantation, *N Engl J Med* 325:1601, 1991.

97. Einsele H, Ehninger G, Hebart H, et al: Polymerase chain reaction monitoring reduces the incidence of cytomegalovirus disease and the duration and side effects of antiviral therapy after bone marrow transplantation, *Blood* 86:2815, 1995.

98. Verdonck LF, Dekker AW, Rozenberg-Arska M, van den

Hoek MR: A risk-adapted approach with a short course of ganciclovir to prevent cytomegalovirus (CMV) pneumonia in CMV-seropositive recipients of allogeneic bone marrow transplants, *Clin Infect Dis* 24:901, 1997.

99. Hibberd PL, Snydman DR: Cytomegalovirus infection in organ transplant recipients, *Infect Dis Clin North Am* 9:863, 1995.

100. Hibberd PL, Tolkoff-Rubin NE, Conti D, et al: Preemptive ganciclovir therapy to prevent cytomegalovirus disease in cytomegalovirus-antibody positive renal transplant recipients, *Ann Intern Med* 123:18, 1995.

101. Merigan TC, Renlund DG, Keay S, et al: A controlled trial of ganciclovir to prevent cytomegalovirus disease after heart transplantation, *N Engl J Med* 326:1182, 1992.

102. van Dorp WT, Vlieger A, Jiwa NM, et al: The polymerase chain reaction, a sensitive and rapid technique for detecting cytomegalovirus infection after renal transplantation, *Transplantation* 54:661, 1992.

103. Storch GA, Buller RS, Bailey TC, et al: Comparison of PCR and pp65 antigenemia assay with quantitative shell vial culture for detection of cytomegalovirus in blood leukocytes from solid-organ transplant recipients, *J Clin Microbiol* 32:997, 1994.

104. Marsano L, Perrillo RP, Flye MW, et al: Comparison of culture and serology for the diagnosis of cytomegalovirus infection in kidney and liver transplant recipients, *J Infect Dis* 161:454, 1990.

105. Pillay D, Ali AA, Liu SF, et al: The prognostic significance of positive CMV cultures during surveillance of renal transplant recipients, *Transplantation* 56:103, 1993.

106. Falagas ME, Snydman DR, Ruthazer R, et al: Surveillance cultures of blood, urine, and throat specimens are not valuable for predicting cytomegalovirus disease in liver transplant recipients, *Clin Infect Dis* 24:824, 1997.

107. Trulock EP: Lung transplantation, *Am J Respir Crit Care Med* 155:789, 1997.

108. Theise ND, Haber MM, Grimes MM: Detection of cytomegalovirus in lung allografts: Comparison of histologic and immunohistochemical findings, *Am J Clin Pathol* 96:762, 1991.

109. Solans EP, Garrity ER Jr, McCabe M, et al: Early diagnosis of cytomegalovirus pneumonitis in lung transplant patients, *Arch Pathol Lab Med* 119:33, 1995.

110. Storch GA, Ettinger NA, Ockner D, et al: Quantitative cultures of the cell fraction and supernatant of bronchoalveolar lavage fluid for the diagnosis of cytomegalovirus pneumonitis in lung transplant recipients, *J Infect Dis* 168:1502, 1993.

111. Paya CV, Hermans PE, Wiesner RH, et al: Cytomegalovirus hepatitis in liver transplantation: prospective analysis of 93 consecutive orthotopic liver transplantations, *J Infect Dis* 160:752, 1989.

112. Rabah R, Jaffe R: Early detection of cytomegalovirus in the allograft liver biopsy: a comparison of methods, *Pediatr Pathol* 7:549, 1987.

113. Paya CV, Holley KE, Wiesner RH, et al: Early diagnosis of cytomegalovirus hepatitis in liver transplant recipients: role of immunostaining, DNA hybridization and culture of hepatic tissue, *Hepatology* 12:119, 1990.

114. Theise ND, Conn M, Thung SN: Localization of cytomegalovirus antigens in liver allografts over time, *Hum Pathol* 24:103, 1993.

115. Naoumov NV, Alexander GJ, O'Grady JG, et al: Rapid diagnosis of cytomegalovirus infection by in-situ hybridisation in liver grafts, *Lancet* 1:1361, 1470 (erratum), 1988.

116. Randhawa PS, Jaffe R, Faruki H, et al: Detection of cytomegalovirus in formalin-fixed paraffin-embedded donor, native and allograft liver tissue using a multiplex polymerase chain reaction–liquid hybridization assay, *Mod Pathol* 7:125, 1994.

117. Wolff MA, Rand KH, Houck HJ, et al: Relationship of the polymerase chain reaction for cytomegalovirus to the development of hepatitis in liver transplant recipients, *Transplantation* 56:572, 1993.

118. Kusne S, Manez R, Frye BL, et al: Use of DNA amplification for diagnosis of cytomegalovirus enteritis after intestinal transplantation, *Gastroenterology* 112:1121, 1997.

119. Drew WL: Cytomegalovirus infection in patients with AIDS, *Clin Infect Dis* 14:608, 1992.

120. Gallant JE, Moore RD, Richman DD, et al: Incidence and natural history of cytomegalovirus disease in patients with advanced human immunodeficiency virus disease treated with zidovudine, *J Infect Dis* 166:1223, 1992.

121. Mintz L, Drew WL, Miner RC, Braff EH: Cytomegalovirus infections in homosexual men. An epidemiological study, *Ann Intern Med* 99:326, 1983.

122. Dodt KK, Jacobsen PH, Hofmann B, et al: Development of cytomegalovirus (CMV) disease may be predicted in HIV-infected patients by CMV polymerase chain reaction and the antigenemia test, *AIDS* 11: F21, 1997.

123. Zurlo JJ, O'Neill D, Polis MA, et al: Lack of clinical utility of cytomegalovirus blood and urine cultures in patients with HIV infection, *Ann Intern Med* 118:12, 1993.

124. Gérard L, Leport C, Flandre P, et al: Cytomegalovirus (CMV) viremia and the CD4+ lymphocyte count as predictors of CMV disease in patients infected with human immunodeficiency virus, *Clin Infect Dis* 24:836, 1997.

125. MacGregor RR, Pakola SJ, Graziani AL, et al: Evidence of active cytomegalovirus infection in clinically stable HIV-infected individuals with CD4+ lymphocytes counts below 100/microliters of blood: features and relation to risk of subsequent CMV retinitis, *J Acquir Immunodef Syndr* 10:324, 1995.

126. Spector SA, McKinley GF, Lalezari JP, et al: Oral ganciclovir for the prevention of cytomegalovirus disease in persons with AIDS, *N Engl J Med* 334:1491, 1996.

127. Wetherill PE, Landry ML, Alcabes P, Friedland G: Use of a quantitative cytomegalovirus (CMV) antigenemia test in evaluating HIV+ patients with and without CMV disease, *J Acquir Immune Defic Syndr* 12:33, 1996.

128. Bek B, Boeckh M, Lepenies J, et al: High-level sensitivity of quantitative pp65 cytomegalovirus (CMV) antigenemia assay for diagnosis of CMV disease in AIDS patients and follow-up, *J Clin Microbiol* 34:457, 1350 (erratum), 1996.

129. Rasmussen L, Morris S, Zipeto D, et al: Quantitation of

human cytomegalovirus DNA from peripheral blood cells of human immunodeficiency virus–infected patients could predict cytomegalovirus retinitis, *J Infect Dis* 171:177, 1994.

130. Gerna G, Parea M, Percivalle E, et al: Human cytomegalovirus viraemia in HIV-1-seropositive patients at various clinical stages of infection, *AIDS* 4:1027, 1990.

131. Spector SA, Wong R, Hsia K, et al: Plasma cytomegalovirus (CMV) DNA load predicts CMV disease and survival in AIDS patients, *J Clin Invest* 101:497, 1998.

132. Dieterich DT, Rahmin M: Cytomegalovirus colitis in AIDS: presentation in 44 patients and a review of the literature, *J Acquir Immune Defic Syndr* 4:S29, 1991.

133. Wilcox CM, Chalasani N, Lazenby A, Schwartz DA: Cytomegalovirus colitis in acquired immunodeficiency syndrome: a clinical and endoscopic study, *Gastrointest Endosc* 48:39, 1998.

134. Goodgame RW: Gastrointestinal cytomegalovirus disease, *Ann Intern Med* 119:924, 1993.

135. Culpepper-Morgan JA, Kotler DP, Scholes JV, Tierney AR: Evaluation of diagnostic criteria for mucosal cytomegalic inclusion disease in the acquired immune deficiency syndrome, *Am J Gastroenterol* 82:1264, 1987.

136. Theise ND, Rotterdam H, Dieterich D: Cytomegalovirus esophagitis in AIDS: diagnosis by endoscopic biopsy, *Am J Gastroenterol* 86:1123, 1991.

137. Francis ND, Boylston AW, Roberts AH, et al: Cytomegalovirus infection in gastrointestinal tracts of patients infected with HIV-1 or AIDS, *J Clin Pathol* 42:1055, 1989.

138. Schwartz DA, Wilcox CM: Atypical cytomegalovirus inclusions in gastrointestinal biopsy specimens from patients with the acquired immunodeficiency syndrome: diagnostic role of in situ nucleic acid hybridization, *Hum Pathol* 23:1019, 1992.

139. Goodgame RW, Genta RM, Estrada R, et al: Frequency of positive tests for cytomegalovirus in AIDS patients: endoscopic lesions compared with normal mucosa, *Am J Gastroenterol* 88:338, 1993.

140. Wilcox CM, Straub RF, Schwartz DA: Prospective evaluation of biopsy number for the diagnosis of viral esophagitis in patients with HIV infection and esophageal ulcer, *Gastrointest Endosc* 44:587, 1996.

141. Robey SS, Gage WR, Kuhajda FP: Comparison of immunoperoxidase and DNA in situ hybridization techniques in the diagnosis of cytomegalovirus colitis, *Am J Clin Pathol* 89:666, 1988.

142. Clayton F, Klein EB, Kotler DP: Correlation of in situ hybridization with histology and viral culture in patients with acquired immunodeficiency syndrome with cytomegalovirus colitis, *Arch Pathol Lab Med* 113:1124, 1989.

143. Wu GD, Shintaku IP, Chien K, Geller SA: A comparison of routine light microscopy, immunohistochemistry, and in situ hybridization for the detection of cytomegalovirus in gastrointestinal biopsies, *Am J Gastroenterol* 84:1517, 1989.

144. Keh WC, Gerber MA: In situ hybridization for cytomegalovirus DNA in AIDS patients, *Am J Pathol* 131:490, 1988.

145. Myerson D, Hackman RC, Nelson JA, et al: Widespread presence of histologically occult cytomegalovirus, *Hum Pathol* 15:430, 1984.

146. Roberts WH, Hammond S, Sneddon JM, et al: In situ DNA hybridization for cytomegalovirus in colonoscopic biopsies, *Arch Pathol Lab Med* 112:1106, 1988.

147. Cotte L, Drouet E, Bissuel F, et al: Diagnostic value of amplification of human cytomegalovirus DNA from gastrointestinal biopsies from human immunodeficiency virus–infected patients, *J Clin Microbiol* 31:2066, 1993.

148. Bonacini M, Young T, Laine L: The causes of esophageal symptoms in human immunodeficiency virus infection: a prospective study of 110 patients, *Arch Intern Med* 151:1567, 1991.

149. Wilcox CM, Diehl DL, Cello JP, et al: Cytomegalovirus esophagitis in patients with AIDS: a clinical, endoscopic, and pathologic correlation, *Ann Intern Med* 113:589, 1990.

150. Wallace JM, Hannah J: Cytomegalovirus pneumonitis in patients with AIDS: findings in an autopsy series, *Chest* 92:198, 1987.

151. Jacobson MA, Mills J, Rush J, et al: Morbidity and mortality of patients with AIDS and first-episode *Pneumocystis carinii* pneumonia unaffected by concomitant pulmonary cytomegalovirus infection, *Am Rev Respir Dis* 144:6, 1991.

152. Salomon N, Gomez T, Perlman DC, et al: Clinical features and outcomes of HIV-related cytomegalovirus pneumonia, *AIDS* 11:319, 1997.

153. Rodriguez-Barradas MC, Stool E, Musher DM, et al: Diagnosing and treating cytomegalovirus pneumonia in patients with AIDS, *Clin Infect Dis* 23:76, 1996.

154. Waxman AB, Goldie SJ, Brett-Smith H, Matthay RA: Cytomegalovirus as a primary pulmonary pathogen in AIDS, *Chest* 111:128, 1997.

155. Gal AA, Klatt EC, Koss MN, et al: The effectiveness of bronchoscopy in the diagnosis of *Pneumocystis carinii* and cytomegalovirus pulmonary infections in acquired immunodeficiency syndrome, *Arch Pathol Lab Med* 111:238, 1987.

156. Uberti-Foppa C, Lillo F, Terreni MR, et al: Cytomegalovirus pneumonia in AIDS patients: value of cytomegalovirus culture from BAL fluid and correlation with lung disease, *Chest* 113:919, 1998.

157. Miles PR, Baughman RP, Linnemann CC Jr: Cytomegalovirus in the bronchoalveolar lavage fluid of patients with AIDS, *Chest* 97:1072, 1990.

158. Millar AB, Patou G, Miller RF, et al: Cytomegalovirus in the lungs of patients with AIDS: respiratory pathogen or passenger? *Am Rev Respir Dis* 141:1474, 1990.

159. Hansen KK, Vestbo J, Benfield T, et al: Rapid detection of cytomegalovirus in bronchoalveolar lavage fluid and serum samples by polymerase chain reaction: correlation of virus isolation and clinical outcome for patients with human immunodeficiency virus infection, *Clin Infect Dis* 24:878, 1997.

160. Rose DN, Sacks HS: Cost-effectiveness of cytomegalovirus (CMV) disease prevention in patients with AIDS: oral ganciclovir and CMV polymerase chain reaction testing, *AIDS* 11:883, 1997.

161. Shinkai M, Bozzette SA, Powderly W, et al: Utility of urine and leukocyte cultures and plasma DNA polymerase chain reaction for identification of AIDS patients at risk for developing human cytomegalovirus disease, *J Infect Dis* 175:302, 1997.

162. Francisci D, Tosti A, Baldelli F, et al: The pp65 antigen-emia test as a predictor of cytomegalovirus-induced end-organ disease in patients with AIDS, *AIDS* 11:1341, 1997.

163. Chadwick EG, Connor EJ, Hanson IC, et al: Tumors of smooth-muscle origin in HIV-infected children, *JAMA* 263:3182, 1990.

164. Lee ES, Locker J, Nalesnik M, et al: The association of Epstein-Barr virus with smooth-muscle tumors occurring after organ transplantation, *N Engl J Med* 332:19, 1995.

165. Henle W, Henle G: Epstein-Barr virus-specific serology in immunologically compromised individuals, *Cancer Res* 41:4222, 1981.

166. Rickinson AB, Kieff E: Epstein-Barr virus. In Fields BN, Knipe DM, Howley PM, editors: *Fields virology*, ed 3, Philadelphia, 1996, Lippincott-Raven.

167. Ho M, Miller G, Atchison RW, et al: Epstein-Barr virus infections and DNA hybridization studies in post-transplantation lymphoma and lymphoproliferative lesions: the role of primary infection, *J Infect Dis* 152:876, 1985.

168. Raab-Traub N, Flynn K: The structure of the termini of the Epstein-Barr virus as a marker of clonal cellular proliferation, *Cell* 47:883, 1986.

169. Lones MA, Shintaku IP, Weiss LM, et al: Posttransplant lymphoproliferative disorder in liver allograft biopsies: a comparison of three methods for the demonstration of Epstein-Barr virus, *Hum Pathol* 28:533, 1997.

170. Young L, Alfieri C, Hennessy K, et al: Expression of Epstein-Barr virus transformation-associated genes in tissues of patients with EBV lymphoproliferative disease, *N Engl J Med* 321:1080, 1989.

171. Cen H, Williams PA, McWilliams HP, et al: Evidence for restricted Epstein-Barr virus latent gene expression and anti-EBNA antibody response in solid organ transplant recipients with posttransplant lymphoproliferative disorders, *Blood* 81:1393, 1993.

172. Rea D, Delecluse HJ, Hamilton-Dutoit SJ, et al: Epstein-Barr virus latent and replicative gene expression in post-transplant lymphoproliferative disorders and AIDS-related non-Hodgkin's lymphomas: French Study Group of Pathology for HIV-associated Tumors, *Ann Oncol* 5 Suppl 1:113, 1994.

173. Delecluse HJ, Kremmer E, Rouault JP, et al: The expression of Epstein-Barr virus latent proteins is related to the pathological features of post-transplant lymphoproliferative disorders, *Am J Pathol* 146:1113, 1995.

174. Oudejans JJ, Jiwa M, van den Brule AJ, et al: Detection of heterogeneous Epstein-Barr virus gene expression patterns within individual post-transplantation lymphoproliferative disorders, *Am J Pathol* 147:923, 1995.

174a. Randhawa PS, Jaffe R, Demetris AJ, et al: Expression of Epstein-Barr virus-encoded small RNA (by the EBER-1 gene) in liver specimens from transplant recipients with posttransplantation lymphoproliferative disease, *N Eng J Med* 327:1710, 1992.

175. Shin SS, Berry GJ, Weiss LM: Infectious mononucleosis: diagnosis by in situ hybridization in two cases with atypical features, *Am J Surg Pathol* 15:625, 1991.

176. Isaacson PG, Schmid C, Pan L, et al: Epstein-Barr virus latent membrane protein expression by Hodgkin and Reed-Sternberg-like cells in acute infectious mononucleosis, *J Pathol* 167:267, 1992.

177. Niedobitek G, Herbst H, Young LS, et al: Patterns of Epstein-Barr virus infection in non-neoplastic lymphoid tissue, *Blood* 79:2520, 1992.

178. Chang KL, Chen YY, Shibata D, Weiss LM: Description of an in situ hybridization methodology for detection of Epstein-Barr virus RNA in paraffin-embedded tissues, with a survey of normal and neoplastic tissues, *Diagn Mol Pathol* 1:246, 1992.

179. Alshak NS, Jiminez AM, Gedebou M, et al: Epstein-Barr virus infection in liver transplantation patients: correlation of histopathology and semiquantitative Epstein-Barr virus–DNA recovery using polymerase chain reaction, *Hum Pathol* 24:1306, 1993.

180. Kenagy DN, Schlesinger Y, Weck K, et al: Epstein-Barr virus DNA in peripheral blood leukocytes of patients with posttransplant lymphoproliferative disease, *Transplantation* 60:547, 1995.

181. Riddler SA, Breinig MC, McKnight JL: Increased levels of circulating Epstein-Barr virus (EBV)–infected lymphocytes and decreased EBV nuclear antigen antibody responses are associated with the development of posttransplant lymphoproliferative disease in solid-organ transplant recipients, *Blood* 84:972, 1994.

182. Rowe DT, Qu L, Reyes J, et al: Use of quantitative competitive PCR to measure Epstein-Barr virus genome load in the peripheral blood of pediatric transplant patients with lymphoproliferative disorders, *J Clin Microbiol* 35:1612, 1997.

183. Lucas KG, Burton RL, Zimmerman SE, et al: Semi-quantitative Epstein-Barr virus (EBV) polymerase chain reaction for the determination of patients at risk for EBV-induced lymphoproliferative disease after stem cell transplantation, *Blood* 91:3654, 1998.

184. Yoshikawa T, Suga S, Asano Y, et al: Human herpesvirus-6 infection in bone marrow transplantation, *Blood* 78:1381, 1991.

185. Kadakia MP, Rybka WB, Stewart JA, et al: Human herpesvirus 6: infection and disease following autologous and allogeneic bone marrow transplantation, *Blood* 87:5341, 1996.

186. Frenkel N, Katsafanas GC, Wyatt LS, et al: Bone marrow transplant recipients harbor the B variant of human herpesvirus 6, *Bone Marrow Transplant* 14:839, 1994.

187. Appleton AL, Sviland L, Peiris JSM, et al: Human herpes virus-6 infection in marrow graft recipients: role in pathogenesis of graft-versus-host disease, *Bone Marrow Transplant* 16:777, 1995.

188. Wang F-Z, Dahl H, Brytting M, et al: Lymphotropic herpesviruses in allogeneic bone marrow transplantation, *Blood* 88:3615, 1996.

189. Cone RW, Hackman RC, Huang M-LW, et al: Human herpesvirus 6 in lung tissue from patients with pneumonitis after bone marrow transplantation, *N Engl J Med* 329:156, 1993.

190. Wilborn F, Brinkmann V, Schmidt CA, et al: Herpesvirus type 6 in patients undergoing bone marrow transplantation: serologic features and detection by polymerase chain reaction, *Blood* 83:3052, 1994.

191. Okuno T, Higashi K, Shiraki K, et al: Human herpesvi-

rus 6 infection in renal transplantation, *Transplantation* 49:519, 1990.

192. Yoshikawa T, Suga S, Asano Y, et al: A prospective study of human herpesvirus-6 infection in renal transplantation, *Transplantation* 54:879, 1992.

193. Dockrell DH, Prada J, Jones MF, et al: Seroconversion to human herpesvirus 6 following liver transplantation is a marker of cytomegalovirus disease, *J Infect Dis* 176:1135, 1997.

194. Herbein G, Strasswimmer J, Altieri M, et al: Longitudinal study of human herpesvirus 6 infection in organ transplant recipients, *Clin Infect Dis* 22:171, 1995.

195. Osman HKE, Peiris JSM, Taylor CE, et al: "Cytomegalovirus disease" in renal allograft recipients: is human herpesvirus 7 a co-factor for disease progression? *J Med Virol* 48:295, 1996.

196. Schmidt CA, Wilbron F, Weiss K, et al: A prospective study of human herpesvirus 6 detected by polymerase chain reaction after liver transplantation, *Transplantation* 61:662, 1996.

197. Drobyski WR, Dunne WM, Burd EM, et al: Human herpesvirus-6 (HHV-6) infection in allogeneic bone marrow transplant recipients: evidence of a marrow-suppressive role for HHV-6 in vivo, *J Infect Dis* 167:735, 1993.

198. Drobyski WR, Knox KK, Majewski D, Carrigan DR: Fatal encephalitis due to variant B human herpesvirus-6 infection in a bone marrow-transplant recipient, *N Engl J Med* 3:1356, 1994.

199. Singh N, Carrigan DR, Gayowski T, Marino IR: Human herpesvirus-6 infection in liver transplant recipients: documentation of pathogenicity, *Transplantation* 64:674, 1997.

200. Singh N, Carrigan DR, Gayowski T, et al: Variant B human herpesvirus-6 associated febrile dermatosis with thrombocytopenia and encephalopathy in a liver transplant recipient, *Transplantation* 60:1355, 1995.

201. Randhawa PS, Jenkins FJ, Nalesnik MA, et al: Herpesvirus 6 variant A infection after heart transplantation with giant cell transformation in bile ductular and gastroduodenal epithelium, *Am J Surg Pathol* 21:847, 1997.

202. Lautenschlager I, Höckerstedt K, Linnavuori K, Taskinen E: Human herpesvirus-6 infection after liver transplantation, *Clin Infect Dis* 26:702, 1998.

203. Hall CB, Long CE, Schnabel KC, et al: Human herpesvirus-6 infection in children, *N Engl J Med* 331:432, 1994.

204. Wilborn F, Schmidt CA, Zimmermann R, et al: Detection of human herpesvirus 6 by polymerase chain reaction in blood donors: random tests and prospective longitudinal studies, *Br J Hematol* 88:187, 1994.

205. Aberle SW, Mandl CW, Kunz C, Popow-Kraupp T: Presence of human herpesvirus 6 variants A and B in saliva and peripheral blood mononuclear cells of healthy adults, *J Clin Microbiol* 34:3223, 1996.

206. Kidd IM, Clark DA, Ait-Khaled M, et al: Measurement of human herpesvirus 7 load in peripheral blood and saliva of healthy subjects by quantitative polymerase chain reaction, *J Infect Dis* 174, 1996.

207. Fabio G, Knight SN, et al: Prospective study of human herpesvirus 6, human herpesvirus 7, and cytomega-

lovirus infections in human immunodeficiency virus–positive patients, *J Clin Microbiol* 35:2657, 1997.

208. Fairfax MR, Schacker T, Cone RW, et al: Human herpesvirus 6 DNA in blood cells of human immunodeficiency virus–infected men: correlation of high levels with high CD4 cell counts, *J Infect Dis* 169:1342, 1993.

209. Caserta MT, Hall CB, Schnabel K, et al: Primary human herpesvirus 7 infection: a comparison of human herpesvirus 7 and human herpesvirus 6 infections in children, *J Pediatr* 133:386, 1998.

210. Adler SP, McVoy M, Chou S, et al: Antibodies induced by a primary cytomegalovirus infection react with human herpesvirus 6 proteins, *J Infect Dis* 168:1119, 1993.

211. Ward KN, Sheldon MJ, Gray JJ: Primary and recurrent cytomegalovirus infections have different effects on human herpesvirus-6 antibodies in immunosuppressed organ graft recipients: absence of virus cross-reactivity and evidence for virus interaction, *J Med Virol* 34:258, 1991.

212. Irving WL, Ratnamohan M, Hueston LC, et al: Dual antibody rises to cytomegalovirus and human herpesvirus type 6: frequency of occurrence in CMV infections and evidence for genuine reactivity to both viruses, *J Infect Dis* 161:910, 1990.

213. Chang Y, Cesarman E, Pessin MS, et al: Identification of herpesvirus-like DNA sequences in AIDS-associated Kaposi's sarcoma, *Science* 266:1865, 1994.

214. Moore PS, Chang Y: Detection of herpesvirus-like DNA sequences in Kaposi's sarcoma in patients with and without HIV infection, *N Engl J Med* 332:1181, 1995.

215. Cathomas G, Tamm M, McGandy CE, et al: Transplantation-associated malignancies: restriction of human herpes virus 8 to Kaposi's sarcoma, *Transplantation* 64:175, 1997.

216. Soulier J, Grollet L, Oksenhendler E, et al: Kaposi's sarcoma–associated herpesvirus-like DNA sequences in multicentric Castleman's disease, *Blood* 86:1276, 1995.

217. Cesarman E, Chang Y, Moore PS, et al: Kaposi's sarcoma–associated herpesvirus-like DNA sequences in AIDS-related body-cavity-based lymphomas, *N Engl J Med* 332:1186, 1995.

218. Rettig MB, Ma HJ, Vescio RA, et al: Kaposi's sarcoma–associated herpesvirus infection of bone marrow dendritic cells from multiple myeloma patients, *Science* 276:1851, 1997.

219. Memar OM, Rady PL, Goldblum RM, et al: Human herpesvirus 8 DNA sequences in blistering skin from patients with pemphigus, *Arch Dermatol* 133:1247, 1997.

220. Di Alberti L, Piattelli A, Artese L, et al: Human herpesvirus 8 variants in sarcoid tissues, *Lancet* 350:1655, 1997.

221. Ganem D: Human herpesvirus 8 and its role in the genesis of Kaposi's sarcoma. In Remington JS, Swartz MN, editors: *Current clinical topics in infectious diseases 18,* Boston, 1998, Blackwell Science.

222. Martin JN, Ganem DE, Osmond DH, et al: Sexual transmission and the natural history of human herpesvirus 8 infection, *N Engl J Med* 338:948, 1998.

223. Regamey N, Tamm M, Wernli M, et al: Transmission of

human herpesvirus 8 infection from renal-transplant donors to recipients, *N Engl J Med* 339:1358, 1998.

224. Renne R, Zhong W, Herndier B, et al: Lytic growth of Kaposi's sarcoma–associated herpesvirus (human herpesvirus 8) in culture, *Nat Med* 2:342, 1996.

225. Foreman KE, Friborg J Jr., Kong WP, et al: Propagation of a human herpesvirus from AIDS-associated Kaposi's sarcoma, *N Engl J Med* 336:163, 1997.

226. Moore PS, Kingsley LA, Holmberg SD, et al: Kaposi's sarcoma–associated herpesvirus infection prior to onset of Kaposi's sarcoma, *AIDS* 10:175, 1996.

227. Gao SJ, Kingsley L, Hoover DR, et al: Seroconversion to antibodies against Kaposi's sarcoma-associated herpesvirus-related latent nuclear antigens before the development of Kaposi's sarcoma, *N Engl J Med* 335:233, 1996.

228. Whitby D, Howard MR, Tenant-Flowers M, et al: Detection of Kaposi sarcoma associated herpesvirus in peripheral blood of HIV-infected individuals and progression to Kaposi's sarcoma, *Lancet* 346:799, 1995.

229. Humphrey RW, O'Brien TR, Newcomb FM, et al: Kaposi's sarcoma (KS)–associated herpesvirus-like DNA sequences in peripheral blood mononuclear cells: association with KS and persistence in patients receiving anti-herpesvirus drugs, *Blood* 88:297, 1996.

230. Ambroziak JA, Blackbourn DJ, Herndier BG, et al: Herpes-like sequences in HIV-infected and uninfected Kaposi's sarcoma patients, *Science* 268:582, 1995.

231. Diamond C, Brodie SJ, Krieger JN, et al: Human herpesvirus 8 in the prostate glands of men with Kaposi's sarcoma, *J Virol* 72:6223, 1998.

232. Howard MR, Whitby D, Bahadur G, et al: Detection of human herpesvirus 8 DNA in semen from HIV-infected individuals but not healthy semen donors, *AIDS* 11:F15, 1997.

233. Blackbourn DJ, Lennette ET, Ambroziak J, et al: Human herpesvirus 8 detection in nasal secretions and saliva, *J Infect Dis* 177:213, 1998.

234. Luppi M, Barozzi P, Marasca R, et al: Polymerase chain reaction detection of human herpesvirus 8 sequences in primary central nervous system lymphomas, *J Infect Dis* 177:520, 1998.

235. Kedes DH, Operskalski E, Busch M, et al: The seroepidemiology of human herpesvirus 8 (Kaposi's sarcoma–associated herpesvirus): distribution of infection in KS risk groups and evidence for sexual transmission, *Nat Med* 2:918, 1041 (erratum), 1996.

236. Kedes DH, Lagunoff M, Renne R, Ganem D: Identification of the gene encoding the major latency-associated nuclear antigen of the Kaposi's sarcoma–associated herpesvirus, *J Clin Invest* 100:2606, 1997.

237. Gao SJ, Kingsley L, Li M, et al: KSHV antibodies among Americans, Italians and Ugandans with and without Kaposi's sarcoma, *Nat Med* 2:925, 1996.

238. Kedes DH, Ganem D, Ameli N, et al: The prevalence of serum antibody to human herpesvirus 8 (Kaposi sarcoma–associated herpesvirus) among HIV-seropositive and high-risk HIV-seronegative women, *JAMA* 277:478, 1997.

239. Simpson GR, Schulz TF, Whitby D, et al: Prevalence of Kaposi's sarcoma associated herpesvirus infection measured by antibodies to recombinant capsid protein and latent immunofluorescence antigen, *Lancet* 348:1133, 1996.

240. Rabkin CS, Schulz TF, Whitby D, et al: Interassay correlation of human herpesvirus 8 serologic tests: HHV-8 Interlaboratory Collaborative Group, *J Infect Dis* 178:304, 1998.

241. Hierholzer JC: Adenoviruses in the immunocompromised host, *Clin Microbiol Rev* 5:262, 1992

242. Shields AF, Hackman RC, Fife KH, et al: Adenovirus infections in patients undergoing bone-marrow transplantation, *N Engl J Med* 312:529, 1985.

243. Flomenberg P, Babbitt J, Drobyski WR, et al: Increasing incidence of adenovirus disease in bone marrow transplant recipients, *J Infect Dis* 169:775, 1994.

244. Michaels MG, Green M, Wald ER, Starzl TE: Adenovirus infection in pediatric liver transplant recipients, *J Infect Dis* 165:170, 1992.

245. Cames B, Rahier J, Burtomboy G, et al: Acute adenovirus hepatitis in liver transplant recipients, *J Pediatr* 120:33, 1992.

246. Khoo SH, Bailey AS, de Jong JC, Mandal BK: Adenovirus infections in human immunodeficiency virus–positive patients: clinical features and molecular epidemiology, *J Infect Dis* 172:629, 1995.

247. Ferdman RM, Ross L, Inderlied C, Church JA: Adenovirus viremia in human immunodeficiency virus–infected children, *Pediatr Infect Dis J* 16:413, 1997.

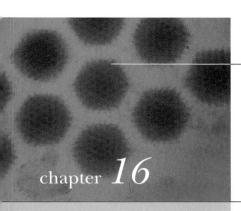

chapter *16*

Gregory A. Storch

Viral Hemorrhagic Fevers and Other Geographically Localized Viral Infections

OVERVIEW

In the current era of rapid global travel, patients can present for medical care with infections acquired thousands of miles away. Therefore clinicians and laboratorians must be prepared to respond to infections acquired anywhere on earth. The most dramatic example is the *viral hemorrhagic fevers*, which are endemic in many tropical countries. Introduction of these infections into Temperate Zone countries will likely increase in the future as global communication and transportation increasingly shrink the globe.

This chapter focuses on viral hemorrhagic fevers and tropical viral febrile illnesses such as dengue. *Hantavirus pulmonary syndrome, Colorado tick fever*, and *alphavirus infections* are also included because of shared virologic and ecologic characteristics. The viruses involved are all ribonucleic acid (RNA) viruses but are otherwise diverse, including members of the families Arenaviridae, Filoviridae, Flaviviridae, Bunyaviridae, Togaviridae, and Reoviridae. Most have animal reservoirs and are transmitted by mosquitoes or ticks. All are characteristic of specific geographic areas, and a key clinical question is where has the patient been before onset of illness.

VIRAL HEMORRHAGIC FEVERS

Viral Agents and Geographic Distribution

The viruses that cause hemorrhagic fever are diverse, including members of the families Filoviridae, Arenaviridae, Flaviviridae, and Bunyaviridae (Table 16–1). All the viruses except dengue virus have an animal reservoir, and several are transmitted by arthropod vectors. All are geographically restricted, and the most important risk factor for human infection is presence in the endemic area (Table 16–2).

Travel to the endemic area is not always required for exposure, since infection has occurred as a result of exposure to materials imported from an endemic area. Dramatic examples were the original outbreak of Marburg disease in Germany and Yugoslavia, resulting from exposure to monkey and monkey kidney cells imported from Uganda. Similarly, cases of Lassa fever have occurred in laboratory workers or health care workers in developed countries caring for patients (or their specimens) with imported illness.

Clinical Manifestations

The clinical manifestations of the hemorrhagic fevers caused by different viruses have considerable overlap. Most begin with the insidious onset of fever, myalgias, and malaise, but yellow fever, Crimean-Congo hemorrhagic fever (CCHF), and Rift Valley fever may have abrupt onsets.[1] Bradycardia, conjunctival injection, and

Table 16.1	Viruses that Cause Hemorrhagic Fever, with Reservoirs and Vectors	
Virus	**Animal reservoir**	**Arthropod vector**
Filoviruses Ebola Marburg	Unknown	Unknown
Arenaviruses Lassa fever Junin Machupo Guanarito Sabiá	Mice	None
Yellow fever	Nonhuman primates	*Haemogogus* and *Aedes* mosquitoes
Dengue	None	*Aedes aegypti* and *Aedes albopictus*
Kyasanur Forest	Nonhuman primates, birds, livestock	Ixodid ticks
Omsk hemorrhagic fever	Rodents	Ixodid ticks
Hantaviruses Hantaan Seoul Puumala	Mice and rats	None
Rift Valley fever	Livestock	Mosquitoes (multiple species)
Crimean-Congo hemorrhagic fever	Livestock, crows, hares	*Hyalomma* ticks

diffuse erythema of the skin may be present. Gastrointestinal (GI) symptoms may include pain, nausea, and vomiting. Pharyngitis may be prominent in Lassa fever. In Marburg and Ebola virus diseases a maculopapular rash may occur on the fifth day of illness.[2]

A *capillary leak syndrome* with hemoconcentration may occur with any of the viral hemorrhagic fevers. Petechiae are the earliest sign of hemorrhagic diathesis, followed by bleeding from the gums, vagina, GI tract, and urinary tract. Leukopenia is often present, but an elevated white blood cell (WBC) count can occur in Lassa fever, dengue hemorrhagic fever, and hemorrhagic fever with renal syndrome (HFRS).[1] Liver enzymes may be abnormal, and coagulation factors may be decreased, with prolongation of the prothrombin time and partial thromboplastin time. Jaundice occurs in yellow fever and Rift Valley fever.[1] Oliguria and decreased renal function are prominent in HFRS. Other diagnoses typically considered in patients with viral hemorrhagic fevers include meningococcemia, rickettsial infection, leptospirosis, malaria, typhoid fever, bacterial sepsis, infectious mononucleosis, and viral exanthematous disease.

The management of viral hemorrhagic fever includes fluids, blood transfusion as necessary, and support for failing organ systems. Ribavirin is effective in Lassa fever and also in HFRS.[1]

Diagnostic Considerations

The diagnosis of viral hemorrhagic fever should be considered in three groups of patients: (1) those who have been in an endemic area within three weeks of onset of fever, (2) those who have had contact with blood or other body fluids or secretions or excretions of persons or animals with viral hemorrhagic fever, and (3) those who worked in a laboratory that handles hemorrhagic fever viruses.[3] All suspected cases of viral hemorrhagic fever should be reported immediately to the Centers for Disease Control and Prevention (CDC, Atlanta, 404-639-1511; 4:30 PM to 8 AM: 404-639-2888) and to the appropriate local and state health departments. Consultation with the CDC will guide specific specimen acquisition and transport.

Laboratory tests for these agents are performed only in *biosafety level 4* (BSL-4) laboratories, those equipped for the highest level of biologic containment.[3a] BSL-4 laboratories are available in the United States only at the CDC and the U.S. Army Medical Research Institute of Infectious Diseases (Frederick, Md, 301-619-2833).

The testing of chemistry and hematology specimens from patients with suspected viral hemorrhagic fever is problematic. Current CDC recommendations include (1) minimizing laboratory testing, (2) using proper precautions in obtaining specimens with care not to con-

Table 16.2 Viral Hemorrhagic Fevers According to Geographic Region

Region	Virus	Family	Comments
Africa	Ebola	Filoviridae	Outbreaks in Zaire, Sudan, Ivory Coast, and Gabon
	Marburg	Filoviridae	Source of human cases unknown, but some evidence points to acquisition in Uganda, Kenya, and Zimbabwe
	Lassa fever	Arenaviridae	Endemic in west sub-Saharian region, especially Sierra Leone, Nigeria, Guinea, and Liberia
	Yellow fever	Flaviviridae	Sub-Saharan region
	Rift Valley fever	Bunyaviridae	Outbreaks in Kenya, South Africa, Egypt, and Mauritania
	CCHF	Bunyaviridae	Human cases reported from South Africa, Mauritania, Senegal, Uganda, and Zaire Virus also isolated in Nigeria, Central African Republic, Kenya, Upper Volta, Madagascar, and Ethiopia
Central and South America	Junin	Arenaviridae	Argentinian hemorrhagic fever
	Machupo	Arenaviridae	Bolivian hemorrhagic fever
	Guanarito	Arenaviridae	Venezuelan hemorrhagic fever
	Sabiá	Arenaviridae	Brazil
	Yellow fever	Flaviviridae	Tropical regions
	Dengue	Flaviviridae	Dengue hemorrhagic fever outbreaks reported from Cuba, Venezuela, Columbia, Brazil, and Nicaragua
Former Soviet Union	HFRS	Bunyaviridae	Eastern Russia, Balkans
	CCHF	Bunyaviridae	Human cases reported from Albania, Bulgaria, Yugoslavia, Russia, and Central Asian Republics
	Omsk hemorrhagic fever	Flaviviridae	Siberia
Middle East	CCHF	Bunyaviridae	Human cases reported from Iraq, Saudi Arabia, Dubai, and Oman. Virus also isolated in Iran
Asia	Dengue	Flaviviridae	Southeast Asia
	HFRS	Bunyaviridae	Pakistan, western China
	Kyasanur Forest	Flaviviridae	India
South Pacific	Dengue	Flaviviridae	Dengue hemorrhagic fever

CCHF, Crimean-Congo (Congo-Crimean) hemorrhagic fever; *HFRS,* hemorrhagic fever with renal syndrome.

taminate the external surfaces of containers, (3) placing specimens in sealed plastic bags, and (4) employing direct transport in clearly labeled, durable, leak-proof containers. In the laboratory, specimens should be handled in a class II biologic safety cabinet with biosafety level 3 practices. Before testing, serum should be treated by addition of 10 μL of 10% Triton X-100 per milliliter of serum for 1 hour. Automated analyzers should be disinfected after use by using procedures recommended by the manufacturer or with 500 parts per million sodium hypochlorite (1:100 dilution of household bleach).[3] Blood smears (e.g., for malaria) are not infectious after fixation in solvents.

In a recent case of Sabiá virus infection managed in a U.S. hospital, chemistry samples were processed in a negative-pressure room and spun in a sealed centrifuge. Hematology specimens were processed in a Coulter counter that did not require removal of the top of the tube, and effluents were treated with sodium hypochlorite and then autoclaved. The Coulter counter was also cleaned after use with several cycles of diluted bleach.[4]

A detailed travel history is essential to narrow the list of causes of a suspected viral hemorrhagic fever (see Table 16–2). Travel in Africa should prompt consideration of Marburg, Ebola, Lassa fever, yellow fever, Rift Valley fever, and CCHF. Travel in South or Central America should suggest the South American arenaviruses (Junin, Machupo, Guanarito, Sabiá), yellow fever, and dengue hemorrhagic fever. Travel in the former Soviet Union should suggest HFRS (Hantaan, Seoul, Dobrava, and Puumula viruses) and CCHF. Exposure to CCHF can also occur in the Middle East. Travel in Asia should prompt consideration of dengue hemorrhagic fever, HFRS, and CCHF. Travel in the Indian subcontinent should suggest exposure to Kyasanur Forest virus and CCHF. Travel in the South Pacific should prompt

consideration of dengue hemorrhagic fever. Because patterns of viral endemicity may change, consultation with experts (e.g., CDC) is strongly recommended.

The tests and specimens used to diagnose viral hemorrhagic fevers vary according to the disease suspected, but important generalizations can be made. *Serology*, especially directed at detection of virus-specific immunoglobulin M (IgM), is often useful. Some patients, however, may present for care or even die before an antibody response has occurred, and tests for the virus itself must be used. Cell culture or suckling-mouse inoculation can be used for many of these viruses. Blood (serum, plasma, or whole blood) is usually the best specimen. *Antigen detection assays* that can be performed on blood specimens are available for a number of the agents. *Immunohistochemistry* (IHC) can be performed on tissues obtained from fatal cases. *Reverse-transcription polymerase chain reaction* (RT-PCR) is gradually being implemented as a rapid means of testing blood samples for evidence of specific viral RNA. Table 16–3 summarizes recommended tests for the diagnosis of viral hemorrhagic fevers.

Ebola and Marburg Diseases

Ebola and Marburg viruses are members of the negative-strand RNA virus family *Filoviridae*. Ebola virus is divided into four subtypes: Zaire, Sudan, Ivory Coast, and Reston. Figure 16–1 shows the source and location of outbreaks caused by Ebola and Marburg viruses.[5]

The first recognized cases of Marburg virus disease occurred in Marburg and Frankfurt (West Germany) and in Belgrade (Yugoslavia) in 1967. The source was African green monkey kidneys imported from Uganda for use in laboratories. Thirty-one human cases occurred, including six secondary cases. The disease has

Table 16.3 Tests Used for Laboratory Diagnosis of Acute Viral Hemorrhagic Fevers

Test	Specimen	Comments
Culture	Blood (serum, plasma, or whole blood), cerebrospinal fluid (for arenavirus infections), tissue (from fatal cases)	Vero cells, mouse inoculation
Electron microscopy	Blood (serum, plasma, or whole blood), urine, tissue	Useful in filovirus infections
Antigen detection	Blood (serum, plasma, or whole blood)	Highest sensitivity early in illness.
Immunohistochemistry	Tissue	Liver and spleen are often useful. Skin may be useful in filovirus infections. Kidney should be examined in hemorrhagic fever with renal syndrome.
Reverse-transcription polymerase chain reaction	Blood (serum, plasma, or whole blood) tissue	Highest sensitivity early in illness
IgM serology	Serum	May not be present early in illness

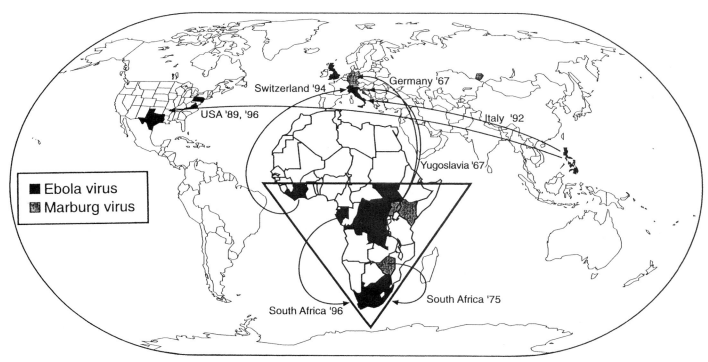

Figure 16.1 Marburg and Ebola virus outbreaks, 1967 to 1997. (From Bremen JG, van der Groen G, Peters CJ, Heymann DL: *J Infect Dis* 176:1059, 1997.)

subsequently been reported from Johannesburg (South Africa) in an individual who had traveled in Zimbabwe and from Kenya.[2]

Ebola virus disease has occurred in explosive outbreaks in Zaire and Sudan with extremely high fatality rates. The virus appeared to spread from person-to-person contact. Some cases resulted from the reuse of syringes contaminated with blood from persons infected with the virus. Ebola cases have occurred in medical personnel caring for infected patients. A recent outbreak among monkeys in a primate-handling center in Reston, Va, was widely publicized. Despite extensive spread among monkeys, only four human cases occurred, all asymptomatic.[2]

No animal or insect reservoir for either Marburg or Ebola virus has been confirmed. Patient management involves general supportive measures with appropriate precautions to minimize the risk of nosocomial transmission.[3] Therapy with immune plasma has been used in some patients.

Diagnostic studies in possible Marburg and Ebola virus cases should be undertaken only in BSL-4 laboratories. Serologic tests for filovirus-specific IgM antibodies provide the best opportunity for establishing a rapid diagnosis and are usually positive within a few days of hospitalization.[2] Diagnosis early in the course of the illness, before an antibody response, can be accomplished using a variety of techniques. Culture is particularly important for characterizing the causative agent. Filoviruses can be cultured from serum using Vero cells.

Electron microscopy has also been used to provide a rapid diagnosis by visualizing the characteristic morphology of the filoviruses directly in serum, urine, or tissue (Figure 16–2). Viral antigen can be detected by fluorescent antibody (FA) staining of impression smears prepared from involved tissues and by IHC performed on formalin-fixed tissue.[6] Antigen capture enzyme immunoassay (EIA) can also be used to detect viral antigen in blood specimens.

Lassa and South American Hemorrhagic Fevers

Lassa fever and the South American hemorrhagic fevers are caused by arenaviruses, which are single-strand RNA viruses in the family Arenaviridae. The arenaviruses are separated into two groups, *Old World* (Lassa fever virus, lymphocytic choriomeningitis virus) and *New World*, or *Tacaribe complex* (Junin, Machupo, Guanarito, and Sabiá viruses). Each arenavirus is associated with a specific rodent host in which the virus causes chronic infection that serves to maintain the virus in nature. Humans are incidental hosts, becoming infected only when they come into contact with virus-containing secretions from infected rodents. The route of exposure is thought to be by aerosol. The distribution of each virus and the circumstances of human exposure are governed by the associated rodent. Figures 16–3 and 16–4 show the geographic distribution of the arenaviruses.

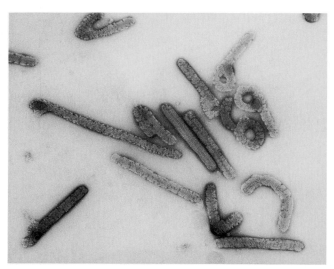

Figure 16.2 Negative-stain electron micrograph of Marburg virus. (×100,000.) (Courtesy R. Regnery and E. Palmer, Centers for Disease Control and Prevention, Atlanta.)

Lassa fever. Lassa fever is endemic in West Africa, where it is associated with rodents of the genus *Mastomys*, which live in close association with human dwellings. Human-to-human transmission has occurred, including a number of episodes of nosocomial spread. The incubation period is 5 to 16 days. Early clinical manifestations are nonspecific and include fever, malaise, sore throat, headache, and chest and back pain. Later manifestations include conjunctival injection, facial and neck edema, maculopapular rash (especially evident in white patients), respiratory and GI symptoms, neurologic manifestations, pleural and pericardial effu-

sions, mucosal bleeding, and shock. Deafness is an important complication.

The hemogram may reveal an elevated hematocrit, normal to moderately increased WBC count, and normal to moderately decreased platelet count.[7] Proteinuria and elevation of serum transaminases are common. An aspartate aminotransferase level greater than 150 U/ml correlates with a high fatality rate.[8] The mortality rate of untreated hospitalized patients is approximately 15%.[7] Therapy with intravenous (IV) ribavirin is effective but must be started early in the illness, highlighting the need for rapid diagnostic capability.[9]

South American hemorrhagic fevers. Argentinian hemorrhagic fever caused by *Junin virus*, Bolivian hemorrhagic fever caused by *Machupo virus*, and Venezuelan hemorrhagic fever caused by *Guanarito virus* are the three best known South American hemorrhagic fevers. Each is associated with a rodent found in rural areas. The clinical features of Argentinian hemorrhagic fever have been described best and include an incubation period of 1 to 2 weeks, followed by fever, malaise, myalgias, dizziness, headache, GI manifestations, flushing of the face and chest, and conjunctival suffusion. Neurologic manifestations are common, including tremors, disorientation, ataxia, and hyporeflexia. Thrombocytopenia, leukopenia, and proteinuria are usually present with full-blown disease. Bleeding manifestations include petechiae, bleeding gums, and mucosal hemorrhage. Hypotension and shock occur in severe cases. Immune plasma and IV ribavirin have been used successfully to treat Argentinian hemorrhagic fever.[7]

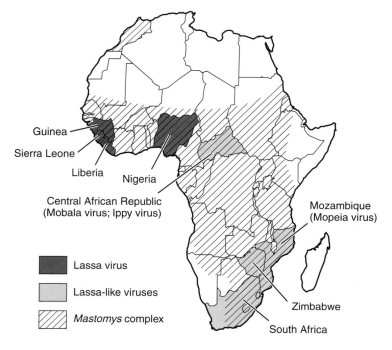

Guinea
Sierra Leone
Liberia
Nigeria
Central African Republic
(Mobala virus; Ippy virus)
Mozambique
(Mopeia virus)
Zimbabwe
South Africa

■ Lassa virus
▨ Lassa-like viruses
▨ *Mastomys* complex

Figure 16.3 Distribution of Old World arenaviruses and genus *Mastomys*. (From Peters CJ: In Richman DD, Whitley RJ, Hayden FG, editors: *Clinical virology*, New York, 1997, Churchill Livingstone.)

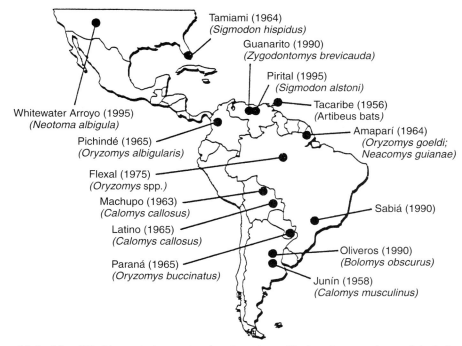

Figure 16.4   New World arenaviruses in the Americas. Circles denote place of isolation and approximate areas of known distribution. (From Peters CJ: In Richman DD, Whitley RJ, Hayden FG, editors: *Clinical virology*, New York, 1997, Churchill Livingstone.)

Diagnostic tests. Patients with Lassa fever are usually viremic when they are admitted to the hospital but may not yet have detectable levels of anti–Lassa fever virus antibodies. Thus early diagnosis is best made by direct detection of virus, using culture, antigen detection, or RT-PCR. Lassa fever virus can be readily cultured from serum samples in Vero cells, but several days are required, as well as BSL-4 containment facilities. Culture of throat wash material is less likely to yield virus than serum, and recovery of virus from urine is unusual.[8] RT-PCR performed on serum, plasma, or whole blood also provides sensitive detection early in the illness. Virtually all patients have detectable viral RNA in blood by the third day of admission.[10] Because different strains of Lassa fever virus exist, the ability of an RT-PCR assay to detect multiple strains is important. Therefore, culture should be used in addition to RT-PCR when possible, especially in evaluating cases from outside the most highly endemic areas.

Tests for detection of Lassa fever virus antigen in serum have been described[11] but are less sensitive than RT-PCR. Lassa fever virus antigens have been detected in fresh tissue by fluorescent antibody (FA) staining and by IHC in formalin-fixed tissue. Detection of Lassa fever virus antibodies is also important but may not be helpful during the first few days of illness.[8, 10] Both indirect immunofluorescence and EIA assays have been used to detect Lassa fever virus-specific IgM and IgG antiviral antibodies. Virus-specific IgM antibodies are usually detectable in the second week of illness.[8, 12]

The principles of diagnosis of the South American hemorrhagic fevers are the same as those for Lassa fever, although the levels of viremia may be lower with the New World arenaviruses. Cocultivation of leukocytes in cell culture can increase the sensitivity of recovery of virus compared with culture of whole blood.[13] An RT-PCR assay to detect Junin virus RNA in blood samples has been described and should provide a rapid diagnosis.[14] Machupo virus has been detected in serum by isolation and with an antigen detection assay.[15] A case of Sabiá virus infection in a laboratory worker was diagnosed by culture and by RT-PCR performed on an acute blood sample. In this case, Sabiá virus-specific IgM antibodies were not detected until day 35 of illness, possibly because of the early use of ribavirin, which also rendered cultures negative.[4]

Dengue

Dengue virus is a positive-sense, single-stranded RNA virus that is a member of the family Flaviviridae. Four antigenically distinct serotypes exist, designated dengue 1 to 4. Infection with one of the types provides enduring immunity against that type but only short-lived immunity against the other types.[16] Dengue virus is transmitted by mosquitoes; the principal vectors are *Aedes aegypti*, a domestic mosquito that tends to breed around human habitations, and *Aedes albopictus*, which has recently become reestablished in the United States. Dengue is distributed throughout the tropical regions of the world (Figure 16–5, *A*). The disease is extremely common, with an estimated 100 million cases per year worldwide.[17] Approximately 100 to 200 cases are imported into the United States each year.

In the endemic areas, dengue is largely a disease of childhood, but persons of any age who enter an endemic region can become infected. The incubation period is 2 to 7 days. Clinical manifestations include high fever, facial flushing, retroorbital headache, and myalgias, often responsible for severe back pain. The severity of the myalgias has given dengue the name "breakbone fever." A maculopapular rash often occurs, starting on the first or second day of illness. Leukopenia and thrombocytopenia are common.[18] No specific antiviral therapy is available.

Dengue hemorrhagic fever. Dengue can be complicated by hemorrhagic manifestations (dengue hemor-

rhagic fever) and a tendency to develop shock (*dengue shock syndrome*). Dengue hemorrhagic fever/dengue shock syndrome occurs when an individual who has experienced infection with one dengue serotype becomes infected with another serotype. This entity has occurred in Southeast Asia, the South Pacific, Central America, and the northern part of South America. Dengue hemorrhagic fever begins like classic dengue, but the illness worsens on the second to fifth day at about the time of defervescence. Hemorrhagic manifestations include petechiae, ecchymoses, oozing from venipuncture sites, epistaxis, and GI hemorrhage. Hemoconcentration and thrombocytopenia are present, pleural effusions are common, and shock may occur.[18]

Diagnostic tests. Dengue virus replicates in cells of the macrophage-monocyte lineage, and viremia is present

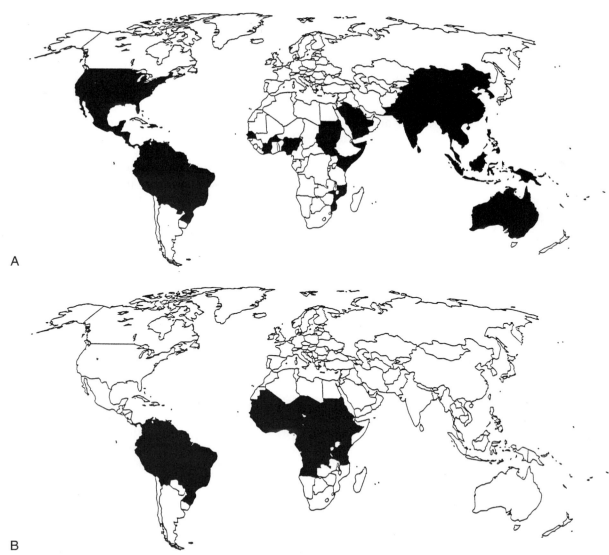

Figure 16.5   Distribution of dengue (**A**) and yellow fever (**B**). (From Monath TP, Tsai TF: In Richman DD, Whitley RJ, Hayden FG, editors: *Clinical virology*, New York, 1997, Churchill Livingstone.)

for the first 3 to 5 days of illness, terminating at about the same time the patient defervesces.[19] Dengue-specific antibodies become detectable within a few days after defervescence. Thus diagnosis early in illness, while the patient is febrile, can be made by direct detection of virus from serum or plasma, using culture or RT-PCR.

Dengue virus can be cultured in a variety of cell types. The most sensitive are mosquito cell lines, but mammalian cells (e.g., LLC-MK2, Vero, BHK-21) can also be used. Intrathoracic injection of mosquitoes is more sensitive than cell culture.[20] Viral isolation is most likely to be successful from specimens obtained very early in the illness. RT-PCR provides an alternative method for rapid diagnosis early in the illness. RT-PCR assays can detect all four serotypes of dengue and can also identify which virus is responsible for the illness.[21, 22] Both culture and RT-PCR rapidly become negative about the time of defervescence.[22]

Serologic tests are useful for the diagnosis of dengue, especially after defervescence. The hemagglutination inhibition assay using goose erythrocytes has been widely used and is still the reference test for distinguishing between primary and secondary infection. Currently, EIA methods are the assays of choice because they allow detection of dengue-specific IgM antibodies. Dengue-specific antibodies are produced in secondary as well as primary infections and are usually detectable by the third afebrile day.[23] Many hospitalized patients are positive at admission, but for maximum sensitivity, at least one specimen should be obtained after the patient defervesces. Use of all four dengue serotype antigens in the assay ensures detection of antibodies made in response to any serotype. The ratio of IgM to IgG antibodies helps determine whether infection is primary or secondary.[23] Alternatively, a negative hemagglutination titer in an acute specimen suggests the infection is primary, whereas a high titer suggests it is secondary. In some parts of the world, cross-reactions with other flaviviruses can be a source of confusion. In Asia the ratio of dengue antibodies to Japanese encephalitis antibodies helps distinguish the antibody response to these two viruses.[23]

Yellow Fever

As with dengue virus, yellow fever virus is a member of the Flaviviridae family. Yellow fever occurs in sub-Saharan Africa and South America, exhibiting two different patterns of transmission (Figure 16–5, *B*). In the *jungle cycle*, mosquitoes of a number of different species transmit infection among nonhuman primates, and humans are infected incidentally. In the *urban cycle*, peridomestic *Aedes aegypti* mosquitoes transmit infection from one human to another. Both cycles occur in Africa, whereas only the jungle cycle currently occurs in South America, where most cases occur between January and March. In Africa, cases occur during the late

rainy season and early dry season.[18] The frequency of the disease has increased in recent years.[24]

Disease manifestations in yellow fever result from infection of Kupffer cells and hepatocytes in the midzone of hepatic lobules. Clinical findings include abrupt onset of fever, malaise, headache, and back pain. These symptoms may subside, but one or several days later the patient experiences return of fever with jaundice and renal dysfunction.[18] Hepatic and renal function deteriorate, and hemorrhagic manifestations may occur. Thrombocytopenia and evidence of disseminated intravascular coagulation (DIC) may be present.

Diagnostic tests. The diagnosis can be confirmed by virus isolation, detection of yellow fever virus RNA by RT-PCR, IHC, or serology. Viremia occurs early in the illness, and the diagnosis can be made by culturing the virus from the blood. During this phase, RT-PCR can detect yellow fever virus RNA in serum,[25] but experience with this technique is limited. Yellow fever antigens can also be detected in blood samples using radioimmunoassay (RIA) or EIA[26] and in hepatic tissue obtained at autopsy using IHC.[25] The detection of yellow fever virus–specific IgM antibodies in serum can provide a rapid diagnosis in patients who survive past the first week. Seroconversion or a rising titer demonstrated in serial specimens can also be diagnostic.

Kyasanur Forest Disease and Omsk Hemorrhagic Fever

Kyasanur Forest disease and Omsk hemorrhagic fever are flavivirus diseases that can have hemorrhagic manifestations. Kyasanur Forest virus is a member of the tick-borne encephalitis complex, is transmitted by ixodid ticks, and occurs in western India. Manifestations of the disease in humans include fever, headache, myalgias, cough, bradycardia, dehydration, GI symptoms, leukopenia, hemorrhagic manifestations, and shock. Meningoencephalitis occurs in some patients.[18] Omsk hemorrhagic fever occurs in Siberia. The causative virus is transmitted by ixodid ticks. The disease is similar to Kyasanur Forest disease. The laboratory diagnosis of both diseases can be made by isolation of virus from blood or by serology.[18]

Hemorrhagic Fever with Renal Syndrome

HFRS is common in the Far East, Russia, and parts of Europe, with 150,000 to 200,000 hospitalized cases reported each year.[27] The disease is caused by several different Old World hantaviruses, all of which are negative-sense, single-stranded RNA viruses, classified in the genus *Hantavirus* in the family Bunyaviridae. A severe form of the disease known as Korean hemorrhagic fever is common in Korea and China and is caused by *Hantaan virus. Seoul virus* and *Dobrava-Belgrade*

Table 16.4	Hantaviruses that Cause Hemorrhagic Fever with Renal Syndrome	
Virus	**Reservoir**	**Geographic distribution**
Hantaan	Field mouse	China, Korea, Russia east of the Urals
Seoul	Brown rat	Worldwide
Dobrava-Belgrade	Field mouse	Balkans and nearby regions
Puumala	Vole	Scandinavia, Russia west of the Urals, Eastern Europe

virus cause a similar but somewhat milder illness. *Puumala virus* is the cause of nephropathia epidemica, a milder form of disease that occurs in Europe and usually does not involve hemorrhagic manifestations.

The natural hosts for hantaviruses are rodents, which experience chronic infection without adverse effects. Each virus is associated with a specific rodent species. Humans become infected when they are exposed to infected rodent excretions. No insect vector is involved in virus transmission. No human-to-human transmission is known to occur, although an exception may be the Andes hantavirus discovered recently in Argentina, which may spread from person to person.[28] Table 16–4 shows the geographic distribution of disease caused by the Old World hantaviruses.[29] Infection occurs in those whose residence or occupation brings them into contact with infected rodents. Most cases occur in adults 15 to 40 years of age, and cases in younger children are unusual.

The pathogenesis of hantavirus infections is related to widespread infection of endothelial cells. In HFRS this involvement is most intense in the kidney, whereas in hantavirus pulmonary syndrome (see later discussion), the involvement is most intense in the lungs. The severe form of HFRS associated with Hantaan virus is divided into five stages: febrile, hypotensive, oliguric, diuretic, and convalescent. After an incubation period that can range from 4 days to 6 weeks, fever begins, accompanied by malaise, myalgias, headache, abdominal pain, facial flushing, and conjunctival injection. Petechiae may be present within several days. The fever typically lasts 3 to 7 days. Toward the end of the febrile period, other manifestations of hantavirus infection occur, including hypotension, sometimes with shock; increased hemorrhagic manifestations; and oliguric renal failure. The hemogram reveals an unusual but characteristic profile: hemoconcentration, thrombocytopenia, elevated WBC count with immature forms, and presence of immunoblasts. The fatality rate in recent experience is 5% to 7%.[30] Ribavirin has been effective for the treatment of the Korean hemorrhagic fever.[31]

Diagnostic tests. The laboratory diagnosis of hantavirus infection differs from most of the other infections discussed in this chapter. Hantaviruses are extremely difficult to grow in the laboratory, and therefore serology is the mainstay of diagnosis. IgG and IgM antibodies to the causative hantavirus are uniformly present when renal involvement is clinically evident.[30] IgM antibodies can be detected by the IgM capture EIA technique. In the United States, these assays are available only through reference laboratories and the CDC. RT-PCR has been used to detect Puumula virus RNA in urine sediment, whereas detection in peripheral blood mononuclear cells has been insensitive.[32]

Rift Valley Fever

Rift Valley fever is endemic in sub-Saharan Africa and has also occurred in Egypt. Rift Valley fever virus is a member of the *Phlebovirus* genus within the family Bunyaviridae. As with all the Bunyaviridae other than the hantaviruses, the virus is transmitted by insect vectors. A number of different mosquito genera have been implicated. The disease affects cattle, sheep, and goats, with a high fatality rate, especially for young animals. High rates of abortion occur in these animals during epizootics, and abortions in animals can signal the presence of a Rift Valley fever outbreak.

Humans can become infected if they are in areas where animal illness is occurring. Human disease is characterized by a short incubation period of 2 to 6 days, followed by a viremic illness with nonspecific symptoms of fever, malaise, and myalgias. Most infected individuals recover uneventfully, but a small proportion progress to a hemorrhagic phase marked by petechiae, GI bleeding, jaundice, and shock.[30] A late postviremic phase of the illness is associated with encephalitis and vision loss caused by retinitis and uveitis characterized by macular and paramacular lesions. Several Rift Valley fever vaccines have been used in both animals and humans.

Diagnostic tests. Rift Valley fever should be suspected in patients with a compatible illness who have traveled in the endemic area or who have been exposed to the virus in a laboratory. During the early phase, laboratory diagnosis is made by detecting the virus, which may be present in the blood in high titer. This can be accomplished by viral isolation through inoculation of cell cultures or suckling mice. In addition, EIA has been used to detect viral antigen in blood.[33] RT-PCR has been used to detect viral RNA in blood specimens from recent cases.[34] During the later stages of illness, especially in patients with retinitis or encephalitis, virus may no longer be detectable in blood. In these patients, the diagnosis is best made by detection of virus-specific IgM antibodies.[35] Alternatively, acute and convalescent serum specimens can be used to show a diagnostic rise in titer using one of a variety of serologic tests to measure the virus-specific IgG antibody response.

Crimean-Congo Hemorrhagic Fever

CCHF is a severe hemorrhagic disease caused by a virus in the genus *Nairovirus* of the Bunyaviridae family. The disease has occurred in Africa, Eastern Europe, the Middle East, and western Asia. Infection may occur in multiple animals, including cows, sheep, goats, hares, and other herbivores. The virus is transmitted to humans by the bite of a *Hyalomma* tick or by direct contact with the tissues of infected animals. Numerous episodes of nosocomial transmission have occurred.

CCHF is characterized by an incubation period of 2 to 12 days, followed by an acute febrile illness that may include facial flushing and conjunctival injection. Hepatomegaly is present in about half of cases at this stage.[30] After 3 to 6 days, hemorrhagic manifestations occur, including petechiae, ecchymoses, epistaxis, GI hemorrhage, and hematuria. Hepatic necrosis and renal failure may occur. The overall fatality rate is 13% to 50%. Laboratory abnormalities include thrombocytopenia, leukopenia or leukocytosis, elevated serum transaminase levels, and evidence of DIC. Ribavirin may have some efficacy for treatment.

Diagnostic tests.   CCHF should be suspected in patients with a consistent illness who have been in the endemic area or have contact with animal tissues or laboratory specimens from the endemic area. Patients are viremic during the first few days of illness, and laboratory diagnosis at this stage is directed at direct detection of the virus in blood. The virus can be cultured by inoculation of Vero or CER cell cultures or suckling mice. Cell culture yields a more rapid result, although mouse inoculation is more sensitive.[36] An antigen detection EIA can be used to detect viral antigen in blood,[37] and RT-PCR can be used to detect viral RNA.[38] These procedures should be undertaken only in a BSL-4 laboratory. IHC and in situ hybridization can also be used to detect viral antigen or RNA in tissues obtained early in the illness.[39] Later in the illness, serologic testing for IgM or IgG antibodies to the virus can be used to make a diagnosis.[38] Fatal cases may be seronegative at the time of death, requiring direct demonstration of virus to make a diagnosis.[40, 41]

HANTAVIRUS PULMONARY SYNDROME

Hantavirus pulmonary syndrome (HPS) was first recognized in 1993 in the Four Corners region of the southwestern United States. The illness was quickly linked to a newly discovered hantavirus now known as *sin nombre virus*. The rodent associated with sin nombre virus is the deer mouse, *Peromyscus maniculatus*. Since 1993, cases of HPS have been documented in most of the states west of the Mississippi River, and evidence of sin nombre virus infection of deer mice has been found in an even wider distribution. In addition, cases of HPS related to several different new hantaviruses (New York, Black Creek Canal, Bayou, Andes, Laguna Negra) have also been recognized in the United States and in Paraguay, Argentina, and Chile (Table 16–5) No insect vector has been implicated, and transmission is believed to result from aerosolization of infected rodent excretions. In the Four Corners outbreak of HPS, most cases occurred in adults with exposure to deer mouse habitats. Sin nombre virus has not been associated with human-to-human transmission, but such transmission may have occurred with the newly discovered Andes virus.[28]

The incubation period of HPS is believed to be 1 to 4 weeks. The prodromal phase is characterized by fever, chills, and myalgias. GI manifestations may be prominent, whereas upper respiratory tract symptoms other than cough are unusual. Important laboratory clues during this phase include thrombocytopenia (less than 150,000 cells/mm^3), elevated serum lactate dehydrogenase and serum transaminases, and decreased serum bicarbonate. After several days of prodromal symptoms,

Table 16.5	Hantaviruses that Cause Hantavirus Pulmonary Syndrome	
Virus	**Reservoir**	**Geographic distribution***
Sin nombre	Deer mouse	United States and Canada, excluding southeastern and eastern seaboard
New York	White-footed mouse	Eastern United States, Canada, and Mexico
Black Creek Canal	Cotton rat	Southeast United States, Central America, northern South America
Bayou	Rice rat	Central and southeastern United States
Andes	Pygmy rice rat	Argentina, Chile
Laguna Negra	Vesper mouse	Paraguay, Argentina, Bolivia, Uruguay, Brazil

*Distribution of implicated rodent.

hypotension and pulmonary edema develop rapidly. These manifestations result from hantavirus infection of endothelial cells, especially those in the pulmonary capillary bed, with resulting capillary leakage. Characteristic hematologic findings during this period include (1) elevated hematocrit, reflecting hemoconcentration; (2) immature circulating leukocytes, including metamyelocytes, myelocytes, and promyelocytes; and (3) circulating plasmacytoid immunoblasts. The immunoblasts often make up 10% or more of circulating lymphocytes. Once pulmonary edema occurs, the fatality rate is high, but recovery is rapid for those who survive the pulmonary edema phase.

Ribavirin has been used to treat patients with HPS, but its efficacy is not established; it is currently being evaluated in a prospective clinical trial.

In disease caused by the more recently discovered New World hantaviruses, renal and skeletal muscle involvement manifested by elevation of serum creatine kinase appears to be more common than in HPS caused by sin nombre virus.[27]

Diagnostic Tests

As with the Old World hantaviruses, sin nombre virus and the other New World hantaviruses are difficult to culture in the laboratory, and therefore viral culture is not used to diagnose HPS. Detection of antibodies to sin nombre virus is the mainstay of diagnosis. Several different assay formats have been used, including IgM capture EIA,[42] indirect immunofluorescence, and Western blot for detection of virus-specific IgG and IgM antibodies.

In a *strip immunoblot assay*, synthetic peptide and recombinant hantavirus antigens are immobilized on a nitrocellulose strip and allowed to react with the patient's serum. The antigens include the nucleocapsid protein (N) and the G1 glycoprotein (G1) of sin nombre virus (Figure 16–6). Patients with past or present infection with any hantavirus have antibodies to N, whereas only those with recent sin nombre virus infection have antibodies to G1. Thus, even though the assay is not a virus-specific IgM antibody assay, it can distinguish between acute and past infection, as well as between infection with sin nombre virus and other hantaviruses. The assay requires no sophisticated instrumentation and is suitable for use in small hospital laboratories.[43]

The sensitivity of the virus-specific IgM antibody assays and the strip immunoassay are almost 100% for patients in the symptomatic phase of HPS.[43, 44]

RT-PCR has also been used to detect sin nombre virus in peripheral blood mononuclear cells (PBMCs) and in serum or plasma. Hantavirus RNA is detectable in 100% of samples of PBMCs and approximately 70% of plasma or serum samples from patients during the acute illness.[44] RT-PCR can also be used to detect hantavirus RNA in tissue samples.

Hantavirus antigens can be detected in formalin-fixed tissue using IHC. This can be particularly useful for analysis of fatal cases.

Hantavirus diagnostic tests are available through most state health department laboratories and the

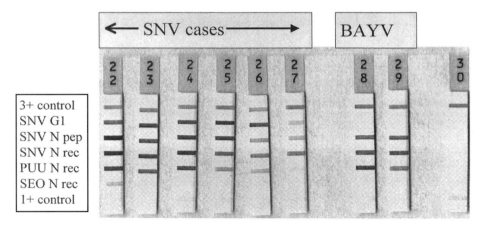

Figure 16.6 Strip immunoblot assay showing diagnostic antibody pattern present in patients with hantavirus pulmonary syndrome caused by sin nombre virus (*SNV*) and Bayou virus (*BAYV*). Antigens placed on each strip are (1) a synthetic peptide corresponding to portion of G1 glycoprotein of SNV, (2) a synthetic peptide corresponding to portion of nucleocapsid (*N*) protein of SNV, (3) a recombinant SNV N protein, and (4) recombinant N proteins from Puumula (*PUU*) and Seoul (*SEO*) hantaviruses. (Courtesy B. Hjelle, Department of Pathology, University of New Mexico, Albuquerque.)

Table 16.6	Alphaviruses that Cause Fever, Rash, and Polyarthropathy*			
Virus	**Region**	**Mosquito vector**	**Animal host**	
Chikungunya	Asia, sub-Saharan Africa	*Aedes aegypti*	None	
O'nyong-nyong	Uganda	*Anopheles*	None	
Sindbis	Europe, Asia, Africa, Australia	*Culex*	Birds	
Mayaro	Central and South America	*Haemogogus*	Primates	
Ross River	Australia	*Aedes, Culex*	Kangaroos, wallabies	

*Contents from Tsai TF, Monath TP: Flaviviruses. In Richman DD, Whitley RJ, Hayden FG, editors, *Clinical Virology*, Churchill Livingstone, New York, 1997.

CDC. Testing is also available through the University of New Mexico (http://thor.unm.edu).

COLORADO TICK FEVER

The virus that causes Colorado tick fever is classified in the genus *Coltivirus* within the family Reoviridae. Like other members of the family, the coltiviruses have a segmented, double-stranded RNA genome. Colorado tick fever virus is found in the western United States and southwestern Canada. It is transmitted to humans from the wood tick, *Dermacentor andersoni*, and is maintained in nature through small mammals, including ground squirrels and chipmunks.

During human infection the virus replicates in hematopoietic cells and can be found for prolonged periods in circulating erythrocytes.[45] Most cases of Colorado tick fever occur between March and October, when exposure to infected ticks is most likely. The incubation period is usually about 4 days but ranges from 1 to 14 days.[46] Typical symptoms include fever, headache, myalgias, and lethargy. Abdominal pain and stiff neck may occur. Approximately half of patients have a biphasic fever consisting of 2 to 3 days of fever, defervescence, and fever for several more days. Petechial rash and central nervous system (CNS) involvement occur in some patients. Mild leukopenia is common, sometimes with thrombocytopenia. A mononuclear pleocytosis may be present with CNS involvement. The differential diagnosis includes Rocky Mountain spotted fever, ehrlichiosis, tick-borne relapsing fever, and enteroviral infection.

Diagnostic Tests

The laboratory diagnosis of Colorado tick fever can be made in several ways. The virus can be readily cultured from a blood clot by inoculation of suckling mice or by cell culture (e.g., Vero, BHK-21). This method is sensitive but requires 4 to 8 days to detect the virus. Cultures can remain positive for weeks after infection.

In one large series, 46% of patients were viremic 4 weeks after onset.[46] A rapid diagnosis can be made by FA staining to detect viral antigen in circulating erythrocytes.[47] This technique is positive in about 50% of cases and often remains positive even longer than culture.[46]

Recently, RT-PCR has been used to detect Colorado tick fever virus RNA. One study found that viral RNA was detectable in serum samples from the day of onset through day 8 of symptoms and was negative in all but one sample obtained after that time.[48] Use of erythrocytes or whole blood may increase the sensitivity of detection.

Diagnosis can also be made serologically using IgM-specific EIA or the plaque reduction neutralization assay. Virus-specific IgM antibodies become detectable approximately 1 to 2 weeks after onset of symptoms and decline after approximately 45 days.[48, 49]

Diagnostic tests for Colorado tick fever are available through the Arbovirus Disease Branch of the Division of Vector-Borne Infections of the CDC at Fort Collins, Colorado.

ALPHAVIRUS INFECTIONS

The alphaviruses are a large and diverse group of positive-strand RNA viruses in the family Togaviridae. Most are transmitted by mosquitoes or other arthropods, and humans are incidental hosts. Several alphaviruses, including eastern, western, and Venezuelan equine encephalitis viruses, are important causes of encephalitis (see Chapter 3). Other alphaviruses cause febrile illnesses with rash and polyarthropathy, which is often the dominant clinical manifestation (Table 16–6).

Diagnostic Tests

Many of the alphaviruses, especially those that do not cause encephalitis, can be isolated in cultures of blood using Vero and BHK-21 cells as well as mosquito cell lines. RT-PCR has been used to detect alphavirus RNA, but experience is limited. A semi-nested PCR assay that detects all known alphaviruses has been described, but clinical application has not yet been reported.[50]

Most often the diagnosis is made serologically by detection of virus-specific IgM antibodies,[51] seroconversion, or a rising titer of IgG antibodies. Persistence of virus-specific IgM antibodies has been noted in some patients, especially those with chronic joint symptoms.[52] Some serologic cross-reaction can occur between closely related alphaviruses.

References

1. Johnson KM: Hemorrhagic fevers: a comparative appraisal. In Richman DD, Whitley RJ, Hayden FG, editors: *Clinical virology,* New York, 1997, Churchill Livingstone.

2. Huggins JW: Filoviridae. In Richman DD, Whitley RJ, Hayden FG, editors*: Clinical virology,* New York, 1997, Churchill Livingstone.

3. Centers for Disease Control and Prevention: Update: management of patients with suspected viral hemorrhagic fever—United States, *MMWR* 44:475, 1995.

3a. Centers for Disease Control and National Institutes of Health: *Biosafety in microbiological and biomedical laboratories,* ed 3, U.S. Government Printing Office, Washington, DC, 1993.

4. Barry M, Russi M, Armstrong L, et al: Brief report: treatment of a laboratory-acquired Sabiá virus infection, *N Engl J Med* 333:294, 1995.

5. Bremen JG, van der Groen G, Peters CJ, Heymann DL: International Colloquium on Ebola Virus Research: summary report, *J Infect Dis* 176:1058, 1997.

6. Wulff H, Slenczka W, Gear JHS: Early detection of antigen and estimation of virus yield in specimens from patients with Marburg virus disease, *Bull World Health Organ* 56:633, 1978.

7. Peters CJ: Arenaviruses. In Richman DD, Whitley RJ, Hayden FG, editors: *Clinical virology,* New York, 1997, Churchill Livingstone.

8. Johnson KM, McCormick JB, Webb PA, et al: Clinical virology of Lassa fever in hospitalized patients. *J Infect Dis* 155:456, 1987.

9. McCormick JB, King IJ, Webb PA, et al: Lassa fever: effective therapy with ribavirin, *N Engl J Med* 314:20, 1986.

10. Demby AH, Chamberlain J, Brown DWG, Clegg CS: Early diagnosis of Lassa fever by reverse transcription-PCR, *J Clin Microbiol* 32:2898, 1994.

11. Niklasson BS, Jahrling PB, Peters CJ: Detection of Lassa virus antigens and Lassa virus–specific immunoglobulins G and M by enzyme-linked immunosorbent assay, *J Clin Microbiol* 20:239, 1984.

12. Wulff H, Johnson KM: Immunoglobulin M and G responses measured by immunofluorescence in patients with Lassa or Marburg virus infections, *Bull World Health Organ* 57:631, 1979.

13. Ambrosio A, Enría D, Maiztegui J: Junin virus isolation from lymphomononuclear cells of patients with Argentinian hemorrhagic fever, *Intervirology* 25:97, 1986.

14. Lozano ME, Enría D, Maiztegui JI, et al: Rapid diagnosis of Argentine hemorrhagic fever by reverse transcriptase PCR-based assay, *J Clin Microbiol* 33:1327, 1995.

15. Kilgore PE, Ksiazek TG, Rollin PE, et al: Treatment of Bolivian hemorrhagic fever with intravenous ribavirin, *Clin Infect Dis* 24:718, 1997.

16. Sabin AB: Research on dengue during World War II, *Am J Trop Med Hyg* 1:30, 1952.

17. Kalayanarooj S, Vaughn DW, Nimmannitya S, et al: Early clinical and laboratory indicators of acute dengue illness, *J Infect Dis* 176:313, 1997.

18. Monath TP, Tsai TF: Flaviviruses. In Richman DD, Whitley RJ, Hayden FG, editors: *Clinical virology,* New York, 1997, Churchill Livingstone.

19. Vaughn DW, Green S, Kalayanarooj S, et al: Dengue in the early febrile phase: viremia and antibody responses, *J Infect Dis* 176:322, 1997.

20. Guzmán MG, Kourí G: Advances in dengue diagnosis, *Clin Lab Diagn Immunol* 3:621, 1996.

21. Lanciotti RS, Calisher CH, Gubler DJ, et al: Rapid detection and typing of dengue viruses from clinical samples by using reverse transcription–polymerase chain reaction, *J Clin Microbiol* 30:545, 1992.

22. Sudiro TM, Ishiko H, Green S, et al: Rapid diagnosis of dengue viremia by reverse-transcriptase–polymerase chain reaction using 3'-noncoding region universal primers, *Am J Trop Med Hyg* 56:424, 1997.

23. Innis BL, Nisalak A, Nimmannitya S, et al: An enzyme-linked immunosorbent assay to characterize dengue infections where dengue and Japanese encephalitis cocirculate, *Am J Trop Med Hyg* 40:418, 1989.

24. Robertson SE, Hull BP, Tomori O, et al: Yellow fever: a decade of reemergence, *JAMA* 276:1157, 1996.

25. Deubel V, Huerre M, Cathomas G, et al: Molecular detection and characterization of yellow fever virus in blood and liver specimens from a non-vaccinated fatal human case, *J Med Virol* 53:212, 1997.

26. Monath TP, Hill LJ, Brown NV, et al: Sensitive and specific monoclonal immunoassay for detecting yellow fever virus in laboratory and clinical specimens, *J Clin Microbiol* 23:129, 1986.

27. Schmaljohn C, Hjelle B: Hantaviruses: a global disease problem, *Emerg Infect Dis* 3:95, 1997.

28. Wells RM, Sosa Estani S, Yadon ZE, et al: An unusual hantavirus outbreak in southern Argentina: person-to-person transmission? *Emerg Infect Dis* 3:171, 1997.

29. Young SA: Hantaviruses. In Rose NR, Conway de Macario E, Folds JD, et al, editors: *Manual of clinical laboratory immunology,* ed 5, Washington, DC, 1997, ASM Press.

30. Mertz GJ: Bunyaviridae: bunyaviruses, phleboviruses, nairoviruses, and hantaviruses. In Richman DD, Whitley RJ, Hayden FG, editors: *Clinical virology,* New York, 1997, Churchill Livingstone.

31. Huggins JW, Hsiang CM, Cosgriff TM, et al: Prospective, double-blind, concurrent, placebo-controlled clinical trial of intravenous ribavirin therapy of hemorrhagic fever with renal syndrome, *J Infect Dis* 164:1119, 1991.

32. Plyusnin A, Hörling J, Kanerva M, et al: Puumala han-

tavirus genome in patients with nephropathia epidemica: correlation of PCR positivity with HLA haplotype and link to viral sequences in local rodents, *J Clin Microbiol* 35:1090, 1997.

33. Niklasson B, Grandien M, Peters CJ, Gargan TP II: Detection of Rift Valley fever virus antigen by enzyme-linked immunosorbent assay, *J Clin Microbiol* 17:1026, 1983.

34. Centers for Disease Control and Prevention: Rift Valley fever—East Africa, 1997-1998, *MMWR* 47:261, 1998.

35. Niklasson B, Peters CJ, Grandien M, Wood O: Detection of human immunoglobulins G and M antibodies to Rift Valley fever virus by enzyme-linked immunosorbent assay, *J Clin Microbiol* 19:225, 1984.

36. Shepard AJ, Swanepoel R, Leman PA, Shepard SP: Comparison of methods for isolation and titration of Crimean-Congo hemorrhagic fever virus, *J Clin Microbiol* 24:654, 1986.

37. Logan TM, Linthicum KJ, Moulton JR, Ksiazek TG: Antigen-capture enzyme-linked immunosorbent assay for detection and quantification of Crimean-Congo hemorrhagic fever virus in the tick, *Hyalomma truncatum, J Virol Methods* 42:33, 1993.

38. Rodriguez LL, Maupin GO, Ksiazek TG, et al: Molecular investigation of a multisource outbreak of Crimean-Congo hemorrhagic fever in the United Arab Emirates, *Am J Trop Med Hyg* 57:512, 1997.

39. Burt FJ, Swanepoel R, Shieh W-J, et al: Immunohistochemical and in situ localization of Crimean-Congo hemorrhagic fever (CCHF) virus in human tissues and implications for CCHF pathogenesis, *Arch Pathol Lab Med* 121:839, 1997.

40. Swanepoel R, Shepard AJ, Leman PA, et al: Epidemiologic and clinical features of Crimean-Congo hemorrhagic fever in southern Africa, *Am J Trop Med Hyg* 36:120, 1987.

41. Khan AS, Maupin GO, Rollin PE, et al: An outbeak of Crimean-Congo hemorrhagic fever in the United Arab Emirates, 1994-1995, *Am J Trop Med Hyg* 57:519, 1997.

42. Ksiazek TG, Peters CJ, Rollin PE, et al: Identification of a new North American hantavirus that causes acute pulmonary insufficiency, *Am J Trop Med Hyg* 52:117, 1995.

43. Hjelle B, Jenison S, Torrez-Martinez N, et al: Rapid and specific detection of sin nombre virus antibodies in patients with hantavirus pulmonary syndrome by a strip immunoblot assay suitable for field diagnosis, *J Clin Microbiol* 35:600, 1997.

44. Hjelle B, Spiropoulou CF, Torrez-Martinez N, et al: Detection of Muerto Canyon virus RNA in peripheral blood mononuclear cells from patients with hantavirus pulmonary syndrome, *J Infect Dis* 170:1013, 1994.

45. Emmons RW, Oshiro LS, Johnson HN, Lennette EH: Extra-erythrocytic location of Colorado tick fever virus, *J Gen Virol* 17:185, 1972.

46. Goodpasture HC, Poland JD, Francy B, et al: Colorado tick fever: clinical, epidemiologic, and laboratory aspects of 228 cases in Colorado in 1973-1974, *Ann Intern Med* 88:303, 1978.

47. Emmons RW, Lennette EH: Immunofluorescent staining in the laboratory diagnosis of Colorado tick fever, *J Lab Clin Med* 68:923, 1966.

48. Johnson AJ, Karabatsos N, Lanciotti RS: Detection of Colorado tick fever virus by using reverse transcription PCR and application of the technique in laboratory diagnosis, *J Clin Microbiol* 35:1203, 1997.

49. Calisher CH, Poland JD, Calisher SB, Warmoth LA: Diagnosis of Colorado tick fever virus infection by enzyme immunoassays for immunoglobulin M and G antibodies, *J Clin Microbiol* 22:84, 1985.

50. Pfeffer M, Proebster B, Kinney RM, Kaaden OR: Genus-specific detection of alphaviruses by a semi-nested reverse transcription–polymerase chain reaction, *Am J Trop Med Hyg* 57:709, 1997.

51. Calisher CH, El-Kafrawi AO, Al-Deen Mahmud MI, et al: Complex-specific immunoglobulin M antibody patterns in humans infected with alphaviruses, *J Clin Microbiol* 23:155, 1986.

52. Niklasson B, Espmark A, Lundström J: Occurrence of arthralgia and specific IgM antibodies three to four years after Ockelbo disease, *J Infect Dis* 157:832, 1988.

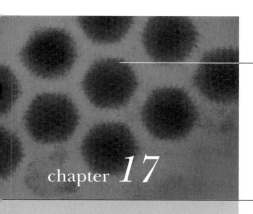

Max Arens

Human Immunodeficiency Virus (HIV) and Other Human Retroviruses

OVERVIEW

This chapter reviews the diagnosis of infections caused by human retroviruses. This group includes human immunodeficiency virus (HIV) types 1 and 2 and human T-cell lymphotropic (leukemia) viruses (HTLV) types I and II. Besides HIV-2 and HTLV-I/II testing, sections focus on HIV antibody testing, p24 antigen assays, culture-based assays for infectious virus, DNA polymerase chain reaction (PCR), and plasma HIV RNA (viral load) assays. Chapter 18 discusses HIV susceptibility testing.

VIROLOGY

Human immunodeficiency virus (HIV) is one of a group of ribonucleic acid (RNA) viruses known as *retroviruses* because during the process of replication, they produce a deoxyribonucleic acid (DNA) copy from the genomic RNA of the virus. The DNA copy becomes integrated into the genome of the infected cell and serves as a template for the synthesis of viral RNA. Some

of this RNA is incorporated into new viral particles, and some becomes the template for the synthesis of viral proteins.

The sequence of the entire HIV genome has been determined, and 11 genes have been identified. Among these are *gag*, which encodes the viral core proteins; *pol*, which encodes the viral polymerase, including protease, reverse transcriptase, and integrase functions; and *env*, which encodes the viral envelope protein. The viral proteins are designated according to their function but also by their molecular weight. For example, *p24* is the main viral core protein, with a molecular weight of 24,000 daltons. Figure 17–1 and Color Plate 17–1 show the viral genes and the proteins they encode.

Two distinct HIV species (serotypes) have been identified, types 1 (HIV-1) and 2 (HIV-2). These viruses are members of the genus *Lentivirus* within the family Retroviridae. The only other known pathogenic human retroviruses, human T-cell lymphotropic (leukemia) virus types I and II (HTLV-I, and HTLV-II) are more distantly related members of the same family. HIV-1 is subdivided into two genetic groups, designated *M* (major) and *O* (outlier). Group M viruses have been found worldwide, whereas group O viruses have been

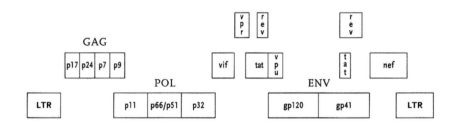

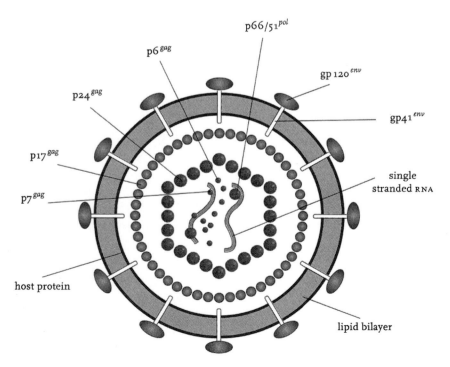

Figure 17.1 HIV genes and proteins they encode. *Gag, pol,* and *env* genes code for structural proteins that are part of virion. Long terminal repeat (*LTR*) gene contains regulatory sequences. All other genes encode proteins that are important in regulation of gene expression. (From Goudsmit J: *Prevention and clinical management of AIDS: the NASBA experience in HIV-1 quantification,* Amsterdam, 1996, Academic Medical Center.)

detected only in Africa and Europe. Group M viruses are divided into eight subtypes, or clades, designated *A* through *H*. Subtype B is the predominant subtype in North America.

HIV ANTIBODY ASSAYS

Infection with HIV is an example of persistent viral infection. Once an individual is infected, ongoing viral replication persists for the person's life. Virtually all infected individuals produce antibodies to HIV. Therefore the presence of HIV antibodies indicates active HIV infection. HIV antibody assays are the primary tools for diagnosing HIV infection in patients seen in all settings, except newborns born to HIV-infected mothers and acutely infected patients who may not have yet developed an antibody response. These special groups are discussed later in this chapter.

Almost all HIV antibody testing is performed using two tests; the *enzyme-linked immunosorbent assay* (ELISA) and the *Western blot*. The ELISA serves as a screening assay. Current instrumentation allows large laboratories to perform hundreds of ELISA assays per day at a cost of several dollars per sample. The usual algorithm for testing specimens for HIV antibodies is to start by performing the ELISA. If the initial ELISA is negative, the specimen is negative for HIV antibodies, and no further testing is performed. If the initial ELISA is positive, the ELISA is repeated in duplicate. If the two repeat tests are negative, the specimen is considered negative for HIV antibodies. If one or both of the repeat ELISAs is positive, the ELISA result is considered positive.

The U.S. Public Health Service (PHS) recommends that no positive ELISA results be given to patients or clients until the ELISA has been repeatedly reactive and a supplemental, more specific test has been used to confirm the ELISA result. The most widely used supplemental test method is the Western blot. The combination of ELISA and Western blot testing for HIV antibodies has extremely high sensitivity and specificity and a positive predictive value of almost 100%.[1]

Enzyme-linked Immunosorbent Assay

The ELISA is based on the ability of an HIV antigen, bound to a solid phase (e.g., plastic bead, microtiter tray), to capture HIV antibodies in the serum or plasma being tested (see Figure 1–15). The captured antibodies are then detected by reaction with enzyme-conjugated antibodies against human immunoglobulins. The presence of the bound enzyme is detected by reaction with a substrate, which is converted from colorless to colored as a result of catalysis by the enzyme. The optical density (OD) of the resulting colored solution is measured in a spectrophotometer and recorded as a positive result if the OD is above a calculated cutoff value for that

Table 17.1	Currently FDA-Licensed HIV ELISAs		
Manufacturer	**Trade Names**	**Detects**	**Antigens**
Abbott Laboratories	HIVAB HIV-1 EIA	HIV-1	Lysate and purified antigens
Abbott Laboratories	HIVAB HIV-1/HIV-2 (rDNA) EIA	HIV-1/2	Recombinant proteins
Murex Diagnostics	Murex SUDS HIV-1	HIV-1	Purified antigens and synthetic peptides
Organon Teknika	Vironostika HIV-1 MicroELISA System	HIV-1	Lysate
Sanofi/Genetic Systems	Genetic Systems HIV-1/HIV-2 Peptide EIA	HIV-1/2	Synthetic peptides
Sanofi/Genetic Systems	Genetic Systems HIV-2 EIA	HIV-2	Lysate

particular run. The antigen preparation used largely determines the assay's specificity.

A variety of HIV ELISAs are currently marketed in the United States. These assays vary in the antigen used and in the configuration of the assay. Table 17–1 lists the HIV assays currently approved by the U.S. Food and Drug Administration (FDA) for donor screening of serum or plasma. Some of the assays are designed for the simultaneous detection of both HIV-1 and HIV-2. Use of tests with this capability is currently required in the United States for screening of all blood donors. Other tests use only an HIV-1 antigen to bind antibodies in the patient's serum. These tests are positive in approximately 60% to 90% of patients infected with HIV-2.

The high purity of the antigens used in some currently available ELISAs is in contrast to the earliest versions, in which the antigen used was prepared from partially purified preparations of HIV grown in cells of human origin. These cells contained human leukocyte antigen (HLA) class II antigens, which led to false-positive tests when used to test serum from individuals with antibodies to HLA antigens. This particular problem has been minimized if not eliminated with third-generation assays, in which all antigens are either purified or recombinant.

Second- and third-generation assays. Several changes have been introduced into second-generation and third-generation ELISAs, which have been commercially available since 1992. The viral *lysate* (HIV-infected cells that have been lysed by a detergent-containing buffer) has been fortified or replaced with purified or recombinant antigens or synthetic peptides. Also, because of the threat of a worldwide HIV-2 epidemic concurrent with the ongoing HIV-1 epidemic, it became advisable to test blood products for HIV-2. This goal was met by the addition of an HIV-2 gp36 recombinant protein to the solid-phase capture antigen of third-generation assays, thus allowing simultaneous testing for these two viruses on the same serum sample with no additional expenditure of time or resources. The FDA has recommended that all blood donated in the United States after June 1, 1992, be tested in this manner.

Some of the third-generation assays have adopted a *double-antigen sandwich* (DAGS) technology to improve the sensitivity for detection of early infection.[2] The DAGS procedure employs a set of antigens bound to the solid phase that serve to capture HIV antibodies. The same set of antigens are enzyme conjugated and used to detect the captured antibodies. The presence of enzyme after the final washing step is revealed by reaction with the substrate. This configuration allows these assays to detect antibodies of both immunoglobulin G (IgG) and immunoglobulin M (IgM) classes, presumably allowing earlier detection of seroconversion. Some third-generation assays (especially a viral peptide assay) has demonstrated an unacceptably high false-positive rate (low specificities and low positive predictive values) when used to test populations with low seroprevalence.[3]

Sensitivity and specificity. Current HIV ELISAs, whether lysate based or second or third generation, are highly sensitive and specific for detecting antibodies to HIV-1. Sensitivity and specificity are both greater than 99%. Even with such excellent test parameters, however, a high proportion of all positive tests from low-risk populations are false positives. This is a consequence of a low percentage of unavoidable false-positive reactions combined with an even lower percentage of true positives. This phenomenon is also expressed as *Bayes' theorem*, which states that the positive predictive value of a test (the percentage of positive tests that are true positives) is a function of the prevalence of the disease in the population. If the prevalence is high, most positive tests will be true positives, but if the prevalence is very low, most positive tests will be false positives, even if the specificity of the test is very high. For this reason, performance of a supplemental test for HIV is important to corroborate positive test results (see later discussion).

Box 17–1 lists causes of false-positive and false-negative ELISA results. Certain immunizations (e.g., influenza vaccine) have been associated with transient false-positive ELISAs.

Box 17.1 Causes of False-Positive and False-Negative HIV ELISA

False positive
Antibodies to HLA antigens
Multiple transfusions
Recent influenza immunization
Improper specimen handling (e.g., heating)
Unknown

False negative
Recent infection (window phase)
Hypogammaglobulinemia
Advanced infection (extremely rare)
HIV-2 (applies only to test kits specific for HIV-1)
Unusual HIV-1 serotype (e.g., group O)

False-negative results. False-negative ELISAs fall into three main categories. The first occurs when testing is performed either very early or very late after infection. Figure 17–2 shows the time that elapses between infection and appearance of detectable HIV antibodies in the serum. It is estimated that current ELISAs first become positive approximately 22 days after infection (95% confidence interval, 9 to 34 days; see Table 17–2). Therefore, if testing is performed earlier after infection, the test will be negative even though HIV infection is present. This is important because acutely infected individuals may have clinical symptoms and may be evaluated during this so-called window period (see Sidebar on diagnosis of the acute retroviral syndrome). Thus a negative HIV ELISA should not be used to rule out HIV when acute infection is being considered. Window periods as long as several years from infection to appearance of HIV antibodies have been reported, but this situation is apparently rare. Also in rare reports, HIV antibody tests became negative very late in the course of infection. Although the antibody level declines with far-advanced HIV infection, it rarely drops below the level of detection of current assays.

A second category of false-negative ELISA involves patients who never develop an HIV antibody response. Rare patients with congenital hypogammaglobulinemia may fall into this category. Also in rare situations, patients repeatedly test negative over a long period but ultimately are shown to be infected.[4, 5]

Finally, the increasing genetic diversity of HIV has led to the evolution of HIV-1 strains that may not be detected by some ELISAs[6-8] (see Sidebar on diagnosis of HIV infection in African patients). Most HIV isolates that are nonreactive or poorly reactive with antibody ELISA and Western blot kits are classified as group O. Lysate-based antibody screening kits are more efficient in detecting group O than kits that use recombinant antigens or synthetic peptides, which are more re-

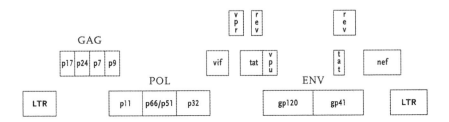

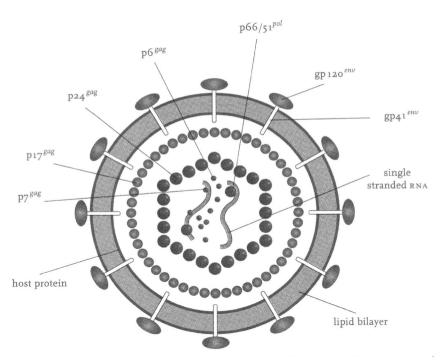

Color Plate 17–1 HIV genes and proteins they encode. *Gag, pol,* and *env* genes code for structural proteins that are part of virion. Long terminal repeat (LTR) gene contains regulatory sequences. All other genes encode proteins that are important in regulation of gene expression. (From Goudsmit J: *Prevention and clinical management of AIDS: the NASBA experience in HIV-1 quantification,* Amsterdam, 1996, Academic Medical Center.)

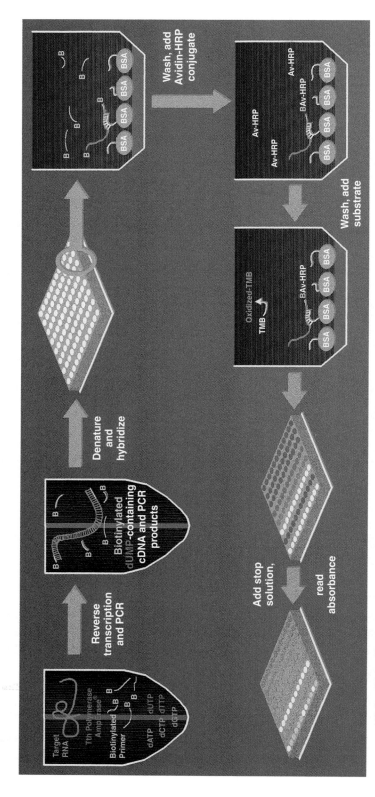

Color Plate 17-2 Amplicor HIV-1 Monitor test format. See text for details. *HRP,* Horseradish peroxidase; *BSA,* bovine serum albumin; *TMB,* 3,3′,5,5′–tetramethylbenzidine. AmpErase, uracil N-glycosylase, a system for preventing PCR product carryover (see Chapter 1 for more details). (Courtesy Roche Molecular Systems, Pleasanton, Calif.)

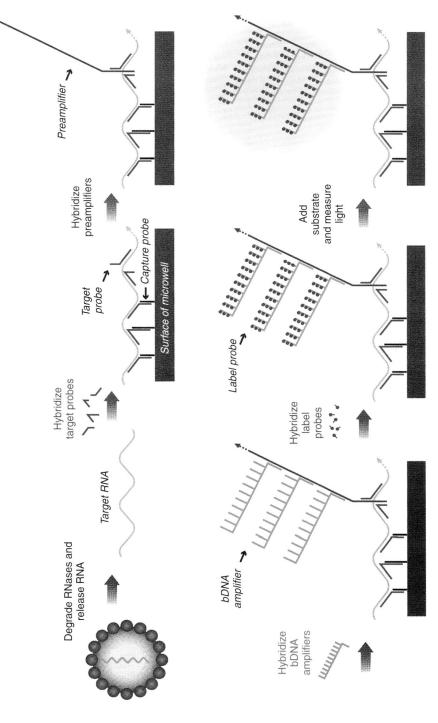

Color Plate 17–3 Quantiplex bDNA version 2.0 test format. See text for details. (Courtesy Bayer Diagnostics, Emeryville, Calif.)

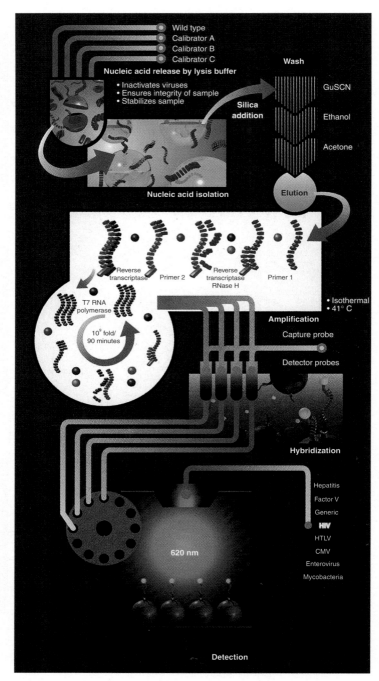

Color Plate 17–4 NucliSens amplification process. See text for details. (Courtesy Organon Teknika, Durham, NC.)

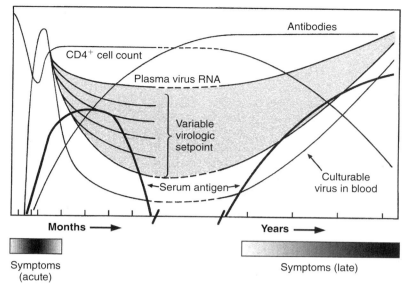

Figure 17.2   Virologic and immunologic course of HIV disease, with markers of HIV disease shown over time. Clinical symptoms may be present during acute phase of illness and again later in disease when immunosuppression manifests as opportunistic infections. *HIV RNA* is first marker to appear and often rises to very high levels before arriving at a patient-specific set point, usually about 10,000 to 100,000 copies/ml plasma. In untreated patients, RNA levels may be unchanged for years but will rise significantly late in disease. Infectious virus may be cultured from blood during most of disease course, except possibly at nadir of viral load. *p24 Antigen* is detectable early in infection but often disappears as antibodies are made and viral load decreases. Antigen may be detectable again later in infection. *Antibodies* are last marker to appear and rise rapidly over first few months of infection. CD4+ cell counts usually drop rapidly during first several weeks after infection, then rise almost to baseline levels, but decline as disease progresses.

stricted in the antibodies they detect (see Table 17–1).[8] The immunologic reactivity of group O strains varies from strain to strain; in one study, some group O strains were reactive with most ELISAs, and others were not reactive with any ELISA tested.[9] The presence of group O variants in Los Angeles and New York City has raised concern that some infections may go undetected for years, even with adequate testing procedures in place for protection of individuals and the blood supply.[10]

Rapid Tests

Certain situations may dictate the use of a testing format other than the traditional ELISA for HIV-1. Some small

Table 17.2	Time from Infection to Detection of HIV-1 Markers

Marker	Mean time to detection	95% confidence interval
Antibody	22 days	9-34 days
p24 antigen	16 days	3-30 days
DNA (by PCR)	16 days	3-30 days
RNA	11 days	1-25 days

Modified from Busch MP, Lee LL, Satten GA, et al: *Transfusion* 35:91, 1995.

laboratories may not have the testing volume to justify a plate washer and reader. Laboratories in undeveloped countries may not have access to ELISA kits. Murex Diagnostics (Norcross, Ga) has developed a rapid microfiltration assay called *Single Use Diagnostic System* (SUDS) that is rapid, accurate, and very simple. The solid-phase capture reagent is a mixture of latex particles coated with affinity-purified p24 antigen and gp41 transmembrane synthetic peptide. The SUDS cartridge filters, concentrates, and absorbs all liquid reagents added during the test. The test is performed in about 10 minutes at room temperature, and specialized instruments are not required. This assay is FDA approved and has sensitivity and specificity similar to traditional ELISA assays when used properly and read by an experienced technician.

According to the Centers for Disease Control and Prevention (CDC), use of rapid on-site testing with reporting of preliminary results is appropriate when a high percentage of patients do not return for test results.[11]

Urine and Saliva Tests

The detection of antibodies to HIV in body fluids other than blood can be useful, especially in screening programs. Antibodies are present in urine but are of low titer. One test (Calypte Biochemical, Berkeley, Calif) is currently FDA approved for the detection of HIV antibodies in urine. Antibodies are also found in oral mucosal transudate (OMT) and are useful for diagnostic purposes. The FDA has approved a collection device called OraSure (manufactured by Epitope, Beaverton, Ore; sold by Organon Teknika, Durham, NC) that absorbs OMT when placed between the lower cheek and gum (Figure 17–3). This absorbent pad is then placed into a preservative and can be mailed at ambient temperature for testing. The accuracy of testing OMT for HIV antibodies, following the ELISA/Western blot algorithm outlined next, is excellent, with sensitivities and specificities similar to testing of serum or plasma.[12]

Western Blot

The standard for supplemental testing is the Western blot (WB) or immunoblot. The WB differs from the ELISA in the method used to present the antigen to the serum specimen. The WB is essentially an ELISA performed on a membrane. The procedure includes preparation of membrane strips containing the antigen, typically prepared long before the test is done and stored until use. To prepare the membrane strips, a partially purified virus preparation (HIV-infected cells lysed with a mild detergent-containing buffer and purified by sedimentation in a gradient) from HIV grown in cell culture is subjected to gel electrophoresis, resulting in separation of the viral proteins. The membrane is cut into strips, each containing the full array of HIV antigens. To perform the test, a membrane strip is exposed to the serum specimen so that antibodies in the specimen can bind to the separated HIV antigens. Bound antibodies from the serum are de-

tected by overlaying an antihuman immunoglobulin that is labeled with an enzyme such as horseradish peroxidase. Finally, the antigen-antibody complex is detected by adding a substrate that changes color and precipitates onto the paper when it interacts with the enzyme. The result identifies the specific HIV antigens recognized by antibodies in the serum specimen (see Figure 17–4).

The WB is read by visually comparing the strip with a positive control strip showing the full array of HIV antigens. The test is classified as *reactive* (HIV antibodies present), *indeterminate* (presence of HIV antibodies cannot be considered definite but cannot be excluded), or *negative* (HIV antibodies absent). A patient's WB is considered reactive when antibodies recognizing a minimum number of HIV antigens are present. Different criteria have been proposed for accepting a WB as "reactive."[13, 14] Since late 1990 the criteria used most widely in the United States are those established by the Association of State and Territorial Public Health Laboratory Directors (ASTPHLD) and the CDC. According to these criteria, a WB is reactive if bands corresponding to two of the HIV proteins p24, gp41, or gp120/160 are present. Blots with no bands are considered negative. When one or more bands are present (including bands that do not correspond to HIV proteins) but the bands do not meet the criteria for being considered positive, the blot is considered indeterminate. These criteria are used in all commercial WB assay kits currently licensed by the FDA.

Indeterminate blots. Indeterminate WBs are very common; as many as 15% to 20% of serum specimens from non–HIV-infected individuals may produce indetermi-

---

Sidebar Diagnosis of the Acute Retroviral Syndrome

Some patients infected with HIV experience a symptomatic illness shortly after becoming infected. The symptoms are similar to those of infectious mononucleosis (see Chapter 12). Laboratory diagnosis may be complicated because symptoms may occur before HIV antibodies are present. However, the level of HIV in plasma is typically very high at the same time. Therefore, direct tests for the presence of HIV such as the p24 antigen test and plasma viral load assays are more likely to yield a diagnosis. Viral load assays are the first tests to become positive after HIV infection (see Table 17–2) and for that reason should be the preferred test. Indeed, a recent study showed that testing for plasma HIV RNA was more

sensitive than the p24 antigen assay in patients with the acute retroviral syndrome.* However, it is very important to be aware that viral load assays were not designed for the diagnosis of HIV, and false positive results have occurred in individuals who are not infected with HIV. The false positive results were recognizable, because the levels of HIV RNA were low (less than 2000 copies per ml).† If plasma HIV RNA assays are used during the acute retroviral syndrome, the diagnosis of HIV should be confirmed with other diagnostic tests, including p24 antigen assay, PCR, or HIV antibody ELISA, performed several weeks later when seroconversion has occurred.

---

*Abstract #178, 6th Conference on Retroviruses and Opportunistic Infections, Hecht FM, Rawal BD, Kahn JO et al: Chicago, Jan. 31-Feb. 4, 1999, page 101.
†Rich JD, Merriman NA, Mylonakis E et al: Misdiagnosis of HIV infection by HIV-1 plasma viral load testing, Ann Intern Med 130:37, 1999.

Sidebar   Diagnosis of HIV Infection in African Patients

Patients from Africa or with an epidemiologic link to Africa may present with symptoms consistent with HIV infection. For example, African children with lymphadenopathy and poor growth may be infected with HIV but the diagnosis may not be straightforward. Since the epidemic in the U.S. and other western countries is, at present, caused almost exclusively by HIV-1, the diagnostic reagents and tools in use are optimized to detect HIV-1. However, the epidemic in Africa includes infections with HIV-2 and with HIV-1 variants that are among the group O strains. Standard assay methods used in the U.S. may not detect either of these infections. The table below shows which methods are useful for diagnosis of African infections and which are not.

Test:	HIV-2	HIV-1 group O
HIV-1 antibody (lysate)	Variable[1]	Variable
HIV-1/2 antibody (3rd gen)	Yes	Variable
HIV-2 antibody ELISA	Yes	No
HIV-1 western blot	Some bands[2]	Some bands[2]
HIV-2 western blot	Yes	Some bands[2]
HIV-1 p24 antigen	Variable[3]	Variable[3]
HIV-1 DNA PCR	No[4]	Variable[5]
Amplicor HIV-1 Monitor v 1.0 (Roche)[6]	No	Some subtypes[6]
Amplicor HIV-1 Monitor v 1.5 (Roche)[6]	No	Additional subtypes[6]
Quantiplex HIV RNA (bDNA; Chiron)	No	Yes
Nuclisens (NASBA; Organon Teknika)	No	Some subtypes
HIV lymphocyte co-culture; detect by p24	Variable[3]	Variable[3]
HIV lymphocyte co-culture; detect by RT	Yes	Yes

[1]The lysate-based HIV-1 EIA systems detect about 60-90% of HIV-2-positive sera.
[2]Antibodies against *pol* and *gag* are more likely to crossreact than antibodies against *env* since *env* is highly variable among different strains due to immunologic pressure. Since most criteria for positivity require 2 *env* bands (gp120/160 and gp41), these blots are not likely to meet the criteria for a positive.
[3]The Organon Teknika antigen assay has the broadest reactivity among all the commercial antigen assays. It will detect all HIV-1 variants, HIV-2 and even simian immunodeficiency virus (SIV). Abbott HIVAG-1 Monoclonal and Coulter Corp. (also a monoclonal-based assay) HIV-1 p24 kits will not detect HIV-2 but Coulter will detect many HIV-1 variants. The Coulter kit for detection of SIV p27 core antigen will detect HIV-2 core antigen (p26).
[4]Specialty Laboratories, Inc. and ViroMED Laboratories, Inc. offer PCR tests for HIV-2.
[5]Roche Amplicor kit which is commercially available is used by Specialty Labs and by ViroMED Labs and does not detect members of HIV-1 group O. ViroMED also offers an assay developed in-house which uses multiple primer sets and will detect all known group O variants.
[6]The original HIV Amplicor (stock#83088 in the US) was developed and optimized for group M, subtype B isolates and also efficiently detects subtypes C and D. Subtypes A, E and F and all group O isolates are underestimated by 10- to 500-fold with this assay. A more accurate estimation of viral loads using the Amplicor assay can be obtained by lowering the annealing temperature to 50 C or by the introduction of a second pair of primers that target the *pol* region of HIV-1 which is more highly conserved than *gag*. A new version of the Amplicor kit with the new primer pair is in development.

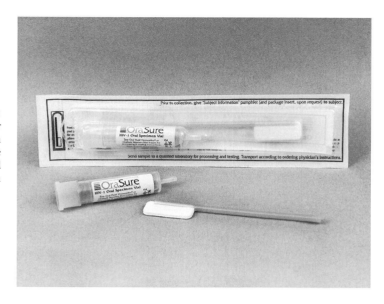

Figure 17.3 OraSure device (Epitope, Beaverton, Ore) for collection of oral mucosal transudate (OMT). Filter pad is placed between lower cheek and gum for collection of OMT, then placed into syringe containing preservative and elution buffer for shipping. Antibodies are extracted into buffer and tested by ELISA and, if positive, Western blot.

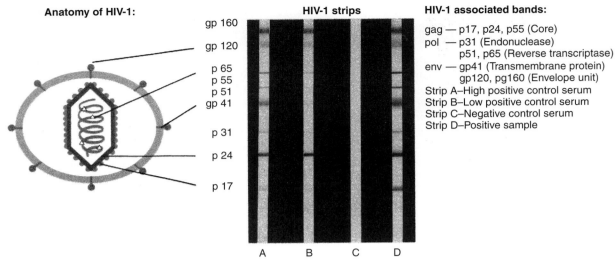

Figure 17.4 HIV-1 Western blots. Examples are shown in center, with viral antigens identified by molecular weight at left and association with specific structural genes or enzymatic functions at right. (Courtesy Organon Teknika, Durham, NC.)

nate blots. This is one reason why the WB is not suitable as a screening test for HIV antibodies. In two studies, no indeterminate WBs from low-risk blood donors signified an HIV infection.[15, 16] However, indeterminate patterns can occur in very early or far-advanced HIV infection. Therefore those WBs containing one or more bands corresponding to an HIV protein must be viewed with some suspicion and adjudicated (Box 17-2). In contrast, WBs classified as indeterminate because of the presence of bands that do not correspond to HIV proteins essentially never signify HIV infection.

Although the sequence of ELISA and HIV testing is highly satisfactory in most patients, the occurrence of positive ELISAs followed by indeterminate WBs can create considerable anxiety. The infection status of many individuals with indeterminate WBs can be resolved by repeating the ELISA and WB after 3 to 6 months to rule out the possibility that the indeterminate blot is the result of very early HIV infection. A more rapid alternative is to perform PCR to detect HIV DNA or an assay to detect plasma HIV RNA (see below). Both these tests become positive in 1 to 4 weeks after infection in virtually all individuals recently infected with HIV (Table 17–2). Thus, since these markers would be detectable well before antibodies appear, a negative PCR for HIV DNA or a negative assay for plasma HIV RNA rules out HIV infection as the cause of an indeterminate WB and almost rules out infection altogether unless the most recent exposure was within the previous 4 weeks.

p24 ANTIGEN ASSAY

In some HIV-infected patients, the HIV p24 antigen, which corresponds to the viral core protein, can be detected directly in plasma using ELISAs designed for antigen detection. Figure 17–2 shows the timing of p24 antigenemia in relation to the natural history of HIV infection. The mean time from infection to first detection of p24 antigen is 16 days, 6 days less than for HIV antibodies.[17] Thus the assay can be used for the diagnosis of acute HIV infection. Other uses include blood donor screening, diagnosis of HIV infection in infants born to HIV-infected mothers, and assessment of prognosis and response to antiretroviral therapy.[18-20] The latter two uses have been almost completely supplanted by quantitative plasma HIV RNA assays because (1) p24 antigen can be detected in the plasma of only approximately 50% of HIV-infected individuals and (2) plasma HIV RNA level is a better predictor of clinical outcome and provides a better assessment of the response to therapy.

Box 17.2 Adjudication of Indeterminate HIV-1 Western Blots

1. Carefully evaluate patient history and risk of HIV-1 or HIV-2 infection with regard to intravenous drug use, sexual contact and promiscuity, travel to Western Africa, and related factors.
2. Consider testing with HIV-2 ELISA if initial testing was performed using an ELISA specific for HIV-1. This is especially important if the indeterminate HIV-1 western blot contains *gag* and *pol* bonds.
3. Perform HIV DNA polymerase chain reaction, quantitative HIV RNA, p24 antigen assay, or HIV lymphocyte co-culture.
4. Repeat HIV antibody ELISA and Western blot in 3 to 6 months.

The specificity of the p24 antigen assay is virtually 100%. This level of specificity depends on the use of a neutralization procedure to confirm an initial positive test. In the neutralization procedure the serum specimen is reacted with an anti–p24 antibody and then retested. The original test is considered neutralizable (truly positive for p24 antigen) if the level of p24 antigen is reduced by the antibody pretreatment.

The Organon Teknika HIV-1 p24 test kit has been reported to detect p24 antigen from HIV-1 group O in culture supernatants. The same kit also detects in culture supernatants the p26 antigen from HIV-2 and the protein corresponding to p24 from the simian immunodeficiency virus (SIV).[21] A commercial antigen kit made for the detection of SIV (Coulter, Hialeah, Fla) will react with HIV-2.

The ability of p24 antigen assays to detect p24 antigenemia is reduced if the patient also has antibodies to p24 antigen, because of the formation of antigen-antibody complexes. Treatment of the serum with acid, base, or heat can dissociate the immune complexes, making more p24 antigen accessible to the detection assay. Use of one of these *immune complex dissociation* (ICD) *procedures* greatly increases the sensitivity of the p24 antigen assay in certain situations. For example, in detecting HIV infection in infants born to HIV-infected mothers, the ICD procedure increased the sensitivity of the p24 antigen assay from approximately 18% to 89.5% in one study.[22] ICD is not required when testing for acute infection because HIV antibodies are not yet present. (See Sidebar on safety of the U.S. blood supply.)[23-25]

CULTURE

HIV was discovered when it was cultured from the lymphocytes of patients with AIDS. Isolation of the virus in culture has been a mainstay of both research and clinical efforts to understand the virus and the disease. With optimal methods the virus can be grown from up to 97% of patients with asymptomatic HIV infection and 100% of AIDS patients.[26] At present, however, viral cultures are almost never needed for the diagnosis or management of patients with HIV infection. The ability to culture the virus remains critical for research studies, including efforts to determine the susceptibility of HIV to antiretroviral drugs. Viral culture is also important to understand unusual cases with conflicting or confusing HIV test results and to discover new variants of HIV or even new human retroviruses.

Procedure

The basic procedure for culturing HIV is referred to as *co-cultivation* because it involves the use of peripheral blood mononuclear cells (PBMCs) from an uninfected individual (the donor) together with PBMCs from the individual being cultured. PBMCs are purified from the

---

Sidebar   Safety of the U.S. Blood Supply

All blood donors in the United States are asked not to give blood if they have any risk factors for HIV infection. In addition, the blood from all donors is tested for HIV antibodies, using an assay that detects HIV-1 and HIV-2. Since March 1, 1996, all donors are also tested for p24 antigen. Positive units are confirmed by Western blot or p24 antigen neutralization. Confirmed positive units are destroyed, and the donors are notified that they are probably infected with HIV and permanently deferred from further donation.[23] The main limitation of this system is donation of blood during the interval between infection and test positivity, the window period. Thus the length of the window period is a critical issue for the safety of the blood supply. For current antibody ELISAs the window period is estimated to be 22 days (95% confidence interval, 9 to 34 days).[17, 24] The window period for the p24 antigen test is estimated to be 16 days.[17]

Before implementation of routine p24 antigen testing, the risk of an HIV-infectious donation being available for transfusion in the United States was estimated at 1 in 450,000 to 660,000 units, or 18 to 27 HIV-infectious donations per year in the United States among the approximately 12 million units donated.[23, 25] It was estimated that p24 antigen testing would remove 4 to 6 infectious units that would otherwise have been available for transfusion, thus lowering the risk of an HIV-infectious donation being used for transfusion to about 1 in 545,000 to 923,000.[25] Some blood banks have implemented nucleic acid testing on pooled blood samples to determine if this risk can be lowered even further.

---

donor blood and stimulated with phytohemagglutinin for 1 to 3 days. Interleukin-2 (IL-2) is sometimes included in this reaction. PBMCs from the individual being cultured are then added to the stimulated donor cells in a mixture containing the tissue culture media RPMI 1640 supplemented with 10% to 20% fetal bovine serum, glutamine, IL-2, and antibiotics. Fresh donor cells are added at weekly intervals. The growth of the virus is detected by performing a p24 antigen assay on the culture media every 3 to 4 days.[27] An alternative method of detection is to assay the media for the presence of reverse transcriptase activity.

HIV culture has been adapted to a microculture technique that requires less blood and uses less reagents.[28] This technique has been performed on plasma or whole blood instead of PBMCs.[28-30]

Quantitative Culture

Quantitative modifications of the HIV culture method have also been applied to plasma or PBMCs.[31-32] In a small longitudinal study on the relationship among viral burden, CD4+ cell counts, and clinical status throughout the course of infection, an increase in cultivable viral burden was demonstrated before or during a decrease in CD4+ T cells.[33] The need for these quantitative culture assays in patient care or in clinical trials has been virtually completely replaced by plasma HIV RNA assays.

Syncytium-inducing Phenotype

Studies directed at growth of HIV in a continuous cell line (as opposed to isolation in primary human lymphocytes, as described earlier) revealed that some isolates caused the formation of *syncytia*, or multinucleated giant cells, in the MT-2 cell line (Figure 17–5). Subsequently, this cell line has been used as a means for demonstrating the *syncytium-inducing* (SI) *phenotype*, which was shown in cross-sectional and longitudinal studies to be associated with rapid disease progression.[33-35] In cross-sectional studies, patients with SI virus were demographically similar to those with non-SI (NSI) virus but had lower CD4+ cell counts and were more likely to have acquired immunodeficiency syndrome (AIDS) and detectable p24 antigen. Longitudinal observations over a mean of 3.3 years showed that the median decline in CD4+ cell counts for patients with NSI virus was 15 cells/year versus 56 cells/year for those with SI virus.[36] Thus conversion of an HIV-infected patient to the SI phenotype is a poor prognostic marker and may lead to an approximately threefold more rapid decline in CD4+ cell counts and more rapid clinical deterioration. The underlying genetic basis of the SI phenotype is related to changes in the V3 loop of the *env* gene, but the pathophysiology of this process is not understood.[37] This assay is generally available only in research laboratories and is not widely used in clinical practice.

DNA POLYMERASE CHAIN REACTION

During the replication cycle of HIV, a DNA copy of the viral RNA, termed *proviral DNA*, is produced and integrated into the host cell chromosome. Conventional DNA PCR can be used to detect HIV proviral DNA in the blood of virtually all HIV-infected individuals. In fact, the detection of HIV DNA was one of the first applications of PCR to diagnostic virology.[38] The main role for HIV DNA PCR is for diagnosis of HIV infection when synthesis of HIV antibodies is masked (neonatal infection) or not present.[4] HIV DNA PCR also has numerous research applications. Quantitative modifications of the assay are research tools without current clinical application.[39, 40]

Different regions of the HIV genome have been used as the target for HIV PCR. The most frequently used region is *gag;* however, primer sets from other regions may also be useful (Figure 17–6). Since HIV replicates in CD4+ PBMCs, HIV DNA PCR is usually performed on DNA extracted from purified PBMCs or from whole blood.[26, 41-44] In one study the sensitivity of PCR was 97% using one primer pair. The sensitivity of HIV culture in the same study was also 97%. Both methods had specificities of 100%.[26] A metaanalysis of 96 studies of PCR for detection of HIV proviral DNA in PBMCs noted that the sensitivity and specificity of PCR were affected by the criteria used to consider a PCR reaction as positive (e.g., one or multiple primer sets). If sensitivity and specificity were equally weighted in importance, the sensitivity and specificity of reported PCR reactions were 97.0% and 98.1%, respectively. The authors concluded that the sensitivity and specificity of DNA PCR are less than 100% even with exquisite analytic sensitivity and PCR results should be evaluated in the context of patient risk, history and relevant clinical findings.

PCR testing largely remains nonstandardized, and the performance of PCR assays may vary greatly among laboratories.[44] A commercial PCR assay for HIV DNA called Amplicor HIV-1 Test has been developed (Roche Molecular Systems, Pleasanton, CA), but is not yet licensed.

Diagnosis of Infected Infants

Currently the most important use of PCR for HIV proviral DNA is in the diagnosis of HIV infection in infants born to HIV-infected mothers.[45-51] In two

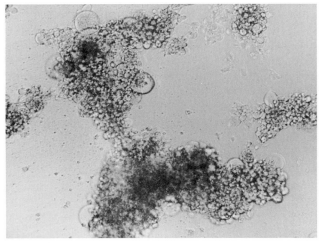

Figure 17.5 Culture of MT-2 cells infected with syncytial-inducing (SI) strain of HIV-1 at day 10 after infection. Multinucleated giant cells are characteristic of SI phenotype in this cell line.

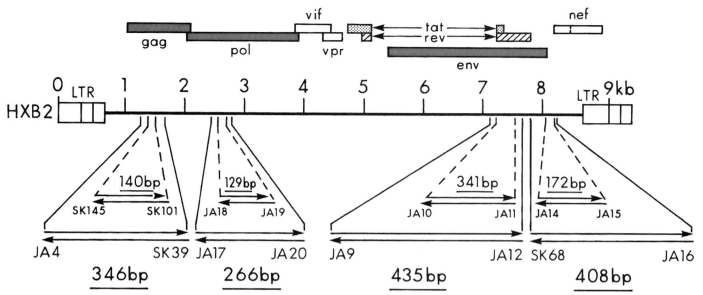

Figure 17.6   HIV-1 genome and targets for DNA polymerase chain reaction (PCR). Four nested sets of primers shown may be used in detection of proviral DNA purified from patient peripheral blood mononuclear cells (PBMCs) or whole blood. See text for details. *LTR*, Long terminal repeat gene; *bp*, base pairs. (JA primers from Albert J and Fenyo EM: Simple, sensitive, and specific detection of human immunodeficiency virus type 1 in clinical specimens by polymerase chain reaction with nested primers, *J Clin Micro* 28:1560-1564, 1990).

studies using the Amplicor assay, the sensitivity of DNA PCR for diagnosis of HIV in exposed infants was 50% during the first month of life, 96% at ages 1 to 6 months, and 98% in infants and children over 6 months of age.[50, 51] The specificity was greater than 99%. In both studies the Amplicor assay was more sensitive than co-culture in detection of HIV-1 in infected infants. Other advantages of PCR are that it can be performed on a relatively small volume of blood (about 200 μl), the result is available rapidly, and performance of the assay does not require the level of biologic containment necessary for culture of HIV.

Current PHS recommendations state that a presumptive determination of HIV infection status can be based on the results of two PCR assays, both performed at age 1 month or older, including one performed at age 4 months or older (see Sidebar).[52] A metaanalysis of 32 studies for the diagnosis of HIV infection in infants found a median sensitivity for PCR of 91.6% (range 31% to 100%) and a median specificity of 100% (range 50% to 100%).[53] These ranges underscore the caution necessary in using PCR studies, since testing performed under "field conditions" may yield highly varied results. The summary sensitivity and specificity were significantly higher for older infants (98.2%) than for neonates (less than 30 days old, 93.3%). With these parameters a negative PCR result is associated with a probability of greater than 97% that HIV infection is not present.[53]

PLASMA HIV RNA (VIRAL LOAD) ASSAYS

In concert with the development of more potent drugs to treat HIV, the recent development of assays that provide a quantitative measurement of HIV RNA in patient plasma (viral load) has revolutionized the approach to management of patients with HIV infection. In addition, these assays have led to major advances in the understanding of the pathophysiology of HIV-associated disease. The level of plasma HIV RNA is believed to reflect replication of HIV throughout the body. Measurement of this level has been shown to have prognostic value beyond that obtained from the CD4+ count.[56] Changes in the level of plasma HIV RNA reflect the response to antiretroviral drugs, and decreased levels are associated with a decreased risk of disease progression. An increase in level while the patient is receiving therapy indicates noncompliance or resistance to the antiretroviral regimen. The availability of plasma HIV RNA assays now allows physicians to individualize and optimize treatment regimens.

The plasma HIV RNA level or viral load reflects the natural history of HIV infection (see Figure 17–2). Levels become detectable approximately 11 days after infection and reach extremely high levels shortly thereafter. During the following weeks to months, an interaction between HIV and the individual's immune system leads to a "set point" or stable level of plasma HIV RNA that persists for some time. The set point is generally reached 6 to 9 months after infection; measurement of viral load before the set point has been reached may not provide an accurate prognosis. After

the set point has been reached, the level is relatively stable, usually showing a gradual increase in the absence of treatment. Late in the course of HIV infection, the level may increase more rapidly.

Therapy with antiretroviral agents greatly decreases the level of plasma HIV RNA. Decreases of 100-fold (2 logs) or greater are common with potent combinations of drugs. Patients treated with an inadequate drug or regimen will soon experience increased levels that may reach or exceed the pretreatment baseline. On the other hand, patients successfully treated will have viral loads that fall beneath the lower limit of detection of the assay and will persist at this undetectable level for prolonged periods. The current approach to therapy in most patients is to make the viral load undetectable and to maintain that state for as long as possible.

Methodologies

Three different technologies are currently available for the quantitative measurement of HIV RNA: (1) target amplification using reverse-transcription polymerase chain reaction (RT-PCR), (2) signal amplification using branched-chain DNA (bDNA) technology, and (3) target amplification using nucleic acid sequence–based amplification (NASBA). Each of these methods is commercially available or under commercial development (Table 17–3). Other methods for quantitating plasma HIV RNA are at earlier stages of development.

Reverse-transcription PCR

A commercial RT-PCR assay called the *Amplicor HIV-1 Monitor* (Roche Molecular Systems, Branchburg, NJ) was the first to be licensed by the FDA for quantitative measurement of HIV RNA levels in plasma (Figure 17–7 and Color Plate 17–2). The assay works by amplifying HIV RNA present in plasma and detecting it using an enzymatic technique. Viral RNA is liberated from viral particles in the plasma by treatment with guanidinium thiocyanate and precipitated with isopropanol. Because PCR works only on DNA and not directly on RNA, the HIV RNA target must be converted to the complementary strand of DNA (cDNA) before PCR can occur. This is accomplished by incubating the purified RNA from the patient's plasma specimen with the enzyme *rTth*, which has reverse transcriptase activity along with necessary reagents, including a specific oligonucleotide primer required to initiate DNA synthesis. After synthesis of the cDNA copy, PCR is performed using conventional methods. The primers are labeled with biotin, resulting in the production of a biotinylated PCR product. The PCR product is denatured, and one of the strands is captured in a well of a 96-well microtiter tray by an HIV-specific oligonucleotide probe that has been bound to the plastic well. The captured strand of the PCR product is detected by adding streptavidin–horse-

---

Sidebar Diagnosis of HIV Infection in the Infant Born to an HIV-Infected Mother

Studies report that 13% to 40% of infants born to HIV-infected mothers become infected with HIV. This percentage range can be reduced by approximately 75% with antiretroviral therapy for the mother and infant.[55]

The laboratory diagnosis of infection in these infants is complicated by passively transferred HIV antibodies of maternal origin in the infant's blood. These antibodies usually disappear by age 9 months but may persist for up to 18 months (or occasionally even longer). Accordingly, during the period when maternal antibodies are still present, direct demonstration of the presence of HIV is required to document infection of the infant. A variety of laboratory tests has been used to accomplish this task, including viral culture, DNA PCR and plasma HIV RNA assays, p24 antigen assays, and assays to detect immunoglobulin A (IgA) HIV antibodies or ex vivo HIV antibody synthesis by infant lymphocytes. DNA PCR and viral culture have emerged as the most sensitive assays. Recent work suggests that the plasma HIV RNA assays may be equally sensitive, but experience is still too limited to draw strong conclusions.

Studies also report that many infants are infected late in gestation or during delivery. Therefore all assays that detect HIV directly are probably less sensitive during the first month of life than later, when levels of viremia are higher. Some experts recommend obtaining a specimen for viral culture and PCR within the first 24 hours of life, since infants who are positive at that time are considered to have been infected in utero and may have more rapid progression (see text for current PHS recommendations).[52]

Diagnosis of vertically transmitted HIV should not be based on a single specimen. If culture or PCR is positive, one of the two tests should be repeated on a second specimen and the diagnosis of infection accepted only if the second specimen also yields a positive result. If the second specimen is negative, further testing is required. This approach should still be considered a presumptive determination. All infants born to HIV-infected mothers should also be followed with HIV antibody tests to be sure that they lose those antibodies by approximately age 18 months.[54, 55]

Table 17.3	Comparisions of Three Commercial HIV RNA Assays		
Factor	**PCR**	**NASBA**	**bDNA**
Standard sample volume	200 μl	100 μl	1000 μl
Lower limit of detection (ultrasensitive)	400 c/ml* (40 c/ml)	400 c/ml (80 c/ml of input[#])	500 c/ml (50 c/ml)
Upper limit of detection	750,000 c/ml	10^7 c/ml	800,000 c/ml
Within-run CV[†]	≤30%	≤30%	≤20%
Detects uncommon subtypes	Few[‡]	Some	All
Potential for contamination	Some	Some	None
Specimen anticoagulant[§]	EDTA	EDTA	EDTA
	ACD	ACD	ACD
		Heparin	Heparin
Use of specimens other than plasma	Some	All	Some
Subsequent use of extracted RNA	No	Yes	No
Same-day results	Yes	Yes	No

*Copies of RNA/ml of specimen.
[†]Coefficient of variation (From Revets H, Marissens D, deWit S, et al: *J Clin Micro* 34:1058-1064, 1996.)
[‡]Primer modifications for detection of subtypes A, E, and F have been submitted to FDA.
[§]*EDTA*, Ethylenediaminetetraacetic acid; *ACD*, acid citrate dextrose.
[#]With an input of 2 ml, the lower limit of detection is 40 c/ml.

radish peroxidase, which binds to the biotinylated PCR strand. The final step is the addition of a peroxidase substrate that undergoes a color change if peroxidase is present.

Quantitative results are achieved by comparing the strength of the reaction (measured as optical density using a spectrophotometer) with that of an internal standard that is amplified in parallel (in same reaction tube) with the patient's plasma RNA. The internal standard has the same primer binding sites as the target HIV RNA so that it will be amplified by the same primers. However, the sequence of the internal portion of the quantitative standard differs from the target so that it can be captured using a different capture probe. This is carried out in wells adjacent to those used to detect the amplified HIV target from the patient's plasma.

Branched-chain DNA

The bDNA assay developed by Bayer Diagnostics (Emeryville, Calif) is called *Quantiplex*. The bDNA assay differs fundamentally from RT-PCR and NASBA (see following discussion) in that it is based on signal amplification rather than target amplification (Figure 17–8 and Color Plate 17–3). First, virus from the patient's plasma specimen is pelleted by centrifugation and disrupted to release the viral RNA, which is captured by hybridization to numerous probes bound to the wells of a 96-well plate. The captured RNA is then allowed to hybridize with bDNA (amplifier probes), which is then further hybridized to enzyme-conjugated probes. The final step is the addition of a chemiluminescent substrate. The resulting chemiluminescent reaction is read in a luminometer.

Quantitative results are generated using a set of four standards to generate a standard curve. All reactions before the last are nonenzymatic hybridizations and are inherently quantitative, thus accounting for the generally high reproducibility of this method (low coefficient of variation, CV).

Nucleic Acid Sequence–based Amplification

The NASBA assay developed by Organon Teknika (Durham, NC) is called *NucliSens*. As with RT-PCR, NASBA involves enzymatic amplification of target RNA. However, the NASBA assay has several differences (Figure 17–9 and Color Plate 17–4).

In addition to reverse transcriptase, NASBA uses two other enzymes, ribonuclease (RNase) H and T7 RNA polymerase, and two specific oligonucleotide primers to achieve amplification of target RNA. Primer 1 binds to the target and acts as primer for the reverse transcriptase to create a cDNA copy of the target HIV RNA. Primer 1 also contains a sequence that allows introduction of a T7 RNA polymerase promoter onto the cDNA copy. The RNA portion of the RNA-DNA hybrid is degraded by the RNase H included in the reaction mixture, leaving a single-stranded DNA copy that now includes the T7 RNA polymerase promoter. Primer 2 binds to this DNA copy and initiates synthesis of the second strand of DNA by reverse transcriptase, which can carry out synthesis using a DNA template as well as an RNA template. The resulting double-stranded DNA copy, with an active T7 promoter, is used by T7 RNA polymerase as a template for transcription of multiple RNA copies, which themselves serve as templates for synthesis of cDNA and are thus cycled back into the previous reactions. The entire process is isothermal,

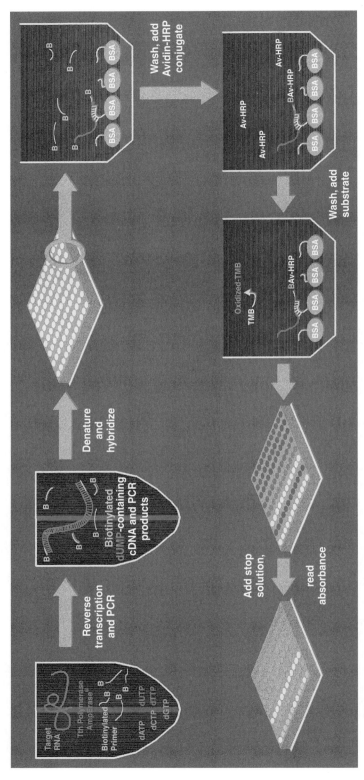

Figure 17.7 Amplicor HIV-1 Monitor test format. See text for details. *HRP,* Horseradish peroxidase; *BSA,* bovine serum albumin; *TMB,* 3,3′,5,5′–tetramethylbenzidine. AmpErase, uracil N-glycosylase, a system for preventing PCR product carryover (see Chapter 1 for more details). (Courtesy Roche Molecular Systems, Pleasanton, Calif.)

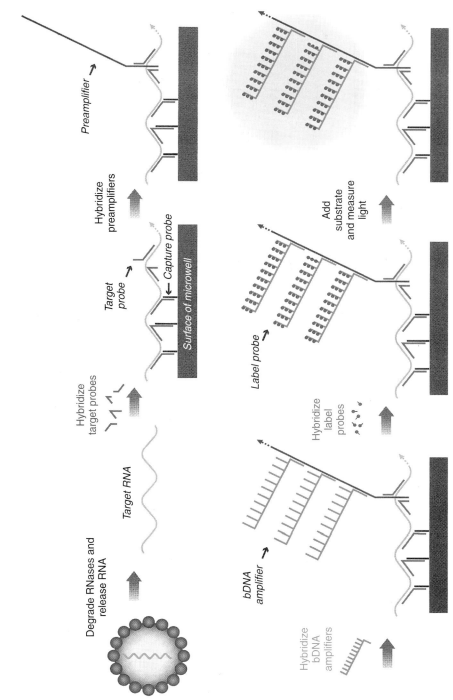

Figure 17.8 Quantiplex bDNA version 2.0 test format. See text for details. (Courtesy Bayer Diagnostics, Emeryville, Calif.)

Degrade RNases and release RNA

Target RNA

Hybridize target probes

Target probe

Capture probe

Surface of microwell

Hybridize preamplifiers

Preamplifier

bDNA amplifier

Hybridize bDNA amplifiers

Label probe

Hybridize label probes

Add substrate and measure light

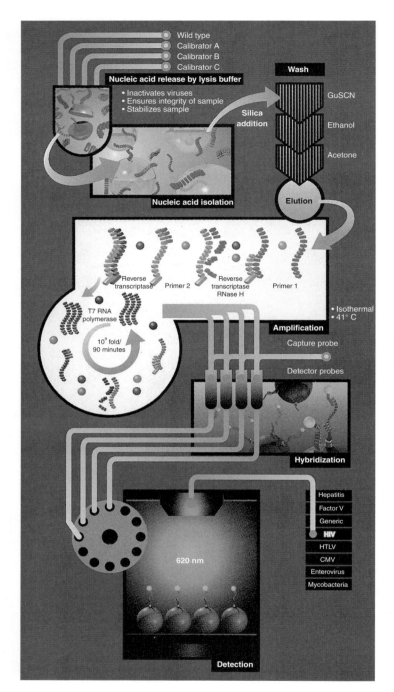

Figure 17.9 NucliSens amplification process. See text for details. (Courtesy Organon Teknika, Durham, NC.)

and detection of the RNA product is through electrochemiluminescent (ECL) probe.

Quantitative results are generated using a standard curve from three internal calibrators included in each tube. The three calibrators are amplified simultaneously with the wild-type target. After amplification the reaction products are split into four separate tubes, and each component (target and three calibrators) is detected separately by specific ECL probes. The extraction procedure used in the NASBA assay is an adaptation of a procedure known to remove enzyme inhibitors and to produce intact, pure nucleic acid that can be used for other procedures (e.g., sequencing) and quantitation.[57, 58]

Comparability of Assays

Although all three assays are considered accurate, results from the three may not be identical. In various comparative studies, HIV RNA values measured by RT-PCR have been up to twofold higher than those measured by bDNA on the same specimens.[59, 60, 60a, 60b] The difference is related to the manufacturers' standards because it is largely eliminated if a common external standard is used to "correct" each assay.[60] To achieve the most accurate comparison of test values, patients should have serial assays performed by the same test method.

Transport and processing. Transport and processing of the blood specimen to separate and remove the plasma are critical issues for HIV viral load testing. Virions and viral RNA are relatively unstable in whole blood and will be lost at a rapid rate if the plasma is not separated and frozen. The usual requirement is that the blood be processed and plasma frozen (preferably at $-70°C$) within 6 hours of the blood draw, but this should be performed sooner if possible. Repeated thaw and refreezing of the plasma (up to three times) will not greatly reduce the recovery of RNA.

Ultrasensitive assays. With the advent of combination therapy for HIV disease, the aim of therapy is to minimize the viral load. The current versions of the three commercially available assays discussed all have lower limits of detection of about 400 to 500 RNA copies/ml when run as standard protocols. Because physicians and patients are interested in viral loads between zero and 500 c/ml, manufacturers and some reference laboratories have developed "ultrasensitive" protocols that can measure RNA levels down to about 25 to 50 copies/ml. The assay methods are the same as in the standard assays, but the new protocols require a larger sample volume to boost the overall sensitivity. The ultrasensitive bDNA and RT-PCR assays are available only at certain reference laboratories but the NucliSens assay can be adapted by any user simply by including a larger volume of plasma in the reaction.

Diagnostic Recommendations

The International Aids Society–USA and PHS have made recommendations for use of plasma HIV RNA assays.[61] Plasma HIV RNA should be measured in all patients with HIV infection. The plasma HIV RNA level measures the magnitude of viral replication and predicts future damage to the immune system. Viral load testing should be done with measurement of the CD4+ T-cell count, which measures the current status of the immune system and predicts the short-term risk of opportunistic infections.

To minimize the effect of assay variability, baseline viral load testing should consist of measurements on two different specimens obtained within 1 to 2 weeks of each other. Because immunizations and opportunistic infections stimulate the immune system and increase the viral load, the testing should be done at least 4 weeks after such a stimulus. Initial treatment decisions are based on the level of HIV RNA as well as CD4+ count and clinical findings, and antiretroviral drug treatment should be considered for all patients with detectable

viral loads. If patients are not being treated, plasma HIV RNA levels should be measured every 3 to 4 months, and a rising level is an indication to begin treatment.

When antiretroviral treatment is started, the plasma HIV RNA should be measured after 1 month. With potent antiretroviral drug regimens, sharp drops in viral load of as much as 100-fold may be apparent at this time. A slower, second phase of decline may not be measurable until 12 to 16 weeks after starting therapy, so plasma HIV RNA should be measured then as well. Thereafter, viral load measurements should be repeated at 3- or 4-month intervals. If the viral load rises by more than threefold ($0.5 \log_{10}$), the change should be considered significant and a sign of possible noncompliance or antiretroviral resistance. Finally, a clinical event or a decline in CD4+ cell count should trigger a viral load measurement that can be used to make a decision to continue, initiate, or change therapy. At low levels of viral load (e.g., 100 to 10,000 copies/ml), changes greater than $0.5 \log_{10}$ may be explained by assay variability. After changes in regimen, viral load should be repeated as described after initiating treatment for the first time. At critical decision points, plasma HIV RNA assays should be repeated at 1-month intervals.

Table 17–4 lists indications for plasma HIV RNA testing.

A recent study has documented the usefulness of quantitative RNA assays as a tool in the diagnosis of neonatal infections. The results indicated that HIV RNA was detected earlier and more reliably than HIV DNA in all neonates but especially in infants more than 14 days to 3 months old. After 14 days of age, 98% of ultimately positive infants were positive for plasma HIV RNA.[54]

Plasma HIV RNA has been measured in pregnant women in studies of vertical transmission.[62, 63] In one study, transmission occurred in 12% of cases when maternal load was less than 1000 copies/ml and in 29% when greater than 10,000 copies/ml.[63] No value beneath which transmission did not occur has been identified but the lowest possible level is desirable during pregnancy, labor, and delivery.

Table 17–5 summarizes recommended laboratory tests for various aspects of HIV diagnosis or prognosis.

DIAGNOSTIC TESTING FOR HIV-2

HIV-2 is similar to but distinct from HIV-1. These viruses share approximately 60% genome homology in the relatively conserved *gag* and *pol* genes but only 30% to 40% homology in other genes. HIV-2 also causes AIDS, but the rate of progression of HIV-2 tends to be slower than with HIV-1, with an average interval from infection to AIDS of 19 years in the absence of treatment versus 10 years for HIV-1. HIV-2 is rare in the United States and most cases have had direct connection with West Africa

Table 17.4	Indications for Plasma HIV RNA Testing*	
Clinical indication	**Information**	**Use**
Initial evaluation of newly diagnosed HIV infection	Baseline viral load "set point"	Decision to start or defer therapy
Every 3-4 months in patients not receiving therapy	Changes in viral load	Decision to start therapy
4 weeks after initiation of antiretroviral therapy	Initial assessment of drug efficacy	Decision to continue or change therapy
3-4 months after start of therapy	Maximal effect of therapy	Decision to continue or change therapy
Every 3-4 months in patients receiving therapy	Durability of antiretroviral effect	Decision to continue or change therapy
Clinical event or decline in CD4+ T cells	Association with changing or stable viral load	Decision to continue, initiate, or change therapy
Syndrome consistent with acute HIV infection	Establishes diagnosis when HIV antibody test is negative	Diagnosis†

Modified from Carpenter CC, Fischl M, Hammer S, et al: *JAMA* 277:1962, 1997.
*Acute illness (e.g., bacterial pneumonia, tuberculosis, herpes simplex) and immunization can cause increases in plasma HIV RNA for 2 to 4 weeks; viral load testing should not be performed during this time.
All plasma HIV RNA results should be verified with a repeat determination before starting or making changes in therapy.
HIV RNA should be measured using the same laboratory and the same assay.
†A positive test for plasma HIV RNA should not be used as the sole evidence for the diagnosis of HIV infection because positive tests have occurred in individuals without HIV infection.

such as being a West African native, having traveled to West Africa, or having a West African sexual contact.[64] HIV-2 cases are more common in Europe than in the United States.

Enzyme-linked Immunosorbent Assay

As with HIV-1, the basic diagnostic test for HIV-2 infection is an ELISA to detect HIV-2 antibodies. Since

Table 17.5	Laboratory Tests Used for Different Aspects of HIV Diagnosis and Prognosis
Need	**Recommended tests**
Diagnosis of HIV infection (excluding infants and acute infections)	ELISA/Western blot
Acute HIV infection	p24 Antigen or DNA PCR or plasma RNA
Indeterminate Western blot	DNA PCR or plasma RNA
Infant born to HIV-infected mother	DNA PCR (plasma RNA can also be used)
Prognosis	Plasma RNA
Response to therapy	Plasma RNA
Blood donor screening	ELISA/Western blot, p24 antigen, plasma RNA

A positive test for plasma HIV RNA should not be used as the sole evidence for the diagnosis of HIV infection because positive tests have occurred in individuals without HIV infection.

June 1992, by FDA mandate, all donated blood is tested for HIV-2 antibodies before use. Accordingly, many HIV antibody ELISAs currently in use in the United States test simultaneously for HIV-1 and HIV-2. HIV-1–specific ELISAs yield a reactive result with approximately two thirds of specimens that contain HIV-2 antibodies.[65] In addition, one HIV-2-specific ELISA is produced commercially (Sanofi Genetic Systems, Redmond, Wash), and testing with this kit is available through many reference laboratories and at the Abbott Virology Reference Laboratory, Abbott Park, IL. The HIV-2-specific ELISA is used mainly for adjudication of results when the HIV-1/2 ELISA is positive and the HIV-1 Western blot (WB) is negative or indeterminate.

Western Blot

Two HIV-2 WB kits are manufactured by Cambridge BioTech (Worcester, Mass; marketed by bioMerieux Vitek) and GeneLabs Diagnostics (distributed by Cellular Products, Buffalo, NY). HIV-2 supplemental testing using these kits is available through many of the major reference laboratories. Neither kit is FDA licensed at present.

A standard algorithm applied to specimens that are reactive with an HIV-1/2 ELISA, but with a negative or indeterminate HIV-1 WB result, is to test them using the HIV-2–specific ELISA. If the specimen is nonreactive in that test, it can be considered negative for HIV-2 antibodies. If the HIV-2 ELISA is reactive on two of three determinations, the specimen must be tested using an HIV-2 WB. The criterion for considering a WB positive for HIV-2 antibodies is the presence of bands corresponding to gp105 (the viral envelope protein) and one of the following: p26, p31, or p55/58/68. This algorithm is the most efficient method for establishing a definitive diagnosis of HIV-2 infection. An alternative would be to perform an HIV-2–specific PCR. This testing is available only in selected reference laboratories.

Testing of serum specimens that contain HIV-2 antibodies with an HIV-1 WB often reveals antibodies against *pol* or *gag* proteins (p55, p24, p17; p66, p51, p31) because those are the most likely to cross-react between the two viruses.[65] Thus an indeterminate HIV-1 WB with *pol* and/or *gag* bands but not *env* bands may represent HIV-2 antibodies. HIV-2–specific antibody testing is indicated to confirm the presence of HIV-2 infection.

Other Tests

Certain HIV p24 antigen assays designed for the detection of HIV-1–associated p24 antigen can also be used for detection of *p26*, the corresponding protein of HIV-2. Tests that detect HIV-2 p26 are the Abbott polyclonal-based p24 antigen assay and the Organon Teknika p24 antigen kit, which has multiple monoclonal antibodies for capture onto the solid phase. In addition, a test to detect the p27 antigen of the simian immunodeficiency virus (SIV) (Coulter Corporation, Hialeah, FL) also detects HIV-2 p26.

Standard co-cultivation used for growth of HIV-1 will also permit growth of HIV-2. The presence of HIV-2 in the culture, however, will be detected only if a p24 antigen assay that detects HIV p26 is used. Alternative approaches would be to detect retroviral growth through the use of the HIV bDNA assay, which detects both HIV-1 and HIV-2, or an assay for reverse transcriptase activity in the culture supernatant.

HIV-2 can be detected by HIV-1 DNA PCR assays if the primers bind to gene segments that are identical or very similar in HIV-1 and HIV-2. Plasma HIV-2 RNA is not detected by the Roche Monitor RT-PCR or by Organon Teknika Nuclisens, and is detectable but not accurately quantitated by the Bayer Diagnostics bDNA assay.

DIAGNOSTIC TESTING FOR HTLV-I AND HTLV-II

As with HIV-1 and HIV-2, human T-cell lymphotropic (leukemia) virus (HTLV) types I and II are exogenous type C retroviruses that cause chronic infections in humans. The viruses share 60% nucleotide homology with each other. Both have a tropism for CD4+ lymphocytes and are believed to have similar modes of

transmission. HTLV-I has been linked to *adult T-cell leukemia* (ATL) and *HTLV-associated myelopathy* (HAM). HTLV-II has not yet been linked conclusively to any disease.

The prevalence of infection with HTLV-I is 1% to 5% in the Caribbean, southern Japan, some areas of Africa, Central and South America, and the southeastern United States. In the United States, HTLV-I has been found in intravenous drug users, prostitutes, patients with ATL and healthy individuals. HTLV-II has recently been identified in Indian tribes of North, Central, and South America.

HTLV-I causes ATL in only 2% to 4% of infected individuals after a long latency period of approximately 30 years. Currently, no prognostic indicators exist to predict which infected individuals will ultimately develop disease. The lifetime risk of HAM is probably lower, about 0.25% to 3%.

As for HIV-1 and HIV-2, the primary test for infection with HTLV-I or HTLV-II is an ELISA that detects antibodies to these viruses. Since 1988, all U.S. blood donors have been tested for HTLV-I/II infection by ELISA. Commercial ELISAs are manufactured with a lysate prepared from cells infected with HTLV-I, but they detect HTLV-II equally well because of extensive antigenic cross-reactivity.[66] Thus specimens that test positive with this assay are properly referred to as *HTLV-I/II positive.*

Because of the possibility of false-positive ELISA results, specimens that are repeatedly positive by ELISA must undergo supplemental testing using WB or radioimmunoprecipitation assay (RIPA). The standard algorithm is to start with an HTLV WB. The criterion for a positive WB is the presence of bands corresponding to the *gag* gene product (p24) and an *env* gene product (gp46, gp61/68, or both). If bands are present that do not fulfill the criterion for positivity, the blot is called indeterminate and a RIPA must be performed. The specimen is considered positive for HTLV-I/II antibodies if antibodies to p24 and to one or more *env* proteins are detected separately or together by the two assays.

Positive specimens require additional testing to make the important distinction between HTLV types I and II so that the patient can be properly counseled about potential for disease. ELISA assays based on synthetic peptide or recombinant protein antigens and PCR may be used to differentiate between HTLV-I and HTLV-II but are only available in research laboratories.[67] A blood donor who is found to have a positive ELISA for HTLV-I/II that is confirmed by supplemental testing is notified and permanently deferred from future blood donations. HTLV-I/II antibody ELISA and WB assays are available in many reference laboratories.

Individuals infected with HTLV-I/II do not test positive with HIV-1 or HIV-2 ELISAs or WBs, HIV-1 p24 antigen assays, or assays for HIV DNA or RNA unless they are also infected with HIV.

References

1. Burke DS, Brundage JF, Redfield RR, et al: Measurement of the false positive rate in a screening program for human immunodeficiency virus infections, *N Engl J Med* 319:961, 1988.

2. Buergisser P, Simon F, Wernli M, et al: Multicenter evaluation of new double-antigen sandwich enzyme immunoassay for measurement of anti–human immunodeficiency virus type 1 and type 2 antibodies, *J Clin Microbiol* 34:634, 1996.

3. Behets F, Disasi A, Ryder W, et al: Comparison of five commercial enzyme-linked immunosorbent assays and western immunoblotting for human immunodeficiency virus antibody detection in serum samples from central Africa, *J Clin Microbiol* 29:2280, 1991.

4. Centers for Disease Control and Prevention: Persistent lack of detectable HIV-1 antibody in a person with HIV infection—Utah, 1995, *MMWR* 45(9):181, 1996.

5. Martin-Rico P, Pedersen C, Skinhoj P, et al: Rapid development of AIDS in an HIV-1-antibody–negative homosexual man, *AIDS* 9:95, 1995.

6. Hu DJ, Dondero TJ, Rayfield MA, et al: The emerging genetic diversity of HIV, *JAMA* 275:210, 1996.

7. Brodine SK, Mascola JR, Weiss PJ, et al: Detection of diverse HIV-1 genetic subtypes in the USA, *Lancet* 346:1198, 1995.

8. Schable C, Zekeng L, Pau C-P, et al: Sensitivity of United States HIV antibody tests for detection of HIV-1 group O infections, *Lancet* 344:1333, 1994.

9. Guertler LG, Zekeng L, Simon F, et al: Reactivity of five anti-HIV-1 subtype O specimens with six different anti-HIV screening ELISAs and three immunoblots, *J Virol Methods* 51:177, 1995.

10. Centers for Disease Control and Prevention: Identification of HIV-1 group O infection, *MMWR* 45(26):1, 1996.

11. Centers for Disease Control: Update: HIV counseling and testing using rapid tests—United States, 1995, *MMWR* 47(11):211, 1998.

12. Gallo D, George JR, Fitchen JH, et al: Evaluation of a system using oral mucosal transudate for HIV-1 antibody screening and confirmatory testing, *JAMA* 277:254, 1997.

13. Centers for Disease Control and Prevention: Interpretation and use of the Western blot assay for serodiagnosis of human immunodeficiency virus type 1 infections, *MMWR* 38(suppl 7):1, 1989.

14. Centers for Disease Control and Prevention: Interpretive criteria used to report Western blot results for HIV-1 antibody testing: United States, *MMWR* 40(40):692, 1991.

15. Jackson JB, MacDonald KL, Cadwell J, et al: Absence of HIV infection in blood donors with indeterminate Western blot tests for antibody to HIV-1, *N Engl J Med* 322:217, 1990.

16. Jackson JB, Hanson MR, Johnson GM, et al: Long-term follow-up of blood donors with indeterminate human immunodeficiency virus type 1 results on Western blot, *Transfusion* 35:98, 1995.

17. Busch MP, Lee LL, Satten GA, et al: Time course of detection of viral and serologic markers preceding human immunodeficiency virus type 1 seroconversion: implications for screening of blood and tissue donors, *Transfusion* 35:91, 1995.

18. Henrard DR, Phillips JF, Muenz LR, et al: Natural history of HIV-1 cell-free viremia, *JAMA* 274:554, 1995.

19. Jackson GG, Paul DA, Falk LA, et al: Human immunodeficiency virus (HIV) antigenemia (p24) in the acquired immunodeficiency syndrome (AIDS) and the effect of treatment with zidovudine (AZT), *Ann Intern Med* 108:175, 1988.

20. Spear JB, Benson CA, Pottage JC, et al: Rapid rebound of serum human immunodeficiency virus antigen after discontinuing zidovudine therapy, *J Infect Dis* 158:1132, 1988.

21. Holody T, Lockwood D, Kay JWD: Detection of retroviral antigens in supernatants of HIV-1 group M clades, HIV-1 group O, HIV-2, and SIV with OTC's HIV-1 p24 antigen test. Presented at the 12th Annual Conference on Human Retrovirus Testing, Houston, February 1995.

22. Quinn TC, Kline R, Moss MW, et al: Acid dissociation of immune complexes improves diagnostic utility of p24 antigen detection in perinatally acquired human immunodeficiency virus infection, *J Infect Dis* 167:1193, 1993.

23. Centers for Disease Control and Prevention: U.S. Public Health Service Guidelines for Testing and Counseling Blood and Plasma Donors for human immunodeficiency virus type 1 antigen, *MMWR* 45(RR-2):1, 1996.

24. Petersen LR, Satten GA, Dodd R, et al: Duration of time from onset of human immunodeficiency virus type 1 infectiousness to development of detectable antibody, *Transfusion* 34:283, 1994.

25. Lackritz EM, Satten GA, Aberle-Grasse J, et al: Estimated risk of transmission of the human immunodeficiency virus by screened blood in the United States, *N Engl J Med* 333:1721, 1995.

26. Jackson JB, Kwok SY, Sninsky JJ, et al: Human immunodeficiency virus type 1 detected in all seropositive symptomatic and asymptomatic individuals, *J Clin Microbiol* 28:16, 1990.

27. Division of AIDS, National Institute of Allergy and Infectious Diseases: *DAIDS Virology Manual for HIV Laboratories*, Pub No NIH-97-3828, Washington, DC, 1997, US Department of Health and Human Services.

28. Erice A, Sannerud KJ, Leske VL, et al: Sensitive microculture method for isolation of human immunodeficiency virus type 1 from blood leukocytes, *J Clin Microbiol* 30:444, 1992.

29. Alimenti A, O'Neill M, Sullivan JL, Luzuriaga K: Diagnosis of vertical human immunodeficiency virus type 1 infection by whole blood culture, *J Infect Dis* 166:1146, 1992.

30. Lewis DL, Arens M: Resistance of microorganisms to disinfection in dental and medical devices, *Nat Med* 1:956, 1995.

31. Lathey JL, Fiscus SA, Rasheed S, et al: Optimization of quantitative culture assay for human immunodeficiency virus from plasma, *J Clin Microbiol* 32:3064, 1994.

32. Dimitrov DH, Melnick JL, Hollinger FB: Microculture assay for isolation of human immunodeficiency vi-

rus type 1 and for titration of infected peripheral blood mononuclear cells, *J Clin Microbiol* 28:34, 1990.

33. Conor RJ, Mohri H, Cao Y, Ho DD: Increased viral burden and cytopathicity correlate temporally with CD4+ T-lymphocyte decline and clinical progression in human immunodeficiency virus type 1–infected individuals, *J Virol* 67:1172, 1993.

34. Japour AJ, Fiscus SA, Arduino J-M, et al: Standardized microtiter assay for determination of syncytium-inducing phenotypes of clinical human immunodeficiency virus type 1 isolates, *J Clin Microbiol* 32:2291, 1994.

35. Bozzette SA, McCutchan JA, Spector SA, et al: A cross-sectional comparison of persons with syncytium- and non-syncytium-inducing human immunodeficiency virus, *J Infect Dis* 168:1374, 1993.

36. Richman DD, Bozzette SA: The impact of syncytium-inducing phenotype of human immunodeficiency virus on disease progression, *J Infect Dis* 169:968, 1994.

37. De Jong J-J, De Ronde A, Keulen W, et al: Minimal requirements for the human immunodeficiency virus type 1 V3 domain to support the syncytium-inducing phenotype: analysis by single amino acid substitution, *J Virol* 66:6777, 1992.

38. Kwok S, Mack DH, Mullis KB, et al: Identification of human immunodeficiency virus sequences by using in vitro enzymatic amplification and oligomer cleavage detection, *J Virol* 61:690, 1987.

39. Abbott MA, Poiesz BJ, Byrne BC, et al: Enzymatic gene amplification: qualitative and quantitative methods for detecting proviral DNA amplified in vitro, *J Infect Dis* 158:1158, 1988.

40. Dickover RE, Donovan RM, Goldstein E, et al: Quantitation of human immunodeficiency virus DNA by using the polymerase chain reaction, *J Clin Microbiol* 28:2130, 1990.

41. Albert J, Fenyo EM: Simple, sensitive, and specific detection of human immunodeficiency virus type 1 in clinical specimens by polymerase chain reaction with nested primers, *J Clin Microbiol* 28:560, 1990.

42. Michael NL, Vahey M, Burke DS, Redfield RR: Viral DNA and mRNA expression correlate with the stage of human immunodeficiency virus (HIV) type 1 infection in humans: evidence for viral replication in all stages of HIV disease, *J Virol* 66:310, 1992.

43. Whetsell AJ, Drew JB, Milman G, et al: Comparison of three nonradioisotopic polymerase chain reaction–based methods for detection of human immunodeficiency virus type 1, *J Clin Microbiol* 30:845, 1992.

44. Owens DK, Holodniy M, Garber AM, et al: Polymerase chain reaction for the diagnosis of HIV infection in adults, *Ann Intern Med* 124:803, 1996.

45. Chadwick EG, Yogev R, Kwok S, et al: Enzymatic amplification of the human immunodeficiency virus in peripheral blood mononuclear cells from pediatric patients, *J Infect Dis* 160:954, 1989.

46. Rogers MF, Ou C-Y, Rayfield M, et al: Use of the polymerase chain reaction for early detection of the proviral sequences of human immunodeficiency virus in infants born to seropositive mothers, *N Engl J Med* 320:1649, 1989.

47. Williams P, Simmonds P, Yap PL, et al: The polymerase chain reaction in the diagnosis of vertically transmitted HIV infection, *AIDS* 4:393, 1990.

48. Scarlatti G, Lombardi V, Plebani A, et al: Polymerase chain reaction, virus isolation and antigen assay in HIV-1-antibody–positive mothers and their children, *AIDS* 5:1173, 1991.

49. Weintrub PS, Ulrich PP, Edwards JR, et al: Use of polymerase chain reaction for the early detection of HIV infection in the infants of HIV-seropositive women, *AIDS* 5:881, 1991.

50. Kovacs A, Xu J, Rasheed S, et al: Comparison of a rapid nonisotopic polymerase chain reaction assay with four commonly used methods for the early diagnosis of human immunodeficiency virus type 1 infection in neonates and children, *Pediatr Infect Dis J* 14:948, 1995.

51. Bremer JW, Lew JF, Cooper E, et al: Diagnosis of infection with human immunodeficiency virus type 1 by a DNA polymerase chain reaction assay among infants enrolled in the women and infants' transmission study, *J Pediatr* 129:198, 1996.

52. Centers for Disease Control and Prevention: 1994 revised classification system for human immunodeficiency virus infection in children less than 13 years of age, *MMWR* 43(RR-12):1, 1994.

53. Owens DK, Holodniy M, McDonald TW, et al: A meta-analytic evaluation of the polymerase chain reaction for the diagnosis of HIV infection in infants, *JAMA* 1275:1342, 1996.

54. Stekette RW, Abrams EJ, Thea DM, et al: Early detection of perinatal human immunodeficiency virus (HIV) type 1 infection using HIV RNA amplification and detection, *J Infect Dis* 175:707, 1997.

55. Connor EM, Sperling RS, Gelber R, et al: Reduction of maternal-infant transmission of human immunodeficiency virus type 1 with zidovudine treatment, *N Engl J Med* 331:1173, 1994.

56. Mellors JW, Rinaldo CR Jr, Gupta P, et al: Prognosis in HIV-1 infection predicted by the quantity of virus in plasma, *Science* 272:1167, 1996.

57. Boom R, Sol CJA, Salimans MMM, et al: Rapid and simple method for purification of nucleic acids, *J Clin Microbiol* 28:495, 1990.

58. Shafer RW, Levee DJ, Winters MA, et al: Comparison of QIAamp HCV kit spin columns, silica beads, and phenol-chloroform for recovering human immunodeficiency virus type 1 RNA from plasma, *J Clin Microbiol* 35:520, 1997.

59. Schuurman R, Descamps D, Weverling GJ, et al: Multicenter comparison of three commercial methods for quantification of human immunodeficiency virus type 1 RNA in plasma, *J Clin Microbiol* 34:3016, 1996.

60. Brambilla D, Leung S, Lew J, et al: Absolute copy number and relative change in determinations of human immunodeficiency virus type 1 RNA in plasma: effect of an external standard on kit comparisons, *J Clin Microbiol* 36:311, 1998.

60a. Mellors JW, Muñoz A, Giorgi JV, et al: Plasma viral load and CD4+ lymphocytes as prognostic markers of HIV-1 infection, *Ann Intern Med* 126:946, 1997.

60b. Goetz MB, Moatamed F, Howanitz JH: Measurement of plasma HIV viral load (VL) by bDNA versus RT-PCR (PCR) assays (abstract), *Clin Infect Dis* 25:394, 1997.

61. Carpenter CC, Fischl M, Hammer S, et al: Antiretroviral therapy for HIV infection in 1997: updated recommendations of the International AIDS Society—USA panel, *JAMA* 277:1962, 1997.

62. Thea DM, Steketee RW, Pliner V, et al: The effect of maternal viral load on the risk of perinatal transmission of HIV-1, *AIDS* 11:437, 1997.

63. Mayaux M-J, Dussaix E, Isopet J, et al: Maternal virus load during pregnancy and mother-to-child transmission of human immunodeficiency virus type 1: the French perinatal cohort studies, *J Infect Dis* 175:172, 1997.

64. Centers for Disease Control and Prevention: Update: HIV-2 infection among blood and plasma donors—United States, June 1992-June 1995, *MMWR* 44(32):603, 1995.

65. Denis F, Leonard G, Sangare A, et al: Comparison of 10 enzyme immunoassays for detection of antibody to human immunodeficiency virus type 2 in West African sera, *J Clin Microbiol* 26:1000, 1988.

66. Cossen C, Hagens S, Fukuchi R, et al: Comparison of six commercial human T-cell lymphotropic virus type I (HTLV-I) enzyme immunoassay kits for detection of antibody of HTLV-I and –II, *J Clin Microbiol* 30:724, 1992.

67. Heneine W, Khabbaz RF, Lal RB, Kaplan JE: Sensitive and specific polymerase chain reaction assays for diagnosis of human T-cell lymphotropic virus type I (HTLV-I) and HTLV-II infections in HTLV-I/II-seropositive individuals, *J Clin Microbiol* 30:1605, 1992.

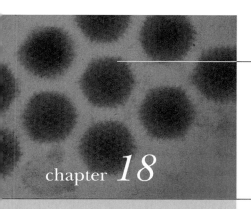

Alejo Erice

Antiviral Susceptibility Testing

OVERVIEW

Until relatively recently, the phenomenon of antiviral resistance had been observed only in the laboratory, where drug-resistant viruses could be obtained under selective drug pressure in vitro. During the last decade, however, infection with viruses resistant to antiviral drugs has become well recognized. Not surprisingly, the emergence of antiviral-resistant viruses has evolved in parallel with the development and availability of more antiviral compounds for clinical use. Most infections caused by resistant viruses have been described in immunocompromised patients and associated with disease progression and failure to respond to antiviral therapy. The recognition that virulent drug-resistant strains could emerge in the clinic has important implications, including the need to develop laboratory methods for determining antiviral susceptibilities that can be used in diagnostic laboratories for detection of resistant viruses.

Laboratory methods to determine susceptibilities of viral isolates to antiviral compounds may be classified as phenotypic and genotypic. *Phenotypic assays* are designed to determine the concentration of an antiviral that would inhibit a virus in culture. Generally, these are culture-based methods in which a known amount of infectious virus is grown in the presence of different concentrations of antiviral agents. Viral production is then plotted against antiviral concentration to determine the *50% inhibitory concentration* (IC_{50}), or the concentration of antiviral agent (expressed in μM or μg/ml) producing 50% inhibition of the virus in culture (Figure 18–1). According to results of phenotypic assays, viruses are classified as susceptible or resistant to a given antiviral compound.

Genotypic assays are designed to determine whether mutations known to confer antiviral resistance are present in the genome of the viruses being studied. Generally, genotypic methods involve molecular technologies to obtain sequence information on target regions of the viral genome. Genotypic assays are useful when the genetic basis for antiviral resistance has been identified and when a predictable relationship exists between the presence or absence of a genetic variant and measurable antiviral resistance. The significance of mutations found in genotypic studies must be further evaluated by assessing the effect of each mutation on the phenotype of recombinant viruses and on the structure and function of mutated viral proteins. These latter studies are required for understanding the mechanisms of antiviral resistance; antiviral susceptibility methods used in diagnostic laboratories are usually limited to phenotypic and genotypic assays.

Clinically, the most relevant question is to determine the pathogenic significance of infections caused by resistant viruses. Although currently available methods can be useful for patient management, further work is necessary to develop rapid and reproducible assays that will permit the timely detection of resistant viral isolates in clinical specimens to guide therapeutic decisions.

HERPES SIMPLEX VIRUS

Antiviral Resistance

Current licensed antivirals for the treatment of infections caused by herpes simplex virus (HSV) types 1 and 2 include acyclovir, famciclovir (the prodrug of penciclovir), and foscarnet (Figure 18–2). All three are inhibitors of the HSV deoxyribonucleic acid (DNA) polymerase, but they have different modes of action (Figure 18–3). *Acyclovir* and *famciclovir* are nucleoside analogs (famciclovir is converted into the active drug *penciclovir* after absorption), whereas *foscarnet* is a pyrophosphate analog. The nucleoside analogs acyclovir and penciclovir require intracellular activation to exert their antiviral activity, whereas foscarnet does not.

Acyclovir is the first line of therapy for HSV infections.[1] Acyclovir is a preferred substrate for the HSV *thymidine kinase* (TK) that phosphorylates acyclovir to acyclovir monophosphate within HSV-infected cells. Acyclovir monophosphate is then progressively transformed by cellular kinases to acyclovir diphosphate and *acyclovir triphosphate* (the active form of acyclovir with antiviral activity). Acyclovir triphosphate competitively inhibits the HSV DNA polymerase and is also incorporated in place of thymidine triphosphate into viral DNA, where it acts as a chain terminator (Figure 18–3).[1] Formation of a complex between the terminated DNA

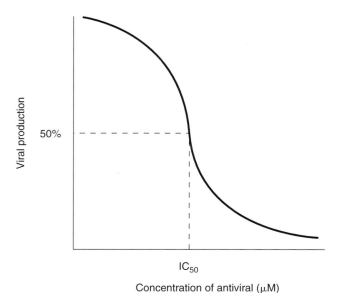

Figure 18.1 Fifty-percent inhibitory concentration (IC_{50}), or concentration of antiviral producing 50% inhibition of virus in culture. In phenotypic assays, IC_{50} is determined by plotting viral production against antiviral concentration.

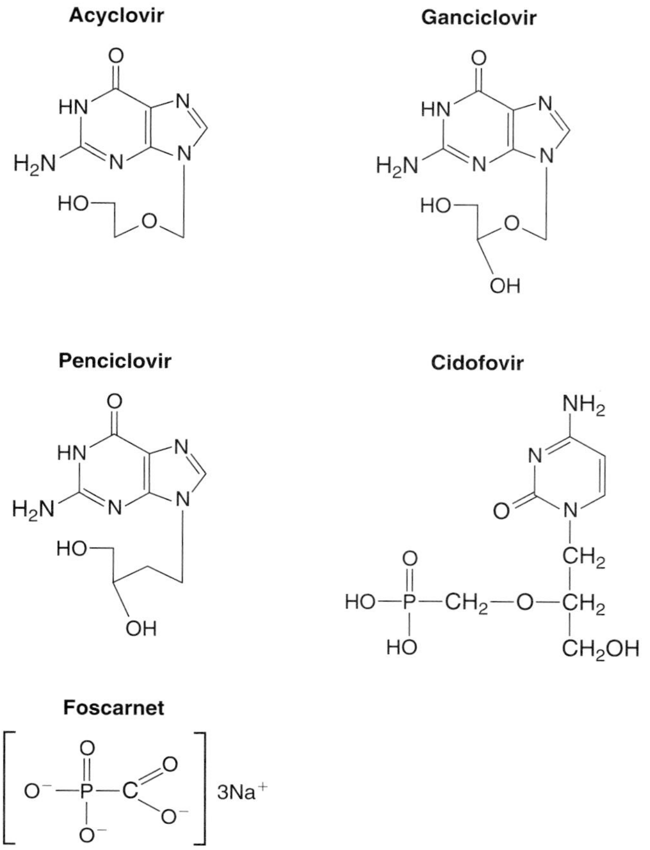

Acyclovir

Ganciclovir

Penciclovir

Cidofovir

Foscarnet

Figure 18.2   Chemical structure of antiviral agents in clinical use for treatment of herpesvirus infections.

template containing acyclovir and the enzyme may lead to irreversible inactivation of the DNA polymerase.

Mechanisms. HSV can become resistant to acyclovir by the following three mechanisms[2, 3]:

1. Absent or decreased production of viral TK (TK⁻ viruses). Acyclovir cannot be phosphorylated in cells infected with TK⁻ viruses.

2. Production of a viral TK with altered substrate specificity (TKᴬ viruses)

3. Altered viral DNA polymerase that is capable of elongating HSV DNA in the presence of high concentrations of acyclovir triphosphate

Because acyclovir and penciclovir require an intact viral TK to exert their antiviral activity, cross-resistance of TK⁻ and TKᴬ viruses to these compounds can be anticipated. Cross-resistance is not universal, however, and TKᴬ viruses can be resistant to acyclovir but fully susceptible to penciclovir. This suggests that the specific sites of interaction of acyclovir and penciclovir with the viral TK may not be identical.[4, 5]

Genetics. Characterization of the sequence of the gene encoding TK in TK⁻ and TKᴬ HSV isolates has demonstrated point mutations and nucleotide deletions located in different regions of the TK gene.[2, 6, 7] These mutations result in the production of aberrant TK proteins that are either truncated or completely absent. Some TK⁻ isolates also have point mutations outside the active TK site.[2] These "off-site" mutations cause functionally significant structural changes in the TK protein.

Resistance of HSV to antiviral agents is also associated with point mutations within conserved regions A, II, III, I, VII, and V of the viral DNA polymerase (Figure 18–4).[8] These mutations may produce cross-resistance between acyclovir and foscarnet, but cross-resistance of HSV DNA polymerase mutants is not uniform. Some foscarnet-resistant HSV isolates containing DNA polymerase mutations are susceptible to penciclovir and acyclovir. This suggests that the specific sites of interaction of the acyclovir and penciclovir triphosphates with viral DNA polymerase differ from that of foscarnet.[9]

Phenotypic Assays

A variety of phenotypic assays have been used to determine antiviral susceptibilities of clinical and laboratory HSV strains, including plaque reduction,[10] dye uptake,[11] EIA-based assays,[12] and assays based on DNA hybridization.[13] Each of these assays measures inhibi-

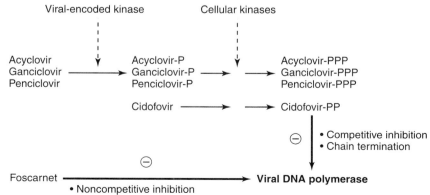

Figure 18.3   Mechanism of action of antiviral agents against herpesviruses (see text). *dNTP,* Deoxynucleotide triphosphate; *PPi,* pyrophosphate.

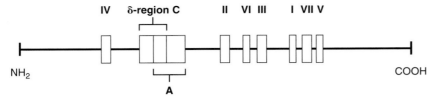

Figure 18.4 Schematic representation of herpesvirus DNA polymerase (UL54). Boxes represent regions of DNA polymerase highly conserved among different herpesviruses. Mutations within or near these regions are associated with antiviral resistance (see text).

Region	Amino acid residues
IV	379 - 421
A	538 - 598
δ-region C	492 - 588
II	696 - 742
VI	771 - 789/790
III	804/805 - 845/846
I	905 - 919/920
VII	962 - 970
V	973/978 - 988

tion of viral growth in the presence of antiviral agents, but by different means. The plaque reduction assay (PRA) and the dye uptake assay (DUA) measure the inhibition of replication of infectious virus. EIA measures the inhibition of synthesis of one or more viral proteins. DNA hybridization assays measure inhibition of viral DNA synthesis.

Plaque reduction. The PRA has been considered the gold standard for antiviral susceptibility testing of HSV and other viruses.[14] A standardized inoculum of a stock virus (previously titrated in cell culture) is inoculated into cultures and incubated in the presence of antiviral agents. Cultures are then observed for the production of viral plaques. The IC_{50} of the isolate is defined as the concentration of antiviral agent causing a 50% reduction in the number of plaques produced. PRAs are labor intensive and involve (1) isolation of the virus in culture, (2) preparation of viral stocks (by sequential passaging of the viral isolate in culture until an adequate amount of virus is present to perform the assay), (3) titration of viral stocks, and (4) the actual antiviral susceptibility testing.

The clinical usefulness of PRAs is limited by the time required to complete the assay (1 to 2 weeks for HSV) and the lack of a standardized method validated across different laboratories. In addition, continuous passaging of the isolates to prepare viral stocks may influence the results of PRAs by selecting viral strains that are not representative of the original population of viruses.

A modified PRA determines antiviral susceptibilities of HSV isolates by using a cell line that expresses ß-galactosidase only after cells have been infected with virus (see also Chapter 1).[15] A similar assay has been successfully used as a rapid screening method for detection of acyclovir-resistant HSV isolates.[16]

Dye uptake. The DUA measures the amount of neutral red dye taken up by viable (noninfected) cells in viral cultures.[11] A standardized inoculum of HSV is inoculated into cell cultures and incubated in the presence of

antiviral agents. After 2 to 3 days, neutral red dye is added to the cultures. After a short incubation time the neutral red dye incorporated by noninfected cells is measured colorimetrically. The IC_{50} of the isolate is defined as the concentration of antiviral agent that reduces the amount of dye uptake by 50%.[11, 14]

The DUA has the same limitations as the PRA, with a turnaround time of at least 2 weeks. DUA reportedly is useful for detection of mixed populations of acyclovir-resistant and susceptible viruses.

DNA hybridization. In these assays, IC_{50} values of HSV isolates are determined by measuring the effect of antiviral agents on HSV DNA synthesis in culture. Previously used dot blot hybridization assays that employed ^{32}P-labeled HSV DNA probes have been replaced by more convenient commercial assays such as the Hybriwix assay (Diagnostic Hybrids, Athens, OH).[13]

The *Hybriwix* assay is the only HSV susceptibility assay that is currently commercially available to laboratories in kit form.[13] Cell cultures are inoculated with sufficient virus to produce 50% to 100% cytopathic effect (CPE) after 48 hours. In practice, a 10-fold or 100-fold dilution of an HSV-infected cell culture producing 100% CPE is used. Cultures are incubated in the presence of different concentrations of antivirals for 48 to 72 hours. Then cells are lysed, and whole genomic DNA is extracted and transferred by capillary action onto negatively charged nylon membranes. Membranes are hybridized to a ^{125}I-labeled HSV probe and counted in a gamma counter for 2 minutes. Mean hybridization values in counts per minute (cpm) for each concentration of antiviral are then calculated. The IC_{50} is defined as the concentration of antiviral agent that reduces viral nucleic acid hybridization values by 50% compared with hybridization values of controls (infected cells incubated in the absence of antiviral drug).

Enzyme immunoassay-based methods. In EIAs, IC_{50} values are determined by measuring the effect of antiviral agents on the quantity of viral antigen produced in cell cultures infected with HSV isolates.[12] EIA is performed after infection of cell cultures with HSV and a 24-hour or 48-hour incubation period in the presence of antiviral agents. Cells are then washed, fixed, and incubated sequentially with an anti-HSV antibody and a peroxidase-conjugated secondary antibody. The color generated, measured spectrophotometrically as optical density, is proportional to the amount of viral antigen produced. The IC_{50} is defined as the concentration of antiviral agent that reduces the optical density by 50% compared with cultures with no antiviral drug.

Diagnostic considerations. Interpretation of results of antiviral resistance studies is difficult. The different susceptibility assays are not well standardized, and disparate results can be obtained using different methods. Variables that affect results of susceptibility testing include type of cell culture, size of the viral inoculum, method used, and the laboratory performing the assay. For example, IC_{50} values obtained with DUA are five to ten times higher than those obtained with PRA for the same isolate,[17] whereas results obtained with EIA-based and DNA hybridization assays correlate well with PRA results. When feasible, a baseline viral isolate from the same patient should be tested in parallel with the suspected resistant isolate. Unfortunately, baseline isolates often are not available. Antiviral susceptibility assays should include well-characterized susceptible and resistant reference isolates.

Antiviral susceptibility assays should always be interpreted in the context of the clinical findings. Clinically, resistance should be suspected when viruses are persistently isolated from patients receiving appropriate antiviral therapy. However, clinical failure may or may not be caused by resistant viruses. Infections caused by resistant HSV isolates are characterized by enlarging, nonhealing, and deep ulcerative lesions from which the virus is persistently isolated during antiviral therapy (Figure 18–5).[18] These infections should be suspected

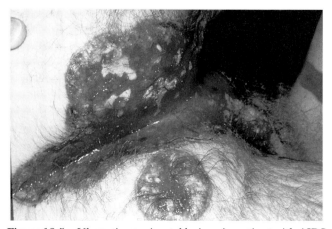

Figure 18.5 Ulcerative perirectal lesions in patient with AIDS caused by an acyclovir-resistant herpes simplex virus strain. (From Engel JP, Englund JA, Fletcher CV, Hill EL: *JAMA* 263:1662, 1990.)

| Table 18.1 | Fifty-Percent Inhibitory Concentrations (IC_{50}) Denoting Antiviral Resistance of Clinical HSV Isolates |

Antiviral	Method	IC_{50} (μM)	Reference(s)
Acyclovir	PRA	>8	1
		>12	14
		≥8	19
	DUA	>12	19, 20
		>12	14
	DNA	≥9	21, 22
		≥8	13
Foscarnet	PRA	≥330	19
	DUA	≥330	23

PRA, Plaque reduction assay; *DUA*, dye uptake assay; *DNA*, DNA hybridization assay.

in individuals who have received prolonged antiviral therapy.

Table 18–1[1, 13, 14, 19-23] lists IC_{50} values that denote resistance of clinical HSV isolates to acyclovir and foscarnet.

Genotypic Assays

Although the regions of the HSV TK and DNA polymerase containing mutations associated with antiviral resistance have been identified, the specific locations of the different mutations vary among resistant HSV strains.[3, 6-8] This heterogeneity has complicated the development of molecular methods for detection of antiviral-resistant HSV mutants in clinical laboratories. Genotypic characterization of antiviral-resistant HSV isolates requires amplification and characterization of TK and DNA polymerase sequences using various methodologies. Although these methods are crucial for understanding the mechanisms of resistance of HSV to antiviral agents, they are presently available only in research laboratories. Rapid molecular methods for detection of mutant HSV isolates resistant to antiviral drugs are not yet available in clinical laboratories.

VARICELLA-ZOSTER VIRUS

Antiviral Resistance

Mechanisms and genetics. Antiviral agents currently licensed for the treatment of infections caused by varicella-zoster virus (VZV) include acyclovir, famciclovir (the prodrug of penciclovir), and foscarnet (see Figure 18–2). All these are active inhibitors of the VZV DNA polymerase.

As with HSV-resistant isolates, most of the acyclovir-resistant VZV isolates have been TK⁻ or TKᴬ.[6] Strains of VZV that are cross-resistant to acyclovir and foscarnet, suggesting an alteration in the viral DNA polymerase, have also been recovered from patients but are less common.

Characterization of TK sequences of TK⁻ and TKᴬ VZV strains resistant to acyclovir and penciclovir has demonstrated nonuniform mutations within the TK gene, including single nucleotide substitutions and nucleotide deletions and insertions. These changes result in the production of aberrant TK proteins that are either truncated or completely absent. The heterogeneity of the mutations found in the TK gene of acyclovir-resistant VZV strains is much greater than that observed in HSV.[24, 25]

Mutations associated with antiviral resistance have been found within conserved regions of the catalytic domain of the VZV DNA polymerase (see Figure 18–4). These point mutations have been associated with cross-resistance to acyclovir and foscarnet.

Phenotypic Assays

A variety of phenotypic assays have been used to determine antiviral susceptibilities of clinical and laboratory VZV strains. These are identical to the methods described for HSV isolates and include PRA, DUA, EIA-based methods, and DNA hybridization assays.[14, 26, 27] Because VZV grows much more slowly than HSV, VZV susceptibility tests take longer to perform than those for HSV.

A specific drug concentration that defines resistance to acyclovir is not presently available. Laboratories instead compare the IC_{50} of the isolate to that of a pretherapy isolate or an isolate known to be susceptible Table 18–2.

Infections caused by resistant VZV isolates are characterized by persistent disseminated hyperkeratotic papules that fail to heal during antiviral therapy (Figure 18–6).[28] These infections are almost exclusively found in patients with AIDS who have received long-term therapy with acyclovir.

Genotypic Assays

Because of genetic heterogeneity,[24, 25] genotypic characterization of antiviral-resistant VZV isolates would

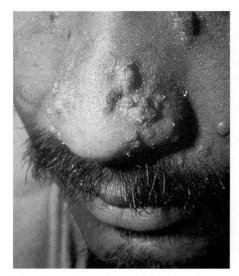

Figure 18.6 Hyperkeratotic papules on face of patient caused by acyclovir-resistant varicella-zoster virus. (From Jacobson MA, Berger TG, Fikrigs, et al: *Ann Intern Med* 112:187, 1990.)

require amplification and characterization of TK (and DNA polymerase) sequences of the virus using different methodologies. Although these methods are crucial for understanding the mechanisms of resistance of VZV to antiviral agents, they are presently available only in research laboratories. Rapid molecular methods for detection of mutant VZV isolates resistant to antivirals are not yet available in clinical laboratories.

CYTOMEGALOVIRUS

Antiviral Resistance

Antiviral drugs currently available for the treatment of CMV infections include ganciclovir, foscarnet, and cidofovir (see Figure 18–2).[29-31] As with acyclovir and penciclovir, *ganciclovir* is a nucleoside derivative that must be phosphorylated to ganciclovir triphosphate to exert its antiviral activity. Within CMV-infected cells, the *UL97 gene* of CMV encodes a protein kinase that phosphorylates ganciclovir to ganciclovir monophosphate, with cellular kinases performing further phos-

Table 18.2	Fifty-Percent Inhibitory Concentrations (IC_{50}) Denoting Antiviral Resistance of Clinical Varicella-Zoster Isolates		
Antiviral	**Method**	**IC_{50} (μM)**	**Reference**
Acyclovir	PRA	≥3-4 times increase compared with control or pretherapy isolate	27
	DNA	>10	25
		≥3-4 times increase compared with control or pretherapy isolate	27
Foscarnet	DNA	>500	25

PRA, Plaque reduction assay; *DNA*, DNA hybridization assay.

phorylation to the triphosphate form. Ganciclovir triphosphate inhibits the CMV DNA polymerase by competing with it for the natural substrate deoxyguanosine triphosphate. In addition, incorporation of ganciclovir triphosphate into viral DNA causes a slowing and subsequent cessation of CMV DNA chain elongation (see Figure 18–3).

Foscarnet reversibly and noncompetitively inhibits the activity of the CMV DNA polymerase. Foscarnet does not require intracellular activation to exert its antiviral activity.

Cidofovir is a nucleoside phosphonate analog that must be phosphorylated to its diphosphoryl derivative by cellular phosphorylating enzymes. Cidofovir diphosphate is a competitive inhibitor of the CMV DNA polymerase. Similar to ganciclovir, the incorporation of cidofovir diphosphate into viral DNA causes a slowing and subsequent cessation of CMV DNA chain elongation.

Studies done in the last 5 years have contributed significantly to understanding the mechanisms of resistance of CMV to antiviral drugs. Ganciclovir-resistant clinical isolates may contain UL97 mutations, UL54 (DNA polymerase) mutations, or mutations in both viral genes (Tables 18–3 and 18–4).[32-51] The functional consequence of UL97 mutations is impaired phosphorylation of ganciclovir in virus-infected cells, with the consequent lack of synthesis of ganciclovir triphosphate. CMV isolates containing UL97 mutations alone are susceptible to foscarnet and cidofovir. Resistance of CMV to foscarnet or cidofovir is associated with amino acid substitutions in conserved regions of the viral DNA polymerase (UL54).[52-54]

Most CMV isolates with mutations in UL54 are resistant to ganciclovir and have variable cross-resistance patterns to foscarnet and cidofovir. Mutations in UL54 regions IV and δ-region C and in region V cause resistance to ganciclovir and cidofovir. Mutations in conserved regions II and VI cause resistance to foscarnet. Mutations in conserved region III are associated with various antiviral susceptibility profiles. Mutations outside conserved regions of UL54 are not associated with significant changes in antiviral susceptibilities of CMV. Multiple UL54 mutations are additive and cause resistance to multiple antivirals (Figure 18–3).

Phenotypic Assays

A variety of phenotypic assays have been used in different studies to determine antiviral susceptibilities of clinical and laboratory CMV strains. Results from studies using these assays are difficult to compare because no standardized phenotypic assay exists and different criteria were used to define CMV resistance.

Plaque reduction. As with HSV and VZV, the PRA remains the gold standard for antiviral susceptibility

Table 18.3	UL97 Mutations in Clinical CMV Isolates Resistant to Ganciclovir	
UL97 mutation	Amino acid change	Proven role in recombinant virus*
M460V	Methionine to valine	X
M460I	Methionine to isoleucine	X
N510S	Aspartic acid to serine	
H520Q	Histidine to glutamine to threonine	X
A590T	Alanine to threonine	
A591D	Alanine to aspartic acid	
A591V	Alanine to valine	
C592G	Cysteine to glycine	
A594V	Alanine to valine	X
A594T	Alanine to threonine	
del 591-594	Deletion of alanine-alanine-cysteine-arginine	X
L595S	Leucine to serine	X
L595F	Leucine to phenylalanine	X
L595T	Leucine to threonine	
del 595	Deletion of leucine	X
L595W	Leucine to tryptophan	
E596G	Glutamic acid to glycine	
E596D	Glutamic acid to aspartic acid	
N597I	Asparagine to isoleucine	
G598V	Glycine to valine	
K599M	Lysine to methionine	
del 600	Deletion of leucine	
C603W	Cysteine to tryptophan	X
C607Y	Cysteine to tyrosine	X
C603Y	Cysteine to tyrosine	
A606D	Alanine to aspartic acid	
V665I	Valine to isoleucine	

*Experiments with recombinant viruses have proved that the mutation confers drug resistance.

testing (Figure 18–7).[14] The principle of this assay is the same as for HSV and VZV. The practical difficulties are even more pronounced for CMV, however, because of its slow and sometimes unpredictable growth in cell culture. A minimum of 4 to 6 weeks is required to complete the assay. In addition, the continuous passaging of the isolates to prepare viral stocks required for the assay may influence the results of PRAs by selecting

Table 18.4 UL54 (DNA Polymerase) Mutations in Clinical CMV Isolates Resistant to Antivirals

Region	UL54 mutation	Amino acid change	Viral phenotype*			Proven role in recombinant virus†
			Ganciclovir	Foscarnet	Cidofovir	
IV	N408D	Asparagine to aspartic acid	R	S	R	
	F412C	Phenylalanine to cysteine	R	S	R	X
	D413E	Aspartic acid to glutamic acid	R	S	R	
δ-region C	L501F	Leucine to phenylalanine	R	S	R	
	L501I	Leucine to isoleucine	R	S	R	X
	T503I	Threonine to isoleucine	R	S	R	
	K513R	Lysine to arginine	R	S	R	
	K513E	Lysine to glutamic acid	R	S	R	
	P522A	Proline to alanine	R	S	ND	
II	T700A	Threonine to alanine	S	R	S	X
	V715M	Valine to methionine	S	R	S	X
	I722V	Isoleucine to valine	R	S	R	
VI	V781I	Valine to isoleucine	R	R	S	
III	L802M	Leucine to methionine	R	R	S	X
	A809V	Alanine to valine	R	R	S	X
	G841A	Glycine to alanine	R	S	ND	
Other	S676G	Serine to glycine	R	S	R	
	G678S	Glycine to serine	R	S	R	
	Y751H	Tyrosine to histidine	R	S	R	

*R, Resistant; S, sensitive; ND, not done.
†Experiments with recombinant viruses have proved that the mutation confers drug resistance.

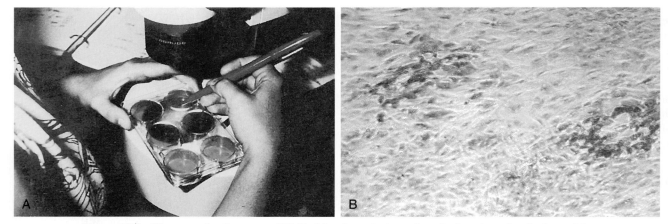

Figure 18.7 Plaque reduction assay (PRA). After inoculation of stock virus (previously titrated in cell culture) in cell monolayers, cultures are overlaid with semisolid culture medium containing antiviral agents. After incubation, the length of which varies according to virus being tested, cells are fixed and stained with crystal violet or methylene blue. Cultures are then observed under a microscope at low power for presence of plaques. Plaques are counted and plotted against concentration of antiviral agent to determine IC_{50} of isolate. **A,** Tissue culture plate with methylene blue–stained cells. Plaques identified and marked under microscope are being counted. **B,** Plaques representing fibroblasts infected with cytomegalovirus (CMV). After staining with methylene blue, CMV-infected cells appear dark blue.

CMV strains that are not representative of the original population of viruses.

DNA hybridization. The DNA hybridization assay described for HSV can also be used with a CMV-specific probe to determine the IC_{50} for CMV.[55] As with PRAs, DNA hybridization assays require isolation of CMV strains, sequential passaging of the isolates in culture for preparation of viral stocks, titration of viral stocks, and susceptibility testing. In addition, DNA hybridization assays are further complicated by the use of radiolabeled probes. Good correlation exists between DNA hybridization and PRA results.

Other methods. Other culture-based methods have been used to determine antiviral susceptibilities of CMV isolates. The principle is the same as in PRAs, but viral production is measured by using immunofluorescence, immunoperoxidase, EIA, or flow cytometry methodologies for detection and quantitation of cells expressing CMV antigens (immediate-early, early, or late).[56-60] Dose inhibition curves are then constructed to determine IC_{50} values of the isolates studied. These assays are also laborious and have the same limitations as PRAs.

To reduce turnaround time in identifying antiviral-resistant CMV isolates, efforts have been made to develop rapid screening assays, as well as methods that can be applied to determine susceptibilities directly in clinical specimens or in primary cultures. A modified PRA has been used for susceptibility testing of CMV isolates directly in primary cultures of clinical speci-

mens after a single replication cycle of the virus. This method provided susceptibility results in 5 days, clearly differentiated between susceptible and resistant CMV isolates, and compared favorably with conventional PRA.[61] In another study, blood leukocytes from patients with documented CMV viremia were used as inoculum in a modified PRA.[62] This method provided results within 4 to 6 days and reliably detected ganciclovir-resistant and foscarnet-resistant CMV isolates. The level of CMV viremia in patients, however, is often too low to allow this assay to be applied.

Additional studies are needed to evaluate the applicability and reproducibility of these rapid phenotypic assays across different laboratories.

Diagnostic considerations. Results of CMV susceptibility studies are difficult to interpret because of the variety of phenotypic assays used in different studies and the different criteria applied to define CMV resistance. Despite these limitations, a ganciclovir IC_{50} of greater than 12 µM, a foscarnet IC_{50} above 400 µM, and a cidofovir IC_{50} above 2 µM have been proposed as the cutoff values that define resistance of CMV to these compounds.[63, 64] More recently, a more accurate cutoff of greater than 4 µM has been set to define resistance to cidofovir.[65] CMV strains with a ganciclovir IC_{50} between 6 and 12 µM are considered "intermediate" phenotypes and have decreased susceptibility to ganciclovir.

Antiviral susceptibility testing of CMV isolates must be standardized, and consensus methodologies should be used. Table 18–5 summarizes published IC_{50} values

Table 18.5   Antiviral Susceptibilities (in µM) of Reference CMV Strains

Method	Ganciclovir IC_{50} AD169*	759rD100†	Foscarnet IC_{50} AD169	759rD100	Cidofovir IC_{50} AD169	759rD100	Reference
PRA	3.1	—	—	—	—	—	70
PRA	1	12	150	150	—	—	69
PRA	4.9	35	64	24	0.6	—	72
PRA	4	—	210	—	0.54	—	73
PRA	10	—	250	—	1	—	67
PRA	5.3	58.9‡	—	—	—	—	61
PRA	2.5	55	—	—	—	—	68
PRA	10	—	200	—	0.5	—	66
PRA	—	—	—	—	0.6	—	74
DNA	1.7	39	50	35	0.49	1.5	72
DNA	0.7	19	—	—	—	—	71
Dot blot	2.6	—	110	—	—	—	73
LARA	6.5	31.6‡	—	—	—	—	61
EIA	5.4	—	150	—	—	—	57
EIA	6.25	—	210	—	1	—	67

IC_{50}, 50% inhibitory concentration; *PRA*, plaque reduction assay; *DNA*, DNA hybridization assay; *LARA*, late antigen reduction assay; *EIA*, enzyme immunoassay.
*Susceptible CMV strain that contains UL97 and DNA polymerase wild-type sequences.
†Ganciclovir-resistant CMV strain that contains a UL97 deletion and a DNA polymerase mutation.
‡Ganciclovir-resistant strain RCL1 was used.

obtained for well-characterized reference CMV strains in different laboratories using a variety of phenotypic assays.[57, 61, 66-74] These results indicate that significant variability exists among methods and laboratories. To reduce this variability and to reach a consensus on the definition of drug resistance in CMV, the AIDS Clinical Trials Group (ACTG) has evaluated a consensus PRA by testing a panel of well-characterized clinical and laboratory CMV strains in 13 U.S. laboratories. Results indicate that susceptible and resistant CMV isolates *can* be readily distinguished by the consensus assay.[63]

Genotypic Assays

The recognition that specific mutations in the UL97 and DNA polymerase genes of CMV are associated with resistance to antiviral compounds has led to the development of genotypic methods for detection of mutant CMV isolates. Screening assays have been developed to take advantage of the strong clustering of mutations at specific UL97 codons in ganciclovir-resistant CMV isolates. These assays are based on *restriction enzyme analysis* of selected polymerase chain reaction (PCR) products amplified from CMV-infected cell cultures.[36]

Mutations at codons 460 and 594 result in the loss of naturally occurring restriction enzyme sites, whereas mutations at codons 520 and 595 create additional restriction sites. The presence of mutations is determined by distinctive restriction patterns visualized by gel electrophoresis (Table 18–6 and Figure 18–8). This screening method can detect mutants when they reach 10% of the viral population in a clinical isolate, and in one study it identified 78% of the isolates resistant to ganciclovir in phenotypic assays.[37]

A major advantage of restriction digest analysis is that provisional susceptibility information can be obtained in less than 2 days and it can be applied directly to clinical samples, including blood leukocytes, plasma, cerebrospinal fluid, and aqueous humor. A disadvantage is that this method may not detect specific mutations involving base changes if they do not change the restriction enzyme pattern. In addition, it will "miss" ganciclovir-resistant CMV isolates containing DNA polymerase mutations with wild-type UL97 sequences.[40] Therefore, although a positive result is virtually diagnostic of ganciclovir resistance, a negative result does not necessarily indicate that a virus is susceptible.

DNA polymerase mutations are detected by sequencing the relevant portions of the polymerase gene. This procedure is currently performed only in a few research laboratories. Analysis of PCR fragments has been used in the detection of the ganciclovir resistance mutation L501F and the ganciclovir/foscarnet resistance mutation A809V in the DNA polymerase region of clinical CMV isolates.[39, 43]

Studies combining both genotypic and phenotypic assays to characterize selected CMV strains are crucial to further the understanding of CMV resistance. Specifically, phenotypic assays are important (1) to detect resistant viruses from patients treated with new antiviral compounds, (2) to define cross-resistance patterns, and (3) to determine the importance of individual mutations in the CMV genome by assessing their effect on the phenotype of mutant viruses. Identification of mutations conferring high level of resistance to antiviral agents (in phenotypic assays) would help in the design of rapid assays targeted to detect highly-resistant CMV isolates.

HUMAN IMMUNODEFICIENCY VIRUS

Antiviral Resistance

Antiretroviral agents currently available for the treatment of human immunodeficiency virus (HIV) infection include inhibitors of the viral *reverse transcriptase* (RT) and inhibitors of the viral *protease*.[75, 76]

RT inhibitors include nucleoside analogs and nonnucleoside compounds (Table 18–7). Nucleoside RT inhibitors require intracellular activation to their tri-

Table 18.6 Restriction Digest Screening for UL97 Mutations Related to Ganciclovir Resistance

Enzyme	UL97 codon	Fragments (base pairs)*	
		Wild-type sequence	Mutant sequence
Nla III	460	198, 168, 126, 9	324, 168, 9
Alu I	520	295, 189, 17	268, 189, 27, 17
Hha I	594	50, 38, 18, 12	62, 38, 18
Mse I	595	76, 42	46, 42, 30
Taq I	595	99, 19	71, 28, 19

*Fragments underlined are normally seen in polyacrylamide gels after ethidium bromide staining.

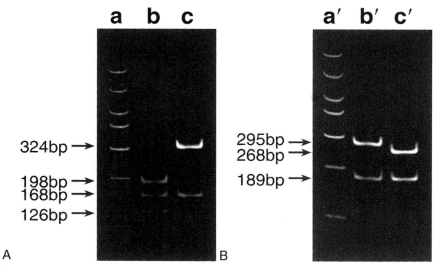

Figure 18.8   Diagnosis of cytomegalovirus (CMV) UL97 mutations by restriction endonuclease analysis. Lanes show digests of UL97 polymerase chain reaction (PCR) amplification products after electrophoresis and ethidium bromide staining. Digestion of V460 mutants with *Nla* III results in fragments with sizes of 324, 168, and 9 base pairs (*bp*). Digestion of Q520 mutants with *Alu* I results in fragments with sizes of 268, 189, 27, and 17 bp. **A,** Lane *a*, 100-bp ladder; lane *b*, laboratory strain AD169 (wild type); lane *c*, clinical isolate with V460 mutation. **B,** Lane *a′*, 100-bp ladder; lane *b′*, laboratory strain AD169 (wild type); lane *c′*, clinical isolate with Q520 mutation. (Data courtesy Wuyi Li, University of Minnesota.)

phosphate (nucleotide) derivatives to exert their anti-HIV activity. This intracellular activation is mediated by cellular enzymes and not by viral-encoded kinases. The nucleotide derivatives then act as competitive substrates and faulty substrates for the HIV RT. This results in inhibition of viral RT and premature termination of elongation of unintegrated proviral HIV DNA.[76] Nonnucleoside RT inhibitors are structurally diverse but have similar mechanism of actions. They do not require intracellular activation to exert their antiviral activity. The binding of nonnucleoside inhibitors to HIV reverse RT-unintegrated proviral HIV DNA complex causes a spatial distortion of the RT's active site. This results in the inefficient incorporation of nucleotides to the elongating proviral DNA chain.[76]

Protease inhibitors do not require intracellular activation to exert their antiviral activity. These compounds bind to the active site of the HIV protease and inhibit its activity. This inhibition prevents the cleavage of polypeptide precursors into the individual proteins of mature infectious virions and results in the release of immature and noninfectious viral particles.[76]

Resistance of clinical HIV isolates to approved therapeutic agents has been recognized since shortly after the initial trials with antiretroviral drugs and is considered a major factor in therapeutic failure with HIV infection.[77, 78] Resistance of clinical HIV strains to RT inhibitors has been associated with specific mutations in the RT coding region of the virus (Table 18–8). The vast majority of the mutations have been found in samples from HIV-infected patients receiving monotherapy. Combination antiretroviral therapy may select for HIV strains containing complex mutational patterns that differ from those selected during monotherapy and may cause broad cross-resistance to all nucleoside RT inhibitors.[79, 80]

The association of the RT mutations with antiretroviral resistance has been confirmed by site-directed mutagenesis studies. Constructed infectious molecular clones of HIV acquire resistance to a specific compound after the introduction of specific mutations into their

Table 18.7	Anti-HIV Compounds
Reverse transcriptase inhibitors	**Protease inhibitors**
Nucleoside analogs	Indinavir
Zidovudine (ZDV, AZT)	Ritonavir
Didanosine (ddI)	Saquinavir
Zalcitabine (ddC)	Nelfinavir
Lamivudine (3TC)	Amprenavir
Stavudine (d4T)	
Abacavir	
Nonnucleoside inhibitors	
Nevirapine	
Delaviridine	
Efavirenz	

Table 18.8   Mutations in HIV Reverse Transcriptase Coding Region Conferring Antiretroviral Resistance

Antiviral	Mutation	Amino acid change
Zidovudine	M41L	Methionine to leucine
	D67N	Aspartic acid to asparagine
	K70R	Lysine to arginine
	L210W	Leucine to tryptophan
	T215Y	Threonine to tyrosine
	T215F	Threonine to phenylalanine
	K219Q	Lysine to glutamine
Didanosine	K65R	Lysine to arginine
	L74V	Leucine to valine
	M184V	Methionine to valine
Zalcitabine	K65R	Lysine to arginine
	T69D	Threonine to aspartic acid
	L74V	Leucine to valine
Lamivudine	M184V	Methionine to valine
Stavudine	V75T/M/S/A	Valine to threonine/methionine/serine/alanine
	T69D/N	Threonine to aspartic acid/asparagine
Abacavir	K65R	Lysine to arginine
	L74V	Leucine to valine
	M184V	Methionine to valine
Multinucleoside resistance	A62V	Alanine to valine
	V75I	Valine to isoleucine
	F77L	Phenylalanine to leucine
	F116Y	Phenylalanine to tyrosine
	Q151M	Glutamine to methionine
	T69S-X-X	Insertion of 2 amino acids
Nevirapine	K103N	Lysine to asparagine
	V106A	Valine to alanine
	V108I	Valine to isoleucine
	Y181C	Tyrosine to cysteine
	Y181I	Tyrosine to isoleucine
	Y188C	Tyrosine to cysteine
	G190A	Glycine to alanine
Delaviridine	K103N	Lysine to asparagine
	Y181C	Tyrosine to cysteine
	Y181I	Tyrosine to isoleucine
Efavirenz	L100I	Leucine to isoleucine
	K103N	Lysine to asparagine
	V108I	Valine to isoleucine
	Y188L	Tyrosine to leucine
	G190S	Glycine to serine

Modified from Hertogs K, DeButhune MP, Miller V, et al: *Antimicrob Agents Chemother* 42:269, 1998.

RT gene. Interestingly, the effect of RT gene mutations associated with antiretroviral resistance on the function of viral RT is variable. For example, the affinity of the RT of zidovudine-resistant viruses for zidovudine tri- phosphate (the metabolite of zidovudine with anti-HIV activity) is similar to that of the RT of zidovudine-sensitive viruses. In contrast, the affinity of RT of viruses resistant to stavudine is reduced compared with that of wild-type viruses susceptible to this agent. This suggests that the molecular mechanism of HIV resistance to different nucleoside RT inhibitors may vary.

Similarly, resistance of clinical HIV strains to prote-ase inhibitors has been associated with specific mutations in the protease coding region of the virus (Table 18–9).[76, 81, 82] Most HIV strains resistant to the protease inhibitors contain several mutations.

Table 18.9   Mutations in HIV Protease Coding Region Conferring Antiretroviral Resistance

Antiviral	Mutation	Amino acid change
Indinavir	L10I/R/V	Leucine to isoleucine/arginine/valine
	K20M/R	Lysine to methionine/arginine
	L24I/V	Leucine to isoleucine/valine
	V32I	Valine to isoleucine
	M46I/L	Methionine to isoleucine/leucine
	I54V	Isoleucine to valine
	L63P	Leucine to proline
	A71V/T	Alanine to valine/threonine
	G73S	Glycine to serine
	V82A/F/T	Valine to alanine/phenylalanine/threonine
	I84V	Isoleucine to valine
	L90M	Leucine to methionine
Ritonavir	K20M/R	Lysine to methionine/arginine
	V32I	Valine to isoleucine
	L33F	Leucine to phenylalanine
	M36I	Methionine to isoleucine
	M46I/L	Methionine to isoleucine/leucine
	I54V/L	Isoleucine to valine/leucine
	L63P	Leucine to proline
	A71V/T	Alanine to valine/threonine
	V82A/F/T	Valine to alanine/phenylalanine/threonine
	I84V	Isoleucine to valine/leucine
	L90M	Leucine to methionine
Saquinavir	L10I/R/V	Leucine to isoleucine/arginine/valine
	G48V	Glycine to valine
	I54V/L	Isoleucine to valine/leucine
	L63P	Leucine to proline
	A71V/T	Alanine to valine/threonine
	G73S	Glycine to serine
	V82A/F/T	Valine to alanine/phenylalanine/threonine
	I84V	Isoleucine to valine
	L90M	Leucine to methionine
Nelfinavir	D30N	Aspartic acid to asparagine
	M36I	Methionine to isoleucine
	M46I/L	Methionine to isoleucine/leucine
	L63P	Leucine to proline
	A71V/T	Alanine to valine/threonine
	V77I	Valine to isoleucine
	I84V	Isoleucine to valine
	N88D	Asparagine to aspartic acid
	L90M	Leucine to methionine
Amprenavir	L10I/R/V	Leucine to isoleucine/arginine/valine
	M46I/L	Methionine to isoleucine/leucine
	I47V	Isoleucine to valine
	I50V	Isoleucine to valine

Phenotypic Assays

Phenotypic assays define whether a particular strain of HIV is sensitive or resistant to an antiretroviral agent by determining its IC_{50}.

Plaque reduction. The PRA was used in early studies of HIV resistance to zidovudine and is based on the inhibition of plaque formation in monolayers of HeLa CD4 cells infected with cell-free HIV.[83, 84] The HeLa CD4 cell line was constructed by transfecting the gene encoding CD4 into HeLa cells so that those cells would express the CD4 antigen on their surface, thereby making the cells susceptible to infection with HIV.

A standardized inoculum of virus is used to infect HeLa CD4 cells in tissue culture plates. After adsorption of the virus, culture medium containing different concentrations of the antiretroviral drug being tested is added to the cultures. After a 3-day incubation period, cells are fixed and stained for the visualization of plaques consisting of foci of multinucleated giant cells. IC_{50} values are determined from plots of the percentage of plaque reduction versus the concentration of antiretroviral agent. Although inexpensive and reproducible, PRA can be used only for HIV isolates exhibiting a syncytium-inducing (SI) phenotype, since only these isolates replicate in HeLa CD4 cells.[83, 84]

Peripheral blood mononuclear cell-(PBMC)-based assays. Susceptibility assays that employ peripheral blood mononuclear cells (PBMCs) permit evaluation of most clinical HIV isolates. A variety of PBMC-based assays have been used in different laboratories. A standardized method for zidovudine susceptibilities using PBMC was developed and validated by laboratories of the ACTG and the U.S. Department of Defense.[85] This is considered the reference method for testing zidovudine susceptibility of clinical HIV strains and has been used to evaluate resistance to this compound in prospective and retrospective studies. It measures the degree of drug inhibition on HIV antigen production in PBMCs after acute infection with a viral isolate.

In this assay, stocks of clinical HIV strains are prepared in co-cultures of patients' PBMCs and phytohemagglutinin-stimulated PBMCs from healthy, HIV-seronegative donors. Titers of these viral stocks are determined by cell dilution cultures (using phytohemagglutinin-stimulated donor PBMCs), and a standardized inoculum of virus is used to infect PBMCs, which are then placed in tissue culture plates and incubated in culture medium containing no drug or different concentrations of zidovudine. Each concentration of zidovudine is tested in triplicate. After a 7-day incubation period, HIV p24 antigen concentrations in cell-free culture supernatant fluids are measured to determine the concentration of zidovudine causing a 50% reduction in HIV p24 antigen concentration relative to the value of controls (IC_{50}). A simplified version of this assay using fewer concentrations of zidovudine and fewer replicates has been standardized among ACTG laboratories.[86]

IC_{50} values defining resistance to zidovudine have been well established by using the consensus ACTG–Department of Defense assay. HIV isolates with IC_{50} values of 0.1 μM or less are considered sensitive to zidovudine, those with IC_{50} values of between 0.1 and 1.0 μM are considered intermediate, and those with IC_{50} values of 1.0 μM or greater are considered resistant to zidovudine.[85] The applicability of this method to determine susceptibilities of HIV isolates to other RT inhibitors and to protease inhibitors requires further studies.

At present, no consensus IC_{50} cutoff values define resistance of clinical HIV isolates to antiretroviral agents other than zidovudine. Phenotypic susceptibility testing remains cumbersome and expensive and is generally performed only by a few highly specialized laboratories.

Genotypic Assays

Genotypic assays determine whether mutations associated with antiretroviral resistance are present in the RT or protease coding regions of HIV. Shortly after the description of the first HIV isolates resistant to zidovudine, a variety of molecular methods were developed with the purpose of revealing mutations associated with resistance to this compound. A common set of mutations in the RT region of HIV are associated with resistance to zidovudine (see Table 18–8), which prompted the development of selective PCR assays for rapid detection of mutant isolates.[87]

In selective PCR assays, a fragment of the HIV RT region (encompassing the regions containing the most mutations associated with resistance to zidovudine) is amplified using PCR performed on cellular DNA from PBMCs obtained directly from the patient, from infected PBMCs in culture, or from cell-free virus circulating in plasma or serum fractions from infected patients. The amplified product is then used in a second PCR reaction employing primer pairs that bind differently to wild-type or mutant sequences at the codons of interest. The product of this second PCR reaction is detected after gel electrophoresis and ethidium bromide staining. For each codon analyzed, the presence of wild-type sequences is indicated by the generation of a PCR product only with the set of wild-type primers or when the band with the highest intensity is obtained with wild-type primers. Conversely, an isolate is considered to contain mutant sequences when a PCR product is generated only with the set of mutant primers or when the band with the highest intensity is obtained with mutant primers. Samples are considered to contain a mixture of wild-type and mutant viruses when two bands of similar intensity are obtained with wild-type and mutant primers.

A major limitation of the selective PCR method is that it provides limited information concerning the genotype of HIV strains from antiretroviral-treated patients. A similar targeted genotypic method based on the hybridization of HIV PCR products to oligonucleotide probes immobilized in lines on a paper strip (line probe assay, or LIPA) is now commercially available.[88]

The finding of a large variety of mutations in the RT and protease regions of HIV isolates from patients treated with multiple antiretrovirals over time, coupled with the complexity of mutations conferring resistance to protease inhibitors, has prompted the use of laboratory methods that provide complete sequence information of these regions of the HIV genome. Manual and automated sequencing methodologies are now typically used to analyze HIV RT and protease sequences amplified directly from plasma and other clinical samples. Application of these methodologies is being incorporated rapidly into the standard of care of HIV-infected patients.

Recombinant Virus Assays

Phenotypic assays based on recombinant DNA technology have been recently developed and are commercially available.[89, 90] In these assays, total ribonucleic acid (RNA) is extracted from plasma. After reverse transcription to generate complementary DNA, HIV RT and protease sequences are amplified by PCR. Amplified products are inserted into an HIV vector that is then used in drug susceptibility assays. An advantage of these assays is that they use uncultured plasma, obviating the need to grow HIV from PBMCs. Because the recombinant virus contains the same RT and protease sequences as the virus circulating in plasma, results of recombinant virus assays truly represent a patient's HIV susceptibility to antiviral agents.

Clinical Applications

Although HIV resistance assays require validation, standardization, and a better defined clinical role, phenotypic and genotypic testing for HIV resistance to antiretroviral drugs may prove useful in patient management.[91] Whereas testing for drug resistance before the start of antiretroviral therapy in untreated patients is not recommended at present, it should be considered in the design of initial antiretroviral regimens if an increased prevalence of resistance is seen in a particular population. Accumulating evidence suggests that phenotypic or genotypic resistance at baseline predicts a poor virologic response to treatment. Thus resistance testing will likely be useful for identifying antiretroviral

agents that might not be effective in treatment regimens.[91] Preliminary studies suggest that the use of genotypic resistance assays to design therapeutic alternatives in patients failing combination therapy is associated with short term virologic benefit.[91a] Additional studies are urgently needed to define the clinical applications and provide guidelines for interpreting the results of the widely used phenotypic and genotypic assays for HIV resistance.

RESPIRATORY VIRUSES

Antiviral drugs clinically available for the treatment of viral respiratory infections include amantadine and rimantadine for the treatment and prophylaxis of *influenza A* infections and ribavirin for the treatment of *respiratory syncytial virus* (RSV) infections. *Amantadine* and *rimantadine* inhibit the replication of influenza A by interfering with the function of the hydrophobic transmembrane protein M2. The M2 protein facilitates viral uncoating during the early steps in the replication cycle of the influenza virus.

The mechanism of action of *ribavirin* is complex and multifactorial. Ribavirin is triphosphorylated by cellular enzymes. Ribavirin triphosphate inhibits viral RNA polymerase activity and interferes with capping and elongation of messenger RNA.

Resistant influenza A strains may appear among patients treated with amantadine and their close contacts, indicating that amantadine-resistant viruses can be associated with failure of prophylaxis and can be transmitted to contacts.[92, 93] Amantadine-resistant influenza strains are cross-resistant to rimantadine. Amantadine-resistant and rimantadine-resistant influenza isolates remain susceptible to ribavirin. Ribavirin-resistant influenza or RSV isolates have not been isolated from patients treated with these compounds. Resistance of influenza isolates to amantadine or rimantadine is associated with single amino acid substitutions at one of four positions (26, 27, 30, or 31) in the M2 protein.[94, 95]

Laboratory methods to determine susceptibilities of influenza isolates include PRAs and EIA-based methods.[96, 97] A rapid genotypic assay based on amplification of M2 sequences followed by restriction enzyme analysis has been developed and may be used for detection of resistant viruses directly in clinical materials.[98] These assays are currently available only in a few research laboratories.

References

1. Balfour HH: Acyclovir. In Peterson PK, Verhoef J, editors: *Antimicrobial agents annual,* ed 3, New York, 1988, Elsevier Science.

2. Crumpacker CS, Schnipper LE, Chartrand P, Knopf KW: Genetic mechanisms of resistance to acyclovir in herpes simplex virus, *Am J Med* (Acyclovir Symposium): 361, 1982.

3. Chatis PA, Crumpacker CS: Resistance of herpesviruses to antiviral drugs, *Antimicrob Agents Chemother* 36:1589, 1992.

4. Earnshaw DL, Bacon TH, Darlinson SJ, et al: Mode of antiviral action of penciclovir in MRC-5 cells infected with herpes simplex virus type 1 (HSV-1), HSV-2, and varicella-zoster virus, *Antimicrob Agents Chemother* 36:2747, 1992.

5. Safrin S, Phan L: In vitro activity of penciclovir against clinical isolates of acyclovir-resistant and foscarnet-resistant herpes simplex virus, *Antimicrob Agents Chemother* 37:2241, 1993.

6. Field AK, Biron KK: "The end of innocence" revisited: resistance of herpesviruses to antiviral drugs, *Clin Microbiol Rev* 7:1, 1994.

7. Gaudreau A, Hill E, Balfour HH, et al: Phenotypic and genotypic characterization of acyclovir-resistant herpes simplex viruses from immunocompromised patients, *J Infect Dis* 178:297, 1998.

8. Biron KK: Cytomegalovirus: genetics of drug resistance. In Mills J, editor: *Antiviral chemotherapy,* ed 4, New York, 1996, Plenum.

9. Boyd MR, Safrin S, Kern ER: Penciclovir: a review of its spectrum of activity, selectivity, and cross-resistance pattern, *Antiviral Chem Chemother* Suppl 1:S3, 1993.

10. McLaren C, Sibrack CD, Barry DW: Spectrum of sensitivity to acyclovir of herpes simplex virus clinical isolates, *Am J Med* (Acyclovir Symposium):376, 1982.

11. McLaren C, Ellis MN, Hunter GA: A colorimetric assay for the measurement of the sensitivity of herpes simplex viruses to antiviral agents, *Antiviral Res* 3:223, 1983.

12. Rabalais GP, Levin MJ, Berkowitz FE: Rapid herpes simplex virus susceptibility testing using an enzyme-linked immunosorbent assay performed in situ on fixed virus-infected monolayers, *Antimicrob Agents Chemother* 31:946, 1987.

13. Swierkosz EM, Scholl DR, Brown JL, et al: Improved DNA hybridization method for detection of acyclovir-resistant herpes simplex virus, *Antimicrob Agents Chemother* 31:1465, 1987.

14. Kimberlin DW, Spector SA, Hill EL, et al: Assays for antiviral drug resistance, *Antiviral Res* 26:403, 1995.

15. Tebas P, Stabell ES, Olivo PD: Antiviral susceptibility testing with a cell line that expresses ß-galactosidase after infection with herpes simplex virus, *Antimicrob Agents Chemother* 39:1287, 1995.

16. Tebas P, Scholl D, Jollick J, et al: A rapid assay to screen for drug-resistant herpes simplex virus, *J Infect Dis* 177:217, 1998.

17. Dekker C, Ellis MN, McLaren C, et al: Virus resistance in clinical practice, *J Antimicrob Chemother* 15(suppl B):137, 1983.

18. Safrin S, Crumpacker CS, Chatis P, et al: A controlled trial comparing foscarnet with vidarabine for acyclovir-resistant mucocutaneous herpes simplex in the acquired immunodeficiency syndrome, *N Engl J Med* 325:551, 1991.

19. Safrin S, Kemmerly S, Plotkin B, et al: Foscarnet-resistant herpes simplex virus infection in patients with AIDS, *J Infect Dis* 169:193, 1994.

20. Barry DW, Nusinoff-Lehrman S, Ellis MN, et al: Viral resistance, clinical experience, *Scand J Infect Dis suppl* 47:S155, 1985.

21. Englund JA, Zimmerman ME, Swierkosz EM, et al: Herpes simplex virus resistant to acyclovir, *Ann Intern Med* 112:416, 1990.

22. Boivin G, Erice A, Crane DD, et al: Acyclovir susceptibilities of herpes simplex virus strains isolated from solid organ transplant recipients after acyclovir or ganciclovir prophylaxis, *Antimicrob Agents Chemother* 37:357, 1993.

23. Safrin S, Assaykeen T, Follansbee S, Mills J: Foscarnet therapy for acyclovir-resistant mucocutaneous herpes simplex virus infection in 26 AIDS patients: preliminary data, *J Infect Dis* 161:1078, 1990.

24. Talarico CL, Phelps WC, Biron KK: Analysis of the thymidine kinase genes from acyclovir-resistant mutants of varicella-zoster virus isolated from patients with AIDS, *J Virol* 67:1024, 1993.

25. Boivin G, Edelman CK, Pedneault L, et al: Phenotypic and genotypic characterization of acyclovir-resistant varicella-zoster viruses isolated from persons with AIDS, *J Infect Dis* 170:68, 1994.

26. Berkowitz FE, Levin MJ: Use of an enzyme-linked immunosorbent assay performed directly on fixed infected cell monolayers for evaluating drugs against varicella-zoster virus, *Antimicrob Agents Chemother* 28:207, 1985.

27. Swierkosz EM, Hodinka RL: Antiviral agents and susceptibility test. In Murray PR, et al, editors: *Manual of clinical microbiology,* ed 7, Washington DC, 1999, ASM Press.

28. Jacobson MA, Berger TG, Fikrig S, et al: Acyclovir-resistant varicella zoster virus infection after chronic oral acyclovir therapy in patients with the acquired immunodeficiency syndrome, *Ann Intern Med* 112:187, 1990.

29. Crumpacker CS: Ganciclovir, *N Eng J Med* 335:721, 1996.

30. Chrisp P, Clissold SP: Foscarnet: a review of its antiviral activity, pharmacokinetic properties, and therapeutic use in immuncompromised patients with CMV retinitis, *Drugs* 41:104, 1991.

31. Lalezari JP, Drew WL, Glutzer E, et al: (S)-1-[3-hydroxy-2-(phosphonyl-methoxy)propyl]cytosine (cidofovir): results of a phase I/II study of a novel nucleotide analogue, *J Infect Dis* 171:788, 1995.

32. Alain S, Honderlick P, Grenet D, et al: Failure of ganciclovir treatment associated with selection of a ganciclovir-resistant cytomegalovirus strain in a lung transplant recipient, *Transplantation* 63:1533, 1997.

33. Baldanti F, Silini E, Sarasini A, et al: A three-nucleotide deletion in the UL97 open reading frame is responsible for the ganciclovir resistance of a human cytomegalovirus clinical isolate, *J Virol* 69:796, 1995.

34. Baldanti F, Underwood MR, Stanat SC, et al: Single amino acid changes in the DNA polymerase confer foscarnet resistance and slow-growth phenotype, while mutations in the UL97-encoded phosphotransferase

confer ganciclovir resistance in three double-resistant human cytomegalovirus strains recovered from patients with AIDS, *J Virol* 70:1390, 1996.

35. Baldanti F, Underwood MR, Talarico CL, et al: The Cys607Tyr change in the UL97 phosphotransferase confers ganciclovir resistance to two human cytomegalovirus strains recovered from two immunocompromised individuals, *Antimicrob Agents Chemother* 42:444, 1998.

36. Chou S, Erice A, Jordan MC, et al: Analysis of the UL97 phosphotransferase coding sequence in clinical cytomegalovirus isolates and identification of mutations conferring ganciclovir resistance, *J Infect Dis* 171:576, 1995.

37. Chou S, Guentzel S, Michels KR, et al: Frequency of UL97 phosphotransferase mutations related to ganciclovir resistance in clinical cytomegalovirus isolates, *J Infect Dis* 172:239, 1995.

38. Chou S, Marousek G, Guentzel S, et al: Evolution of mutations conferring multidrug resistance during prophylaxis and therapy for cytomegalovirus disease, *J Infect Dis* 176:786, 1997.

39. Chou S, Marousek G, Parenti DM, et al: Mutation in region II of the DNA polymerase gene conferring foscarnet resistance in cytomegalovirus isolates from 3 subjects receiving prolonged antiviral therapy, *J Infect Dis* 178:526, 1998.

40. Erice A, Gil-Roda C, Pérez J, et al: Antiviral susceptibilities and analysis of UL97 and DNA polymerase sequences of clinical cytomegalovirus isolates from immunocompromised patients, *J Infect Dis* 175:1087, 1997.

41. Erice A, Borrell N, Li W, et al: Ganciclovir susceptibilities and analysis of UL97 region in cytomegalovirus isolates from bone marrow recipients with CMV disease after antiviral prophylaxis, *J Infect Dis* 178:531, 1998.

42. Hanson MN, Preheim LC, Chou S, et al: Novel mutation in the UL97 gene of a clinical cytomegalovirus strain conferring resistance to ganciclovir, *Antimicrob Agents Chemother* 39:1204, 1995.

43. Harada K, Eizuru Y, Isashiki Y, et al: Genetic analysis of a clinical isolate of human cytomegalovirus exhibiting resistance against both ganciclovir and cidofovir, *Arch Virol* 142:215, 1997.

44. Lurain NS, Ammons HC, Kapell KS, et al: Molecular analysis of human cytomegalovirus strains from two lung transplant recipients with the same donor, *Transplantation* 62:497, 1996.

45. Smith IL, Shinkai M, Freeman WR, et al: Polyradiculopathy associated with ganciclovir-resistant cytomegalovirus in an AIDS patient: phenotypic and genotypic characterization of sequential virus isolates, *J Infect Dis* 173:1481, 1996.

46. Smith IL, Cherrington JM, Jiles RE, et al: High-level resistance of cytomegalovirus to ganciclovir is associated with alterations in both the UL97 and DNA polymerase genes, *J Infect Dis* 176:69, 1997.

47. Smith IL, Taskintuna I, Rahhal FM, et al: Clinical failure of CMV retinitis with intravitreal cidofovir is associated with antiviral resistance, *Arch Ophthalmol* 116:178, 1998.

48. Smith IL, Hong C, Pilcher ML, et al: Development of resistant cytomegalovirus genotypes during oral ganciclovir prophylaxis/preemptive therapy. Presented at the 38th Interscience Conference on Antimicrobial Agents and Chemotherapy, San Diego, September 1998.

49. Wolf DG, Smith IL, Lee DJ, et al: Mutations in human cytomegalovirus UL97 gene confer clinical resistance to ganciclovir and can be detected directly in patient plasma, *J Clin Invest* 95:257, 1995.

50. Wolf DG, Lee DJ, Spector SA, et al: Detection of human cytomegalovirus mutations associated with ganciclovir resistance in cerebrospinal fluid of AIDS patients with central nervous system disease, *Antimicrob Agents Chemother* 39:2552, 1995.

51. Wolf DG, Yaniv I, Honigman A, et al: Early emergence of ganciclovir-resistant human cytomegalovirus strains in children with primary combined immunodeficiency, *J Infect Dis* 178:535, 1998.

52. Lurain NS, Thompson KD, Holmes EW, et al: Point mutations in the DNA polymerase gene of human cytomegalovirus that result in resistance to antiviral agents, *J Virol* 66:7146, 1992.

53. Sullivan V, Biron KK, Talarico CL, et al: A point mutation in the human cytomegalovirus DNA polymerase gene confers resistance to ganciclovir and phosphonylmethoxyalkyl derivatives, *Antimicrob Agents Chemother* 37:19, 1993.

54. Cihlar T, Fuller MD, Cherrington JM: Characterization of drug resistance-associated mutations in the human cytomegalovirus DNA polymerase gene by using recombinant mutant viruses generated from overlapping DNA fragments, *J Virol* 72:5927, 1998.

55. Dankner WM, Scholl D, Stanat SC, et al: Rapid antiviral DNA–DNA hybridization assay for human cytomegalovirus, *J Virol Methods* 28:293, 1990.

56. Telenti A, Smith TF: Screening with a shell vial assay for antiviral activity against cytomegalovirus, *Diagn Microbiol Infect Dis* 12:5, 1989.

57. Tatarowicz WA, Lurain NS, Thompson KD: In situ ELISA for the evaluation of antiviral compounds effective against human cytomegalovirus, *J Virol Methods* 35:207, 1991.

58. Gerna G, Baldanti F, Zavattoni M, et al: Monitoring of ganciclovir sensitivity of multiple human cytomegalovirus strains coinfecting blood of an AIDS patient by an immediate-early antigen plaque assay, *Antiviral Res* 19:333, 1992.

59. Weinberg A, Schneider SA, Bate BJ, Clark JC: Antigen reduction assay for cytomegalovirus susceptibility to antivirals. Presented at the 34th Interscience Conference on Antimicrobial Agents and Chemotherapy, Orlando Fla, October 1994.

60. McSharry JM, Lurain NS, Drusano GL, et al: Flow cytometry determination of ganciclovir susceptibilities of human cytomegalovirus isolates, *J Clin Microbiol* 36:958, 1998.

61. Pepin JM, Simon F, Dussault A, et al: Rapid determination of human cytomegalovirus susceptibility to ganciclovir directly from clinical specimen primocultures, *J Clin Microbiol* 30:2917, 1992.

62. Gerna G, Sarasini A, Percivalle E, et al: Rapid screen-

ing for resistance to ganciclovir and foscarnet of primary isolates of human cytomegalovirus from culture-positive blood samples, *J Clin Microbiol* 33:738, 1995.

63. Crumpacker C: Drug resistance in cytomegalovirus: current knowledge and implications for patient management, *J Acquir Immune Defic Syndr* 12(suppl):S1, 1996.

64. Drew WL, Miner R, Saleh E: Antiviral susceptibility testing of cytomegalovirus: criteria for detecting resistance to antivirals, *Clin Diagn Virol* 1:179, 1993.

65. Cherrington JM, Fuller MD, Lamy PD, et al: In vitro antiviral susceptibilities of isolates from CMV retinitis patients receiving first or second line cidofovir therapy: relationship to clinical outcome, *J Infect Dis* 178:1821, 1998.

66. Lurain NS, Spafford LE, Thompson KD: Mutation in the UL97 open reading frame of human cytomegalovirus strains resistant to ganciclovir, *J Virol* 68:4427, 1994.

67. Lurain NS, Thompson KD, Holmes EW, Read GS: Point mutations in the DNA polymerase gene of human cytomegalovirus that result in resistance to antiviral agents, *J Virol* 66:7146, 1992.

68. Sullivan V, Biron KK, Talarico C, et al: A point mutation in the human cytomegalovirus DNA polymerase gene confers resistance to ganciclovir and phosphonylmethoxyalkyl derivatives, *Antimicrob Agents Chemother* 37:19, 1993.

69. Biron KK, Fyfe JA, Stanat SC, et al: A human cytomegalovirus mutant resistant to the nucleoside analog 9-{[2-hydroxy-1 (hydroxymethyl)ethoxy]methyl} guanine (BW B759U) induces reduced levels of BW B759U triphosphate, *Proc Natl Acad Sci USA* 83:8769, 1986.

70. Cole NL, Balfour HH Jr; In vitro susceptibility of cytomegalovirus isolates from immunocompromised patients to acyclovir and ganciclovir, *Diagn Microbiol Infect Dis* 6:255, 1987.

71. Boivin G, Erice A, Crane DD, et al: Ganciclovir susceptibilities of cytomegalovirus (CMV) isolates from solid organ transplant recipients with CMV viremia after antiviral prophylaxis, *J Infect Dis* 168:332, 1993.

72. Stanat SC, Reardon JE, Erice A, et al: Ganciclovir-resistant cytomegalovirus clinical isolates: mode of resistance to ganciclovir, *Antimicrob Agents Chemother* 35:2191, 1991.

73. Sullivan V, Coen DM: Isolation of foscarnet-resistant human cytomegalovirus patterns of resistance and sensitivity to other antiviral drugs, *J Infect Dis* 164:781, 1991.

74. Cherrington JM, Miner R, Hitchcock MJ, et al: Susceptibility of human cytomegalovirus to cidofovir is unchanged after limited in vivo exposure to various clinical regimens of drug, *J Infect Dis* 173:987, 1996.

75. Connolly JC, Hammer SM: Antiretroviral therapy: reverse transcriptase inhibition, *Antimicrob Agents Chemother* 36:245, 1992.

76. Hammer SM, Inouye RT: Antiviral agents. In Richman DD, Whitley RJ, Hayden FG, editors: *Clinical virology*, New York, 1997, Churchill Livingstone.

77. Richman DD: Resistance of clinical isolates of human immunodeficiency virus to antiretroviral agents, *Antimicrob Agents Chemother* 37:1207, 1993.

78. Erice A, Balfour HH: Resistance of human immunodeficiency virus type 1 to antiretroviral agents: a review, *Clin Infect Dis* 18:149, 1994.

79. Shafer RW, Kozal MJ, Winters MA, et al: Combination therapy with zidovudine and didanosine selects for drug-resistant human immunodeficiency virus type 1 strains with unique patterns of *pol* gene mutations, *J Infect Dis* 169:722, 1994.

80. Bloor S, Hertogs K, Desmet RL, et al: Virological basis for HIV-1 resistance to stavudine investigated by analysis of clinical samples, Presented at the Second International Workshop on HIV Drug Resistance & Treatment Strategies, Lake Maggore, Italy, June 1998.

81. Condra JH, Schleif WA, Blahy OM, et al: In vivo emergence of HIV-1 variants resistant to multiple protease inhibitors, *Nature* 374:569, 1995.

82. Condra JH, Holder DJ, Schleif WA, et al: Genetic correlates of in vivo viral resistance to indinavir, a human immunodeficiency virus type 1 protease inhibitor, *J Virol* 70:8270, 1996.

83. Chesebro B, Wehrly K: Development of a quantitative sensitive focal assay for human immunodeficiency virus infectivity, *J Virol* 62:3779, 1988.

84. Larder BA, Kemp SD: Multiple mutations in HIV-1 reverse transcriptase confer high-level resistance to zidovudine (AZT), *Science* 246:1155, 1989.

85. Japour AJ, Mayers DL, Johnson VA, et al: Standardized peripheral blood mononuclear cell culture assay for determination of drug susceptibilities of clinical human immunodeficiency virus type 1 isolates, *Antimicrob Agents Chemother* 37:1095, 1993.

86. Marschner IA, Mayers DL, Erice A, et al: Standardized peripheral blood mononuclear cell culture assay for determination of drug susceptibilities of clinical human immunodeficiency virus type 1 isolates: effect of reducing the number of replicates and concentrations, *J Clin Microbiol* 35:756, 1997.

87. Larder BA, Kellam P, Kemp SD: Zidovudine resistance predicted by direct detection of mutations in DNA from HIV-infected lymphocytes, *AIDS* 5:137, 1991.

88. Stuyver L, Wyseur A, Rombout A, et al: Line probe assay for rapid detection of drug-selected mutations in the human immunodeficiency virus type 1 reverse transcriptase gene, *Antimicrob Agents Chemother* 41:284, 1997.

89. Hertogs K, DeBethune MP, Miller V, et al: A rapid method for simultaneous detection of phenotypic resistance to inhibitors of protease and reverse transcriptase in recombinant human immunodeficiency virus type 1 isolates from patients treated with antiretroviral drugs, *Antimicrob Agents Chemother* 42:269, 1998.

90. Kellam P, Larder BA: Recombinant virus assay: a rapid phenotypic assay for assessment of drug susceptibility of human immunodeficiency virus type 1 isolates, *Antimicrob Agents Chemother* 38:23, 1994.

91. Hirsch MS, Conway B, D'Aquila RT, et al: Antiretroviral drug resistance testing in adults with HIV infection, *JAMA* 279:1984, 1998.

91a. Durant J, Clevenbergh P, Halfon P, et al: Drug-resistance genotyping in HIV-1 therapy: the VIRADAPT randomized controlled trial, *Lancet* 353: 2195, 1999.

92. Degelau J, Somani SK, Cooper SL, et al: Amantadine-resistant influenza A virus in a nursing facility, *Arch Intern Med* 152:390, 1992.

93. Hayden FG, Sporber SJ, Belshe RB, et al: Recovery of drug-resistant influenza A virus during therapeutic use of rimantadine, *Antimicrob Agents Chemother* 35:1741, 1991.

94. Belshe RB, Smith MH, Hall CB, et al: Genetic basis of resistance to rimantadine emerging during treatment of influenza virus infection, *J Virol* 62:1508, 1988.

95. Hay AJ, Zambon MS, Wolstenholm AJ, et al: Molecular basis of resistance of influenza virus to amantadine, *J Antimicrob Chemother* 18(suppl B):19, 1986.

96. Hayden FG, Cote KM, Douglas GD: Plaque inhibition assay for drug susceptibility testing of influenza viruses, *Antimicrob Agents Chemother* 17:865, 1980.

97. Belshe RB, Burk B, Newman F, et al: Resistance of influenza A virus to amantadine and rimantadine: results of one decade of surveillance, *J Infect Dis* 159:430, 1989.

98. Klimov AI, Rocha E, Hayden FG, et al: Prolonged shedding of amantadine-resistant influenza A viruses by immunodeficient patients: detection by polymerase chain reaction-restriction analysis, *J Infect Dis* 172:1352, 1995.

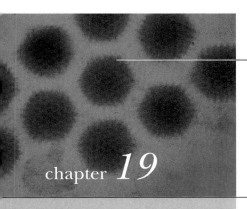

chapter *19*

Max Arens

Subtyping and Genomic Analysis of Viruses

OVERVIEW

Typing or subtyping and fingerprinting of the genomes of microorganisms is useful for many purposes. *Typing* refers to separation based on large genetic differences among members of a single virus species. Detection of stable distinctions within a group of viruses identified by typing is referred to as *subtyping*. Typing and subtyping were traditionally performed using serologic methods that depended on antigenic distinctions. Thus they tended to be directed at viral proteins that were subjected to immunologic pressure. These serotyping systems are still widely used but are increasingly being supplemented or even replaced by molecular typing methods. The distinctions revealed by typing and subtyping are often important for understanding epidemiologic patterns of viruses and certain aspects of pathogenesis, such as immunity and reinfection.

Viral fingerprinting refers to methods that detect distinctions smaller than those detected by typing and subtyping. Fingerprinting may allow recognition of individual isolates of certain viruses, especially ribonucleic acid (RNA) viruses, that tend to have more genomic variability than deoxyribonucleic acid (DNA) viruses. Recognition of these fine distinctions may be important for understanding the biology of viruses and can be the basis for studies of molecular epidemiology.

In general, typing, subtyping, or fingerprinting are more demanding for viruses than more complex organisms such as bacteria, simply because viruses are generally more difficult to manipulate in the laboratory. Numerous methods are now available, however, and most are not carried out in routine diagnostic laboratories but may be available in research laboratories with special interest in a specific virus. The methods vary in the level of resolution they can achieve and the classes of virus they can detect. Thus the information required and the virus analyzed determine the choice of method. Rapid advances in molecular biology, especially in automated nucleotide sequencing, will make molecular methods more widely available in the future.

Table 19–1 summarizes molecular methods for subtyping and fingerprinting of viral genomes. Table 19–2 lists subtyping and molecular fingerprinting methods used for medically important viruses.

SEROTYPING

The traditional method for typing and subtyping viruses is serotyping, which involves using well-defined antibodies to define stable antigenic differences. Some virus species cannot be subtyped by serologic methods simply because significant antigenic differences do not exist. Serologic methods have been used to define major viral groups (i.e., types), such as influenza types A to C, parainfluenza types 1 to 4, poliovirus types 1 to 3,

herpes simplex virus types 1 (HSV-1) and 2 (HSV-2), adenovirus types 1 to 49, and more than 100 rhinovirus types. Depending on the availability of antisera, finer distinctions can be made, such as hepatitis B virus (HBV) subtypes *ayw*, *ayr*, *adw*, and *adr*. The availability of monoclonal antibodies has made it possible to create even finer distinctions. For example, a large panel of monoclonal antibodies to rabies virus has allowed definition of viral differences characteristic of the host species (e.g., raccoon, skunk, bat).[53] This system has been very useful in understanding the epidemiology of animal rabies and identifying the source of human cases.

Antibody-based virus typing is carried out using a variety of assay formats. Traditional methods include complement fixation, hemagglutination inhibition, hemadsorption inhibition, and neutralization. Currently, *fluorescent antibody* (FA) *staining* and *enzyme immunoassay* (EIA) are the most widely used methods. In general, serotyping has been useful for making relatively large distinctions among viruses, but it may not be able to distinguish among individual isolates within a serotype. The need for this capability provides the impetus for the molecular methods described next.

RESTRICTION FRAGMENT LENGTH POLYMORPHISM

Typing or subtyping of viruses by detection of restriction fragment length polymorphisms is a versatile and widely used method. Its basis is the activity of *restriction endonucleases*, which are enzymes that cleave DNA at specific four-nucleotide or six-nucleotide recognition sequences. The presence of nucleotide differences (i.e., mutations) at restriction endonuclease cleavage sites in different strains of virus results in different patterns of fragments after digestion of viral DNA with the restriction endonuclease. This phenomenon is termed *restriction fragment length polymorphism* (RFLP). The technique requires (1) fairly large amounts of purified or partially purified viral DNA, (2) a set of restriction enzymes with which to cut the DNA, (3) the ability to separate the DNA fragments by electrophoresis, and (4) a method for documenting the results. The results are usually displayed as patterns of bands in an agarose gel stained with ethidium bromide (Figure 19–1).

The RFLP typing method is directly applicable to DNA viruses but may be used with an RNA viral genome if it is first converted to complementary DNA (cDNA) in a reverse-transcription reaction. Viruses with large DNA genomes (e.g., cytomegalovirus [CMV]) may have 20 to 50 bands, whereas viruses with smaller genomes (e.g., adenoviruses) have only five or 10 bands. The method is often not applicable to viruses with very small genomes because of an insufficient number of bands. The restriction enzyme used for the digestion is an

Table 19.1   Molecular Methods for Characterization of Viruses

Method	Restriction enzyme	Probe	Basis for distinctions	Level of resolution	Advantages	Disadvantages
Restriction fragment length polymorphism (RFLP)	Yes	No	Restriction sites	Subtypes	Simple; wide applicability	Samples only the restriction sites; difficult to use with RNA viruses
Southern blot	Yes	Yes	Restriction sites Probe sites	Subtypes	Wide applicability Can analyze complex genome	Samples only the restriction sites and probe sites; technically complex; may require radioisotopes
Oligonucleotide fingerprint analysis	No	No	RNase T1 cleavage sites	Subtypes Quasispecies	Directly applicable to RNA viruses Can detect point mutations	Complex electrophoresis procedure
Analysis of polymerase chain reaction (PCR) products: Reverse hybridization (RH) DNA enzyme immunoassay (DEIA)	No	Yes	Probe sites	Subtypes	Simple; commercially available	Accuracy depends on appropriate choice of probes and stability of the nucleotide sequence of the probe target
Ribonuclease protection assay	No	Yes	Probe sites	Subtypes	Readily applicable to RNA viruses	Requires a radioactive probe; technically difficult
Single-strand conformation polymorphism (SSCP)	No	No	Mobility differences	Subtypes	Detects a few mutations in a large number of bases	Identifies the presence but not the location of mutations
Heteroduplex mobility assay (HMA)	No	No	Mobility of hetero- vs homo- duplexes	Quasispecies	Can visualize many quasispecies	Cannot distinguish quasispecies with <2%-3% nucleotide differences
Nucleotide sequencing	No	No	Nucleotide sequence	Single genome (if cloned)	Wide applicability Can identify single nucleotide mutation	Technically complex; produces large amounts of data; automated sequencing requires expensive equipment
Genome segment length polymorphism (electropherotyping)	No	No	Segment length	Subtypes	Simple technique for segmented genomes	Cannot detect mutations but only variations in segment length; only applicable to viruses with segmented genomes

important factor in the resultant number of bands. No easy way exists, and generally there is no need, to correlate the pattern (e.g., a missing band or an extra band) with mutations at specific locations in the genome without extensive molecular hybridization studies or even sequencing of the genomes being compared. A significant limitation is that the RFLP method cannot detect a mutation unless it falls within the recognition sequence of the restriction endonuclease being used for DNA digestion. If different serotypes of a virus are known, as with HSV and adenoviruses, RFLP analysis of the DNA will identify the serotype as well as the subtype.

Cytomegalovirus

CMV was the first virus to be subjected to RFLP analysis of viral genomic DNA for epidemiologic purposes. Kilpatrick et al[3] demonstrated the usefulness of this method by digestion of 11 human strains of CMV. They

Table 19.2 Application of Molecular Subtyping and Fingerprinting Methods to Specific Viruses

Virus	Method	References
Adenovirus	RFLP	1, 2
Cytomegalovirus (CMV)	RFLP	3-11
	PCR-RFLP	
	Southern blot	
	Glycoprotein B genotyping	
Dengue	Nucleotide sequencing	12
Epstein-Barr (EBV)	RFLP	13-16
	Analysis of termini	
Enterovirus	RFLP	17-27
	RT-PCR RFLP	
	Oligonucleotide fingerprint analysis	
	SSCP	
	Nucleotide sequencing	
Hepatitis B (HBV)	Southern blot	28
	SSCP	
	PCR-SSCP	
	Nucleotide sequencing	
Hepatitis C (HCV)	SSCP	29-33
	PCR-SSCP	
	RH	
	DEIA	
	Nucleotide sequencing	
Human immunodeficiency (HIV)	HMA	34-39
	HTA	
	Nucleotide sequencing	
Herpes simplex (HSV)	RFLP	40-42
	PCR-RFLP	
	Southern blot	
Influenza	Ribonuclease protection assay	43-46
	HMA	
	Nucleotide sequencing	
Polyomavirus JC	Nucleotide sequencing	47
Measles	RT-PCR	48
	RFLP	
Parainfluenza	Serotyping	49-51
	Sequencing	
Parvovirus B19	SSCP	52
	PCR-SSCP	
Rabies	Monoclonal antibody typing	53-55
	Nucleotide sequencing	
Respiratory syncytial (RSV)	Ribonuclease protection assay	56-58
	PCR-RFLP	
	Nucleotide sequencing	
Rhinovirus	Serotyping	59-62
	Nucleotide sequencing	
Rotavirus	Genome segment length polymorphism	63-65
Small, round-structured viruses (Norwalk-like viruses)	Southern blot	66-68
	Nucleotide sequencing	
Varicella-zoster (VZV)	RFLP	69, 70
	Long PCR-RFLP	

See Table 19-1 for abbreviations. *RT,* Reverse transcription; *HTA,* heteroduplex tracking assay.

observed that each strain had a unique pattern of fragments when separated by electrophoresis in an agarose gel. Subsequent studies have documented a number of interesting observations regarding epidemiology of CMV. Huang et al[4] showed that five of six congenitally infected babies had the same strain of CMV as their mothers and thus concluded that endogenous CMV is the most frequent cause of intrauterine transmission.

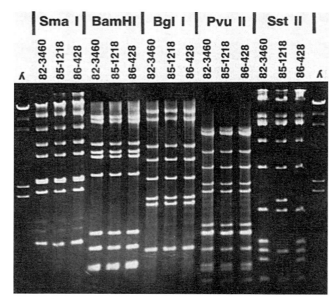

Figure 19.1 Agarose gel electrophoresis of DNA fragments from restriction enzyme digestion of adenovirus type 7b isolates from St. Louis. DNA was digested, subjected to electrophoresis in agarose containing ethidium bromide, and photographed under ultraviolet light. Three different isolates were digested with five different restriction enzymes, shown across top of figure. Digestion with Sst II revealed differences in pattern of 85-1218 isolate. Lambda (λ) DNA markers are in first and last lanes. (From Arens M, Dilworth V: *J Clin Microbiol* 26:1604, 1998.)

Spector and Spector[5] used the RFLP technique to study the epidemiologic relationships of three CMV isolates from two twins and their mother. They showed that the infants were infected with two different strains of virus during an extended hospitalization after birth (twin A was infected at 9 weeks of age and twin B at 6 weeks). The mother, who was CMV negative before and shortly after giving birth, became infected at 6 months postpartum with the strain carried by twin A. In another study at a nursery, RFLP analysis of CMV strains isolated from the urine of eight infants demonstrated that one had transmitted CMV to two other infants, apparently through fomites. The two infants began shedding CMV on the same day, 22 days after the index case was transferred into the intensive care nursery.[71]

Herpes Simplex

Buchman et al[40] analyzed 14 isolates of HSV and showed that among more than 50 total restriction enzyme cleavage sites, variability was present in at least 16. An RFLP analysis concluded that two HSV-1 isolates had been introduced independently into a pediatric intensive care unit. RFLP analysis of the isolates in an outbreak of HSV encephalitis in Boston showed that all isolates from seven patients had different restriction patterns and thus were not epidemiologically linked.[72]

Adenovirus

RFLP analysis has been used in extensive studies of the molecular epidemiology of adenoviruses over the past 20 years[73-76] (see Figure 19–1). Wadell[73] compiled a compendium on the subject, and Wigand and Adrian[74] devised a system for classification of the genome types and their relation to serotypes. One analysis described a population of adenovirus genotypes that was especially homogeneous[75] compared with other analyses of the same genotypes in other locations. Another analysis explored the possibility that the pathology of adenovirus disease is related to the genotype of the virus.[2]

SOUTHERN BLOT

The classic Southern blot[77] is a modification of RFLP analysis. After viral DNA is digested with a restriction enzyme, the resulting fragments are subjected to electrophoresis in an agarose gel, transferred onto a nitrocellulose sheet, and then hybridized with a labeled probe consisting of the entire genome or a specific segment of the genome. Some or all of the restriction enzyme digestion fragments are visualized, depending on whether they hybridize with the probe. The advantage of Southern blot is that with appropriate probe selection, relatively simple and straightforward typing schemes of very complex genomes can be achieved. Disadvantages are that it is relatively cumbersome to perform in the laboratory and that it detects only a small proportion of existing variability, depending on the specific restriction endonuclease and detection probe used.

Southern blot is often used to detect PCR products and can be used to perform subtyping when variable restriction enzyme cleavage sites exist within the amplified segment (see next section).

Cytomegalovirus

Southern blot analysis[78] and conventional RFLP analysis[79] have demonstrated that a single patient can be infected with multiple strains of CMV. In a landmark report on the transmission of CMV in renal transplantation, Chou[80] showed that 15 distinct strains (genotypes) of CMV were isolated from 19 organ recipients; four of the 19 had paired isolates with the same genotype. In all four pairs of recipients with a common donor, both recipients shed the same strain of CMV, suggesting that both acquired it from the donor. Also, seropositive recipients could be reinfected by a new strain of CMV after transplantation (Figure 19–2). Similar analyses performed on bone marrow transplant recipients demonstrated that some CMV infections after transplant are caused by strains of virus present before the transplant.[81]

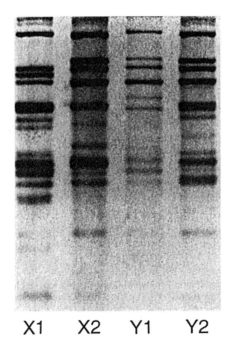

Figure 19.2 Southern blot analysis of cytomegalovius (CMV) isolates from two seropositive patients who shed a new strain of CMV after kidney transplantation. Patterns for isolates X1 and Y1 (obtained before transplant) are clearly different from patterns for X2 and Y2, which were isolated from patients X and Y after transplant. (From Chou S: *N Eng J Med* 314:1422, 1986.)

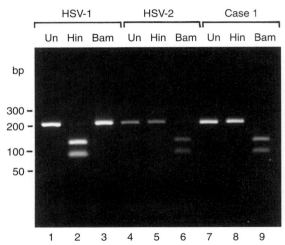

Figure 19.3 Typing of herpes simplex virus (HSV) by restriction endonuclease digestion of PCR products. Both HSV-1 and HSV-2 are amplified by same PCR reaction, yielding a product of 211 base pairs (*bp*). Product from amplification of HSV-1 is digested by restriction endonuclease *Hinf* I (Hin) but not by *Bam*HI (Bam). Product from amplification of HSV-2 is digested by *Bam*HI but not by *Hinf* I. Figure shows digestion of amplification products from control strains of HSV-1 and HSV-2 and from a patient. Digestion pattern of patient's amplification product indicates that patient was infected with HSV-2. (From Schlesinger Y, Tebas P, Gaudreault-Keener M, et al: *Clin Infect Dis* 20:842, 1995.)

PCR PRODUCT ANALYSIS

The polymerase chain reaction (PCR) can be used to amplify regions of viral genomes that provide information for typing and subtyping. A variety of methods are available for characterizing PCR products to highlight sequence differences that are significant for genotyping or fingerprinting purposes.

PCR-RFLP

The RFLP method can be applied to analysis of DNA sequences that have been amplified by PCR. Advantages of using PCR products for analysis include (1) the availability of large amounts of DNA for analysis and (2) the possibility of application to RNA viruses by use of reverse-transcription PCR (RT-PCR). The restriction enzyme cleavage products can be visualized by gel electrophoresis and ethidium bromide staining or by Southern blot. A relative disadvantage of PCR-based analysis is that the number of restriction enzyme sites is inevitably limited by the relatively short sequences that can be amplified by PCR. Therefore this method is more applicable to delineating relatively large subtype differences, rather than molecular fingerprinting of the full genomes of individual viral isolates.

Herpes simplex, enteroviruses, and measles. PCR-RFLP is useful for subtyping HSV. HSV-1 and HSV-2 can be amplified by the same PCR reaction and distin-

guished from one another by different patterns of restriction endonuclease digestion (Figure 19–3).[42]

In the differentiation of enterovirus serotypes, Kuan[17] used RT-PCR to amplify a 297-bp (base pair) amplicon (amplified product) from the 5′ noncoding region of the virus that was cleaved by restriction endonucleases and analyzed on an agarose gel. Fragment patterns were characteristic of the serotype, as shown by comparison with prototype strains.

The same technique has been applied to epidemiologic studies of measles virus, another RNA virus. Katayama et al[48] documented the changing distribution of measles genotypes in Japan through amplification of the hemagglutinin and nucleoprotein genes, followed by digestion of amplified product, which allowed strain typing of the isolate.

Varicella-zoster. PCR-RFLP has been applied to discriminate between wild-type varicella-zoster virus (VZV) and the VZV vaccine strain.[69] This assay replaced a much more technically demanding RFLP analysis of whole-virus genomic DNA. Since VZV is extremely stable genetically, it has been difficult to apply PCR-RFLP to establish a subtyping system because of the lack of sufficient differences in digestion patterns to make distinctions. *Long PCR* has alleviated this problem by allowing amplification of DNA products from 6.8 to 11.4 kb (kilobases). When digested with the appropriate restriction enzyme, these products have shown differences among various isolates. Forty VZV isolates from

Japan were classified into 17 groups after the long PCR-RFLP analysis.[70]

Cytomegalovirus. PCR-RFLP analysis of the *glycoprotein B* (gB) gene of CMV has been used to establish a typing scheme that may yield insights into pathogenesis. CMV gB is the major target of neutralizing antibodies in infected patients. RFLP analysis of a large portion of the gene has resulted in identification of five distinct genotypes,[8, 11] which have also been sequenced. The various gB genotypes have distinct geographic and demographic features. CMV gB type 1 is most common among Caucasians,[82] and gB type 2 is most common among Japanese.[11] CMV gB type 4 was more prevalent in Italians than Californians infected with human immunodeficiency virus (HIV)[9]. Some evidence suggests that the gB genotype might confer increased virulence, since one study associated gB type 2 with symptomatic infection in stem cell transplant patients.[10]

Reverse Hybridization

The reverse hybridization method (or line probe assay) is based on a system in which PCR products amplified from test specimens are hybridized to probes bound to membrane strips in a parallel-line configuration.

Hepatitis C. An assay using RT-PCR and reverse hybridization for genotyping and subtyping analysis of hepatitis C virus (HCV) is commercially available (Inno-LiPA HCV, Innogenetics, Duluth, Ga). HCV RNA is extracted from serum, and a segment of the genome from the 5′ noncoding region is amplified by a nested RT-PCR using biotinylated primers. The PCR products are hybridized to probes on the membrane strips, and hybrids are detected by alkaline phosphatase–conjugated streptavidin (see Chapter 1). Reaction of the amplified fragment with the specific probes results in formation of lines on the strip, allowing identification of HCV genotypes 1 to 6 and also the major subtypes. The recently described Vietnamese genotypes 7 to 9[83] cannot be identified with the current assay.

This assay has been evaluated for its usefulness in genotyping of HCV.[84] HCV RNA was amplified from the serum of 61 HCV-positive patients and analyzed by reverse hybridization. Results were compared to genotyping based on sequencing of the 5′ noncoding region and the nonstructural 5 region. The reverse hybridization assay was able to identify correctly all the HCV genotypes (1, 2, and 3) and subtypes 2a, 2b, and 3a. The assay incorrectly identified the subtype of one of 11 HCV-1a viruses as HCV-1b, three of 31 HCV-1b viruses as HCV 1a, and four of four HCV-2c viruses as HCV-2a. Subsequent evaluations by the same group[31] and another group[33] concluded that this particular reverse hybridization assay misinterpreted 2% to 10% of the HCV-1a and HCV-1b subtypes and that it could not be used for differentiation of HCV-2a and HCV-2c. The

shortcomings of this assay apparently result from the choice of probes. The distinction between subtypes 1a and 1b depends on a single nucleotide difference at position -99 in the 5′ noncoding region and subtypes 2a and 2c are identical in the region of the assay probes.

DNA Enzyme Immunoassay

The DNA enzyme immunoassay (DEIA) is a sensitive hybridization-based system used for detection of PCR products. PCR or RT-PCR products are denatured by heating and hybridized to probes bound to microtiter plates. The resulting double-stranded DNA hybrids are then detected by a murine monoclonal antibody. Bound antibody is detected using a rabbit antibody to mouse immunoglobulin conjugated to horseradish peroxidase, followed by addition of the appropriate enzyme substrate.

Hepatitis C. DEIA has been used for typing of HCV. A commercial assay (GEN-ETI-K DEIA, DIASorin, Stillwater, Minn) includes six different probes directed against the HCV core region. In a recent evaluation and direct comparison of the reverse hybridization assay (LiPA-II) and the DEIA assay,[33] 112 of 120 evaluable samples (93.3%) yielded concordant results. Of the eight subtyping discrepancies, all were in genotypes 1 and 2 and were misassigned by the reverse hybridization assay, apparently because of the suboptimal probe positions discussed earlier.

Both reverse hybridization and DEIA appear to be excellent choices for the determination of HCV genotype and reasonable choices for the determination of subtype. DEIA has a higher accuracy for subtyping, however, especially for identifying HCV-1 and HCV-2 subtypes.

SINGLE-STRAND CONFORMATION POLYMORPHISM ANALYSIS

Single-strand conformation polymorphism (SSCP) analysis is the method by which Orita et al[85] demonstrated that a single nucleotide substitution was sufficient to cause a mobility shift of a fragment of single-stranded DNA in a neutral polyacrylamide gel. Initially the general procedure was to use RFLP fragments from genomic DNA, one from the wild-type genome and one from a possible mutant. The fragments were denatured by alkali treatment, and mobilities of the fragments were compared after electrophoresis in a neutral polyacrylamide gel. More recently, modifications have been made to accommodate PCR amplification of a specific region of wild-type or mutant genomes before denaturation and separation on a neutral gel.[86] In either case, if one or more mutations is present in the segment of the mutant genome being tested, that segment is likely to run at a different position in the gel than the same segment from the wild-type genome. The altered electrophoretic pattern is caused by changes in the secondary structure of the restriction fragment or the PCR amplicon.[85]

The separation of the wild-type and mutant fragments depends on several environmental factors, including temperature of the gel during electrophoresis, concentration of the electrophoresis buffer, and presence of denaturing agents in the gel. One major advantage of SSCP analysis is that it can "screen" the entire genetic makeup of several hundred base pairs of DNA, whereas RFLP samples only a few bases (those making up the restriction sites).

Human Parvovirus B19

An analysis of genetic variability in the nonstructural gene of human parvovirus B19 by PCR-SSCP revealed the presence of six genotypes among 50 samples of virus from several countries.[52] Sequencing of this region confirmed the presence of mutations in the different genotypes, and all were silent mutations. Good correlation was found between the SSCP genotype and the country from which the virus was obtained. Also, within Japan, genotypes 1, 2, 3, and 4 were circulating between 1981 and 1987 in about equal numbers, but between 1990 and 1994, 90% of those tested were type 3.

Hepatitis B

An epidemiologic investigation into an outbreak of HBV infection in a pediatric oncology unit was based on the ability to distinguish genotypes of the virus by PCR-SSCP.[28] PCR was used to amplify a 189-bp product from the hypervariable (pre-S1) region of the genome. This product was denatured and subjected to electrophoresis in neutral polyacrylamide gels. Forty unrelated controls all had distinct patterns in gels, and all but six of the 58 oncology patients had patterns that fell into five different groups. This extensive investigation revealed that several HBV isolates had been introduced independently into the unit and that some had been spread extensively.

Hepatitis C

SSCP analysis has also been applied to HCV.[29] A nested RT-PCR assay was used to amplify a 289-bp amplicon from the conserved 5′ noncoding region, which was analyzed in nondenaturing polyacrylamide gels (Figure 19–4). This method was able to identify correctly the strain type of 73 HCV-positive samples that had been genotyped by sequencing and dideoxy fingerprinting. The PCR-SSCP method was more rapid and less expensive than either of the established methods but provided the same information on strain typing.

OLIGONUCLEOTIDE FINGERPRINT ANALYSIS

Molecular fingerprinting is more difficult for RNA viruses than for DNA viruses because of the lack of sequence-specific enzymes that cleave RNA in the way that restriction endonucleases cleave DNA at specific four-base or six-base sequences. An early approach to this problem was oligonucleotide fingerprinting, a powerful but technically complex method first described by DeWachter and Fiers[87] in 1972. The method employs ribonuclease (RNase) T1, an endonuclease purified from *Aspergillus oryzae* that cleaves single-stranded RNA on the 3′ side of G residues. A large number of fragments are produced and analyzed by two-dimensional electrophoresis. The virus must be labeled with ^{32}P before enzyme cleavage, allowing detection of the digestion products by autoradiography. The cleavage products make up approximately 10% of the viral genome[25] and appear as a fan-shaped array of spots distributed according to their size and composition.[87]

Before RT-PCR and nucleotide sequencing became widely available, this procedure was considered the most sensitive method available for fingerprinting RNA

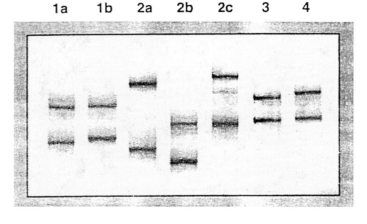

1a   1b   2a   2b   2c   3   4

Figure 19.4 Single-strand conformation polymorphism (SSCP). RT-PCR products from the 5′ noncoding region from various hepatitis C virus (HCV) genotypes were electrophoresed in 11.5% polyacrylamide gel and visualized by silver staining. HCV types (*numbers*) and subtypes (*letters*) are shown across top of figure. (From Lareu RR, Swanson NR, Fox SA: *J Virol Methods* 64:11, 1997.)

viruses. Oligonucleotide fingerprint analysis has been used for poliovirus,[23, 24] influenza virus,[46] vesicular stomatitis virus,[88] and enteroviruses.[19, 22, 89]

Poliovirus

Oligonucleotide fingerprint analysis has been most widely used in the study of molecular variation among the enteroviruses, particularly polioviruses. The method was used in the early epidemiologic studies of the distribution of poliovirus subpopulations among infected human communities and in studies undertaken to clarify the molecular evolution of poliovirus during infection and passage through the human intestine. Studies found that the poliovirus genome was quite plastic; the genome underwent continual change during natural epidemic transmission. Within a single epidemic in a confined geographic area, small differences were detected between patterns, and no two patterns were exactly alike.[22] New spots appeared on the autoradiograms, and others disappeared. Even the patterns among infected family members were different. Also, oligonucleotide fingerprinting was able to distinguish poliovirus vaccine strains from circulating "wild" strains, thus providing a timely method for detecting wild-type infections and for tracking possible vaccine revertants of the type 1 oral polio vaccine.

Enterovirus 70

In contrast to the extreme variability of the poliovirus genome, oligonucleotide fingerprint analysis of the genome of enterovirus 70 (EV 70), the cause of epidemic acute hemorrhagic conjunctivitis around the world, is quite stable. Only one basic genotype of EV 70 appears to be in circulation worldwide, and isolates from one year to the next and from one geographic region to the next have very similar patterns. Numerous intervening infections that linked different isolates did not result in major changes in the fingerprint patterns of EV 70.[25]

RIBONUCLEASE PROTECTION ASSAY

The ribonuclease protection assay developed by Myers et al[90] is an alternative means for fingerprinting RNA genomes. The assay is versatile and can be used to demonstrate the presence and approximate locations of point mutations in DNA or RNA. When applied to the analysis of RNA viruses, it is sometimes called the *RNase mismatch cleavage method.*

A relatively short RNA probe is synthesized in vitro from cloned DNA corresponding to a variable portion of the viral genome. The RNA probe is labeled with a radioisotope, usually ^{32}P, and allowed to hybridize with RNA from the test strain. The resulting heteroduplex

molecules are digested with RNase A, which cleaves only single-stranded RNA. The result is that the labeled RNA probe will be cleaved only in regions where it does not match the sequence of the test strain. The cleavage fragments are separated by gel electrophoresis and visualized by autoradiography. The method is able to detect about half of single-base mutations.[90] The failure to cleave all mismatches may be related to the secondary heteroduplex structure of the probe.

Although the ribonuclease protection assay is technically difficult, it has considerable power to fingerprint RNA viruses in a manner similar to the RFLP for DNA viruses.

Influenza and Respiratory Syncytial Virus

Using a technique developed to demonstrate point mutations in RNA transcripts from the *c-ras* gene,[91] the ribonuclease protection assay was used to investigate genetic relatedness and evolution of field isolates of influenza virus.[43]

Epidemiologic studies of respiratory syncytial virus (RSV) have used a probe corresponding to a segment of the G glycoprotein of RSV. One study showed that epidemiologically linked isolates (coinfected twins, infants infected during a nosocomial outbreak, and institutionalized adults infected during an outbreak) had identical banding patterns, whereas unrelated isolates had different patterns (Figure 19–5). Another study investigated the genetic variability and evolution of the different subtypes of RSV circulating in Spain.[57] Mutations that appeared in early isolates were retained in later isolates, and viruses isolated during a short time span showed highly similar band patterns. Different isolates from the same winter outbreak of RSV showed considerable heterogeneity. The RSV G gene accumulated mutations at a faster rate than other genes.

GENOME SEGMENT LENGTH POLYMORPHISM (ELECTROPHEROTYPING)

Certain RNA viruses, such as rotavirus and the influenza viruses, have segmented genomes. For these viruses, electrophoresis of the viral genomic RNA yields a series of bands. Differences in the migration of the bands can be used for typing and fingerprinting. Electropherotyping has been applied more extensively to analysis of rotavirus genomes because of much greater heterogeneity in the size of the segments, both within a single strain and among different strains.

Rotavirus

Rotaviruses that infect humans fall into groups A, B, and C (groups D to G are not known to infect humans), all of which have 11 segments of ds-RNA, including some of variable length. When total rotavirus RNA is extracted from a clinical sample and subjected to electrophoresis on a polyacrylamide gel,[65] the classic electropherotype pattern of group A rotaviruses reveals four classes, with segments 1 to 4 in the largest class,

segments 5 and 6 in the second class, 7 to 9 in the third class, and 10 and 11 in the smallest class.

The electropherotype of epidemiologically unrelated rotaviruses may vary because of small differences in the lengths of some segments. This observation has been used to study the epidemiology and transmission of rotavirus. Dolan et al[63] developed a simplified method for these analyses in which RNA was extracted directly from clinical specimens, subjected to electrophoresis in Laemmli stacking polyacrylamide gels, and detected using the extremely sensitive silver stain technique. The authors found 10 different electropherotypes among 68 rotavirus-containing specimens and noted that the predominant strain was different in each of three consecutive winter outbreaks. This same basic technique was used to study the molecular epidemiology of rotavirus infection in children in South Africa[92] and to demonstrate the nosocomial transmission of rotavirus in hospitalized patients in Santiago, Chile[64] (Figure 19–6).

HETERODUPLEX ASSAYS

The heteroduplex mobility assay (HMA) and the heteroduplex tracking assay (HTA) are based on mismatches between the strands of double-stranded DNA resulting in bulges that slow the migration of the DNA segment during gel electrophoresis.[93] These assays are used to investigate the genetic variability (at the molecular level) of various strains of a virus or the sequence variability within a single isolate of a virus. Many RNA viruses, including HIV, exist as a population of individual virions whose genomes exhibit sequence variability at multiple positions. The population of viruses with differing genome sequences is referred to as a *quasispecies*.

Heteroduplex Mobility Assay

If PCR or RT-PCR is performed on target material containing sequence variability between the primer binding sites, the amplified product will reflect this sequence variability. Double-stranded DNA products formed by association of exactly complementary strands (*homoduplexes*) will migrate differently in gels than double-stranded products of the same length formed from strands that are not exactly complementary (*heteroduplexes*). Although the difference in migration may not be apparent in agarose gels, it may be visualized in polyacrylamide gels (see Figure 19–4).

In HMA, PCR is performed on two or more viral isolates being analyzed. PCR products from the different isolates are mixed and allowed to anneal. Sequence differences in the PCR products are revealed by one or more heteroduplex bands (Figure 19–7). The relative retardation of gel mobility is proportional to the degree

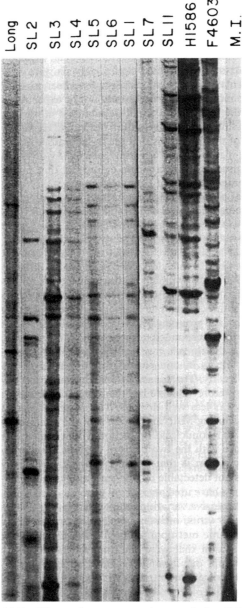

Figure 19.5 Ribonuclease protection analysis of RNA extracted from eight respiratory syncytial virus (RSV) isolates from children infected in St. Louis in a single season and from two isolates from patients in Seattle during a different season. RNA from each isolate was analyzed using a ^{32}P-labeled transcript using T7 polymerase. RNase cleavage products were separated by electrophoresis in 8% polyacrylamide containing 8-M urea. Various lanes are different exposures of same gel. Long strain of RSV and mock-infected cells (M.I.) are controls in first and last lanes, respectively. (From Storch GA, Park CS, Dohner DE: *J Clin Invest* 83:1899, 1989.)

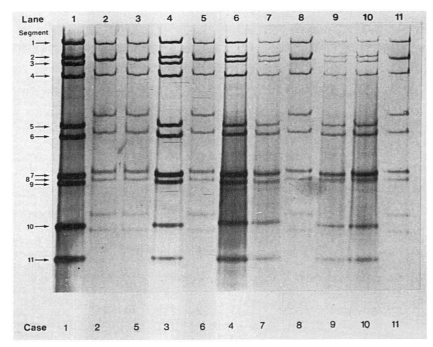

Figure 19.6 Electropherotypes of rotavirus isolates from 11 hospitalized patients in Santiago, Chile. Rotavirus RNA was extracted from stool specimens, subjected to electrophoresis in polyacrylamide gel, and visualized by silver stain for comparison. Eleven gene segments are labeled at left. (From Gaggero A, Avendaño LF, Fernández J, Spencer E: *J Clin Microbiol* 30:3295, 1992.)

of nucleotide sequence difference between the isolates being tested. HMA can detect genetic differences as small as 2% in an amplicon of several hundred base pairs. The major advantage of this technique is that it can be used to screen isolates and determine genetic relatedness without DNA sequencing.

Human immunodeficiency virus. HMA has been used efficiently in the analysis of the relatedness of HIV quasispecies diversity within a single individual and the diversity of HIV strains from around the world. Delwart et al[34] showed that intrasubject relatedness of DNA from the *env* gene (excluding gaps in the sequences) was about 1% to 5%, with corresponding heteroduplex mobilities of 1.0 to 0.9 (ratio of mobility of the heteroduplex to that of the homoduplex). If gaps caused by insertions and deletions were considered in the distance calculations, the DNA distances ranged from 2% to 8% and the heteroduplex mobilities from 1.0 to about 0.45. At the other end of the spectrum, a comparison of U.S. isolates to African isolates revealed DNA distances of approximately 18% to 23% and heteroduplex mobilities of about 0.18 to 0.32. HMA can also provide a rapid identification of the subtype of an HIV strain.[34]

In a separate analysis, Delwart et al[34] plotted pairwise comparisons between viruses from a given geographic region. A very high degree of viral genetic diversity was shown for isolates from Africa, consistent with the notion that the HIV-1 epidemic began on that continent. The divergence of HIV-1 isolates from North America and Europe was limited (i.e., the DNA distances formed a single cluster), whereas the experimen-

tally determined DNA distances from Brazil and from Thailand revealed two distinct clusters, indicating the recent introduction of virus from two divergent sources. Delwart and others[35, 94] have continued to use the HMA and HTA to study HIV-1 evolution in individual patients in vivo and during progression to acquired immunodeficiency syndrome (AIDS).

Influenza. HMA has also been used in combination with *multiplex reverse transcription* (MRT) and *multiplex PCR* (MPCR) to differentiate the hemagglutinin genes of different influenza virus types and subtypes.[44] Three RT primers and seven pairs of PCR primers (for amplification of all known influenza types and subtypes) in the MRT-MPCR method differentiated the strains by type and subtype based on size differences in the amplified products of types A, B, and C. These amplified products were then analyzed by HMA. The amplified product of a clinical strain was mixed with the amplicon of a reference strain, and the resulting mobility shift pattern after electrophoresis indicated the divergence of the amplicon. These assays could be performed in 2 days and thus were a rapid and simple method for identification and genomic analysis of clinical influenza virus strains.

Heteroduplex Tracking Assay

HTA is a variation of the HMA methodology that has been used to characterize the extent of sequence heterogeneity within a specific quasispecies. A radioactive-labeled probe is hybridized with PCR products from an isolate being analyzed. Sequence variabil-

A Observation of the phenomonon

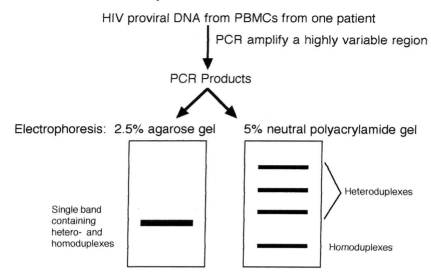

B Experimental measurement of DNA distance from patient A

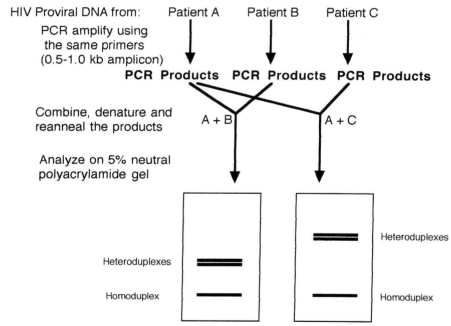

Figure 19.7 Heteroduplex mobility assay (HMA). **A,** Heteroduplexes and homoduplexes may be detected in polyacrylamide but not in agarose gels. The homoduplex band results from association of exactly complementary strands. The heteroduplex bands result from association of complementary strands having at least one nucleotide mismatch. *PMBCs,* Peripheral blood mononuclear cells. **B,** Measurement of DNA sequence divergence of virus isolates from two patients (patients B and C) using a "reference" strain from patient A.

ity within the PCR product results in formation of one or more radiolabeled heteroduplexes from binding of PCR products to the probe. Analysis by gel electrophoresis allows characterization of the presence and extent of sequence heterogeneity, since retardation of the heteroduplex formed by the probe plus the PCR product is proportional to their sequence relatedness.

Human immunodeficiency virus. Recently, using a gp120/V3-specific HTA in which a subtype B consensus *env*-V3 sequence was used as a probe, evolution was measured by divergence from a consensus sequence and correlated with the syncytium-inducing (SI) phenotype of the isolates.[38] The V3-HTA was able to detect 96% of the SI variants tested, and the overall accuracy for identifying SI and non-SI variants was 88%. Thus this assay may be useful for the identification of phenotypic traits in HIV-1 and may obviate the need for costly and time-consuming culture-based procedures used to determine the SI or non-SI phenotype.

NUCLEOTIDE SEQUENCING

The experimental determination of the linear arrangement of bases in a viral genome is the ultimate form of genomic characterization. Sequencing of the genome has the potential to distinguish between parent and progeny virus even if only a single mutation has occurred in the replication process. Automated sequencing instruments have made it easier to obtain sequence data than to carry out some of the methods described earlier.

The volume of data produced can create challenging data management problems. Thus it is often useful to apply sequencing to limited portions of the viral genome that are informative for subtyping purposes. In many cases the comparison includes the regions subjected to immunologic pressure by the host (i.e., the major antigenic epitopes of the surface proteins). In other cases, however, the nontranslated regions of the genomes may be unique for a subtype because they are subject to random mutations that may persist for a long time in the complete absence of immunologic pressure. The use of PCR amplification in conjunction with automated sequencing has streamlined the process so that large amounts of sequence data can be available within a few days. Sequencing can be readily applied to any viral genome segment that can be amplified by PCR.

Human Immunodeficiency Virus

The complete sequence of the HIV-1 genome was published in 1985.[95] Since that time, numerous studies have reported the use of sequencing to define and understand the genetic variability of HIV. Early reports showed a high degree of variation over time in specific genes within a single patient.[37] Other HIV sequencing projects attempted to establish a correlation between sequence heterogeneity in the V3 region of the envelope in sequential specimens and the stage of HIV disease, as determined by CD4+ cell counts.[36] These studies concluded that only a highly restricted subset of virus quasispecies are transmitted to establish infection in a new host.

Sequence divergence between an HIV-infected asymptomatic blood donor and three pediatric recipients was also studied by sequencing the immunodominant *env*-V3 region.[96] The results demonstrated that mutations occur during natural selection within the host only in specific locations surrounding the V3 loop but rarely, if ever, within the loop structure.

The power of sequencing for molecular epidemiology related to a forensic inquiry was demonstrated in a highly publicized investigation of the possible transmission of HIV in a dental practice.[39] A 680-bp segment of the envelope gene was amplified by RT-PCR and sequenced from blood specimens obtained from the dentist, seven of his patients who were found to be HIV positive, and 35 local HIV-infected controls. From the primary sequence, three analyses were performed: DNA distance, phylogenetic trees (Figure 19–8), and amino acid signature patterns. The results showed that the viruses from the dentist and five of the patients were closely related, leading to the conclusion that these patients had been infected (through an unknown mechanism) while receiving care from the dentist.

Influenza

A recent application of sequencing for rapid molecular characterization involved avian influenza A (H5N1) isolated from a child in Hong Kong with fatal influenza.[45] An isolate of this virus was obtained from a tracheal aspirate specimen. The hemagglutinin (HA) and neuraminidase (NA) genes were amplified by RT-PCR and sequenced to confirm the H5N1 genotype. The sequence analysis revealed a multiple basic amino acid insertion upstream from the trypsin cleavage site. This insertion, previously found in highly pathogenic influenza strains, is thought to extend the tissue range of the virus by allowing proteases other than trypsin to cleave the HA protein into HA1 and HA2 domains, thus enabling systemic spread of the virus.

SUMMARY

All the methods described in this chapter have been developed over the past 20 years. They are useful in further subdividing and characterizing the broad groups of viruses that are isolated or detected by routine procedures in the clinical virology laboratory. Molecular virologists have performed subtyping of viruses mainly because of interest in epidemiologic studies. Direct analysis of the viral genome is a reasonable and practical way to approach these issues. The HIV/AIDS epidemic has also been a driving force in molecular genotyping technology to understand better the mechanisms of disease transmission and progression and to characterize antiretroviral resistant isolates.

Many of these methods can be performed with simple equipment in unsophisticated environments, making them useful to clinical as well as research laboratories. Because of rapid technologic advances, nucleotide sequencing and other methods for the molecular analysis of viral genomes will become more widely available and will be used more frequently for practical applications in clinical laboratories.

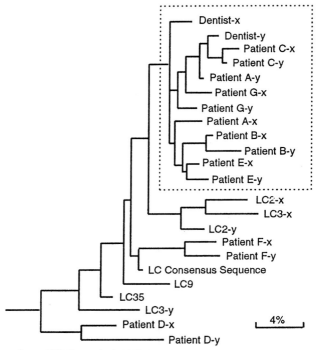

Figure 19.8 Sequencing of HIV proviral DNA in a forensic investigation. This type of analysis is the extreme case of subtyping or quasispecies analysis, since single nucleotide changes over a segment of several hundred bases are compared among HIV isolates. In this phylogenetic tree analysis of HIV-1 *env* region, sequences from a dentist, several of his patients, and local controls (*LC*) were compared. Two most divergent cloned sequences from each person (designated *x* and *y*) were compared to the most divergent cloned sequences from each control, except for LC9 and LC35, from which only a single direct PCR sequence was available. Closely related sequences (*dotted box*) were presumed to be epidemiologically linked (i.e., patients within box probably acquired their infections from the dentist). Controls and patients outside box were not epidemiologically related. (From Ou C-Y, Ciesielski CA, Meyers G, et al: *Science* 256:1167, 1992.)

References

1. Hierholzer JC, Barme M: Counterimmuno-electrophoresis with adenovirus type-specific anti-hemagglutinin sera as a rapid diagnostic method, *J Immunol* 112:987,1974.

2. Li Q, Zheng Q, Liu Y, Wadell G: Molecular epidemiology of adenovirus types 3 and 7 isolated from children with pneumonia in Beijing, *J Med Virol* 49:170, 1996.

3. Kilpatrick BA, Huang E-S, Pagano JS: Analysis of cytomegalovirus genomes with restriction endonucleases Hind III and EcoR-1, *J Virol* 18:1095, 1976.

4. Huang E-S, Alford CA, Reynolds DW, et al: Molecular epidemiology of cytomegalovirus infections in women and their infants, *N Engl J Med* 303:958, 1980.

5. Spector SA, Spector DH: Molecular epidemiology of cytomegalovirus infections in premature twin infants and their mother, *Pediatr Infect Dis* 1:405, 1982.

6. Tolpin MD, Stewart JA, Warren D, et al: Transfusion transmission of cytomegalovirus confirmed by restriction endonuclease analysis, *J Pediatr* 107:953, 1985.

7. Winston DJ, Huang E-S, Miller MJ, et al: Molecular epidemiology of cytomegalovirus infections associated with bone marrow transplantation, *Ann Intern Med* 102:16, 1985.

8. Shepp DH, Match ME, Lipson SM, Pergolizzi RG: A fifth human cytomegalovirus glycoprotein B genotype, *Res Virol* 149:109, 1998.

9. Zipeto D, Hong C, Gerna G: Geographic and demographic differences in the frequency of human cytomegalovirus gB genotypes 1-4 in immunocompromised patients, *AIDS Res Hum Retroviruses* 14:533, 1998.

10. Hebart H, Greif M, Krause H: Interstrain variation of immediate early DNA sequences and glycoprotein B genotypes in cytomegalovirus clinical isolates, *Med Microbiol Immunol* 186:135, 1997.

11. Wada K, Mizuno S, Kato K, et al: Cytomegalovirus glycoprotein B sequence variation among Japanese bone marrow transplant recipients, *Intervirology* 40:215, 1997.

12. Deubel B, Nogueira RM, Drouet MT, et al: Direct sequencing of genomic cDNA fragments amplified by the polymerase chain reaction for molecular epidemiology of dengue-2 viruses, *Arch Virol* 129:197, 1993.

13. Sidagis JK, Ueno M, Tokunaga M, et al: Molecular epidemiology of Epstein-Barr virus (EBV) in EBV-related malignancies, *Int J Cancer* 72:72, 1997.

14. Falk K, Gratama JW, Rowe M, et al: The role of repetitive DNA sequences in the size variation of Epstein-Barr virus (EBV) nuclear antigens, and the identifica-

tion of different EBV isolates using RFLP and PCR analysis, *J Gen Virol* 76:779, 1995.

15. Katz BZ, Niederman JC, Olson BA, Miller G: Fragment length polymorphisms among independent isolates of Epstein-Barr virus from immunocompromised and normal hosts, *J Infect Dis* 157:299, 1988.

16. Raab-Traub N, Flynn K: The structure of the termini of the Epstein-Barr virus as a marker of clonal cellular proliferation, *Cell* 47:883, 1986.

17. Kuan MM: Detection and rapid differentiation of human enteroviruses following genomic amplification, *J Clin Microbiol* 35:2598, 1997.

18. Fujioka S, Koide H, Kitaura Y, et al: Analysis of enterovirus genotypes using single-strand conformation polymorphisms of polymerase chain reaction products, *J Virol Methods* 51:253, 1995.

19. Minor PD, Schild GC, Ferguson M, et al: Genetic and antigenic variation in type 3 polioviruses: characterization of strains by monoclonal antibodies and T1 oligonucleotide mapping, *J Gen Virol* 61:167, 1982.

20. Mulders MN, van Loon AM, van der Avoort HG, et al: Molecular characterization of a wild poliovirus type 3 epidemic in The Netherlands (1992 and 1993), *J Clin Microbiol* 33:3252, 1995.

21. Mulders MN, Lipskaya GY, van der Avoort HG, et al: Molecular epidemiology of wild poliovirus type 1 in Europe, the Middle East, and the Indian subcontinent, *J Infect Dis* 171:1399, 1995.

22. Nottay BK, Kew OM, Hatch MH, et al: Molecular variation of type 1 vaccine-related and wild polioviruses during replication in humans, *Virology* 108:405, 1981.

23. Lee YF, Kitamura N, Nomoto A, Wimmer E: Sequence studies of poliovirus RNA. IV. Nucleotide sequence complexities of poliovirus type 1, type 2 and two type 1 defective interfering particles RNAs, and fingerprint of the poliovirus type 3 genome, *J Gen Virol* 44:311, 1979.

24. Lee YF, Wimmer E: Fingerprinting high molecular weight RNA by two-dimensional electrophoresis: application to poliovirus RNA, *Nucleic Acids Res* 3:1647, 1976.

25. Kew OM, Nottay BK, Hatch MH, et al: Oligonucleotide fingerprint analysis of enterovirus 70 isolates from the 1980 to 1981 pandemic of acute hemorrhagic conjunctivitis: evidence for a close genetic relationship among Asian and American strains, *Infect Immun* 41:631, 1983.

26. Rivera VM, Welsh JD, Maizel JV: Comparative sequence analysis of the 5′ noncoding region of the enteroviruses and rhinoviruses, *Virology* 165:42, 1988.

27. Muir P, Kämmerer U, Korn K, et al: Molecular typing of enteroviruses: current status and future requirements, *Clin Microbiol Rev* 11:202, 1998.

28. Hardie DR, Kannemeyer J, Stannard LM: DNA single strand conformation polymorphism identifies five defined strains of hepatitis B virus (HBV) during an outbreak of HBV infection in an oncology unit, *J Med Virol* 49:49, 1996.

29. Lareu RR, Swanson NR, Fox SA: Rapid and sensitive genotyping of hepatitis C virus by single-strand conformation polymorphism, *J Virol Methods* 64:11, 1997.

30. Biasin MR, Fiordalisi G, Zanella I: A DNA hybridization method for typing hepatitis C virus genotype 2c, *J Virol Methods* 65:307, 1997.

31. Lee J-H, Roth WK, Zeuzem S: Evaluation and comparison of different hepatitis C virus genotyping and serotyping assays, *J Hepatol* 26:1001, 1997.

32. Castelain S, Khorsi H, Zawadzki P, et al: Direct blotting electrophoresis for sequencing and genotyping hepatitis C virus, *J Virol Methods* 65:237, 1997.

33. Pogam SL, Dubois F, Christen R, et al: Comparison of DNA enzyme immunoassay and line probe assays (Inno-LiPA HCV I and II) for hepatitis C virus genotyping, *J Clin Microbiol* 36:1461, 1998.

34. Delwart EL, Shpaer EG, Louwagie J, et al: Genetic relationships determined by a DNA heteroduplex mobility assay: analysis of HIV-1 *env* genes, *Science* 262:1257, 1993.

35. Delwart EL, Sheppard HW, Walker BD, et al: Human immunodeficiency virus type 1 evolution in vivo tracked by DNA heteroduplex mobility assays, *J Virol* 68:6672, 1994.

36. McNearney T, Hornickova Z, Markham R, et al: Relationship of human immunodeficiency virus type 1 sequence heterogeneity to stage of disease, *Proc Natl Acad Sci USA* 89:10247, 1992.

37. Hahn BH, Shaw GM, Taylor ME, et al: Genetic variation in HTLV-III/LAV over time in patients with AIDS or at risk for AIDS, *Science* 232:1548, 1986.

38. Nelson JAE, Fiscus SA, Swanstrom R: Evolutionary variants of the human immunodeficiency virus type 1 V3 region characterized by using a heteroduplex tracking assay, *J Virol* 71:8750, 1997.

39. Ou C-Y, Ciesielski CA, Myers G, et al: Molecular epidemiology of HIV transmission in a dental practice, *Science* 256:1165, 1992.

40. Buchman TG, Roizman B, Adams G, Stover BH: Restriction endonuclease fingerprinting of herpes simplex virus DNA: a novel epidemiological tool applied to a nosocomial outbreak, *J Infect Dis* 138:488, 1978.

41. Buchman TG, Roizman B, Nahmias AJ: Demonstration of exogenous genital reinfection with herpes simplex virus type 2 by restriction endonuclease fingerprinting of viral DNA, *J Infect Dis* 140:295, 1979.

42. Schlesinger Y, Tebas P, Gaudreault-Keener M, et al: Herpes simplex virus type 2 meningitis in the absence of genital lesions: improved recognition with use of the polymerase chain reaction, *Clin Infect Dis* 20:842, 1995.

43. Lopez-Galindez C, Lopez JA, Melero JA, et al: Analysis of genetic variability and mapping of point mutations in influenza virus by the RNase mismatch cleavage method, *Proc Natl Acad Sci USA* 85:3522, 1988.

44. Zou S: A practical approach to genetic screening for influenza virus variants, *J Clin Microbiol* 35:2623, 1997.

45. Subbarao K, Klimov A, Katz J, et al: Characterization of an avian influenza A (H5N1) virus isolated from a child with a fatal respiratory illness, *Science* 279:393, 1998.

46. Young JF, Desselberger U, Palese P: Evolution of human influenza A viruses in nature: sequential mutations in the genomes of new H1N1 isolates, *Cell* 18:73, 1979.

47. Agostini HT, Ryschkewitsch CF, Mory R, et al: JC virus (JCV) genotypes in brain tissue from patients with pro-

gressive multifocal leukoencephalopathy (PML) and in urine from controls without PML: increased frequency of JCV type 2 in PML, *J Infect Dis* 176:1, 1997.

48. Katayama Y, Shibahara K, Kohama T, et al: Molecular epidemiology and changing distribution of genotypes of measles virus field strains in Japan, *J Clin Microbiol* 35:2651, 1997.

49. Komada H, Klippmark E, Orvell C, et al: Immunological relationships between parainfluenza virus type 4 and other paramyxoviruses studied by use of monoclonal antibodies, *Arch Virol* 116:277, 1991.

50. Beraud F, Kessler N, Aymard M: Contribution of monoclonal antibodies to the study of parainfluenza virus antigens, *Dev Biol Standard* 57:257, 1984.

51. Dave VP, Hetherington SV, Portner A, et al: Inter- and intra-patient sequence diversity among parainfluenza virus-type 1 nucleoprotein genes, *Virus Genes* 14:153, 1997.

52. Kerr JR, Curran MD, Moore JE, et al: Genetic diversity in the non-structural gene of parvovirus B19 detected by single-stranded conformational polymorphism assay (SSCP) and partial nucleotide sequencing, *J Virol Methods* 53:213, 1995.

53. Smith JS, Fishbein DB, Rupprecht CE, et al: Unexplained rabies in three immigrants in the United States, *N Engl J Med* 324:205, 1991.

54. Sakamoto S, Ide T, Nakatake H, et al: Studies on the antigenicity and nucleotide sequence of the rabies virus Nishigahara strain, a current seed strain used for dog vaccine production in Japan, *Virus Genes* 8:35, 1994.

55. Smith JS, Orciari LA, Yager PA, et al: Epidemiologic and historical relationships among 87 rabies virus isolates as determined by limited sequence analysis, *J Infect Dis* 166:296, 1992.

56. Storch GA, Park CS, Dohner DE: RNA fingerprinting of respiratory syncytial virus using ribonuclease protection, *J Clin Invest* 83:1894, 1989.

57. Cristina J, López JA, Albó C, et al: Analysis of genetic variability in human respiratory syncytial virus by the RNase A mismatch cleavage method: subtype divergence and heterogeneity, *Virology* 174:126, 1990.

58. Meteyard JD, Young PR: Optimization of PCR and automated sequencing of clinical isolates of respiratory syncytial virus, *J Virol Methods* 50:335, 1994.

59. Horsnell C, Gama RE, Hughes PJ, Stanway G: Molecular relationships between 21 human rhinovirus serotypes, *J Gen Virol* 76:2549, 1995.

60. Duechler M, Skern T, Sommergruber W, et al: Evolutionary relationships within the human rhinovirus genus: comparison of serotypes 89, 2, and 14, *Proc Natl Acad Sci USA* 84:2605, 1987.

61. Hughes PJ, North C, Jellis CH, et al: The nucleotide sequence of human rhinovirus 1B: molecular relationships within the rhinovirus genus, *J Gen Virol* 69:49, 1988.

62. Cooney MK, Fox JP, Kenny GE: Antigenic groupings of 90 rhinovirus serotypes, *Infect Immun* 37:642, 1982.

63. Dolan KT, Twist EM, Horton-Slight P, et al: Epidemiology of rotavirus electropherotypes determined by a simplified diagnostic technique with RNA analysis, *J Clin Microbiol* 21:753, 1985.

64. Gaggero A, Avendaño LF, Fernández J, Spencer E: Nosocomial transmission of rotavirus from patients admitted with diarrhea, *J Clin Microbiol* 30:3294, 1992.

65. Arens M, Swierkosz EM: Detection of rotavirus by hybridization with a nonradioactive synthetic DNA probe and comparison with commercial enzyme immunoassays and silver-stained polyacrylamide gels, *J Clin Microbiol* 27:1277, 1989.

66. Levett PN, Gu M, Luan B, et al: Longitudinal study of molecular epidemiology of small round-structured viruses in a pediatric population, *J Clin Microbiol* 34:1497, 1996.

67. Ando T, Jin Q, Gentsch JR, et al: Epidemiologic applications of novel molecular methods to detect and differentiate small round structured viruses (Norwalk-like viruses), *J Med Virol* 47:145, 1995.

68. Yamazaki K, Oseto M, Seto Y, et al: Reverse transcription–polymerase chain reaction detection and sequence analysis of small round-structured viruses in Japan, *Arch Virol* 12(suppl):271, 1996.

69. LaRussa P, Lungu O, Hardy I, et al: Restriction fragment length polymorphism of polymerase chain reaction products from vaccine and wild-type varicella-zoster virus isolates, *J Virol* 66:1016, 1992.

70. Takayama M, Takayama N, Inoue N, Kameoka Y: Application of long PCR method of identification of variations in nucleotide sequences among varicella-zoster virus isolates, *J Clin Microbiol* 34:2869, 1996.

71. Spector SA: Transmission of cytomegalovirus among infants in hospital documented by restriction-endonuclease-digestion analyses, *Lancet* 1:378, 1983.

72. Hammer SM, Buchman TG, D'Angelo LJ, et al: Temporal cluster of herpes simplex encephalitis: investigation by restriction endonuclease cleavage of viral DNA, *J Infect Dis* 141:436, 1980.

73. Wadell G: Molecular epidemiology of human adenoviruses, *Curr Top Microbiol Immunol* 110:191, 1984.

74. Wigand R, Adrian T: A rational system for classifying and denominating adenovirus genome types, *Res Virol* 142:47, 1991.

75. Arens M, Dilworth V: Remarkably homogeneous population of adenovirus type 3 and 7 genome types, *J Clin Microbiol* 26:1604, 1988.

76. Johansson ME, Andersson MA, Thörner PÅ: Adenoviruses isolated in the Stockholm area during 1987-1992: restriction endonuclease analysis and molecular epidemiology, *Arch Virol* 137:101, 1994.

77. Southern EM: Detection of specific sequences among DNA fragments separated by gel electrophoresis, *J Mol Biol* 98:503, 1975.

78. Drew WL, Sweet ES, Miner RC, Mocarski ES: Multiple infections by cytomegalovirus in patients with acquired immunodeficiency syndrome: documentation by Southern blot hybridization, *J Infect Dis* 50:952, 1984.

79. Spector SA, Hirata KK, Neuman TR: Identification of multiple cytomegalovirus strains in homosexual men with acquired immunodeficiency syndrome, *J Infect Dis* 150:953, 1984.

80. Chou S: Acquisition of donor strains of cytomegalovirus by renal-transplant recipients, *N Engl J Med* 314:1418, 1986.

81. Winston DJ, Huang E-S, Miller MJ, et al: Molecular epi-

demiology of cytomegalovirus infections associated with bone marrow transplantation, *Ann Intern Med* 102: 16, 1985.

82. Chou SW, Dennison KM: Analysis of interstrain variation in cytomegalovirus glycoprotein B sequences encoding neutralization-related epitopes, *J Infect Dis* 163:1229, 1991.

83. Tokita H, Okamoto H, Tsuda F, et al: Hepatitic C virus variants from Vietnam are classifiable into the seventh, eighth and ninth major genetic groups, *Proc Natl Acad Sci USA* 91:11022, 1994.

84. Zeuzem S, Rüster B, Lee J-H, et al: Evaluation of a reverse hybridization assay for genotyping of hepatitis C virus, *J Hepatol* 23:654, 1995.

85. Orita M, Iwahana H, Kanazawa H, et al: Detection of polymorphisms of human DNA by gel electrophoresis as single-strand conformation polymorphisms, *Proc Natl Acad Sci USA* 86:2766, 1989.

86. Hayashi K: PCR-SSCP: a simple and sensitive method for detection of mutations in the genomic DNA, *PCR Methods Applications* 1:34,1991.

87. DeWachter R, Fiers W: Preparative two-dimensional polyacrylamide gel electrophoresis of ^{32}P-labeled RNA, *Anal Biochem* 49:184, 1972.

88. Clewley JP, Bishop DHL, Kang CY, et al: Oligonucleotide finger prints of RNA species obtained from rhabdoviruses belonging to the vesicular stomatitis virus subgroup, *J Virol* 23:152, 1977.

89. Harris TJR, Robson KJH, Brown F: A study of the level of nucleotide sequence conservation between the RNAs of two serotypes of foot and mouth disease virus, *J Gen Virol* 50:403, 1980.

90. Myers RM, Larin Z, Maniatis T: Detection of single base substitutions by ribonuclease cleavage at mismatches in RNA: DNA duplexes, *Science* 230:1242, 1985.

91. Winter E, Yamamoto F, Almoguera C, Perucho M: A method to detect and characterize point mutations in transcribed genes: amplification and overexpression of the mutant *c-Ki-ras* allele in human tumor cells, *Proc Natl Acad Sci USA* 82:7575, 1985.

92. Steele AD: Shift in genomic RNA patterns of human rotaviruses isolated from white children in South Africa, *S Afr Med J* 79:143, 1991.

93. Wang Y-H, Griffith J: Effects of bulge composition and flanking sequence on the kinking of DNA by bulged bases, *Biochemistry* 30:1358, 1991.

94. Delwart EL, Pan H, Sheppard HW, et al: Slower evolution of human immunodeficiency virus type 1 quasispecies during progression to AIDS, *J Virol* 71:7498, 1997.

95. Ratner L, Haseltine W, Patarca R, et al: Complete nucleotide sequence of the AIDS virus, HTLV-III, *Nature* 313:277, 1985.

96. McNearney T, Hornickova Z, Kloster B, et al: Evolution of sequence divergence among human immunodeficiency virus type 1 isolates derived from a blood donor and a recipient, *Pediatr Res* 33:36, 1993.

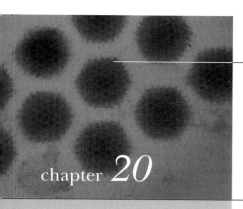

Richard Buller

Discovery of New Viral Pathogens

chapter *20*

OVERVIEW

Recently the term *emerging infections* has gained popularity for describing infectious diseases with increasing incidence, especially those caused by newly recognized pathogens. Viral diseases figure prominently among these infections. The term may conjure up images of infections caused by mutations arising from some primordial pathogenic soup. However, while it is true that some agents, such as the recently described H5N1 avian influenza virus in Hong Kong, may suddenly appear in the human population, most newly described viruses have likely infected humans since antiquity and are recognized due to advances made in techniques used to detect and identify viruses in clinical specimens. Changes in human interactions and in the environment also contribute to the emergence of new pathogens. The newly recognized hantavirus pulmonary syndrome in the southwestern United States is an example of a disease emerging due to ecologic changes.

This chapter discusses viruses discovered in recent years, and the methods used to detect them, along with diagnostic recommendations if a new viral agent is suspected.

HISTORIC BACKGROUND

Historically, *viruses* were initially defined as infectious agents that were able to pass through filters capable of blocking the passage of bacteria. Later, animal inoculation and embryonated hen's eggs were used to grow animal viruses. Not until the late 1940s was the first practical method of cell culture described for an animal virus. The 1950s and 1960s were the heyday of clinical virology, during which cell culture systems were discovered for many of the most common human viral agents. Subsequent to this period, new viral agents were recognized as the result of such diverse methodologies as fortuitous serologic reactions, electron microscopy studies, and sophisticated molecular biology techniques.

Table 20–1 lists viral agents and the methods used for their discovery.

CELL CULTURE

Although the contribution of cell culture to the discovery of new viral agents is primarily associated with the 1950s and 1960s, this technique has continued to yield new viruses into the modern era. The most dramatic recent example is the isolation and growth of the *human immunodeficiency virus* (HIV) in cultures of T lymphocytes in 1983.[29] In the early 1980s a new immunodeficiency syndrome was recognized, primarily in male homosexuals. Termed the acquired immunode-ficiency syndrome (AIDS), the cause was unknown but viruses were suspected. Because the disease resulted in a profound suppression of T-cell–mediated cellular immunity, as well as decreased numbers of certain T-cell subsets, experts in human retroviruses reasoned that T cells might be a target of infection for the unknown virus and that a human retrovirus might be the cause. They applied retroviral culture methods to lymph nodes, and later peripheral blood cells, from patients with AIDS or AIDS-related complex. The procedures included preparing cell suspensions from disrupted lymph nodes or peripheral blood samples and placing the cell suspensions in cell culture medium supplemented with interleukin-2 (IL-2) to stimulate growth of T lymphocytes. After about 2 weeks in culture, reverse transcriptase, an enzyme associated with retroviruses, was detected in culture supernatants. When the original cells were subcultured, particles with the morphology of retroviruses were observed by electron microscopy (EM) in the cultures.[29, 30, 56]

Another more recent example of cell culture providing the first recognition of a virus as a human pathogen was the isolation of *Cache Valley virus* from a patient with fatal encephalitis.[57] The virus, a mosquito-borne member of the Bunyamwera serogroup of arboviruses, had previously been isolated only from vertebrates and mosquitoes, but never from a human. The patient was a previously healthy young man with a severe encephalitic illness. Routine viral cultures of the patient's cerebrospinal fluid and blood were performed, and cytopathic effect (CPE) was noted within a few days in the inoculated cell cultures. EM of the infected cells was performed to uncover the nature of the presumed virus responsible for the CPE and revealed viral particles with the morphologic characteristics of members of the family Bunyaviridae. The virus was positively identified as Cache Valley virus by serologic and molecular methods.

As demonstrated by these two examples, although cell culture lacks the drama of newer molecular methods, its versatility ensures that it will continue to play a role in the future in uncovering new viral agents. As illustrated by the discovery of HIV, knowledge of the location and pathogenesis of the disease can provide important clues regarding the choice of cell culture systems and other methodologies that can be employed to detect a new virus.

SEROLOGY

Human parvovirus B19 (B19) and *hepatitis B virus* (HBV) are examples of viruses whose existence was revealed unexpectedly during the course of serologic studies. In both cases, precipitin lines caused by an antigen-antibody reaction were observed when two human sera were allowed to react.

Table 20.1	Methods Used for Discovery of Human Viral Pathogens	
Virus	**Methods**	**Year**
Adenovirus	Tissue culture	1953[1]
Astrovirus	Electron microscopy	1975[2, 3]
BK (polyomavirus)	Cell culture	1971[4]
Calicivirus	Immune electron microscopy	1972[5]
Coronavirus	Tissue/cell culture	1965-66[9, 10]
Cytomegalovirus	Tissue culture	1956-57[6, 8]
Dengue	Animal inoculation	1945[11]
Ebola	Cell culture, electron microscopy	1977[17]
Enteroviruses		
Poliovirus	Tissue culture	1949[13]
Coxsackievirus	Animal inoculation, cell culture	1949[14, 15]
Echovirus	Animal inoculation, cell culture	1949[15, 16]
Epstein-Barr	Cell culture, electron microscopy	1964[12]
Hepatitis A	Immune electron microscopy	1973[18]
Hepatitis B	Serology (immunoprecipitation)	1965[19]
Hepatitis C	Animal inoculation, cDNA library expression screening	1989[20]
Hepatitis D	Serology (direct immunofluorescence, animal inoculation)	1977[21, 22]
Hepatitis E	Immune electron microscopy, animal inoculation	1984[23, 24]
Hepatitis G	Animal inoculation, cDNA library expression screening	1996[25]
Human herpesvirus 6	Leukocyte culture, serology, electron microscopy	1986[26]
Human herpesvirus 7	Lymphocyte culture, electron microscopy	1990[27]
Human herpesvirus 8	Representational difference analysis	1994[28]
Human immunodeficiency	Lymphocyte culture, electron microscopy, serology	1983-84[29, 30]
Human T-cell leukemia type I	Lymphocyte culture, electron microscopy, serology	1980[31]
Human T-cell leukemia type II	Lymphocyte culture, serology	1982[32]
Influenza	Embryonated hen's egg culture	1933, 1940, 1950[33-36]
JC (polyomavirus)	Electron microscopy, cell culture	1965, 1971[37-39]
Lassa fever	Animal inoculation, cell culture, serology	1970[40]
Measles	Cell culture, serology	1954[41]
Mumps	Chick embryo culture	1945[42]
Parainfluenza	Cell culture, serology	1956, 1958, 1960[45-47]
Parvovirus B19	Serology (immunoprecipitation), immune electron microscopy	1975[48]
Respiratory syncytial	Cell culture, serology	1956[49]
Rhinovirus	Cell culture, serology	1956-57[50-51]
Rotavirus	Electron microscopy	1973[52]
Sin nombre (Four Corners hantavirus)	Serology, consensus primer PCR	1993[53]
Varicella-zoster	Cell culture	1953[54]
Yellow fever	Animal inoculation	1928[55]

cDNA, Complementary strand of deoxyribonucleic acid; PCR, polymerase chain reaction.

With HBV, although it was long appreciated that a form of hepatitis could be spread through exchange of blood products ("serum hepatitis"), none of the attempts to develop an animal model or grow the agent in culture was successful. In 1965 Blumberg et al[19] reported the discovery of a new antigen that they named the "Australia antigen" because they first recognized it in the serum of Australian aborigines. The discovery occurred fortuitously during studies using serum from hemophiliac patients (presumed to contain antibodies to multiple human antigens because of frequent transfusions) to characterize polymorphisms in human serum lipoproteins from diverse populations. A previously unrecognized precipitin line was noted (Figure 20–1). When the precipitin was visualized by EM, viral particles were seen.[58] Detailed epidemiologic studies were required to implicate the new virus in serum hepatitis.

Parvovirus B19 was similarly discovered as a new precipitin line found in studies of electrophoresis to

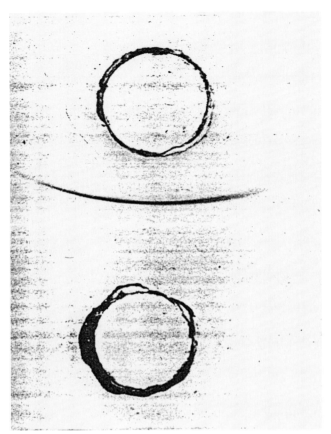

Figure 20.1 Formation of precipitin line between serum from leukemia patient (*top* well) and hemophilia serum (*bottom* well). (From Blumberg BS, Alter HJ, Visnich S: *JAMA* 191:542, 1965.)

screen serum for HBV antigen.[41] Again, EM of the precipitin revealed viral particles, but in this case the particles had the morphology of parvoviruses. Studies over the next several years linked the new virus to erythema infectiosum,[59] aplastic crisis in patients with sickle cell disease and other chronic hemolytic anemias,[60] hydrops fetalis,[61, 62] and acute arthritis.[63]

Three factors likely contributed to HBV and parvovirus B19 being revealed by serologic studies. First, the viruses were previously undiscovered because no practical culture methods existed (or exists) for either of these viruses. Second, infections with these viruses are common, and thus many human sera contain antibodies to these viruses. Third, depending on the virus and the stage of infection, both these viruses at times are found in extremely high titers in the blood, providing a source of viral antigen that could react with the serum being used as a source of antibody. During the course of both serologic studies that uncovered these viruses, fortuitous reaction of serum containing a high titer of viral particles with a serum containing specific antiviral antibodies led to formation of an unanticipated precipitin line. Astute pursuit of the unexpected finding led to discovery of new viruses.

ELECTRON MICROSCOPY

Viruses are classified into taxonomic groups based partly on physical characteristics such as size, shape, symmetry, and presence or absence of a lipid envelope. EM is critical to the determination of these physical characteristics. Because the information can often yield important clues to the nature of an unknown virus, EM has been an important tool in the recognition of some new viral agents.

Immune electron microscopy (IEM) has been an especially useful technique in identifying viruses in stool specimens. IEM involves the addition of specific immune serum to the virus suspension before viewing by EM. Antiviral antibodies in the serum coat the viral particles and cause them to agglutinate, facilitating discrimination of viral particles from artifacts present in stool specimens. In searching for a new virus, convalescent serum from a patient recovering from the disease can be used as the immune serum.

Viruses whose existence was uncovered by EM include hepatitis A virus and several agents of viral gastroenteritis, including rotaviruses, Norwalk, and related viruses.

The identification of *Norwalk virus* as an important agent of viral gastroenteritis illustrates the EM's importance in the field of viral gastroenteritis (see Chapter 5). An outbreak of nonbacterial gastroenteritis occurred in Norwalk, Ohio, in the early 1970s. Stool filtrates prepared from infected patients were given to human volunteers, who then developed a similar disease. Using IEM and convalescent sera from infected individuals, Kapikian et al[5] demonstrated 23-nm viral particles in stool material obtained from the infected volunteers (Figure 20–2). Further studies proved that these particles, later named Norwalk virus, were an important cause of viral gastroenteritis. More recently, molecular

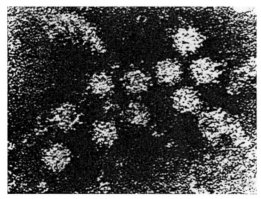

Figure 20.2 Aggregated Norwalk virus particles visible by electron microscopy (× 231,000) after incubation of stool filtrate with serum from a volunteer previously experimentally challenged with Norwalk virus. (From Kapikian AZ, Wyatt RG, Dolin R, et al: *J Virol* 10:1076, 1972.)

methods have revealed that Norwalk virus is a member of the calicivirus family.[64, 65]

The initial visualization of a human *rotavirus* was also made by EM but in a slightly different manner. Rather than by the IEM method used for Norwalk virus, the first viewing of the distinctive wheel-like appearance of a human rotavirus was made when thin sections of duodenal mucosa biopsies from children with diarrhea were examined by EM.[52] Subsequently the virus was detected often on EM examination of stool specimens from infants with diarrhea.[66]

Although EM has been instrumental in the elucidation of several viral diseases, the literature is replete with reports of viral-like particles observed by EM in association with certain diseases. Unlike the evidence linking Norwalk virus and rotaviruses with disease, the significance of many of these reports of viral sightings by EM is uncertain. Therefore EM evidence of a new viral agent should always be interpreted with caution and in conjunction with other data.

MOLECULAR BIOLOGY

Molecular biology techniques are revolutionizing the practice of infectious disease medicine. The application of these methods is having a significant impact not only on the identification of new infectious agents, but on diagnostics and basic research into pathogenesis as well.

Molecular biology techniques are based on principles of nucleic acid biochemistry. Of these principles, the *nucleic acid hybridization reaction* is central to many molecular biology methods. The hybridization reaction refers to the ability of complementary strands of nucleic acid to seek out and bind to each other through hydrogen bonds. The specificity of hybridization can be controlled to allow for either binding of strands not completely complementary or only those strands with 100% complementarity. Hybridization can be confirmed by labeling one of the strands with a radioisotope, enzyme, or dye.

A powerful group of molecular techniques referred to as *amplified nucleic acid reactions*, the best known of which is the polymerase chain reaction (PCR), also have a hybridization reaction at their core (see Chapter 1). A pair of oligonucleotide "primers" is allowed to hybridize with target deoxyribonucleic acid (DNA), after which an enzymatic reaction using DNA polymerase copies the segment of nucleic acid between the binding sites of the primer pair. These reactions cycle many times, resulting in the production of a large quantity of the desired sequence, which can then be used in further studies, such as the determination of the nucleotide sequence. Advances in nucleic acid sequencing technology now allow long pieces of nucleic acid to be rapidly and accurately sequenced. Sequence data are then entered into computer programs that can quickly search large databases looking for similarities or other relationships between the sequence of interest and previously sequenced genes.

Three specific techniques—complementary DNA (cDNA) library screening, representational difference analysis, and PCR using consensus primers—have been used for the discovery of new viral agents (Figure 20–3).

cDNA Library Screening

A cDNA library is produced using either specific or random oligonucleotide primers in conjunction with the enzyme reverse transcriptase to make cDNA copies of a population of ribonucleic acid (RNA) molecules or less often DNA molecules. The cDNA copies are then cloned into plasmid vectors, which in turn are transfected into bacterial hosts. The collection of bacteria carrying a population of cDNA sequences is then referred to as a *library*. Libraries can be screened for the presence of specific sequences through hybridization reactions using labeled probes. Alternately, as discussed next, libraries can be constructed such that cDNA sequences are expressed as proteins, which can then be selected functionally or on the basis of reaction with antibodies.

Hepatitis C virus (HCV) is an example of a virus that was identified by the cDNA library screening method. With the identification of hepatitis A and B viruses and the subsequent development of serologic screening assays for these viruses, it was evident that one or more other viral agents was responsible for most transfusion-associated cases of hepatitis. The unknown agent could be propagated in chimpanzees, but efforts to culture the virus or gain other meaningful information about it were unsuccessful.

HCV was finally identified when a group of investigators applied the cDNA screening method to the problem (Box 20–1).[20] First, plasma from an infected chimpanzee known to contain a high titer of the agent was ultracentrifuged to pellet any putative viral agent. Nucleic acid extracted from the pellet was then enzymatically converted to cDNA, which was cloned into a polypeptide expression vector (bacteriophage lambda gt11). To detect viral polypeptides, the expression library was screened using serum obtained from a patient presumably infected with the non-A non-B hepatitis agent, which was assumed to contain antibodies to the unknown agent. After screening approximately 1 million clones, a clone was identified that produced a polypeptide sequence that reacted with antibodies from the patient's serum.

Further experiments indicated that the original viral nucleic acid was single-stranded RNA and that the virus was related to the flavivirus group.[67] This work also resulted in the identification of HCV antigens used to produce the HCV serologic assay (see Chapter 8).[68]

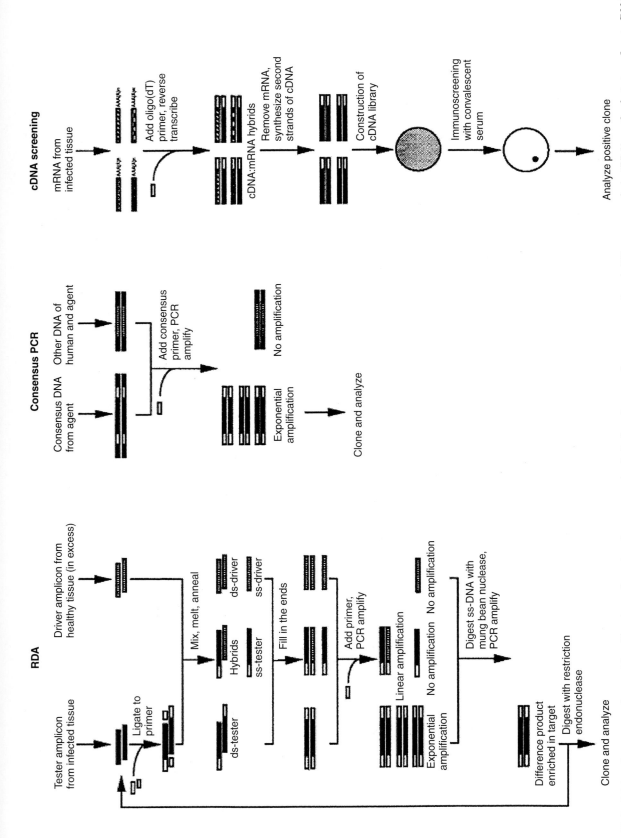

Figure 20.3 Molecular approaches to identification of previously unrecognized viral pathogens. In representational difference analysis (*RDA*) method, *tester* refers to DNA suspected to contain the putative causative agent, and *driver* refers to DNA from normal individual. Tester and driver DNA are each digested with a restriction endonuclease to produce cleavage products. DNA oligonucleotides with sequences corresponding to polymerase chain reaction (*PCR*) primers are enzymatically added by a ligation reaction, and cleavage products from tester and driver DNA are amplified by PCR. After amplification, the oligonucleotides are enzymatically cleaved from the PCR amplification products. The amplified products are referred to as *tester amplicons* and *driver amplicons*. Next, an oligonucleotide corresponding to a different PCR primer is enzymatically ligated only onto the tester DNA. Tester DNA (containing the oligonucleotide) and a large excess of driver DNA (not containing the oligonucleotide) are mixed, and the double-stranded DNA molecules are melted to achieve separation of the strands. Reannealing is allowed to occur, with the expectation that the only double-stranded tester molecules that form will be those that do not correspond to any DNA sequences present in the driver amplicons. The double-stranded tester molecules are the only ones that have both ends consisting of oligonucleotides with PCR primer binding sites. Finally, PCR is performed using the primers corresponding to the oligonucleotides. The only sequences that can undergo exponential amplification are the unique tester sequences. (See text for consensus PCR and cDNA screening methods.) (From Gao SJ, Moore PS: *Emerg Infect Dis* 2:159, 1996.)

Box 20.1   Steps in Discovery of Hepatitis C Virus

1. Identify a high-titer infectious chimpanzee plasma.
2. Concentrate presumed viral particles by ultra-centrifugation.
3. Prepare cDNA library.
   a. Use reverse transcription.
   b. Clone into phage λgt11.
4. Express encoded proteins.
5. Screen expressed proteins for reactivity with a serum from a patient with chronic non-A non-B hepatitis (presumed to contain antibodies to the causative agent).
6. Use the cDNA corresponding to the reactive protein to screen the library for larger overlapping clones.
7. Determine that identified overlapping clone does not hybridize with human or chimpanzee DNA.
8. Determine nucleotide sequence.
9. Characterize causative agent through studies of original infectious plasma and liver from an infected chimpanzee, using the identified clone to detect viral nucleic acid in those specimens.

Modified from Choo QL, Kuo G, Weiner AJ, et al: *Science* 244:359,1989.

The cDNA screening method is a powerful technique, but it is not readily applicable to all searches for an unknown viral agent. With HCV, infected chimpanzee serum provided a source of viral nucleic acid that was reasonably separate from host nucleic acids. More than 1 million clones still had to be screened before a viral sequence was identified. Some viruses, such as Kaposi's sarcoma–associated herpes virus (see following discussion), are intimately associated with host genomic sequences. Application of cDNA screening to the search for such a virus would result in the production of a cDNA library composed primarily of host sequences. Although it might be theoretically possible to identify viral sequences in such a library, the number of clones that would likely have to be screened would be prohibitive. Fortunately, other methods are capable of retrieving low copy numbers of viral nucleic acids from many host sequences.

Representational Difference Analysis

Representational difference analysis (RDA) can selectively amplify rare sequences from a large pool of host sequences. Unlike PCR, which requires some knowledge of the sequence of interest to design primers, RDA requires no prior knowledge of the sequence being sought.[69]

RDA involves isolating nucleic acid from tissue suspected of harboring an unknown virus. The DNA is first digested into fragments using one or more restriction endonucleases. The resulting restriction fragments are modified by attaching (on their ends) short sequences containing binding sites for PCR primers. The collection of fragments is then amplified by PCR, resulting in effective amplification of only those fragments whose size is suitable for PCR amplification. This procedure produces a sampling or "representation" of the genome, and the amplified fragments are referred to as *tester amplicons*. Another collection of DNA fragments is then produced by similar methods from nucleic acid extracted from normal uninfected tissue. This collection is referred to as *driver amplicons*. The sequences corresponding to PCR binding sites are then removed enzymatically, and a segment corresponding to a different PCR primer is ligated only onto the tester amplicons. A large excess of the driver amplicons is then allowed to hybridize with the tester amplicons. Because like sequences hybridize to like sequences and because driver amplicons are present in excess, the resulting mixture will contain mostly hybrids consisting of one modified fragment and one unmodified fragment or two unmodified fragments. Only those sequences found in the infected tissue, presumably from some unknown agent, will form hybrids consisting of two modified fragments. Subjecting the mixture to PCR, using primers hybridizing to the primer binding sequences that had been attached to the fragments, allows exponential amplification of only those duplexes containing two modified fragments. Therefore only sequences unique to the infected tissue are amplified. Any amplified fragments can then be sequenced and the sequences compared to sequence databases.

The Kaposi's sarcoma–associated herpes virus (KSHV), also known as *human herpesvirus type 8* (see Chapter 15), is an example of a previously unknown viral agent identified by RDA. The epidemiology of Kaposi's sarcoma had suggested that an infectious agent was involved in its etiology. Application of RDA to DNA extracted from Kaposi's lesions identified a sequence that had homology to Epstein-Barr virus and a simian herpesvirus.[28] This finding led quickly to identification of the virus as a member of the herpesvirus group. The virus was strongly linked not only to Kaposi's sarcoma,[72] but also to multicentric Castleman's disease[71] and body cavity lymphoma.[72] Subsequently a culture system for the virus was developed.[73, 74]

Consensus Primers

The term *consensus sequence* refers to nucleic acid sequences that are conserved across phylogenetic groups. Such sequences can be used for phylogenetic studies and the identification of novel pathogenic organisms. For example, consensus sequences in ribosomal RNA genes have been exploited for the identification of new bacterial agents of disease.[75] Because certain ribosomal RNA sequences are conserved in all genera of bacteria, PCR primers can be designed that allow amplification of the ribosomal RNA gene from a previously unidentified bacterium that may be present in a clinical specimen. By sequencing the intervening variable sequence present in the PCR product and comparing the sequence to those of previously sequenced bacteria available in sequence data banks, the phylogenetic relationship of the unknown bacterium to known genera can be determined.

Unfortunately, no consensus sequences are found across all groups of viruses, but sequences are found within viral groups. For example, consensus sequences are preserved in human herpesviruses[76] and the enteroviruses.[77] Therefore, if a viral agent is suspected and culture and other laboratory methods are unsuccessful in identifying a virus, PCR primers can be designed that bind to known viral consensus sequences. The primers can then be used to amplify the unknown sequence using one of the available amplification methods, such as PCR. The amplified fragment can then be sequenced and compared to known sequences. Clues to the consensus sequence can be inferred from the nature of the disease or the physical characteristics of viral particles seen on electron micrographs.

The causative agent of hantavirus pulmonary syndrome in the United States, the *sin nombre virus*, is an example of a viral agent discovered by the amplification of viral nucleic acid using primers directed to consensus sequences. The infection caused by this virus was previously unrecognized because of its low prevalence and the lack of available techniques to identify the agent. The syndrome was recognized after a sudden cluster of human cases suggested a hantavirus disease on the basis of clinical and epidemiologic characteristics.[78] The outbreak was eventually attributed to an expansion of the rodent vector population following an increase in food sources for these animals after an unusually wet rainy season. Antibodies cross-reactive with known hantavirus antigens were found initially in the sera of patients with the syndrome. The causative virus was identified by designing PCR primers that corresponded to conserved regions in the genome of known hantaviruses. When applied to specimens from patients with hantavirus pulmonary syndrome, PCR using these consensus sequences amplified a fragment of hantavirus genome that differed from other known hantaviruses.[53]

STEPS IN IDENTIFICATION OF SUSPECTED NEW VIRAL AGENT

Submission of specimens for viral culture is a first step in the identification of a viral agent. If the clinician is fortunate, the virus will grow in cell culture, announcing its presence by the production of CPE. Then the identity of the virus can be determined based on the nature of the CPE or by using monoclonal antibodies directed against specific viral proteins.

In the absence of cytopathology, EM might be used to examine the cell culture because certain viruses grow in culture with no apparent pathology to the cells. If viral particles were observed, the physical parameters of the particles would provide important clues regarding the classification of the unknown virus and would suggest other avenues of identification. For example, if herpesvirus-like particles were observed on EM, one could apply PCR using primers specific for herpesvirus consensus sequences.

Not all viruses can be grown in culture. With culture-negative specimens, one could apply EM directly to specimen material. If viral particles were observed with morphology typical of a group of viruses, the consensus primer PCR approach could be attempted. If, on the other hand, viral-like particles were seen but no particular morphology was discerned, the cDNA library screening approach might be appropriate.

A serologic approach to the identification of an unknown virus could also be taken. Guided by such parameters as clinical illness or EM information, sera from infected patients could be reacted against panels of viral antigens in an effort to uncover a serologic relationship between the antibodies in the patient's serum and known viral antigens. If a serologic reaction were revealed, one could use that information to direct further testing by a molecular method.

When the previous methods fail, molecular methods may be attempted, such as expression library screening, RDA, or PCR using consensus primers. These techniques represent major efforts that are beyond the scope of routine laboratories. Fortunately, emerging infections are receiving much more attention since the AIDS/HIV outbreak. The Centers for Disease Control and Prevention (CDC, Atlanta) has formulated a plan to deal with emerging infectious diseases.[79] This plan calls for collaborative surveillance and research involving state and local health departments. A clinician caring for a patient suspected of being infected with a novel virus should consider contacting a local or state health authority to access this infrastructure.

References

1. Rowe WP, Huebner RJ, Gilmore LK, et al: Isolation of a cytopathogenic agent from human adenoids undergoing spontaneous degeneration in tissue culture, *Proc Soc Exp Biol Med* 84:570, 1953.
2. Rowe WP, Hartley JW, Waterman S, et al: Cytopathogenic agent resembling human salivary gland virus recovered from tissue cultures of human adenoids, *Proc Soc Exp Biol Med* 92:418,1956.

3. Smith MG: Propagation in tissue cultures of a cyto-pathogenic virus from human salivary gland virus (SGV) disease, *Proc Soc Exp Biol Med* 92:424, 1956.

4. Weller TH, Macauley IC, Craig JM, Wirth P: Isolation of intranuclear inclusion producing agents from infants with illnesses resembling cytomegalic inclusion disease, *Proc Soc Exp Biol Med* 94:4, 1957.

5. Tyrrell DAJ, Bynoe ML: Cultivation of a novel type of common-cold virus in organ cultures, *Br Med J* 1:1467, 1965.

6. Hamre D, Procknow JJ: A new virus isolated from the human respiratory tract, *Proc Soc Exp Biol Med* 121:190, 1966.

7. Epstein MA, Achong BG, Barr YM: Virus particles in cultured lymphoblasts from Burkitt's lymphoma, *Lancet* 1:702, 1964,

8. Enders JF, Weller TH, Robbins FC: Cultivation of the Lansing strain of poliomyelitis virus in cultures of various human embryonic tissues, *Science* 109:85, 1949.

9. Dalldorf G, Sickles GM, Plager H, Gifford R: A virus recovered from the feces of "poliomyelitis" patients pathogenic for suckling mice, *J Exp Med* 89:567, 1949.

10. Melnick JL, Shaw EW, Curnen EC: A virus isolated from patients diagnosed as non-paralytic poliomyelitis or aseptic meningitis, *Proc Soc Exp Biol Med* 71:344, 1949.

11. Committee on the ECHO Viruses: Enteric cytopatho-genic human orphan (ECHO) viruses, *Science* 122:1187, 1955.

12. Johnson KM, Lange JV, Webb PA, Murphy FA: Isolation and partial characterisation of a new virus causing acute haemorrhagic fever in Zaire, *Lancet* 1:569, 1977.

13. Feinstone SM, Kapikian AZ, Purcell RH: Viruslike antigen associated with acute illness, *Science* 182:1026, 1973.

14. Blumberg BS, Alter HJ, Visnich S: A "new" antigen in leukemia sera, *JAMA* 191:541, 1965.

15. Choo QL, Kuo G, Weiner AJ, et al: Isolation of a cDNA clone derived from a blood-borne non-A, non-B viral hepatitis genome, *Science* 244:359, 1989.

16. Rizzetto M, Canese MG, Gerin JL, et al: Transmission of the hepatitis B virus–associated delta antigen to chimpanzees, *J Infect Dis* 141:590, 1980.

17. Rizzetto M, Canese MG, Arico S, et al: Immunofluorescence detection of new antigen-antibody system (delta/anti-delta) associated to hepatitis B virus in liver and in serum of HBsAg carriers, *Gut* 18:997, 1977.

18. Kane MA, Bradley DW, Shrestha SM, et al: Epidemic non-A, non-B hepatitis in Nepal: recovery of a possible etiologic agent and transmission studies in marmosets, *JAMA* 252:3140, 1984.

19. Bradley DW, Krawczynski K, Cook EH Jr, et al: Enterically transmitted non-A, non-B hepatitis: serial passage of disease in cynomolgus macaques and tamarins and recovery of disease-associated 27- to 34-nm viruslike particles, *Proc Natl Acad Sci USA* 84:6277, 1987.

20. Linnen J, Wages J Jr, Zhang-Keck ZY, et al: Molecular cloning and disease association of hepatitis G virus: a transfusion-transmissible agent, *Science* 271:505, 1996.

21. Salahuddin SZ, Ablashi DV, Markham PD, et al: Isolation of a new virus, HBLV, in patients with lymphopro-liferative disorders, *Science* 234:596, 1986.

22. Frenkel N, Schirmer EC, Wyatt LS, et al: Isolation of a new herpesvirus from human CD4+ T cells, *Proc Natl Acad Sci USA* 87:748, 87(19):7797 (erratum), 1990.

23. Chang Y, Cesarman E, Pessin MS, et al: Identification of herpesvirus-like DNA sequences in AIDS-associated Kaposi's sarcoma, *Science* 266:1865, 1994.

24. Barre-Sinoussi F, Chermann JC, Rey F, et al: Isolation of a T-lymphotropic retrovirus from a patient at risk for acquired immune deficiency syndrome (AIDS), *Science* 220:868, 1983.

25. Popovic M, Sarngadharan MG, Read E, Gallo RC: Detection, isolation, and continuous production of cyto-pathic retroviruses (HTLV-III) from patients with AIDS and pre-AIDS, *Science* 224:497, 1984.

26. Poiesz BJ, Ruscetti FW, Gazdar AF, et al: Detection and isolation of type C retrovirus particles from fresh and cultured lymphocytes of a patient with cutaneous T-cell lymphoma, *Proc Natl Acad Sci USA* 77:7415, 1980.

27. Kalyanaraman VS, Sarngadharan MG, Robert-Guroff M, et al: A new subtype of human T-cell leukemia virus (HTLV-II) associated with a T-cell variant of hairy cell leukemia, *Science* 218:571, 1982.

28. Smith W, Andrews CH, Laidlaw PP: A virus obtained from influenza patients, *Lancet* 1:66, 1933.

29. Francis TJ: A new type of virus from epidemic influenza, *Science* 92:405, 1940.

30. Taylor RM: A further note on 1233 ("influenza C") virus, *Arch Virusforsch Gesamte* 4:485, 1951.

31. Francis TJ, Quilligan JJ Jr, Minuse E: Identification of another epidemic respiratory disease, *Science* 112:495, 1950.

32. Buckley SM, Casals J: Lassa fever, a new virus disease of man from West Africa. 3. Isolation and characterization of the virus, *Am J Trop Med Hyg* 19:680, 1970.

33. Enders JF, Peebles TC: Propagation in tissue culture of cytopathogenic agents from patients with measles, *Proc Soc Exp Biol Med* 86:277, 1954.

34. Habel K: Cultivation of mumps virus in the developing chick embryo and its application to studies of immunity to mumps in man, *Public Health Rep* 60:201, 1945.

35. Weller TH, Neva FA: Propagation in tissue culture of cytopathic agents from patients with rubella-like illness, *Proc Soc Exp Biol Med* 111:215, 1962.

36. Parkman PD, Buescher EL, Artenstein MS: Recovery of rubella virus from army recruits, *Proc Soc Exp Biol Med* 111:225, 1962.

37. Kapikian AZ, Wyatt RG, Dolin R, et al: Visualization by immune electron microscopy of a 27-nm particle associated with acute infectious nonbacterial gastroenteritis, *J Virol* 10:1075, 1972.

38. Chanock RM: Association of a new type of cytopatho-genic myxovirus with infantile croup, *J Exp Med* 104:555, 1956.

39. Chanock RM, Parrott RH, Cook K, et al: Newly recognized myxoviruses from children with respiratory disease, *N Engl J Med* 258:207, 1958.

40. Johnson KM, Chanock RM, Cook MK, Huebner RJ: Studies of a new human hemadsorption virus. I. Isolation, properties and characterization, *Am J Hyg* 71:81, 1960.

41. Cossart YE, Field AM, Cant B, Widdows D: Parvovirus-like particles in human sera, *Lancet* 1:72, 1975.

42. Morris JA, Blount REJ, Savage RE: Recovery of cytopathogenic agent from chimpanzees with coryza, *Proc Soc Exp Biol Med* 92:544, 1956.

43. Price WH: The isolation of a new virus associated with respiratory clinical disease in humans, *Proc Natl Acad Sci USA* 42:892, 1956.

44. Pelon W, Mogabgab WJ, Phillips IA, Pierce WE: A cytopathogenic agent isolated from naval recruits with mild respiratory illnesses, *Proc Soc Exp Biol Med* 94:262, 1957.

45. Bishop RF, Davidson GP, Holmes IH, Ruck BJ: Evidence for viral gastroenteritis, *N Engl J Med* 289:1096, 1973 (letter).

46. Nichol ST, Spiropoulou CF, Morzunov S, et al: Genetic identification of a hantavirus associated with an outbreak of acute respiratory illness, *Science* 262:914, 1993.

47. Weller TH: Serial propagation *in vitro* of agents producing inclusion bodies derived from varicella and herpes zoster, *Proc Soc Exp Biol Med* 83:340, 1953.

48. Gallo RC, Salahuddin SZ, Popovic M, et al: Frequent detection and isolation of cytopathic retroviruses (HTLV-III) from patients with AIDS and at risk for AIDS, *Science* 224:500, 1984.

49. Sexton DJ, Rollin PE, Breitschwerdt EB, et al: Life-threatening Cache Valley virus infection, *N Engl J Med* 336:547, 1997.

50. Bayer ME, Blumberg BS, Werner B: Particles associated with Australia antigen in the sera of patients with leukaemia, Down's Syndrome and hepatitis, *Nature* 218:1057, 1968.

51. Anderson MJ, Lewis E, Kidd IM, et al: An outbreak of erythema infectiosum associated with human parvovirus infection, *J Hyg (Lond)* 93:85, 1984.

52. Pattison JR, Jones SE, Hodgson J, et al: Parvovirus infections and hypoplastic crisis in sickle-cell anaemia, *Lancet* 1:664, 1981 (letter).

53. Knott PD, Welply GA, Anderson MJ: Serologically proved intrauterine infection with parvovirus, *Br Med J (Clin Res Ed)* 289:1660, 1984.

54. Brown T, Anand A, Ritchie LD, et al: Intrauterine parvovirus infection associated with hydrops fetalis, *Lancet* 2:1033, 1984 (letter).

55. White DG, Woolf AD, Mortimer PP, et al: Human parvovirus arthropathy, *Lancet* 1:419, 1985.

56. Lambden PR, Caul EO, Ashley CR, Clarke IN: Sequence and genome organization of a human small round-structured (Norwalk-like) virus, *Science* 259:516, 1993.

57. Jiang X, Wang M, Wang K, Estes MK: Sequence and genomic organization of Norwalk virus, *Virology* 195:51, 1993.

58. Flewett TH, Bryden AS, Davies H: Virus particles in gastroenteritis, *Lancet* 2:1497, 1973 (letter).

59. Choo QL, Richman KH, Han JH, et al: Genetic organization and diversity of the hepatitis C virus, *Proc Natl Acad Sci USA* 88:2451, 1991.

60. Kuo G, Choo QL, Alter HJ, et al: An assay for circulating antibodies to a major etiologic virus of human non-A, non-B hepatitis, *Science* 244:362, 1989.

61. Lisitsyn N, Wigler M: Cloning the differences between two complex genomes, *Science* 259:946, 1993.

62. Moore PS, Chang Y: Detection of herpesvirus-like DNA sequences in Kaposi's sarcoma in patients with and without HIV infection, *N Engl J Med* 332:1181, 1995.

63. Soulier J, Grollet L, Oksenhendler E, et al: Kaposi's sarcoma–associated herpesvirus-like DNA sequences in multicentric Castleman's disease, *Blood* 86:1276, 1995.

64. Cesarman E, Chang Y, Moore PS, et al: Kaposi's sarcoma–associated herpesvirus-like DNA sequences in AIDS-related body-cavity-based lymphomas, *N Engl J Med* 332:1186, 1995.

65. Renne R, Zhong W, Herndier B, et al: Lytic growth of Kaposi's sarcoma–associated herpesvirus (human herpesvirus 8) in culture, *Nat Med* 2:342, 1996.

66. Foreman KE, Friborg J Jr., Kong WP, et al: Propagation of a human herpesvirus from AIDS-associated Kaposi's sarcoma, *N Engl J Med* 336:163, 1997.

67. Relman DA, Loutit JS, Schmidt TM, et al: The agent of bacillary angiomatosis: an approach to the identification of uncultured pathogens, *N Engl J Med* 323:1573, 1990.

68. Rozenberg F, Lebon P: Amplification and characterization of herpesvirus DNA in cerebrospinal fluid from patients with acute encephalitis, *J Clin Microbiol* 29:2412, 1991.

69. Rotbart HA: Enzymatic RNA amplification of the enteroviruses, *J Clin Microbiol* 28:438, 1990.

70. Centers for Disease Control: Outbreak of acute illness—southwestern United States, 1993, *MMWR* 42:421, 1993.

71. Centers for Disease Control and Prevention: Preventing emerging diseases: a strategy for the 21st century—overview of the updated CDC plan, *MMWR* 47:1, 1998.

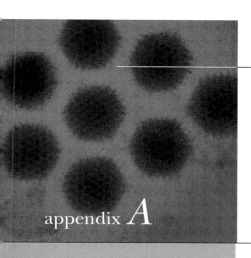

appendix *A*

Likely Viral Agents and Useful Diagnostic Specimens According to Clinical Syndrome

Syndrome	Etiologic agents	Specimen(s)	Test(s)	Comments
Meningitis	*Usual*			
	Enteroviruses (echo, coxsackie)	CSF	RT-PCR, culture	RT-PCR more sensitive than culture
	Unusual			
	HSV-2	CSF	PCR	May be recurrent, genital lesions may be present or absent
	HIV	Plasma	RT-PCR	Diagnosis of HIV should not be based solely on RT-PCR
	EBV	Serum	Serology	
		CSF	PCR	Limited experience
	VZV	CSF	PCR	Cutaneous lesions may be absent
	Mumps	CSF	Culture	Notify laboratory of possible mumps
		Saliva	Culture	Notify laboratory of possible mumps
		Serum	Serology (IgM)	
	LCM virus	CSF	Culture	Reference laboratory
		Serum	Serology	
Encephalitis	*Usual (non–HIV associated)*			
	HSV	CSF	PCR	
	Arboviruses	CSF	Serology (IgM)	
		Serum	Serology (IgM)	
	Usual (HIV–associated)			
	CMV	CSF	PCR	Quantitative testing is useful to identify clinically signifcant infection
	EBV	CSF	PCR	CNS lymphoma
	VZV	CSF	PCR	Past or present zoster is common although cutaneous lesions may be absent
	JC virus	CSF	PCR	Progressive multifocal leuko-encephalopathy
	Unusual (non–HIV associated)			
	VZV	CSF	PCR	Limited experience
	EBV	CSF	PCR	Limited experience
	HHV-6	CSF	PCR	Limited experience, HHV-6 DNA may be detected in children with acute HHV-6 infection (roseola) in the absence of symptomatic neurologic disease
	Enteroviruses	CSF	RT-PCR, culture	
	Mumps	CSF, saliva	Culture	Notify laboratory of possible mumps
		Serum	Serology (IgM)	
	B virus	CSF	Culture, serology	Reference laboratory (see text)

Syndrome	Etiologic agents	Specimen(s)	Test(s)	Comments
		Serum	Serology	Reference laboratory (see text)
		Lesions	Culture	Reference laboratory (see text)
	Rabies	CSF	RT-PCR, culture, serology (after day 8 of illness)	Reference laboratory
		Saliva	RT-PCR, culture	Reference laboratory
		Skin	FA stain	Reference laboratory
		Serum	Serology (after day 8 of illness)	Reference laboratory
Respiratory infection	Influenza, RSV, parainfluenza, adenovirus, rhinovirus	NP aspirate, wash, or swab; sputum; tracheal aspirate; BAL fluid	Culture, FA stain, membrane EIA (RSV and influenza A), optical immunoassay (influenza A and B)	NP specimens preferred in young children. In immunocompromised patients, also consider CMV. FA staining does not detect rhinovirus.
Gastroenteritis	Rotavirus, adenovirus, calcivirus, astrovirus	Stool	EIA (rotavirus, adenovirus, astrovirus), EM	EIA preferred for rotavirus and adenovirus. EIA for astrovirus is investigational.
Skin or mucous membrane lesion	HSV, VZV	Swab	Culture, FA stain	FA stain more sensitive than culture for VZV
	Poxviruses	Swab, biopsy	EM, PCR, culture	Preferred method depends on poxvirus being sought (see text).
	Papillomavirus	Cervical swab, skin biopsy	PCR, hybrid capture assay	
Hepatitis	HAV	Serum	Serology (IgM)	
	HBV	Serum	Serology (HBsAg)	
	HCV	Serum	Serology	Positive EIA should be confirmed with RIBA or RT-PCR.
	HDV	Serum	Serology	Reference laboratory
	HEV	Serum	Serology	Reference laboratory
Myocarditis, pericarditis	Enteroviruses, Adenovirus	Myocardial or pericardial biopsy, pericardial fluid, stool, throat or NP swab, aspirate, or wash	Culture, RT-PCR	Multiple other viruses are rare causes (see text). RT-PCR and PCR are investigational.
Conjunctivitis/ keratitis	Adenovirus, HSV, VZV	Swab	Culture, FA stain, PCR	PCR is investigational.
Retinitis	CMV, VZV, HSV	Vitreous	PCR	Laboratory diagnosis of CMV retinitis usually not required; when required, aqueous fluid may be useful in addition to vitreous.
Hemorrhagic cystitis	BK virus	Urine	PCR	
	Adenovirus	Urine	Culture	

Table continued on following page

Syndrome	Etiologic agents	Specimen(s)	Test(s)	Comments
Infectious mononucleosis	EBV	Serum	Serology (heterophile antibody assay)	Paul-Bunnell heterophile antibody assay, ox-cell hemolysin assay, and mononucleosis slide tests are comparable.
	CMV	Serum	Serology (IgM)	
	HIV	Plasma	RT-PCR	False-positive tests have occurred (see text); positive test should be confirmed by other methods.
Rash	Enterovirus	Stool, throat, or NP	Culture	
	Parvovirus B19 (fifth disease)	Serum	Serology (IgM)	
	HHV-6 (roseola)	Whole blood	Serology plus HHV-6 PCR	Positive PCR performed on leukocytes or whole blood plus negative HHV-6 IgG antibody assay indicates acute infection (investigational).
	Measles	Serum	Serology (IgM)	
		NP swab, aspirate, or wash	FA stain	
	Rubella	Serum	Serology (IgM)	
Congenital infection	***In utero***			
	CMV	Amniotic fluid	Culture or PCR	PCR preferred when specimen must be transported
	Rubella	Fetal blood	Serology (IgM)	
		Amniotic fluid	Culture or RT-PCR	
	Parvovirus B 19	Amniotic fluid	PCR	
	Postpartum			
	CMV	Urine	Culture	Obtain within first week of life to document in utero acquisition
	HSV	Lesion, conjunctiva, throat, urine, blood	Culture	
	Rubella	Pharynx, urine, conjunctiva, stool, CSF, blood	Culture	
		Serum	Serology (IgM)	Should be confirmed by culture whenever possible.
	Parvovirus B19	Serum	Serology (IgM) or PCR	
	HIV	Blood	PCR (DNA)	
Systemic infection in immunocompromised host	CMV	Blood	Culture, pp65 antigenemia assay, PCR, or hybrid capture assay	Diagnosis of localized disease should be made from studies of specimens from site of disease.
HIV	HIV	Serum	HIV antibody assay	

CSF, Cerebrospinal fluid; *RT-PCR,* reverse-transcription polymerase chain reaction; *HSV-2,* herpes simplex virus type 2; *HIV,* human immunodeficiency virus; *EBV,* Epstein-Barr virus; *VZV,* varicella-zoster virus; *IgM,* immunoglobulin M; *LCM,* lymphocytic choriomeningitis; *CMV,* cytomegalovirus; *CNS,* central nervous system; *HHV-6,* human herpesvirus type 6; *FA,* fluorescent antibody; *RSV,* respiratory syncytial virus; *NP,* nasopharyngeal; *EIA,* enzyme immunoassay; *BAL,* bronchoalveolar lavage; *EM,* electron microscopy; *HAV,* hepatitis A virus; *HBsAg,* hepatitis B surface antigen; *RIBA,* recombinant immunoblot assay; *RNA,* ribonucleic acid; *DNA,* deoxyribonucleic acid; *IgG,* immunoglobulin G.

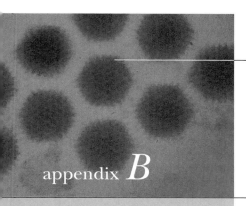

Specimen Collection Guide

General Instructions

Because viral inactivation occurs more rapidly at room temperature, it is always desirable to place specimens on ice as soon as possible after collection. Blood specimens are an exception and can be transported at room temperature. Specimens for which transport to the laboratory may exceed 24 hours should be frozen. Freezing temperature should be −70°C or colder (freezing at −20°C should be avoided). Freezing with dry ice is sufficient until specimens can be placed in a −70°C freezer. Rapid transport to the laboratory is always desirable.

Specimen	Procedure
Nasopharyngeal swab	Use swab with flexible metal shaft and Dacron or rayon tip. Insert swab into posterior nasopharynx. Rub swab against mucosal surface. Leave in place for 10 to 15 seconds if possible. Collection of specimens from both nostrils increases amount of material available for examination. Place swab(s) into vial of transport media. Use scissors to cut shaft so top of vial can be screwed on securely.
Nasopharyngeal aspirate	Requires source of suction (syringe, vacuum pump, or wall suction), specimen trap with two outlets, and catheter (no. 6 to 14 French, depending on size of patient). Without applying suction, insert catheter through nose into posterior nasopharynx (approximately the distance from tip of nose to external opening of ear). Apply gentle suction, leave catheter in place for a few seconds, then withdraw slowly. Suction contents of vial of viral transport media through catheter tubing to assist in moving material from tubing into trap and to add viral transport media to specimen. Cover trap openings so that material will not spill.

Specimen	Procedure
Nasopharyngeal wash	Use rubber bulb (1-2 oz for infants) or syringe to instill 3-5 ml of non-bacteriostatic saline into one nostril while occluding the other. If patient able to cooperate, instruct to close glottis (by making "humming" sound with mouth open). If rubber bulb is used, release pressure on bulb to allow saline and mucus to enter bulb. Remove from nose and squeeze into vial of transport media. If syringe is used, apply suction to syringe to recover saline and nasal secretions. Alternatively, hold sterile container (e.g., urine cup) under patient's nose and ask patient to expel material into it. In either case, add contents of vial of viral transport media to recovered saline-nasal secretions.
Throat swab	Obtain specimen by rubbing swab vigorously over pharynx and tonsils. If commercial swab is used, follow directions for adding transport media to swab. Otherwise, place swab in vial of viral transport media, and cut shaft so top of vial can be screwed on securely.
Throat washing	Have patient gargle with 5-10 ml of phosphate-buffered saline or non-bacteriostatic sterile saline and expel contents of gargle into sterile container (e.g., urine cup). Contents of tube of viral transport media may be added.
Sputum	Have patient expectorate into sterile container. If specimen is to be cultured, add contents of vial of viral transport media, and transport to laboratory. Note that material does not have to possess thick purulent consistency that is desirable for sputum used for bacterial cultures.
Saliva	Used for isolation of mumps virus or cytomegalovirus. Collect saliva by using swab or by having patient spit into sterile container. For mumps virus, swabbing area around Stensen's duct is recommended. Place swab in vial of viral transport media, and cut shaft so top of vial can be screwed on securely. If sterile container is used, add contents of vial of viral transport media unless specimen can be transported immediately to laboratory.

Specimen	Procedure
Tracheal aspirate	Connect specimen trap to wall suction and suction catheter. Insert suction catheter through endotracheal tube and apply suction. Withdraw catheter when specimen has been collected. Place suction catheter in vial of viral transport media, and suction contents through tubing into trap to assist in moving specimen from tubing into trap and to add viral transport media to specimen.
Bronchial wash or bronchoalveolar lavage fluid	Collect at least 5 ml into sterile container, place on ice, and transport immediately to laboratory. Contents of vial of viral transport media may be added.
Blood	Obtain 5-10 ml of blood by vascular puncture or withdrawal through catheter (may be possible to use smaller blood volume for pediatric patients). Appropriate tube is determined by test to be performed, blood component on which test is performed (whole blood, leukocytes [buffy coat], plasma, or serum) and laboratory's preference. Assays performed on blood specimens, including CMV pp65 antigenemia assay, hybrid capture assay, polymerase chain reaction (PCR), reverse-transcription-PCR, and branched DNA assay may have specific collection tube requirements. Communication with laboratory is essential. Whole blood, leukocytes, and plasma require collection into tube containing anticoagulant. Anticoagulants used most often are EDTA (purple-top tube), heparin (green-top tube), acid-citrate-dextrose (ACD) (yellow-top tube), and citrate (blue-top tube). Most serologic procedures, some cultures (e.g., for enteroviruses), and some PCR assays (e.g., for parvovirus B19) are performed on serum. Serum specimens require collection into tube that does not contain anticoagulant (red-top tube). Blood specimens do not have to be placed on ice if transport requires less than 1 day. Note that prolonged transport can severely compromise ability to recover cytomegalovirus in culture from blood specimens.

Specimen	Procedure
Bone marrow	Place in anticoagulated tube used for collection of whole-blood specimens.
Cerebrospinal fluid	Place in sterile tube and transport to laboratory. At least 1 ml is desirable for culture. Culture and PCR can be performed on same specimen. Volume requirements for PCR must be determined by communicating with laboratory.
Stool	For detection of viral causes of acute gastroenteritis, obtain within first few days of illness. Place 2-4 g of stool or approximately 5 ml of liquid stool in sterile container and transport to laboratory. Stool is preferred to rectal swabs. If swab is to be used, insert swab 2-4 cm within anus and rotate to obtain fecal material. Be sure that fecal material is visible on swab.
Tissue	Place in sterile container and moisten with viral transport media or sterile saline.
Urine	Place 1-10 ml in sterile container.
Amniotic fluid	Place at least 2 ml in sterile container.
Miscellaneous fluids	Place 1-10 ml in sterile container.
Miscellaneous swabs	Place swab in vial of viral transport media, cut shaft so that top of vial can be closed securely, and transport to laboratory. If commercial collection swab is used, follow instructions for adding transport media to swab.
Conjunctival swab	Remove any exudate present with initial swab. Rub second swab across conjunctiva, place in vial of viral transport media, and cut shaft so top of vial can be closed securely.
Corneal scraping	Collected by ophthalmologist. Place in vial of viral transport media and transport immediately to laboratory. For fluorescent antibody stains, material may be applied directly to microscope slides.
Skin scraping	If vesicle is present, use sterile scalpel to unroof it. Fluid is useful for viral culture. Collect fluid using swab. Place swab in vial of viral transport media. Use scalpel blade or swab to obtain material from base of lesion, and apply to microscope slide for fluorescent antibody staining. Material from base of lesion can also be added to viral transport media for use in culture.

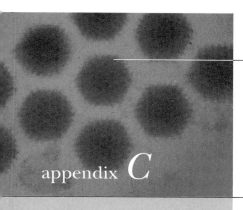

Virology Reference Laboratories

The **Centers for Disease Control and Prevention** (CDC, Atlanta) and many state health department laboratories provide specialized viral diagnostic testing. Contact with the state health department is usually required before submission of specimens to CDC. Many states require that specimens sent to CDC be routed through the state health department laboratory.

Viral diagnostic testing is also performed by the following private commercial laboratories:

ARUP Laboratories
500 Chipeta Way
Salt Lake City, UT 84108
Tel: (800) 522-2787
    (801) 583-2787
Fax: (800) 522-2706
Internet: *www.arup-lab.com*

BBI–North American Clinical Laboratories
75 North Mountain Rd.
New Britain, CT 06053
Tel: (203) 225-1900
    (800) 866-6254
Fax: (203) 223-6279
Internet: *www.bbii.com*

LabCorp
358 South Main St.
Burlington, NC 27215
Tel: (336) 222-7566
Internet: *www.labcorp.com*

Mayo Medical Laboratories
200 First St. SW
Rochester, MN 55905
Tel: (800) 533-1710
Fax: (507) 284-1759

MRL Reference Laboratory
10703 Progress Way
Cypress, CA 90630-4717
Tel: (800) 445-0185
     (714) 220-1900
Fax: (714) 220-9213
Internet: *www.mrlinfo.com*

Quest Laboratories, Inc.
Multiple locations
Internet: *www.questdiagnostics.com*

Specialty Laboratories, Inc.
2211 Michigan Ave.
Santa Monica, CA 90404-3900
Tel: (800) 421-4449
     (310) 828-6543
Fax: (310) 828-6634
E-mail: specialty@specialtylabs.com
Internet: *www.specialtylabs.com*

ViroMed Laboratories, Inc.
6101 Blue Circle Drive
Minneapolis, MN 55343
Tel: (612) 931-0077
     (800) 582-0077
Fax: (612) 939-4215
E-mail: *clientserv@viromedlabs.com*

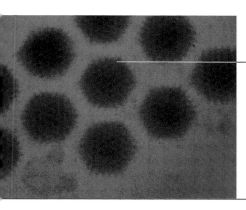

Index

Page numbers in boldface type indicate boxed material; page numbers in italic type indicate references to illustrations and photographs; page numbers followed by 't' indicate tables; underlined page numbers indicate sidebars in the text.